PROTOCOLS

PROTOCOLS

ANDREW HUBERMAN
with JESSICA WAPNER

Cornerstone Press

CORNERSTONE PRESS

UK | USA | Canada | Ireland | Australia
India | New Zealand | South Africa

Cornerstone Press is part of the Penguin Random House group of companies
whose addresses can be found at global.penguinrandomhouse.com

Penguin Random House UK, One Embassy Gardens,
8 Viaduct Gardens, London SW11 7BW

penguin.co.uk

Penguin Random House UK

First published in the US by Simon Element 2026
First published in the UK by Cornerstone Press 2026
001

Interior design by Karla Schweer

Printed and bound in Great Britain by Clays Ltd, Elcograf S.p.A.

The authorised representative in the EEA is Penguin Random House Ireland,
Morrison Chambers, 32 Nassau Street, Dublin D02 YH68

A CIP catalogue record for this book is available from the British Library

ISBN: 978-1-52992-128-1 (hardback)
ISBN: 978-1-52992-129-8 (trade paperback)

Penguin Random House is committed to a sustainable future
for our business, our readers and our planet. This book is made
from Forest Stewardship Council® certified paper.

FSC www.fsc.org MIX Paper FSC® C018179

Disclaimer

For Costello, Zoë, and Strummer, whose only tasks were to sleep well and enough, eat clean but not too much, stay hydrated, view sunlight, and get exercise. And endlessly give and receive love. Must be nice . . .

For everyone else: I wrote this book for you.

Contents

Introduction

Welcome to *Protocols*.

This book is a guide for improving your health and performance. If you're struggling with one or more areas of your health, it can help you. If you're generally feeling good and you want to level up one or more of those areas, it can also help you.

What is a protocol? A protocol is an established formula to help you overcome common obstacles, achieve a specific health or performance goal, or generally improve your day-to-day physical or mental state. Each is simple to implement. Each is designed to take the minimum amount of time to produce the greatest possible results. Each can work the first time, and every time.

As you learn these protocols, you'll discover the science behind why they work and, in doing so, you'll also discover a lot about how your brain and body work. Because each is based on known aspects of our physiology. They work because they are based in how we work. The science is important for at least two reasons that go beyond just substantiation. First, by understanding how a given protocol can, say, improve your sleep or your ability to focus and learn new things, you place yourself in the position to customize it to suit your needs, while still allowing it to produce the effect you want. Second, you'll start to see similar biological themes turning up in what otherwise would seem like disparate systems. Our brains and bodies repurpose a lot of the same mechanisms to allow these systems to work in concert. Knowing some of the science behind each protocol affords you insights not just into how that protocol works, but how different protocols synergize. Practically speaking, that gives you a level of control over your health that simply learning "do protocol A to get effect B" just can't provide. You can determine what works for your needs and your goals in the context of your life, without having to make the pursuit of health a singular focus.

Because let's face it: The real reason to do any of these protocols is to feel and perform better, mentally and physically, and to have more energy so you can go about the rest of your life.

I should say, too, what this book is not. This book is not about "optimization," at least not in the typical sense. That word calls to mind the idea of spending a lot of time perfecting your daily routine. True optimization is about rescuing time—not just by increasing the number of years of your life, but by increasing the number of effective hours of your days (and the number of hours of great sleep at night). Many protocols in this book take only a few minutes to do and can be done whenever you'd like. Others take a bit more time or need to be done within a certain time frame each day or week.

You'll also notice from just these few short paragraphs that I eschew the whole notion of "biohacking." A hack is a shortcut that involves leveraging something toward a typically unrelated goal, like jury-rigging a paperclip and tape to fix broken eyeglasses. Hacks are never long-term solutions. The protocols in this book are the opposite of hacks. They are science-supported tools, grounded in robust physiological mechanisms—neural circuits, hormones, and neurotransmitters that have been hardwired into your brain and body starting from even before you were born. You just need to learn how to access them.

You'll notice that I mostly emphasize the behaviors that can make the greatest difference in your immediate and long-term health. However, because I often get asked which prescription drugs, supplements, and devices are useful to help achieve a given health or performance goal, I discuss those tools too.

Indeed, "What should I take?" is one of the most common questions I get from both men and women. Many people have a perception that the secret to health and performance resides in exogenous molecules—meaning something that comes from outside our body. Make no mistake: Certain pills, powders, or injectables can make a positive difference in health and performance. But because certain behaviors can so potently activate multiple physiological mechanisms, including the release of endogenous molecules—meaning, you guessed it, something that comes from inside our bodies—there is simply no replacement for them. That is why no pill can (or ever will) replace exercise, or sleep, or proper stress control. Even drugs that allow for neuroplasticity, or your brain's capacity to rewire and learn, won't produce learning on their own. Plasticity must be directed toward a particular endpoint. That requires certain behaviors. We must do the right things in the right sequence. Or, as a colleague of mine aptly put it, "better living through chemistry still requires better living."

Which means you don't have to buy anything to achieve your health or performance goals. Some people have disposable income to devote to tools for health and performance. Others do not. I wrote this book for everyone and can assure you that it is (and I believe always will be) a core fact that behavioral tools really move the needle in the right direction. And the right ones can work for everyone. Whether you are young or old, currently fit or out of shape, the protocols in this book can make you feel, look, and think far better, and thereby show up better at work or school or on the field or in the gym, and in your relationships . . . even in your relationship to yourself. I know that statement to be true because literally millions of people have implemented these protocols to great success and continue to do so every day. I also know because I personally use them.

In fact, I discovered many of the protocols in this book because I needed them, in some cases urgently. I, like so many others, have struggled with sleep and stress, finding the "right" diet, knowing the best way to exercise to meet specific goals, and on and on.

But if I have one innate quality, it's curiosity. I love to learn. I also love to share what I learn with others. And what drives my curiosity—at least in the realm of health and performance—is the same thing that likely brought you to this book: I wanted to know the best solutions to those challenges.

There are no tools included in this book that I have not personally tried. Some I have used for brief periods because they are for overcoming a sticking point, and then best set aside. Others are mainstays in my daily life and will remain so until I die because they are so central to my physical and mental health, and my ability to focus and learn effectively as they continue to help me reach my performance goals. I stand by every tool and every concept.

These protocols cover what I know works. Whereas on the *Huberman Lab*, my podcast, I explore and share both topics of which I am certain as well as topics that I'm still exploring—such as peptides or psychedelics—this book focuses mostly on the former. Its chapters on sleep; exercise; stress control; nutrition; light; focus, motivation, and learning; and personal growth are the result of years of research, both in the lab and in life, from experts in every topic, and from my own work. Some protocols are basic; others are more advanced. You'll be able to decide which are best for your needs and goals.

For those of you who are new to my work, I'll share a bit about my background for context and how we—yes, me and you—got here. If you're going to read this book and use these tools, my hope is that you'll come to see that we are collaborators on this journey. Again, I discovered many of the protocols in this book because I need them. If you do too, know that you are not alone.

As of writing this introduction, I'm fifty years old. For the last three decades, I have spent most of my waking hours researching how the nervous system—that is, the brain and the spinal cord—works, develops, and can change, for better or worse. This is referred to as neuroscience. I first learned about the field of neuroscience in college, from Harry Carlisle. He was a physiologist, a neuroscientist, and a professor at my university. I took his course, and there I first learned about brain circuits for motivation, about learning and memory, and on and on. This treasure trove of knowledge simply did not exist anywhere else at that time, not even in textbooks. He taught all of neuroscience but emphasized the neural and hormonal and peptide interactions between the brain and the body. Harry knew how to connect the dots in a way that only a masterful teacher can. During a lecture one day, he paused writing on the chalkboard, turned to face us, and said: "The next time you see someone delusional from schizophrenia, or collapsed from depression, or addicted to speed, consider what it is to try to move, think, or feel a certain way when the neurons—the cells that subserve those efforts—are simply not there, or are broken . . ." Something clicked for me.

In some sense, I was primed for that moment. By nineteen, I had witnessed a lot of people with mental and physical health issues related to the brain. Several had become badly addicted to alcohol and drugs. We now know addiction is a brain issue, but back then, most people thought it was simply a lack-of-willpower issue. Many of the "high functioning" people I grew up around suffered from anxiety or depression. By humanizing science and explaining that what often appears psychological is actually physiological, Harry's course inspired me to become a neuroscientist. Also, what could be more interesting than the brain?

To be fair, becoming a scientist wasn't entirely unexpected. I've always loved observing and learning about animals, including humans. And my father is a scientist—a theoretical physicist. Until I was thirteen, my family ate dinner together every night, and my father's colleagues would sometimes join us. While other families talked about politics or discussed sports over dinner, the only "sport" in my home was science, and the star players were scientists. I heard stories about Richard Feynman and Murray Gell-Mann, famed Nobel Prize–winning physicists, and Ed Wilson, the founder of sociobiology, along with other luminaries. We still laugh about the time when my sister, then a toddler, walked over to one of the most famous Nobel Prize winners, smiled at him, and then threw up on his lap . . . and he was cool about it. And my maternal grandfather was a biochemist. When we visited, he would take me to his lab to help collect data on the metabolism and body composition of rats fed different types of diets.

So it made perfect sense that I would become a scientist, right? Well, yes and no. When I turned fourteen my parents divorced. I harbor no resentment about it, but at the time, the change made things at home and school unravel. Keep in mind, it was the 1980s, when divorce was less common, and I hit puberty at fourteen too, so it's impossible to know if what ensued was fueled by the sudden disruption in my family structure or the surge of hormones in my brain and body. As we say in science: "Bad experiment . . . too many variables to determine causality."

What I do know is that from ages fourteen to nineteen, before I found myself in Harry's course, my life was a blur of wild, eye-opening adventures, painful losses, and at times, full-blown mayhem. I got really into skateboarding—which back then was rather niche. I loved skateboarding for the activity itself, and for the community of eccentric and often unruly characters it attracted. And I loved that it was a daily lesson in discipline, focus, and energy: You try, try, try, fail, fail, fail, almost succeed, then fail one hundred times more before you finally land the trick. Often with plenty of pain all along the way. And skateboarding was 100 percent self-directed. We all pushed each other by example, and encouraged each other too, but there were no coaches, no referees. Indeed, skateboarding was a go-to activity for those of us who wanted to do a sport but for whom parental involvement wasn't necessary or, frankly, wanted. We were completely feral. And "we" were multi-generational and from every background imaginable. Skateboarding has also always been an unusual sport because it has twelve-, thirteen-, and fourteen-year-old kids hanging out with guys (back then it was almost exclusively guys) in their late teens, twenties, and thirties. Some were from the suburbs. Others from cities. And they came from all over the country to the legendary spots we frequented. I became close friends with people from all walks of life. And I got a lot of exposure to drugs, alcohol, sex, and violence. I also missed a lot of school.

I was okay at skateboarding. I picked up a small sponsorship or two. But I was never a contender to turn professional. As much as I may have wanted it and worked at it, I just didn't have the chops. I am blessed to know and remain friends with several of the greats from that time. And I witnessed some truly historic skateboarding. It's impossible to put into words the amount of raw energy and innovation you would find at the now-legendary Embarcadero Plaza ("EMB") in San Francisco or at a contest in San Diego, or in Washington Square Park in New York City in the early 1990s. For that and many other reasons, those years remain among the fondest and most inspiring memories of my childhood. But that's what I was: a child. Marbled into all the amazing experiences were a lot of hard ones too. Now, I want to be careful with what I say next. On the one hand I wouldn't wish a lot of what I experienced in those years on anyone, much less a young kid, but I also wouldn't trade it in either. I was completely free, and yet I felt uncertainty about everything. I got hurt a lot and spent a lot of time on crutches.

My physical injuries led to a few very good decisions, however. They motivated me to go against the convention among skateboarders back then and start running and training with weights. While it might seem commonplace now, in the early 1990s, unless you were a bodybuilder, pre-season football player, or headed to the military, no one lifted weights. Gyms were not a thing. Even weirder was if you were an American kid who meditated, but I started doing that too.

That taught me the basics of exercise- and stress-induced adaptations, and how they are similar and yet different. It goes something like this: Run farther or faster than the last time and the next run becomes easier . . . and unlocks the opportunity to run a little farther and faster, and so on. Lift a weight until you can't do another repetition despite your best effort in one session, and the next session, you can lift the same amount of weight for more repetitions, or move more weight. Set a timer for five minutes, sit still and try to focus on your breathing while the inevitable agitation grows, then subsides, then grows again. The next day, set the timer for six minutes, then seven minutes; and pretty soon twenty minutes is doable.

Another very good decision, though not exactly related to the physical injuries: I started thinking about college. My girlfriend had graduated high school a year ahead of me and moved away to university. I missed her and would visit often. In the end, I mostly applied to college just to be near her. I didn't really expect to get in. But I did.

As you might predict, my first year at college did not go well. I kept up with exercise and meditation, but I missed lectures, and I got into stupid fights. The adage "you get out what you put in" is true. I got what I deserved, which was not a whole lot.

Then came the big turning point. On the Fourth of July, 1994, when a group of us were arriving at a barbecue at our friend's house and saw it was getting robbed, we did what any young male morons would do: We fought the robbers. I don't remember it even being a decision. I just recall running straight into the mix. Anyone who has actually been in a street fight—not a boxing class, or a sanctioned match with gloves and a referee—will tell you that it's not like in the movies. Things can escalate really fast, and people can get hurt, or killed. That fight was ugly. Although luckily no one got badly injured, the police showed up and we all had a lot of explaining to do. The guys who were robbing the house were arrested, not us. In fact, before driving off, the police congratulated me. I felt nauseous. It wasn't that I wished I had gotten in trouble for what had happened; I just realized that I was going nowhere in life, so the accolades felt more like a loser trophy than anything worth celebrating. Somewhere in my gut I knew that regardless of who was at fault, I wasn't making good choices; I knew I was gravitating toward self-destruction.

I spent the rest of that July Fourth weekend in reflection. I was nineteen, and I wasn't good at anything useful. And I wanted to be. So I made the decision to get my life on track by focusing on something I knew had an "if you just show up every day and work hard at it, there is something waiting for you at the end" quality.

I decided to focus on school. I didn't know what I would do with a college degree or even what degree to pursue, but at that point I didn't care. I just needed a path I knew would lead to someplace better than where I was at that moment. I would figure out the ultimate goal later.

Having missed so much of high school, I knew I was coming from behind, so I moved to a studio apartment away from campus. I studied around the clock, stopping only to go to class, eat, sleep, or exercise. To say I was motivated is an understatement—I lived in the constant fear of remaining a directionless loser, and that kept me going. I didn't have solid study habits from high school to rely on. So I brute-forced it. I would set a timer and push myself to study in two-hour blocks, refusing to let myself get up even for a trip to the bathroom. After each block, I would take a short break and then get back to work. After I completed three of those cycles, I would allow myself a nap if I needed it, then I would hammer out three more. I worked alone, in my studio apartment, reading and taking detailed notes on every chapter, passage, and sentence. I drank ungodly amounts of water, yerba maté, black coffee, and Diet Coke with lemon juice. I went to every lecture and office hours. I tested myself on course material in my head while I biked to class and when I lay down to sleep at night. My first and last thoughts of the day were about my course material. I sat in the front row of every lecture. Mind you, I still had no idea what I would declare as my major. No specific subject felt like "the one." I was just clawing my way forward. My girlfriend—who had known me since high school—remarked, "What happened to you?!" She was at once pleased and a bit frustrated with my turnaround. On the one hand, now I was more acceptable to her parents, but I was also a lot less "fun" to be around. Perhaps other guys could go out on Friday and hang out at the beach on Saturday and go to concerts in the park on Sunday and still do well in school. I was not one of them. I was on a mission to right myself. Once a month or so I would go to a party. Friends jokingly called me "Dart" because I would "Irish goodbye" at midnight, to ensure I got enough sleep so I wouldn't blow the next day. I didn't feel I was missing out on anything. By nineteen I had accrued enough wild experiences and parties for several lifetimes. For me, the action was elsewhere.

But soon stress and lack of sleep caught up with me. Also, while fear is a potent motivator, it's not a sustainable one. I started catching colds. I got into a bike accident. Back then no one really talked about stress or the importance of sleep the way they do now, much less why it's important to cycle periods of focused intensity with rest in between in order to avoid burnout. I bumped up my meditation from twenty to thirty minutes a day. That helped reduce my stress and improved my ability to focus for long stretches of studying. I kept up my exercise program of lifting and running three times a week each, but I started approaching my lifting sessions and runs also as forms of meditation.

Something unexpected but really cool happened with that. I found that by putting as much attention as possible on each repetition in the gym, or by letting my mind go blank while I ran, I soon could switch on those brain states of focus and calm when not exercising. It was my first taste of learning how to deliberately access, and shift between, different brain states. I was intrigued. So I started reading about brain states. Which led me to reading about drugs. I was never much into recreational drugs. In high school and college, I drank alcohol and I smoked a bit of weed, and I tried psilocybin and LSD. I confess I didn't like any of it. Caffeine was my drug. I mentioned that to the owner of a Chinese medicine shop in town. She encouraged me to try a few herbs instead of coffee. One made me feel like I was going to have a heart attack (pure ephedra tea? I do not recommend!) but a few others made me both incredibly focused and calm for hours at a time. Cool! . . . but then they quickly stopped working. Not cool. I also tried a mineral that an acupuncturist said would give me much deeper sleep. It gave me lucid dreams, which led me to read a book by a guy named J. Allan Hobson at Harvard about the neurochemistry of sleep and dreaming. That started me on limiting my caffeine at night. But those experiments worked: I began feeling better and performing better in my classes again. I was excited by the idea of how significant shifts in my health and performance could come about from seemingly small behaviors and, in some cases, from ingesting specific compounds.

I also experimented with over-the-counter supplements. A few really worked: For instance, I started taking creatine monohydrate when I was twenty, and it definitely helped to make me stronger. Only now do we know of some of its additional benefits for cognition, especially when mildly sleep-deprived.[1] I tried ginseng and ginkgo but they gave me brutal headaches.

The sum total from all I was doing was that not only did my level of focus and performance in school improve tremendously but my mood improved too. I was sleeping well. I consistently woke up excited for the day. I kept building physical strength. Every Sunday I would go on a long run lasting an hour or more. I had gained a level of control over my life. Studying new information for hours at a time had become a habit, and even an enjoyable one. I had come to associate the frustration of not understanding something at the start of a learning session as a stage to get through, not something to avoid. I never expected to land a skateboarding trick the first time, so why would learning new information be any different? I knew the formula: reps, reps, and more reps until you get it. I was starting to understand the learning process as just that, a process.

And right then is when I found myself in Harry's course in neuroscience. That's when things clicked. I was finally able to bring all the resources of discipline, focus, and energy to a specific, career-related goal: I would become a neuroscientist.

To this day when people ask me how to find their calling, I say whatever you do, don't wait for it to find you. Start working hard now and learn how to take care of your mental and physical health while doing it. It could be school, or a creative pursuit, or starting a business, but stick to that structure. Do *something* hard (for you) that builds on itself every single day. It will ready you for when *the thing* becomes clear.

I've seen so many people work at something like crazy, ignore their physical and mental health, and burn out. Or wait for their calling to beckon them, and have their physical and mental health spiral in the meantime. The key is to make sure the things you do to support your health also prepare you for your calling when it comes. Build mental and physical strength and resilience. And endurance. Master getting a great night's sleep on a regular basis. Work hard in whatever job you do. That's the secret.

I worked hard in Harry's lab during my junior and senior years of college. We ran experiments side by side. I devoured every book I could on the topic of the brain, and physiology too. I went to neuroscience seminars with the grad students and professors. Harry and I even published a paper together. It wasn't a landmark study or anything, but it was solid. And I was the first author on the author line. Which meant I wasn't just another undergrad who volunteered in a lab to get a letter of recommendation for grad school. I was a real scientist. A nascent one, but a scientist nonetheless. "Anyone can read and critique a paper," Harry said, "but once you go through the process of posing a good question, wagering a hypothesis, designing and carrying out experiments, analyzing the data and writing up the findings and your interpretation of them, and you get it peer reviewed and published, you're forever changed. You'll never look at data—or the world—the same way again." I am forever grateful to Harry for giving me that opportunity.

And indeed, I applied everything I learned about the process of doing that study to my pursuit of tools for health and performance: reading, learning, asking questions, testing hypotheses, and gathering data about how different types of exercise, light, nutrition, and so on affected me. I found much of this information shrouded in esoteric names or siloed into subcultures in ways that made it difficult to access. But I had been part of a subculture once before, and I had learned how to navigate it. And because I had grown up among scientists, I knew that this information could be useful to many.

Indeed, I would occasionally spot an intriguing overlap between something I had learned in my biology textbooks and what I happened to stumble upon in my pursuit of tools for health and performance. My once disparate worlds were starting to gradually converge.

And while my life after college may read a bit dry, like a CV, for me it was incredibly exciting. I became obsessed with our biological rhythms, and how they were affected by light. I got my master's degree by mapping the eye-to-brain circuits that help control those rhythms, and published those findings. From age twenty-five to thirty, I completed my PhD in neuroscience, researching the development and neuroplasticity of the brain. A lot of people hate grad school and finish looking a decade older than their biological age. I loved it. I worked for a scientist named Barbara Chapman, who taught me how to ask really good questions and design the right experiments to address them. She gave me a lot of leeway to develop new tools to answer previously hard-to-crack mysteries. I published six first-author papers with Barbara, all in terrific journals, including one in *Science*. None of it was easy. I routinely worked eighty-plus hours a week. It was both mentally and physically demanding. Turns out the skill I learned on road trips long ago—sleeping in cars and vans—served me well. So did all the tools for sleep and focus that I had figured out in college. Because I often slept in the lab. Along the way, I presented at dozens of meetings, an important part of academic training for which I am forever grateful. No one is born a good public speaker. It's a skill. One I got good at only because I had to present data to both friendly faces and expert critics who were anything but soft in their delivery. Nothing went perfectly, but little by little, and with plenty of red-in-the-face gaffes along the way, I was gaining mastery at my craft.

Professionally, it all paid off too. I got a great postdoctoral fellowship at Stanford. There I kept working with complete focus, day and night. I was inspired to do so, because at Stanford everyone was operating at the highest level. It is a truly amazing place.

But the postdoc step is an uncertain one in a scientist's career. There is no degree at the end, no promise of success even if you show up and work extremely hard. The vast majority of postdocs drop out of academic science and many out of science altogether. Also, my project had me competing with a big lab back east and an even bigger lab in Switzerland, and I was a lone postdoc chipping away with the help of two Stanford undergraduates, Nicko Josten and Mike Susman. I felt the pressure of not failing; I didn't want us to get "scooped"—nerd-speak for "beat to the punch"—on publishing. For the first time in a long time, fear and stress reentered the picture. And something else happened too. One day as I was headed into the lab, I found I barely had enough energy to climb two flights of stairs. And I slept fine the night before. I was doing everything "right." Or at least I thought so . . .

So I returned to the process that had served me well in college: I searched for tools on how to healthily increase my mental and physical vigor day in and day out. I read, I self-experimented. I also spoke to people who seemed to have a lot of mental and physical vigor but who came by it through effort and therefore understood the process, not simply because they were gifted with great genetics or were innately high energy. At that point I had no intention of being a public health educator. I just wanted to know what would really help me, a person very willing to put in effort but not a natural in any regard with respect to fitness, learning . . . or really anything.

Though I was, and remain, curious. The adage "seek and you shall find" is true. I found new ways to support my health and performance. Some things have remained the same over the years—for instance, I've hardly ever altered my overall exercise routine, as you'll see. It continues to work well, and not just for me. But other things caused me to make immediate changes to my diet and the way I approach sleep. I adopted a daily practice for something kind of like meditation but which is fundamentally different and quickly restores mental and physical vigor, even when sleep-deprived. And I found new tools for focus. I got good at task switching. All of it helped me complete my postdoctoral training at Stanford with first author papers, a host of invited reviews, and most importantly, the skills and confidence to take the next big step.

I was fortunate. I had made a name for myself in the fields of neural development and neural regeneration. Several figures from my papers were in major textbooks. I accepted a position as a professor at UC San Diego, one of the best neuroscience programs in the world. I was now teaching both undergraduate and graduate students in the classroom and in my lab, writing and reviewing research papers and grants for the National Institutes of Health, and traveling the world to give seminars. I was on journal editorial boards. My lab published a paper in *Nature*—arguably the best and most competitive journal in all of science. And many more in other top-tier journals. At forty, I returned to Stanford, this time as a tenured professor.

So all was fine and good, yes? Alas, no. While I was in grad school, Harry Carlisle—the person who inspired this path and with whom I had become close friends—took his own life. Soon after I started my lab in San Diego, Barbara Chapman died of breast cancer, at fifty. I was devastated.

And then my former postdoc advisor at Stanford, Ben Barres, had a heart attack right in front of me at dinner. He was an MD, and a PhD too, so when he looked up from his salmon filet and said, "I'm having a heart attack," I didn't ask questions. I rushed him to the hospital, where later we learned it wasn't just a heart attack. Ben got diagnosed with pancreatic cancer. He died about a year later.

I was never prepared for this kind of news. And it seemed to be coming from all sides of my life past and present. In one particularly dark month, three close friends of mine from childhood—Aaron King (the famed graffiti artist ORFN whose work showed in the San Francisco Museum of Modern Art), John Eikleberry, and Jonny Farrer—all of whom were kind, creative, brilliant people, died. Stomach cancer, fentanyl overdose, suicide. I was devastated.

At a far less tragic but still concerning level, often when I ran into friends and colleagues I barely recognized them because they were so out of shape. And often in pain. They complained about their backs, or insomnia, or autoimmune issues. They were concerned, too, about the health—both physical and mental—of their kids. Mind you many of these folks were MDs or scientists. They knew the science but that didn't seem to matter. One colleague of mine in San Diego became addicted to pain meds and stopped running his lab. Then he died. No one in our community talked about it. It was as if we thought we were immune to the addictions that stem from the very brain circuits we studied.

It became clear to me that a lot of people were struggling in one or more areas of health, as I once had. It didn't matter if they were doctors, scientists, entrepreneurs, or musicians, male, female, young or old . . . no one was immune.

Of course, I didn't have all the answers. But I had tools I knew were potent and could be valuable to others. And from my research, both in my lab and outside of it, I understood several of the mechanisms behind why those tools worked. I was by no means an expert in all fields of biology, but I was fluent in neuroscience. By the time I was a professor, if I had any questions about a specific field of biology, I knew world-class experts who could give me the answers, if such answers existed. I knew a lot of world-class MDs too. And experts in physical health and performance.

Some of the best tools were little-known variations on the classic "eat right, get sleep, exercise" adage. These variations were rarely discussed but maximized results. Other tools came from experts in the trauma-healing and addiction-recovery communities. Some came from elite athletes or their coaches. Still more came from my most forward-thinking MD colleagues and friends. My benchmark was always the same: If the tools worked for me and for others, did not require a lot of time or money, and were safe, they became part of my arsenal, and I would pass them along to others if I thought they might be of help to them too.

Mind you, all along I was still working in my lab, studying brain development, regeneration, and neuroplasticity. Our work was increasingly focused on remedying diseases, but none of it was related to issues I or family members personally had challenges with. But because I saw that stress was such a pervasive issue, and at the heart of so many of the health and performance challenges that so many scientists and MDs, young and old, were struggling with, I decided to devote a significant fraction of my lab to studying stress, resilience to stress, and real-time stress control. My lab's work became more immediately applicable to more people. And that felt good. Here were more tools for friends, family, and colleagues, and they became part of my arsenal as well.

While I love academic science, it has always been somewhat painful to see incredible data from published findings that I know could be of benefit to the general public kept out of their reach. It's not that the scientific community actively hides their findings. To the contrary. Universities have press offices, and the news outlets have long had health and science sections. But all I had to do was compare what the press said about the work I knew and understood, with what the scientists who actually did the work said and what some of them were starting to do to support their own health and that of their families, to know that there was a gap—a trench, actually—between the two. No one was to blame. There was nothing nefarious going on. It was just how things were. I decided to try to fill that gap.

Which is why in 2019, I started sharing tools for health and the science behind them on social media, and in 2021, I started the *Huberman Lab* podcast. At that time much of the world was locked down. Stress was at an all-time high, so I felt even more compelled to share information I knew could help people. I knew nothing about podcasting, but I grew up with the ultimate example of DIY media: Skateboarders have always filmed their own movies, long before social media or reality TV made it a thing. My close friend from high school Jake Rosenberg filmed us all as kids. He eventually became a legend in skateboarding filmmaking, as well as one of the original contributors to the film editing program Adobe Premiere.

So to start a podcast, I DIY'd it. But not alone. I recruited my friend Rob Mohr, who had a small podcast and knew the basics of the genre. We looped in famed skateboard photographer Mike Blabac, skateboard filmmakers and editors Chris Ray and Martin Fobes, and we did what we knew would work. We recorded a person—me—talking about and living his passion: science and tools for health. I also started interviewing my colleagues from Stanford and beyond on the podcast. (My bulldog-mastiff Costello was asleep under the desk in my recording studio/closet snoring away for many of our first episodes.)

There are three other critical players who make it work. First is Ian Mackey, whom we (ethically) poached from Stanford's media team to come work for the podcast. Another is Greg Annunziata, who was my Uber driver and is now *Huberman Lab* podcast admin. It's not uncommon that people ask me questions about tools for health, but on a short ride to the airport one day, Greg asked the right questions. I immediately recognized that he was as curious as I am. As he dropped me off, I said: "You should come work for me." That was four years ago.

Everyone on the team wanted to learn, and apply, science-based tools for health and performance in their lives. Mike used the tools in this book to bring lifelong blood pressure issues into check and to lose, and keep off, sixty pounds of extra weight. He also quit excessive drinking, something he had done for decades. Ian—once very overweight—is now super fit and thriving in every aspect of life. Another member of the team has multiple sclerosis and, with these tools, has been able to reduce a lot of his symptoms. He has vigor to spare. All of us use protocols for sleep, exercise, nutrition, stress control, and more to navigate extremely demanding yet rewarding family and professional lives. None of us are naturals at this. We are passionate, hardworking, and yes, curious. But we are humans, which means we need tools for health and performance as much as anyone else.

Which brings me to the third essential player here: you.

I wrote this book for you, so you can benefit from the very same tools they use, and many others too. Podcast episodes are great, but what I have striven to do in the pages that follow is provide something different. The format is such that you can skip to any chapter, learn about the information there, and apply it easily. You can also read the book from start to finish. As mentioned before, the scientific themes build on one another, the same way they do in real life, in your body and brain. The protocols are organized in order of importance and impact for each chapter. Each begins with a series of steps that explain what to do. Then comes the science, which explores the mechanisms behind why they work. I also answer questions I'm frequently asked by friends, family, colleagues, and the general public.

One of my hopes is that from reading this book you will start to think about your health in a more scientific way. Try a given protocol, then pay attention to how it shifts your mental and physical health and your performance. I occasionally use the term *anecdata* to refer to these kinds of insights, ones based on a person's experience. Individual experiences are often dismissed because academic science does not generally consider a sample size of one person as evidence—except in formal case studies, of course. And yet, each of our lives is its own kind of laboratory. There is nothing wrong with giving credence to your own experience and to watching how something affects you as a source of data. The key is to become a *systematic observer* of you. See how starting a protocol affects your body, your emotions, or your productivity. Also take note of what happens when you stop doing a protocol—switching to the control arm of an experiment, if you will.

Of course, as you learn about the mechanisms that underlie the various protocols, I also hope you will come to appreciate the astonishingly beautiful thing that is our biology—the cells, organs, and interactions among bodily systems that create our mental and physical life. Surely, we are more than just a bunch of cells and chemicals. But those cells and chemicals are truly magnificent in their arrangements and power. *Protocols* is about tapping into, and leveraging, that power.

And so, we begin.

CHAPTER 1

PROTOCOLS

for SLEEP

Sleep is the subject of the first chapter of this book because sleep profoundly impacts every aspect of our physiology and psychology. Put simply, sleep is the foundation of our mental health, our physical health, and our performance.[1] We win by sleeping.

I came to that realization pretty early but only because I struggled with sleep. As a kid I slept like a log—always a solid eight to nine hours, rarely waking up in the middle of the night even once. As a teen I would stay out late and sleep in on the weekends, as most of us did. I never thought about my sleep.

When I reached my junior year in high school, however, everything changed. I would lie down, fall asleep right away, but then wake up three to four hours later, wide awake. Then I would toss and turn. Eventually I would fall back asleep but then needed to sleep really late into the morning to feel rested. School started at 8:00 a.m., so that wasn't an option most days. That had me falling asleep in class, feeling wide awake in the evening, and then the whole cycle would repeat.

Toward the end of high school when I started getting into fitness, I learned that we recover from exercise during sleep. That was the early 1990s and the public was not yet aware of the importance of sleep. There was some science on it—in fact some of the best work on the role of sleep for health and cognition was coming from the Stanford Sleep Lab just a few miles up the road from where I lived. But it was from a prominent trainer in the world of fitness that I first learned to take sleep seriously. He gave me one mostly good suggestion for sleep, and one terrible one. The mostly good suggestion was to read the work of Allan Hobson—a sleep researcher from Harvard—and I eventually did, although I discovered Allan's focus was mainly on the importance of dreams, which felt like a bit of a tease for someone with sleep issues. The terrible advice he gave me? He told me if I woke up in the middle of the night and couldn't fall back asleep that I should drink a half mug of white wine. I was seventeen! I tried it anyway, and it didn't work for me. Thankfully. We now know alcohol greatly reduces the quality and restorative properties of sleep, even if it does help some people fall asleep.

Eventually I figured out how to master the art of getting a great night's sleep, but it took time. Years, in fact. The science progressed too, of course, and we now know a lot about both the importance of sleep and ways to remedy pretty much any sleep issue. I wish I had the information you are about to read back in high school, and college, and graduate school, and my postdoc. The reality is, the busier we are, the more important sleep is to our health and performance. But no matter how busy or calm our life is, a great night's sleep is crucial to our mind and body.

If you are like the majority of people, and you struggle to get a great night's sleep, you want to remedy that as soon as possible.[2] But even if you are one of those rare individuals who sleeps deeply every night and wakes up feeling fully refreshed every day, there are still ways to improve your sleep and thus, your quality of life. Regardless of which category you fall into, this chapter will help.

I'd like to mention here that this chapter is a long one. We go deep into the science of sleep, but I promise you it's all made accessible. I know that understanding this science will help you get a great night's sleep. I wrote this chapter so you can browse by topic or tool. Start with the parts that interest you most, or the protocols that you think will help you right now.

I prefer to focus on the benefits of doing things correctly, but when it comes to sleep, it's worth thinking a bit about the downsides of getting things wrong too, and learning to avoid those. Sleep deprivation—a term that means getting too little sleep or waking up too many times during the night—has been linked to significantly elevated risk of heart disease, stroke, and numerous hormonal imbalances involving—just to name a handful: cortisol, estrogen, testosterone, and insulin, the latter of which can cause type 2 diabetes.[3] Obesity, mental health issues, physical injuries, cancer, car accidents, depression, hypertension, and age-related dementia have all also been linked to poor sleep.[4] Sleep deprivation doesn't necessarily *directly* create these problems; rather it impairs cellular mechanisms that cascade to produce multiple issues within and between different organs and systems.

To be clear, everyone has a bad night's sleep now and again. But here's a good goal for you: Aim to sleep well 90 to 95 percent of the nights of your life, and allow the remaining 5 to 10 percent of those nights to be bad due to uncontrollable negative circumstances, like a work conflict, or joyful experiences, like a great party. Do your best to make sleep a top priority so that the rest of your life can be that much better.

Perhaps you have heard some of this before. Most people know a bit about the benefits and importance of sleep. As I mentioned above, that is a fairly recent development. It was about a decade ago when Matthew Walker, who formerly directed the Center for Human Sleep Science at the University of California, Berkeley, and is currently at the University of Texas in Dallas, wrote the now famous book, *Why We Sleep*. At that time, the "I'll sleep when I'm dead" or the "I'll catch up on sleep this weekend" mentalities prevailed.[5] Thanks in large part to Matt's book and other public education efforts, people now recognize they *must* sleep, yet the majority of people still don't sleep well and far too many people sleep poorly, with nearly half of adults reporting their sleep satisfaction as an "F"—meaning the lowest possible grade.[6] It is true that we all have slightly different sleep needs.

Some of us consider ourselves morning larks. We prefer to rise early. Others are night owls who prefer to stay up late. These are what sleep researchers call chronotypes: genetically determined features of the chemicals, cells, and circuits that regulate when we prefer to go to sleep and wake up. You can blame your parents for your bedtime (and wake time) preference.

Separate from your chronotype is the total amount of sleep you need. Some of us need six hours to feel fully rested, others need eight, and some people feel great with just five. I should point out, however, that the feel-great-on-five folks are exceedingly rare. Most people need seven to eight.[7] But as mentioned above, according to recent reports from the National Sleep Foundation and the Centers for Disease Control and Prevention (CDC), at least a third of Americans do not get nearly enough sleep—and that statistic is likely to be a vast underestimate given the enormous increase in time spent on social media and online nowadays.[8] In fact, that figure skyrockets to more than 75 percent among high school students. That's right, approximately three-fourths of teens are not getting enough sleep,[9] which is extremely concerning given that our adolescent and teen years are when much of our brain wiring related to mood and behavior regulation, as well as attention and learning, gets solidified. From birth until about age twenty-five is an especially sensitive and time-limited phase, or what is called a *critical period*.[10] And the thing about critical periods is eventually they close: While our brains remain plastic our entire lives, the amount of neuroplasticity possible in those first twenty-five years far exceeds what is possible afterward, so teens can't simply make up for their lost brain wiring later on.[11] We have no idea what the long-term consequences of this kind of chronic sleep deprivation are, but we do know that far too many young people are missing out on sleep at exactly the time when they need it most.

Compulsive overuse of phones and other screen-based technologies at night is a major factor for the poor sleep of adolescents and teens, but also for the poor sleep habits of adults.[12] A central feature of life in the twenty-first century is to always be connected online and by text. So much so that by the classic definition of shift work, many—perhaps even *most* people—worldwide, now meet the definition of a shift worker, that is, awake for two to three hours between 10:00 p.m. and 5:00 a.m. Shift work is not just about staying up late but also involves reduced amounts of exposure to sunlight during the day, lack of sufficient darkness at night, and a nocturally-shifted eating schedule. That has well-established negative health effects, including poor gut health, mental health deficits, and even decreased lifespan.[13] So this is no trivial matter. Smartphone technologies are not to blame per se, but when we use those technologies certainly is. We can scroll 24-7 and unless we resist, the light from our phone, tablet, or computer screen impairs our sleep. Not to mention that the content we absorb on those screens often affects our sleep, too, because of the elevated levels of arousal—aka stress—that content creates. Even if being on our phones or tablets in the hours before sleep doesn't stress us out, it can disrupt our sleep.[14] We rarely hear how texting alters our sleep patterns but I would argue that for many people, it is at least as pernicious as social media in this regard. To be clear, texting is a wonderful tool for communication; it allows us to connect quickly. And social media can be a good source for learning, social connection, and entertainment. The downside, however, is that we can have conversations and observe events at any time of day or night. If we wake up in the middle of the night, we know we should roll over and go back to sleep, but many of us instead start reading and sending texts, or scrolling the internet or browsing social media.

So it comes as no surprise that most of us now qualify as shift workers but very few of us are sacrificing our sleep hours by doing actual work.[15] We have all become so habituated to this new normal of consuming content and communicating at all hours that we don't see how out of sync it really is with our sleep and therefore our health.

The good news is, we can fix our sleep duration, quality, and even determine its timing—regardless of our chronotype—without having to disengage too much from these technologies.

And it's oh-so-worth it because when I say, "We win by sleeping," I am referring to the fact that sleep shapes everything about us—how we look, how we think, and how we feel. But I also mean that if you get your sleep right 90 percent of the time, you'll be absolutely amazed how your appearance, health, and performance will improve. The data say you'll likely live longer as well.[16]

This chapter offers protocols you can easily integrate into your life to get far more restful and restorative sleep. That is, to "sleep better." None take much time, and many of them are downright pleasurable. Let's consider these protocols in order of their importance.

SLEEP PROTOCOL

1

View Sunlight as Soon as Possible After Waking

WHAT TO DO:

- **Get morning sunlight in your eyes as soon as possible after waking.** Go outside and look in the direction of the sun for at least five to ten minutes each morning. Your goal should be to get sunlight in your eyes within the first thirty to sixty minutes of waking up.
- **A few things to keep in mind.** If you wake up before the sun rises, you'll obviously have to wait. If you can view the sun as it comes up across the horizon, great, but that's not vital for this protocol to work.

  Morning sunlight, as we will review, differs in quality from sunlight at other times of the day. It is best viewed by facing the sun without any physical barriers, like awnings or buildings, obscuring your view. Don't wear a brimmed hat, as it blocks some of the light that would otherwise reach your eyes from overhead. Wearing eyeglasses or contacts is fine but, alas, this protocol won't work nearly as well through a window or windshield, as that will filter out many of the relevant wavelengths of light. Skip the sunglasses while doing this protocol. What about clouds? No matter how overcast, there is always some sunlight coming through once the sun is up. In fact, the more accurate way to state this protocol would be "get as-early-in-your-day-as-possible *daylight* in your eyes," but that is a mouthful. The point is that the sun provides daylight even on overcast days. Just compare how bright it is at 8:00 a.m. on an overcast day to midnight the night before. So forget the "there is no sun out in winter where I live" argument. There is daylight, and you want to view it. Indeed, this protocol is especially important on cloudy days.

Caution: Do not stare at the sun. Never force your eyes to stay open. Allow your natural squint and blink reflexes to protect your eyes. If the sun still feels too bright, look a few degrees to the side of the sun.

HOW IT WORKS:

Correctly timed sunlight viewing—especially morning sunlight viewing—is immensely beneficial to our overall health. This simple, zero-cost protocol powerfully affects your daytime mood, focus, and alertness, and improves your sleep, which further improves your health and performance in myriad ways.

The power of this protocol arises from its impact on three synergistic elements: your circadian clock, your eyes (or more specifically, the nerve cells in your eyes that detect sunlight and communicate its presence to your circadian clock), and specific qualities of light that come from the sun, especially when it is low, relative to the horizon. Together, these three elements make up a robust network that drives many of the biological processes in your brain and body.

I first learned about the importance of viewing morning sunlight from one of the world's preeminent sleep researchers, Seiji Nishino, MD, PhD. I was working in his lab at Stanford during a summer home from college, and I noticed he would always stop to face the sun for a few minutes before going into the lab for the day. Even if he arrived at the lab before sunrise (not uncommon for researchers in a sleep lab!), he would make sure to step outside shortly after sunrise and face the sun for a few minutes before returning to work. That was way back in 1996—when our understanding of the mechanisms of human circadian biology was rudimentary compared to now. Seiji explained that viewing morning sunlight felt good, that it gave him more energy for the day, and that it improved his sleep. I started joining him and joked that we resembled the many ground squirrels around us up on their haunches doing the very same thing. Little did I know that the exact same morning sunlight-sensing cells, circuits, and mechanisms were at play in us and those squirrels and, in fact, in every mammal where they have been examined.

I quickly noticed that on days I viewed morning sunlight, I also felt good, had more energy for the day, and slept better at night, so I kept with it. You should experience those benefits, too, because of the way morning sunlight—whether on a clear or cloudy day—kickstarts a powerful set of hormonal and neural mechanisms that positively shift the state of your entire brain and body for many hours afterward. It can work the first time and every time, and once you understand a bit about those mechanisms, it will allow you to easily adjust this protocol to your schedule and circumstances to derive the maximum benefits with minimal time investment.

Your Circadian Clock

Located a few centimeters above the roof of your mouth is a small cluster of neurons called the *suprachiasmatic nucleus*, or SCN.[17] The SCN is your master circadian clock. Its job is to coordinate the activities of all the cells and organs in your body into a coherent twenty-four-hour rhythm so that certain cells and organs in your body are more active, and other cells and organs are less active, depending on the phase of that twenty-four-hour rhythm. The SCN keeps your body and brain on schedule.

The first documented discovery of a circadian clock came not from studies of humans or even of rodents, but of plants. In 1729, a French astronomer named Jean-Jacques d'Ortous de Mairan noticed that a mimosa plant kept in a totally dark room continued to rhythmically fold and unfold its leaves every twenty-four hours, just as if the sun was shining through the window.[18] It was a mystery: If the plant was not unfurling to absorb sun or other light, then what was guiding its movements? About two hundred years later, German biologist Erwin Bünning tracked the movements of bean plant leaves and reported that they followed a cycle lasting 24.4 hours. Observations such as these confirmed that plants had internal, or what scientists call "endogenous," clocks that followed what later became known as . . . a circadian rhythm, named for the Latin *circa diem*, or "around a day." And as decades of research would eventually confirm, the vast majority of organisms on Earth—not just plants but also insects, rodents, reptiles, and all mammals, including humans—have an endogenous timekeeper that keeps a twenty-four-hour circadian rhythm, even in the absence of any external cues about the status of the outside world.[19]

Our core body temperature, the release of certain hormones, and most notably our sleep-wake cycle, all follow a twenty-four-hour circadian rhythm.[20] Even when scientists extracted individual cells from the body, the cells continued to follow this rhythm.[21] And which genes they expressed and when, the proteins downstream of those genes, the cells' enzymatic activities—indeed not just *some* things but nearly everything about cellular function—appeared to vary, not randomly, but rather systematically every twenty-four hours. That was remarkable.

But what is equally remarkable is that all cells in our body can coordinate their individual rhythms in a manner that is timed perfectly with one another—like a well-practiced symphony, except this symphony involves not a few hundred or even a thousand participants, but trillions. And just like a symphony, it is not as if every cell simply needs to start and end its activity at the same time. Some cells need to be active at the same time, or *in-phase* with one another; some need to be active at opposite times, or in *anti-phase*, and still others repeat their cycles of activity faster, then slower, then faster, again with a unique signature and yet, still repeating once every twenty-four hours. And the start and end time of each cell's twenty-four-hour rhythm must be tightly bound to all the other cells of the body, just like the start and end of a symphony. Without this coordination, you end up with noise rather than music, illness rather than wellness. The only difference is the symphony that is your physiology never ceases; it repeats every twenty-four hours, from the day you're born until the day you die.

The basis of that persistent and extraordinarily precise biological coordination remained a mystery until somewhat recently. Clues came from multiple sources. First, studies in which people were placed into constant dark environments—such as caves or windowless bunkers—confirmed the existence of a circadian rhythm in humans. Back in 1938, two physiologists spent a month in Mammoth Cave, Kentucky (perhaps figuring this experiment was best done on themselves before asking anyone else to try it).[22] There, they confirmed that human body temperature has a circadian rhythm whereby it increases upon waking, decreases approximately ten to twelve hours later, drops to its nadir during sleep, then rises once again—all once every twenty-four hours, even though the subjects/researchers had no access to sunlight or other cues about time of day. And other studies confirmed that, in the absence of an alternating pattern of ambient light and darkness, the human body still maintains a circadian rhythm for numerous aspects of our physiology.[23]

In 1966, a German physician named Jürgen Aschoff initiated what became known as the bunker experiment, in which subjects (not researchers this time!) spent several weeks in a sealed bunker, living life as usual but without any windows or other ways to determine the passage of time.[24] They found that subjects generally spent about one-third of each twenty-four-hour period sleeping and two-thirds of it awake, just as most humans living aboveground do. However, the wake-up and to-sleep times of the people in the bunker drifted—they woke up slightly later and went to sleep slightly later each day. Thus, the bunker experiment confirmed the existence of a circadian rhythm, but one that requires some external cue to anchor it. What remained mysterious was the biological basis of the circadian clock—was it a bloodborne factor? In the liver? In the brain? In the pineal gland? Theories abounded but none of them held up to experimentation. And another major question remained: In the environment outside the bunker, which external cues were responsible for setting that clock to a specific start and finish time each day?

Subsequent discoveries, first in rodents and later in humans, revealed the existence of a small cluster—or what is called a "nucleus"—of neurons located a few centimeters above our mouths that had a key part to play. It was later named the suprachiasmatic nucleus (SCN) for "above the chiasm"—the chiasm being the location at the base of the brain where the nerve fibers from both eyes partially cross. As I mentioned earlier, the SCN is the master circadian clock: the structure that coordinates the activities of all our cells and organs. In other words, the SCN is the orchestra conductor that makes sure each cell's twenty-four-hour rhythm starts on time.[25] In 1972, Irving Zucker's lab at UC Berkeley and Robert Moore's lab at the University of Chicago independently discovered that lesions to the SCN render organisms' circadian pattern arrhythmic and disorganized.[26] Naturally occurring SCN lesions caused by tumors eventually showed the SCN is necessary for sleep-wake, hunger, and other bodily rhythms to obey circadian cycles in humans as well.[27] Moreover, animal studies showed that transplanting even just a small number of healthy SCN neurons into an arrhythmic brain restored a coherent twenty-four-hour rhythm, proving the SCN is both necessary and sufficient for endogenous circadian rhythms.[28]

If ever there was a brain structure whose function is beautifully organized to help ensure our survival as a species, it is the SCN. Even the SCN's seeming imperfection turns out to be perfect after all.

Stay with me here. For example, the SCN generates a period—meaning a cycle length—that is close to but not quite twenty-four hours. The SCN's period tends to be a bit longer than that, up to 24.5 hours.[29] By virtue of this, it can shift the start of the circadian rhythm forward or backward according to seasonal changes in day length or other survival-based needs, without making a mess and setting our cells on different schedules.[30] In other words, allowing a little room in its period duration affords us more flexibility and overall precision, not less, which is great because as we all know life is rarely the same from one day to the next. What's more, it is also what allows for *phase shifting*,[31] or the ability to change the start time of the daily cycle. If you're wondering why this doesn't have us waking up later and going to sleep later each day, it's because viewing morning light and evening light nudges your clock back and forth perfectly, to keep it regular. Later I'll explain how you can leverage that to overcome jet lag or any new schedule fast, but for now, all you need to know is that the not-exactly-twenty-four-hour rhythm is a feature, not a flaw.

As you probably already realize from the call to action that is Sleep Protocol 1, our SCN cares about whether it is light or dark out. And of course light-dark cycles are set by the spin of the earth. But how is it that our SCN—a tiny cluster of neurons embedded deep in the darkness of our brains—"knows" about the spin of the earth? Let's consider how to answer that question with insights from planetary science and cosmology.

We're all on this big sphere in space, spinning around at about one thousand miles per hour, causing us to face the sun, then away from the sun, then back toward the sun every twenty-four hours. Because the earth is round, the exact duration of sunlight we can experience each day depends, of course, on where we happen to be on earth. The variability is large, ranging from rather equal light-dark splits at the equator to nearly full days and/or nights of darkness or sunlight exposure at the poles. But no matter where we are on earth, inside each of our brains, our SCN steadily churns out that slightly longer than twenty-four-hour rhythm of coordinated cellular activity across our whole body.

Ultimately it is our SCN that tells us when to sleep and when to wake. We are a diurnal, not a nocturnal, species. We can stay up late and sleep all day if we choose, but even for night owls, all our bodily systems of hormones and neurotransmitters, our immune system, our levels of focus and quality of that focus, all of it, function much better when we live diurnally and wake just before or during the early daylight hours and go to sleep some hours after sundown.[32] (Yes, night owls would be wise to do this too—that is, if mental and physical health are your priority.)

Keep in mind these are independent phenomena; the earth's spin and travel around the sun is not what causes our SCN to have a twenty-four-hour rhythm, nor does it tell us when to sleep and when to wake, but they do need to be linked. So how do we link—or what is called *entrain*—our SCN's rhythm with the light-dark cycle generated by the earth's spin and travel around the sun? Remember, our SCN resides deep in our brain. It lives in the darkness of our skulls. To synchronize our circadian clock with the day-night cycle cast on us by our location on earth, we need a way for the presence or absence of sunlight to be conveyed to the SCN. And the best way to do that is to call upon the one part of our brain that has direct access to sunlight: our eyes.

Your Eyes

Wait, did I say that your eyes are part of your brain? Yes, that is correct. Lining the inside-back part of each of your eyeballs is a thin sheet of brain tissue called the neural retina. Your neural retinas were squeezed out and away from the rest of your brain during the first trimester of your life, while you were still in your mother's womb, and then grew wirelike extensions into the brain proper, forming two optic nerves. Your optic nerves convey electrical signals about the presence or absence of sunlight, objects, faces, moving vehicles, and on and on to different brain areas, including—you guessed it—the SCN.[33]

The connections between your eyes and your brain are truly a spectacular product of biological engineering. First, they solve the problem of how to inform image-forming regions of your brain about "what is out there" in the world, so you can see faces, moving objects, and colors. They also solve the problem of letting your SCN know "*when* it is out there" in the world, by the presence of sunlight. The neurons that convey the presence of sunlight to the SCN are not of the image-forming kind; they don't respond to the shape of the sun, but instead to its brightness and to the specific wavelengths of sunlight that reach your eyes when the sun is low in the sky. We refer to these specific wavelengths as low solar angle sunlight.[34]

Have you ever noticed that low solar angle sunlight appears more yellow than midday sun? Or even orange? Check out a sunrise or sunset and compare the color of sunlight to the color of sunlight at noon. Of course, sunlight doesn't change according to where it is in the sky, but what portions of sunlight are visible to us does.

Sunlight is always full spectrum: It contains all wavelengths of light, red-orange-yellow-green-blue-indigo-violet, or ROYGBIV, just as they taught us in elementary school. The R(ed), O(range), and Y(ellow) are longer wavelengths of light, the G(reen) is medium wavelength, and the B(lue), I(ndigo), and V(iolet) are shorter wavelengths. And of course, the sun emits UV and far-red, or infrared wavelengths, too, but we can't see those (although many other animals and insects can). When the sun is high in the sky, it appears white, because all the wavelengths of light arrive at our eyes at roughly the same intensities. When the sun is low in the sky, we see the sun as more yellow, orange, or red, because molecules in the atmosphere preferentially redirect the shorter blue, indigo, and violet wavelengths of light—a process called Rayleigh scattering. (We'll discuss the properties of light in depth in chapter 5.)

All mammals, us humans included, have evolved a special system of light detection that responds specifically to the presence and contrast of short and long wavelengths of bright light, which is exactly what reaches your eyes if you view sunlight early or late in the day, while the sun is fairly low in the sky. In other words, we all have a sunrise and sunset detecting system in our eyes that communicates the time of day to our SCN.[35]

As I mentioned earlier, this timekeeping eye-to-brain circuit is also a fairly recent discovery. And by recent, I mean *recent*: In the late 1990s, there still wasn't general agreement among circadian biologists whether light—and not some other cue like social interactions—was the dominant force entraining our SCN. Then, in 1998, neuroscientist Ignacio "Iggy" Provencio made a key discovery. Iggy found a molecule in the skin of an African frog species that caused its skin to darken when exposed to sunlight was also present in the eyes of mice.[36] The molecule was an opsin, which is a kind of protein that absorbs light, and when it does, it changes its conformation to set off a signaling cascade.[37] Since the same opsin was known to cause darkening of dermal melanophores in frog skin, Provencio called the mouse retinal opsin *melanopsin*. Other labs confirmed melanopsin-containing cells are abundant in the human retina, too, mostly in the lower portion that views the upper visual field, which, you might have guessed, corresponds to the sky.[38]

So we have a frog-skin-like set of cells in our eyes? Not quite. To explain what makes melanopsin-containing retinal cells so special, first a bit about photoreceptors. Photoreceptors are neurons that convert light into electrical signals the rest of the retina and brain can interpret. But the retinal cells that contain melanopsin are not like other photoreceptors. The melanopsin-containing retinal neurons Iggy discovered turned out to be both photoreceptive and retinal ganglion cells—the neurons that connect the eyes to the brain and the very cells whose wirelike extensions, or axons, make up the optic nerves. Soon after, a group of neuroscientists, David Berson and Felice Dunn at Brown University and Samer Hattar and King Wai-Yau at Johns Hopkins University, along with several of their students and postdocs, confirmed that melanopsin RGCs send their axons to the SCN *and* that they fire electric signals, thereby releasing neurotransmitters, when light is shone on them.[39] Remarkably, they did this when they were isolated from all other retinal cells. As long as the light shone was very bright and long lasting, they fired electrical signals. These cells were therefore named intrinsically photosensitive RGCs (ipRGCs) to differentiate them from the other 99 percent of RGCs that can't respond directly to light on their own. Some years later, work from the Neitz Color Vision Lab at the University of Washington in Seattle and by others showed that the optimal stimulus for ipRGCs isn't just bright light.[40] They discovered that the best way to activate the ipRGCs that connect to the SCN is with sustained very bright light, similar to what we see as blue or green light, contrasted with medium wavelengths of light, or what we typically see as yellow or orange—in other words, features prominent in low solar angle sunlight. The color contrasts in sunrises and sunsets tell your brain about what time it is in the twenty-four-hour cycle. That collection of work, from the discovery of melanopsin to ipRGCs, and how they work, was revelatory. It meant that there was a specific neural circuit extending from the eye to the brain dedicated to entraining the SCN and our circadian rhythms. That circuit is tuned to—neuroscience lingo for "responds to"—the presence of low solar angle sunlight. The SCN then handles the job of body- and brain-wide synchronization of circadian rhythmicity. This sunlight-driven circadian entrainment circuit requires no learning or practice to activate. It is present from birth and functions the first time and every time to control, among other things, your sleep-wake cycle.

The Sun

Which brings us to the final piece of the puzzle—the part that is not hardwired but that you control with your behavior—and that is the call to action of this protocol: exposing your eyes to morning sunlight (or in its absence, to the next best alternative, which I describe below). Doing so activates the ipRGC-to-SCN circadian entrainment circuit and initiates dozens of beneficial processes that get and keep your brain and body going throughout the day. And toward the evening, it puts you in the best possible position to get a great night's sleep.

In fact, we have copious evidence that this is foundational to both our daytime well-being and nighttime sleep. As one small example, a group of architects and neurologists came together in 2014 to investigate how windowless offices affected the people who worked in them.[41] They asked twenty-seven office workers who had either no windows, or work areas situated far from windows, and twenty-two people working in offices with windows, about their well-being and sleep quality. The questionnaire scores were decidedly poorer among the windowless workers. They reported more sleep disturbances and an overall unsatisfactory quality of sleep.

In the early 2000s, a group of chronobiologists (scientists who study biological timing) at the Institute for Medical Psychology, in Munich, Germany, surveyed five hundred people about their sleep times, light exposure, and chronotype—as in, morning person, night owl, et cetera (you'll find out how to determine yours in Sleep Protocol 4).[42] They found that the amount of light exposure during the day correlated with what time people went to bed: More exposure during the day meant earlier bedtimes. This link can be partly explained by external factors, like employment: People whose livelihoods depend on being outdoors are more likely to be early-to-bed types, especially if their work requires them to rise early or is physically demanding. But that doesn't explain the connection entirely. It turns out that it's also due, in part, to the fact that exposure to daylight has a regulating effect on our physiology—causing elevated levels of alertness by a host of different pathways, including hormonal and neural pathways. As one review put it, "In sum, research seems to agree that daylight (at high intensities) is beneficial for sleep."[43]

There are also numerous studies showing that bright-light exposure early in the day—at the intensities that one would get from being outdoors in the morning—is beneficial for everything from mood to hormone health, daytime energy levels, and on and on.[44] But before you say, "Okay, got it!," there's just a bit more to understand about the underlying mechanisms in this protocol, and that's the relationship between sleep and wakefulness. And it will help you get the most out of this protocol, regardless of where you live and the time of year.

Our daytime levels of alertness reflect the quality and duration of our nighttime sleep. That's a giant "duh." We all know that if we sleep poorly, we drag both mentally and physically the next day. We also all know that if we sleep great, we're focused and motivated to do all kinds of things that require energy . . . and that we have the energy to do them.

But what most people do not know is that the relationship between sleep and wakefulness works in the other direction too. When we are alert during the morning and daytime, we are more likely to expend mental and physical energy that in turn helps us sleep at night. Even those of us who sleep well typically find that increasing our daytime physical activity—especially in the hours between sunrise and 2:00 p.m.—leads to significantly better sleep,[45] which in turn leads to more energy the next day, which improves sleep, and so on. Again, you're probably thinking, "This is common knowledge. Do we really need science to explain this?"

Here is the lesser-known fact: Morning sunlight viewing is the best way to increase our morning and daytime energy levels.[46] Not food (although fine to eat early in the day), not caffeine (also fine). It's morning sunlight.

Morning sunlight increases your energy levels through at least three different mechanisms. First, it suppresses any residual melatonin you may have circulating in your brain (Sleep Protocol 3 includes an extensive look at melatonin, a hormone that helps promote sleepiness).[47] As discussed above, when the ipRGCs are activated by sunlight viewing, they send electrical signals to the SCN. The SCN, in turn, stimulates a collection of neurons in the nearby paraventricular nucleus, or PVN. The PVN then sets off a cascade of signals that go through the spinal cord and back up to the pineal gland in the brain, shutting off melatonin production.[48] Voila! You've suppressed the primary hormone that promotes sleepiness by viewing morning sunlight.

Second, bright light reaching your eyes helps suppress the action of adenosine, a chemical that also leads to feelings of sleepiness.[49] Sunlight does this indirectly via its effects on other systems in the brain and body, but nonetheless, it has a potent adenosine-reducing effect. (We'll take a deep dive into adenosine in Sleep Protocol 7). After a full night's sleep, adenosine levels tend to be low, but if you happen to not get enough sleep (as so many of us do), morning light helps reduce any residual adenosine. That both increases your alertness and prevents the residual adenosine from delaying your circadian clock, which would otherwise bias you toward waking up later the next day, then going to sleep later, then waking up even later the following day, and so on (what chronobiologists call a *phase delay*).[50] Such circadian "drift" brought on by mild sleep deprivation is very common. It is best remedied by viewing morning sunlight to reset your circadian rhythm.[51]

Third, we need to talk about cortisol. Because it's often discussed in the context of chronic stress, which is bad, most people think cortisol is "bad" too. But it's not bad. Cortisol is essential to health and your levels of energy—you just don't want your cortisol levels to be elevated at the wrong times.[52]

Your SCN is located in your hypothalamus (H), which is part of a biological circuit that also includes your pituitary gland (P), a small, stalk-like protrusion at the base of your brain that releases hormones into your bloodstream. The circuit also includes your adrenal glands (A), which reside atop your kidneys. This circuit is known as the HPA axis.[53] The HPA axis is one of the main systems that responds to stress (which is why you'll hear more about it in chapter 3). Here's how it works: It starts with signals from the hypothalamus, which then stimulate the release of specific hormones from the pituitary, which in turn stimulate adrenaline and cortisol release from your adrenals.

The HPA axis is also involved in the sleep-wake cycle. When your ipRGCs are activated by low solar angle morning sunlight and your SCN receives the ensuing signal, it alerts your adrenal glands to release adrenaline and cortisol via the HPA axis.[54] Cortisol and adrenaline dramatically increase levels of alertness, the latter likely by activating receptors on your vagus nerve,[55] a large portion of which extends from the organs in your body up into your brain and stimulates areas there such as the locus coeruleus to make norepinephrine, which has the net effect of "waking" you up.[56] Cortisol does a lot of things. It also decreases inflammation and regulates our immune systems to protect against viral and bacterial infections.[57] And it helps regulate our energy levels. Think about cortisol as a wakefulness-promoting hormone, not a stress hormone, if you want to understand what the cortisol in your body is doing most of the time. It's also useful to consider how cortisol ebbs and flows across time due to signals from your circadian clock. By measuring cortisol levels every twenty minutes in human subjects, researchers found cortisol reaches its apex at about sixty minutes or so after you wake up and that it is lowest about four to five hours after you fall asleep.[58] Then it begins to rise sharply across the final two to three hours of your sleep until—boom! You wake up due in large part to what is called the cortisol awakening response (CAR). Yes, reaching a threshold level of cortisol is a major factor in what ultimately rouses you from sleep. As mentioned above, your cortisol continues to rise and peaks about sixty minutes after waking, then slowly drops down as you head into the early and late afternoon. Cortisol levels generally stay low and continue to drop in the evening and at nighttime (assuming it doesn't spike from stress or intense exercise—more on that below), and then it falls to its nadir in those first four to five hours of sleep before starting to rise again toward morning. We return to this *circadian cortisol curve* in chapter 3, and the role it plays in promoting health in women and men of all ages. For now, the key thing to know is that for cortisol to support our health, it needs to peak in the first hour or so after waking; it then needs to drop precipitously in the evening and night and continue falling to reach its nadir in those initial four to five hours of sleep.[59]

Viewing morning sunlight doesn't directly cause the morning peak in cortisol, but it can dramatically amplify its rise by as much as 50 percent.[60] This also helps ensure that this peak comes early in the day and isn't shifted to the afternoon. Late-day elevations in cortisol have negative consequences over time such as sleeplessness, anxiety, and metabolic disease.[61]

A quick note: A morning workout, morning caffeine, and breakfast (provided it isn't a huge and/or carbohydrate-laden one) will all promote wakefulness, too, and thereby contribute to a well-aligned circadian rhythm. But morning sunlight is the most potent lever for increasing morning cortisol and thus energy during your day, and for improving your sleep at night. Don't underestimate its power.

Keep your circadian rhythm attuned to the sun, and all of these mechanisms will work as they should.

COMMON QUESTIONS:

It's often dark when I wake up. What do I do if I have no access to morning sunlight but I want to start my day?

If you wake up before sunrise, and you want to start your day, I suggest turning on as many bright indoor lights in your home—or hotel room, or wherever you may be—as possible. Sunlight cannot be replaced by standard indoor lighting, but turning on indoor lighting first thing won't hurt. Then get outside to view morning sunlight once the sun is up.

If you wake before sunrise every day, or if you live in a part of the world where it is very dark in winter, you may want to invest in a 10,000 lux light to help ensure you get enough light in the morning (lux is a measure of brightness). Most cost about $100, and some are portable for travel. I often wake up before sunrise, and because the ipRGCs can be activated by very bright artificial lights if those bright lights include sufficient short wavelengths, I keep a 10,000 lux lamp in my kitchen and bathroom.[62] It lacks long wavelength light, so I also have a red incandescent light next to it and I turn that on too. I use the red incandescent light from SaunaSpace (no affiliation). I turn them both on first thing in the morning and then I get outside to view morning sunlight once the sun is up. I am well aware these lights are not a replacement for sunlight, but they help bridge the gap until the sun is up. Once the sun is up, you can be sure I go outside to view it!

And I will sometimes keep the 10,000 lux lamp and a red incandescent light on and facing me for an hour or so once I'm back working at my desk or getting ready for the day. Chapter 5 further explains the logic and benefits of this extended morning light exposure. There I also mention options that can be of real help for sleep as well as other aspects of health too, such as metabolic health.

But remember, morning sunlight is the best stimulus for your ipRGCs, SCN, and circadian rhythm, and it costs nothing! Figure out how to view it each morning. Again, you don't need to see it cross the horizon as it rises. If you do, great, but if you wake up after sunrise, that's fine. Do your best to view sunlight within the first thirty to sixty minutes after waking up. Bring your coffee or tea outside with you. Bring your spouse or kids if they're awake. Bring your dog if you have one. Remember, dogs, cats, cows, and other animals have ipRGCs and an SCN, too, and they benefit from morning sunlight in many of the same ways and via the same mechanisms as we do.[63]

What if it's cloudy outside?

To activate your ipRGCs fastest, go outside and face east toward the sun on a nice, clear morning with no clouds in the sky. Obviously, this isn't possible for everyone every day.

Again, fortunately, sparse clouds do not interfere with the interaction between sunlight and our circadian clock. However, if the sky is densely overcast and gray, a 10,000 lux light can be a real help, but still aim for getting more sunlight in your eyes to compensate for the lower intensity of sunlight and reduced yellow-blue contrast exposure you're likely to get on very overcast days. In fact, it's *especially* important that you get sunlight in your eyes on overcast days. This is for three reasons: (1) dense clouds reduce the number of photons reaching your eyes in a given amount of time; (2) they filter out much of the longer (yellow, orange, and red) wavelengths of light, and (3) you are likely to be indoors more on cloudy days, which can cause the SCN to fall out of sync with the solar cycle, which leads to later nights, more artificial light exposure at night, more circadian disruption, and so on.

Aim to extend the sunny, clear day recommendation of a minimum of five to ten minutes, to at least fifteen minutes on cloudy days, and thirty minutes (minimum) on densely overcast days. That may seem like a long time, but remember, you don't need to stand in one place gazing at the sky. Take a walk. Make a call. Listen to a book or podcast or talk to a friend, partner, or other family member. And even if you can't be outside for the full time recommended above, some sunlight hitting your eyes in the morning is better than none. If you miss a day completely due to travel or sickness or other reasons, don't despair—your energy levels that day may be lower because you didn't get the cortisol spike bright morning light causes, but your circadian rhythm is the reflection of your previous three to four days of sunlight viewing activity.

Do I need to worry about sunlight damaging my eyes?

Excessive UV light exposure can cause cataracts and, as we have all heard, skin damage, accelerated skin aging, and some forms of skin cancer, topics I cover in more detail later in the book. But viewing morning sunlight is much safer than viewing overhead midday sunlight—because that Rayleigh scattering of short wavelength light when the sun is low in the sky includes UV and thus reduces your UV exposure significantly. It is when the sun is overhead that the UV index is high. UV light isn't bad, per se, but you don't want too much of it reaching your eyes or skin. Chapter 5 goes into the benefits and drawbacks of UV.

NEVER, EVER force yourself to stare at the sun—or any light source for that matter, at any time of day. Your natural blink and "look away" reflex is a built-in circuit (yes, there is a dedicated circuit for this) to protect your eyes. People with macular degeneration or other eye conditions ought to be especially careful about viewing midday sunlight, and if very sensitive to sunlight, they may want to consult with their ophthalmologist before doing any deliberate sunlight viewing.

What about eyeglasses and contact lenses?

Eyeglasses and contact lenses are both perfectly fine to wear while viewing morning sunlight. Neither one blocks light from reaching your eyes, even if your eyeglasses or contacts have UV filters.

Sunglasses and transition lenses, however, should be avoided while viewing morning sunlight because they block out a lot of the relevant wavelengths that trigger the valuable mechanisms covered in this protocol. Moreover, they reduce the number of photons reaching your eyes. Of course it's fine to wear sunglasses as needed for comfort and safety at other times of day.

What about viewing sunlight through a window or windshield? Is that the same?

People relentlessly ask me this and my response is equally persistent: No, it's not the same. It's far less effective, though better than nothing. But if there is any way to get outside, do. Windows and windshields, especially nowadays, filter the intensities and wavelengths you want for this protocol to work. "How come viewing morning sunlight through eyeglasses or contacts is fine but not windows or windshields?" you may wonder. Because windows do something called spectral filtering: They reduce the amount of light—especially short wavelength light—that would otherwise reach your eyes. Corrective lenses don't; they let far more light through. That's their job. Well, that and to correct any optical errors in the structure of your eyeballs so you can see things clearly. Windows and windshields do neither.

SLEEP PROTOCOL

2

View Sunlight in the Late Afternoon

WHAT TO DO:

- **Get sunlight in your eyes in the late afternoon or early evening.** Ideally, go outside and spend at least ten to fifteen minutes there before the sun sets. If at all possible, face or walk west toward the sun. You do not need to see the sun drop below the horizon. That's a wonderful thing if you can—who doesn't love a sunset? Alas, most of us don't live or work in the right place to do so. Luckily, just going outside and getting some ambient light in your eyes in the late afternoon or early evening is beneficial. Seeing the sunset is a bonus.
- **A few things to keep in mind.** As with the previous protocol, it is best to face the sun directly, not through a window or windshield, and without wearing sunglasses or a brimmed hat. Perhaps you can get an unobscured view by going up to a rooftop or by walking a few blocks from where you work or live. From a health perspective, that is well worth it. Again it's especially important to do this protocol on overcast days.

HOW IT WORKS:

We've already unpacked the basic physiological processes linking your circadian clock, your eyes, and specific qualities of light that drive the sleep-wake cycle. Afternoon sunlight exposure taps into some of the same basic underlying cells, circuits, and mechanisms, but has both distinct and added benefits, including partially protecting you from some of the negative health effects of viewing artificial lights late at night.

Here again we start with the SCN. Earlier I described the SCN as a "cluster of neurons," but that doesn't really do it justice. A key feature of the SCN is that it contains two oscillators, each following a roughly twenty-four-hour rhythm of electrical activity, but offset from one another.[64] It's as if they are singing in a round, with peaks happening at different yet specific moments within the twenty-four-hour cycle. One peak roughly corresponds to morning and the other to evening, and each can be entrained to sunrise and sunset. And they communicate with one another to be sure neither the morning nor the evening oscillator runs too fast or too slow. That helps generate the SCN's coherent daily rhythm that all other cells in the body follow. It also allows us to shift our clock forward or back as the lengths of days and nights change across the seasons.

Here's the best way to think about it: These two oscillators are like bookends buttressing a row of vertically stacked books, making the books less likely to fall over. This is the right analogy given that viewing morning sunlight shifts the phase of our circadian clock forward, making us want to go to sleep earlier and wake up earlier. Viewing late afternoon or early evening sunlight delays the phase of our clock, which, because it shifts the timing of the release of hormones like melatonin, makes us want to go to bed later and wake up later. So viewing both morning and afternoon sunlight thus helps keep us on a regular sleep-wake schedule, because the phase shift effects of morning and evening sunlight offset each other.[65]

Another great reason to view sunlight in the late afternoon or early evening is that it helps buffer us against the negative effects of viewing bright artificial lights at night.[66] In the morning, we need to see a lot of bright light to train our SCN with the solar cycle, and to elevate our levels of alertness. Unless it's a 10,000 lux lamp, most artificial lights and certainly our phone or computer screens just can't do the job at that time. After sundown, however, it takes extremely little bright light to quash our melatonin levels, and shift our circadian clock. And even if we can still fall asleep at night, that sleep is not going to be as high quality.

In fact, studies show that as little as fifteen seconds of bright light can significantly shift our circadian clock.[67] And while most screens are not as bright as the lights used in these studies, our ipRGCs and SCN work to sum photons—that is, add up all the light we see from various sources. And let's face it, most people are looking at their phone and other screens for a lot longer than fifteen seconds after sundown.

To recap: In the morning, you need more bright light in your eyes than a screen or conventional home lighting can provide, and at night you want far less light reaching your eyes than typically comes from a phone or computer screen or conventional home lighting. It all has to do with how our eyes are more sensitive to detecting light at different times of day or night. If that seems inconvenient, you're right; nowadays it is! But the circuits underlying retinal and circadian sensitivity across the twenty-four-hour cycle evolved long before humans had artificial lighting, much less the bright, short-wavelength-enriched LED screens and LED bulbs that we use today.

I, like most people, often wake up once in the middle of the night to use the bathroom. If I had things my way, our circadian system would be buffered from the phase-shifting effects of light at that time, but I wasn't consulted at the design phase, and our ipRGCs are *exquisitely* sensitive to bright light in the middle of the night and wee hours of morning. In fact, our ipRGCs and SCN become increasingly responsive to light with every hour after sundown.[68] If you're wondering if fireplaces, campfires, candlelight, or moonlight are too bright to view after dark, the answer is no. Firelight sources emit very long wavelengths, and moonlight is low lux. Candlelight is typically just 1 lux. A bright, full moon is *less* than 1 lux! Compare those numbers to a typical table lamp, which is 200 to 400 lux, or commonly used overhead indoor LED lighting, which is 500 to 1,000 lux.

So are we to all avoid artificial lighting and opt for candlelight or moonlight?

Maybe, but more on that later. In the meantime, let's acknowledge that most people just won't do that, and even if we opt to at home, we can't control the lighting of most other environments like office cubicles, restaurants, hotels, and the rest.

That is where this protocol can help. Viewing sunlight in the afternoon reduces the sensitivity of neural circuits in your retinas, so that any artificial light you see after dark does not have as strong an effect in disrupting melatonin and other circadian-related molecules and processes in your eyes and brain. This protocol is especially important if your mornings and days are mostly spent under artificial indoor lights, as that will cause any artificial lights you view at night to have an outsized negative effect on your sleep and circadian rhythms.[69] Think of viewing the sunset as your (partial!) nighttime TV-watching or phone-scrolling inoculation. That said, you should still strive to dim the lights in the evening, and make it as dark as possible while you sleep, as discussed in the next protocol.

COMMON QUESTIONS:

What if I can't get myself to a place where I can see sunlight in the late afternoon or early evening?

I understand. Most of us are working, driving, or otherwise occupied indoors when the sun is setting—especially in the fall and winter months. And while sunsets are both beautiful and beneficial, telling your boss "I need to leave to go watch the sunset" is not going to go over well. (Although saying "Let's go watch the sunset together because it's good for our health" might be a good idea, depending on how you frame the question.) If you can't watch the sunset, just try to go outside at some point in the afternoon to get some ambient daylight in your eyes before dark, even if it's just for a stroll around the block, or a few moments on a balcony. Do whatever you can. The ambient light will still serve your SCN, and thus your circadian rhythm, sleep, and health, in numerous beneficial ways.

SLEEP PROTOCOL

3

Avoid Viewing Bright Lights in the Final Hour Before Bedtime

WHAT TO DO:

- **After sundown, limit your nighttime light exposure.** You have a few options for how to do that. Which you use will depend on where you are and what activities you need to carry out.
  - **Option 1: Dim the lights.** After sundown, dim the lights in your home or wherever you are in the hours before sleep.
  - **Option 2: Use red lights at night.** I am a fan of using soft amber or red incandescent (or even amber or red LED lights, which are easier to find nowadays) for indoor lighting after dark as they don't spike cortisol or suppress melatonin as much as many bright white LED lights do.[70] Remember, you want to try to keep your cortisol low in the late evening and especially the final few hours before your bedtime at night. You also want your melatonin elevated then. While this protocol might seem extreme, shifting to amber or red lighting in the final hours before sleep can make a marked difference for some people's ability to fall and stay deeply asleep, which extends to every aspect of next-day energy, mood, and focus.[71]
    - *Consider buying a few high-quality red light bulbs.* Bon Charge makes great LED bulbs that are just the right level of brightness to see, but not so bright as to disrupt circadian rhythms and Ra

Optics has LED bulbs that lack the usual flicker of LEDs and can shift between daytime and "candlelight" mode (I have no affiliation with Bon Charge or Ra Optics, but I use these brands at home, and I travel with one or two of their bulbs when on the road and staying in hotels.) SaunaSpace makes a large, red incandescent bulb that is about the size of a shoebox that can illuminate a medium-sized room. I have one in my living room and another in my bedroom. Incandescent bulbs give off a softer illumination than LED ones, and have some known advantages for mitochondrial health, which I cover in chapter 5.

- *Consider small, portable side table LED lamps or bulbs that can be flipped from bright white to yellow to red, depending on the time of day or night.* Bon Charge makes these. They are great if you need to navigate to the bathroom at night. They charge off your computer or a wall outlet and (hooray) don't require Wi-Fi or an app. I know many people who have solved their "I wake up in the middle of the night to go to the bathroom and then can't fall back asleep" issues by switching to these.

Note: *I am not talking about "red light therapy," and you don't need a fancy red-light panel for this protocol. In fact, red-light panels tend to be very bright—exactly the opposite of what you want to use at night! They have their place, which I will discuss later in this book.*

- **Option 3: Use combination UV, blue, and green light blocking glasses after sundown.** This is the most versatile and cost-effective option. Consider buying a pair of blue and green light blocking glasses if you need to be on a computer, look at a phone, or watch TV at night. They are also helpful when you can't control the lighting because you're out at a restaurant, in an airport, et cetera, at night.

  I helped design ROKA Wind Down glasses, which block the full range of blue and green light, are lightweight, and come in a variety of frames. They are excellent quality.

- **Option 4: Use good ol' candlelight.** Just make sure to blow it out before you go to sleep!

HOW IT WORKS:

Humans are not the strongest or fastest creatures on earth, but we are the best at building technologies. Every technology—the automobile, the smartphone, airplanes, antibiotics—brings the potential for unprecedented power over nature in our daily lives. Artificial lights have vanquished darkness. But in the case of LED lights, in particular, this technology also carries a risk to our circadian cycle, our mitochondria, and thus, our health.

Until about ten years ago, most artificial lighting used incandescent bulbs, which contain more long-wavelength light and a more even distribution of different wavelengths than LED bulbs. Incandescent bulbs have been largely phased out because they are less energy efficient than LED bulbs. Nowadays, most indoor lighting comes from LEDs, which emit a disproportionate amount of short-wavelength light that can potently reduce melatonin levels.[72] Emerging evidence also points to negative effects of LEDs on mitochondrial health (which we'll go into later, in chapter 5).[73]

Those are some of the risks. Now let me explain why bright artificial light at night may also be affecting our mood. Each of us has a brain structure called the habenula that sits at the middle and top part of an egg-shaped brain structure called the thalamus.[74] Your thalamus is a station for routing different types of sensory and motor information to the correct parts of your brain so you can detect and integrate that information into your thoughts and actions. When I was an undergraduate and graduate student taking neuroanatomy, the habenula was listed as having an "unknown function." Recent studies in rodents, fish, and humans finally revealed what it does.[75]

We now know the habenula is part of a network that controls depressive feelings and disappointment.[76] Habenula activation creates those states by altering dopamine and serotonin dynamics in brain areas associated with reward.[77] Why would we harbor such a structure and circuit? The answer is that not all behaviors are meant to be rewarded. Some need to be punished so we are less likely to repeat them. And it turns out that viewing bright light in the "you really should be asleep now" phase of your circadian cycle is one of them. Animal studies and emerging evidence in humans show that viewing bright lights at night causes your ipRGCs to activate a specific region called the perihabenula.[78] That leads to elevated levels of cortisol, reductions in dopamine, next-day anxiety, and deficits in learning—all consequences that appear to be separate from any reductions in total sleep time.[79]

For most people, the "you really should be asleep now" time is somewhere between the hours of 11:00 p.m. and 4:00 a.m. But of course, neither your SCN nor your habenula knows clock time; they only know circadian time, which follows the circadian body temperature, cortisol, and other twenty-four-hour rhythms I described briefly earlier in this chapter. Your body temperature starts to rise in the final two hours before waking, and continues to rise throughout your morning and day until you reach the mid to late afternoon.[80] At that point, it starts to decline. That decline continues as we sleep, reaching its lowest point, called, unimaginatively, your *temperature minimum time* about two to three hours prior to waking.[81] So when I say avoid viewing bright lights from LEDs or other sources at night, I am referring to the time about six to eight hours before your temperature minimum time. This may seem overly technical, but knowing your temperature minimum time can be very valuable. And no, you don't have to measure your body temperature; your temperature minimum is the approximate time in your twenty-four-hour circadian cycle that roughly corresponds to two hours before you typically wake up, alarm clock or no. The exact clock time of course will vary depending on whether you are a morning lark or a night owl, or somewhere in between (more on how to determine that soon). But since most people wake up between 6:00 and 8:00 a.m., their temperature minimum time is between 4:00 and 6:00 a.m. If that's you, assuming you'd like to fall asleep anytime between 10:00 p.m. and midnight, it means you should avoid viewing bright artificial lights between 11:00 p.m. and 4:00 a.m. You would do even better to dim the lights starting around 8:00 or 9:00 p.m. Put simply, to avoid habenula activation and shifting your circadian clock, avoid bright artificial lights in the four to six hours prior to your temperature minimum time.

If you want to figure out your exact temperature minimum time, simply take the average of your wake-up times over the course of three to four days and subtract two hours. Then strive to avoid viewing bright artificial light in the full six-hour period prior to that. I generally wake up at about 6:30 a.m., which means my temperature minimum time is 4:30 a.m., so I avoid viewing bright artificial light between 10:30 p.m. and 4:30 a.m.

I know this all sounds technical, but it's very simple. By doing it, you'll likely enjoy improvements in your sleep and thus daytime mood, focus, and alertness. I acknowledge that many people can fall asleep after being under bright artificial lights in the hours before bedtime, but knowing several such folks, I can assure you even they benefit by adopting this simple (and incidentally cost-saving) change. Bonus: your home feels cozier at night too.

A bit more on those mood improvements: In 2018, a team of researchers, including noted UCLA psychiatrist Peter Whybrow, reviewed the data on the potential link between LED lighting and mental health. They concluded that exposure to blue light, in particular, posed a risk to sleep and other processes governed by the circadian system.[82] There is also evidence suggesting that the way in which artificial lighting at night interferes with this system may lead to depression.[83]

These findings do not mean we should all throw away our LED lights. However, if you can find incandescent lights for your home, they are preferable because they're less disruptive to the circadian system. In a study from 2020, researchers found that incandescent lighting interfered with the production of melatonin far less often than LED or fluorescent lights.[84] (I cover why this is in chapter 5.) If you can't find incandescent bulbs, consider the Bon Charge or Ra Optics bulbs or ROKA Wind Down or other short wavelength (not just "blue") blocking glasses.

Experiment with the options in this protocol to see what works best for you. And no matter what bulbs you choose for your home, still dim them before bed, and keep it dark in the six to eight hours prior to your temperature minimum time. If a light is bright enough, it doesn't matter if it is an LED or incandescent, it will still alter your circadian cycle.[85]

COMMON QUESTIONS:

What if I want to go to a game, concert, party, or movie and view bright lights? Will that destroy my sleep that night?

This is an important question, as we need to live a life that is not just focused on health. From a circadian perspective, no, it will not destroy your sleep. Your natural wake-up and to-sleep times are determined by your genetics, your social activity, your exercise routine, your stress levels, and the average timing and amount of your morning and evening light viewing—especially morning sunlight—in the prior days. As I mentioned earlier, the idea is to strive to get great sleep about 90 percent of the nights of your life, and reserve the remaining about 10 percent for when challenges or fun keep you up late, or even until dawn. Yes, wearing glasses that block UV, blue, AND green wavelength light can help keep your sleep on target, even when you're going out a lot, but who wants to wear those lenses on a first date or on your wedding night? They can be fun to wear to concerts and dinner, but I hate to think that anyone would miss out on the joys of life to avoid bright light exposure to their eyes. That said, if you're getting a lot of screen LED light in your eyes at night because you're scrolling on your phone or computer or watching a big flat-screen monitor, that will take a negative toll on your health. Please adjust this protocol so that it works for you. Also, you shouldn't wear these glasses while driving, for obvious reasons; there are a lot of road signs and lights that you would not be able to see accurately—or at all depending on their color, and you could get into an accident.

What I describe here is what to strive for. Everyone diverges from that now and again. Enjoy your life and meet its moments by prioritizing your health most of the time and not stressing about the occasional night out.

What about kids? Do the same rules about lighting apply?

Yes. They need great sleep even more than we do, given the stage of brain and bodily development they are in. Teens, though, tend to stay up late to socialize online or otherwise. Keep in mind that kids and teens often need eight to ten hours of sleep.[86] But their socialization is vital, too, so you'll have to strike a balance between encouraging a healthy relationship to artificial light, screens, and their social life. That said, if your teen or child is depressed or anxious, it's important to assess their sleep patterns and relationship to light, especially the amount and timing of screen use. I have heard from many parents whose kids had a significant improvement in their mental health with the protocols listed here. Some were only able to convince their teens to use their phones outside in the yard instead of in their rooms in the morning. Others have told me their kids love the morning and evening sunlight viewing for the immediate mental and physical benefits it provides. I won't make this a parenting protocol, but the phrase "be a channel, not a dam" comes to mind as possibly useful in this context.

My infant wakes up frequently throughout the night. Can dim lighting help me cope with interrupted sleep?

Yes. Even if your infant is waking frequently through the night, try to keep the lights as dim as possible during those stretches, and/or use red light bulbs (again, not the same as red light therapy panels). Dimming lights will help you fall back asleep with your infant and will also help your baby's circadian system start to become attuned to the solar cycle. Babies have very different REM and other sleep cycles compared to adults—they naturally get much more REM, but the general effects of light and darkness on their cortisol and melatonin levels are very similar to those of healthy adults. That is one reason why the practice of dividing breastmilk refrigerated for later use into "collected in morning" and "collected at night" is becoming more commonly discussed in health circles. The former contains relatively more cortisol and the latter relatively more melatonin.[87]

SLEEP PROTOCOL

4

Find Your Ideal To-Sleep and Wake-Up Times and Strive to Adhere to Them

WHAT TO DO:

- **Find your chronotype to set your schedule.** Some people sleep better when they stay up late and sleep in late; others feel best when they go to bed early and wake up early; and most people fall somewhere in between, preferring to go to sleep somewhere between 10:00 p.m. and midnight and to wake up between 6:00 and 8:00 a.m.
- **Try to stick to your schedule.** As long as you sleep for at least six to eight hours a night, pick a sleep-wake schedule that works for you. Even shifting slightly closer to your chronotype will afford you much more restorative sleep.

A systematic approach to figuring out your ideal sleep-wake schedule:

Let's get something out of the way. If you've been reading this chapter and thinking, "Hmm, my circadian rhythm is nothing like the one you describe," then maybe you are a night owl. Or maybe you just think you are. Kenneth Wright, whose lab at the University of Colorado Boulder studies circadian rhythms, wanted to figure out how much of people's preference to go to bed long after sundown and sleep in many hours past sunrise was due to a natural inclination, and how much was due to the influence of artificial indoor lighting.[88] He and several colleagues gave participants wrist monitors that measured the intensity and timing of their light exposure throughout the day, as well as their activity patterns, so that they could know when the participants were sleeping. Next, they measured their melatonin levels every hour to see whether the participants' bedtimes matched up with their circadian-driven increases in melatonin—which is a reliable measure of circadian clock output. Finally, the participants were sent packing. They went camping for a week, with only the sun and campfires as their light sources; no flashlights, screens, or other electronic devices permitted.

That one week was all it took for participants to sync sleep-wake cycles to the rising and setting of the sun. Before the outing, some of the participants were convinced they were morning people and others were convinced they were night owls. After a week in the wilderness, those differences faded. They all went to sleep around sunset. The researchers noted that the intensity of the light the participants experienced while camping was four times greater than the intensity of light in their normal lives—a testament to how much time they normally spent indoors. Interestingly, just one weekend spent camping had a similar effect of shifting people's circadian rhythm toward being early risers and people who prefer to go to sleep early. Mind you, those shifts were not just while camping. They persisted *after* they came back. This study was small and in no way does it mean there is no such thing as a night owl. But the rapidity and degree of the change suggest that artificial lighting masks the preference of many people to have a solar-cycle-aligned rhythm.

There are potential health implications tied to shifting toward (or away) from your innate sleep-wake timing. And they suggest that except for bona fide night owls, a more solar-cycle-aligned rhythm is beneficial. A large-scale 2019 study of nearly 700,000 subjects showed a causal link between being a morning person and better mental health—that's right: a causal link.[89] A different study found a higher risk for cardiovascular disease among people who went to sleep later and slept for a long time.[90] Another analysis using data from 6,258 people in Finland found a link between routine late nights and type 2 diabetes.[91] The patterns a night owl keeps have also been linked to depression.[92]

And there are new data showing that even if you prefer to go to bed and sleep late, shifting to becoming an early riser can improve your health.[93] But telling a night owl to become a morning person can be dangerous—people cling to their natural sleep cycles like a pit bull on a rope toy.

Whether you think you're a night owl or not, by systematically experimenting with your to-sleep and wake-up times a bit and by limiting bright artificial light exposure in the final hour or two before sleep, you can determine the ideal sleep-wake schedule for you. Few people can do genetic testing or sleep lab analysis to determine their true chronotype, but there is a simpler way and it's worth exploring.

Here's how:

Unless you are perfectly happy with your sleep, for one week, try getting into bed by 8:30 to 9:00 p.m. If you're not ready for bed at that time, read a book or do another non-screen activity, but turn all the lights out by 9:00 to 9:30 . . . maybe 10:00 p.m. at the latest.

Many people who do this wake up at 6:00 a.m. or even 5:00 a.m. the next day feeling more refreshed than ever before. Those who had previously been going to sleep at 11:00 p.m. or 12:00 a.m. and assumed they needed eight or more hours of sleep to feel rested often find they can feel great with just six or seven hours of sleep if they just get to sleep a bit earlier.

This process aligns your sleep more accurately with your genetically driven cortisol and melatonin rhythms. The genes that determine chronotype impact what are called clock genes, which are located in your SCN, and in almost every other cell of your body too. Your SCN entrains every cell in your body by changing its patterns of clock gene expression, either directly or indirectly, by altering the timing and type of peptides, hormones, and neural signals those cells receive. It's a multipronged and highly distributed network that allows your SCN to do that. That is one reason why once people find their correct sleep schedule, they often notice their digestion and immune systems improve, as well as key biomarkers of metabolism, not just their sleep and mood. It's not unusual to get more deep and REM sleep and awaken feeling substantially more refreshed when you obey your chronotype. Nocturnal growth hormone release[94] is strongly regulated by your circadian clock,[95] and is released in the first hours of sleep. If you are meant to go to sleep between 8:30 and 10:00 p.m. and you stay up late, you miss out on getting some of that growth hormone. And growth hormone is vital for bodily and brain repair, metabolism, and myriad other health functions.[96]

A few things to keep in mind as you try this protocol. If you typically have been going to sleep after 10:30 p.m., dim the lights as described in Sleep Protocol 3. Also, remember that it is perfectly normal to wake up once to go to the bathroom in the middle of the night. If you do, I highly recommend that you do not look at a clock or turn on bright lights. Chances are you'll fall back asleep within thirty minutes or less. No matter when you typically have been going to sleep, eating too close to bedtime and/or drinking caffeine late in the day will mess up this whole experiment—both lead to more frequent nighttime wakings, so don't do either.[97] In general, eating your last bite of food at least two to three hours before bedtime is best, provided you are not experiencing gnawing hunger near bedtime, in which case a small snack one hour before is helpful. Yes, eating too close to bedtime may disrupt sleep, but gnawing hunger will keep you awake, so we need to be practical about this whole "don't eat too close to bedtime" thing.[98] And try not to drink caffeine after 1:00 or 2:00 p.m. (more on the reasons why in Sleep Protocol 11).

If you are not used to going to sleep this early, and you find yourself unable to fall asleep even after several nights, you may just be genetically wired to go to sleep between 10:30 p.m. and midnight. True night owls do exist! There is nothing wrong with that, provided your schedule lets you sleep long enough for you to feel rested the next day. Again, this assumes you are not drinking caffeine after 1:00 or 2:00 p.m., stressed out, or otherwise generating elevated levels of arousal late in the day, all things that can affect your sleep-wake schedule.

Indeed, people prefer different sleep schedules. Approximately 33 percent of people feel great going to sleep between 10:30 p.m. and midnight and waking up between 6:30 and 7:30 a.m.[99] The other

33 percent do best going to sleep between 8:30 and 10:00 p.m. and waking up between 4:30 and 6:30 a.m. The remaining third are bona fide night owls—in the absence of caffeine or work demands, their genetically driven melatonin rhythms and circadian rhythms cause them to be wide awake until 12:30 a.m., 1:00 a.m., or even 2:00 to 3:00 a.m., and they do best waking up between 9:00 and noon.[100] The point is to determine which group you are in, and to do so while not letting other variables screw up your experiment.

It is oh-so-valuable to know what your body and brain need, and thrive on. If you're truly an early or late chronotype, perhaps you can delegate tasks to family members or roommates to meet life's demands. You can select courses and workout times that better match your rhythms. I will even go so far as to say that, because of the way that getting your sleep-wake times right generates outsized positive effects on your health and cognition, you might even be wise to try to build your life around it. Tell your boss you'll have fewer sick days (you will), tell your partner you'll be a better partner (you will), and if you have kids, a better parent (you will). Feel free to cite me during the negotiations. There are aspects of our biology that we can neglect for a while before it causes issues. Chronotype is not one of them. Of course, we can shift our circadian clock for child-rearing, work, or travel, and this book teaches you how to do that more effectively, but we can't disobey our chronotype for more than a few years before it catches up with us, and often it only takes a few weeks of disobeying it before we start to notice mild to severe malaise, irritability, or poor digestion. Fortunately, the reverse is also true. Align better with your chronotype—even by just an hour or two and you'll often feel much better within days.

That said, our ideal sleep timing and total sleep needs do change as we age. Some of that is socially driven, but other aspects are related to changes in our pineal gland—the gland that makes melatonin and other hormones and neurotransmitters.[101]

Also, when we are sick or recovering from an injury or bout of chronic stress, we need more sleep. The point here is to figure out the best sleep schedule for you, this year, and know that it may drift a bit over time, or in specific circumstances.

Key point 1:

Keep in mind that regardless of your ideal sleep-wake schedule, you benefit from being consistent with any sleep-wake schedule. That means going to bed and waking up at the same time, plus or minus thirty minutes, six to seven nights out of the week. Consistent does not mean neurotic. Strive, don't strain, to get things right. Nothing is worse than trying to force yourself to sleep.

Key point 2:

It is very normal to feel very awake about one to three hours before your bedtime. That increase in arousal, sometimes referred to as the "wake maintenance zone," is thought to be an adaptive mechanism for allowing us to secure our physical surroundings and safety prior to sleep, but that is just speculation. A transient increase in alertness—that for some occurs around sunset and for others around one to three hours before their typical bedtime—also may happen; it's well documented in sleep studies, although to my knowledge its physiological basis has not yet been explored in detail.[102] Remember, this is a transient increase, so don't sweat it. Let it pass and embrace the drop in body temperature, the rise in melatonin, and sleepiness that follows.

HOW IT WORKS:

The intricacies of what happens when we sleep—the so-called architecture of sleep—deserves a book of its own, and indeed many have been written about it.

Rarely discussed, however, is how the architecture of each sleep-wake cycle influences our sleeping *and our waking* states. We touched on this topic a bit earlier in this chapter. But now, by exploring the architecture of sleep itself, we can start to understand how the placement of six to eight hours of sleep in each twenty-four-hour cycle, and the consistency of that placement from one day to the next, has a profound effect on exactly what happens while we sleep, and how that impacts whether our sleep is maximally restorative.

The Stages of Sleep

Many people are familiar with the two major types of sleep: rapid eye movement, or REM, sleep, and non-REM sleep. Non-REM sleep is often referred to as deep or slow-wave sleep, but that's oversimplified. Non-REM sleep consists of three distinct phases that we enter, one after the other. These are referred to as N1, N2, and N3 sleep, and only in the N3 stage does actual deep or slow-wave sleep occur. Cycling through N1, to N2, to N3, to REM sleep takes, on average, about ninety minutes. So a person who sleeps for three hours might make it through two cycles, a person who sleeps for six hours experiences four cycles, and a person who sleeps 7.5 hours gets five cycles, and so on.

We enter N1, or *light sleep*, first and it typically lasts five to ten minutes. It is easy to rouse us from N1 sleep. But N1 is not merely a transition stage; during N1, our body starts to generate additional adenosine triphosphate, or ATP, the chemical that fuels all our biological processes. What's more, proteins that have become misshapen or broken during our waking hours get repaired during N1, and proteins that help build memories by reconfiguring our neural circuits are created.[103]

Next we enter N2 sleep, which lasts about twenty minutes. During N2 our body temperature drops, our heart rate slows down, and our brain produces sleep spindles—surges of transient brain activity that help consolidate information we have learned in the days prior.[104] Sleep spindles are vital for learning new cognitive information and motor skills, which both represent types of neuroplasticity.[105] We explore this in greater detail in chapter 6.

N2 has another intriguing feature: PGO waves, which are surges of large-scale brain activity that travel from the pons (P) of the brainstem, to the geniculate (G), a structure in our thalamus (the sensory waystation we discussed earlier), and then to our occipital (O) cortex, which resides in the back of our brain and is involved in, among other things, visual processing. PGO waves trigger the release of massive amounts of glutamate, an excitatory neurotransmitter that is a requisite component of the multistage process of learning, such as in the formation and elimination of synapses.[106]

After N1 and N2 we enter deep sleep, what sleep researchers call *slow-wave sleep*, or N3. This is an extremely restorative stage of sleep. During N3, our brain waves shift to very high amplitude and low frequency, aka *slow*; our heart rate slows way down, and growth hormone is released from our pituitary gland into our bloodstream.[107] What's more, the active repair of our muscle, brain, and other bodily tissues occurs—including our tendons, skin, heart, et cetera.[108] That process involves a lot of protein synthesis, or the repair and regeneration of cells and tissues by use of specific amino acids.[109] Some of that repair and regeneration occurs in response to tissue damage from exercise, but most of it is simple "housekeeping"-based cellular turnover and repair, which is also vital to our health and longevity. N3 is also when *glymphatic washout* of our brain occurs.[110] This process was discovered just in the past fifteen years or so and involves the pulsing of lymph-like fluid through our brain, thereby removing the waste products caused by normal brain metabolism and any cellular debris that accumulated the previous day.[111] This glymphatic clearance is actively governed by multiple brain regions—including the locus coeruleus—that we will talk about more below and in later chapters.

REM sleep, or rapid eye movement sleep, follows N3, but often we cycle from N3 back to N2 for a few minutes or more before advancing into REM sleep. REM sleep is crucial for sorting through all that waking life brings our way by eliminating or strengthening specific neural connections in accordance with what information we need to keep and what we should discard.[112] Thus, think of REM sleep as an experience audit, with only the meaningful experiences surviving the cut.

One more interesting thing about REM: Our body becomes mostly paralyzed during this stage, a phenomenon known as sleep atonia.[113] The most prevalent hypothesis to explain sleep atonia is that it keeps us from acting out our dreams during REM sleep.[114] Our brains are extremely active during REM and the dreams we experience during this stage tend to be vivid and emotionally laden—often marked by flying, swimming, being filled with anxiety or awe, and highly dynamic in how we move through time and space (in the dream of course).[115] The idea is that REM-associated atonia prevents us from acting in accordance with what are essentially in-sleep hallucinations, which would put us in danger.

The relative amount of time we spend in REM sleep increases, and the amount spent in deep N3 sleep decreases, as we complete more sleep cycles across a night of sleep. This means our most vivid dreams tend to occur as we approach morning. A baby's sleep is largely REM sleep, and the amount of REM we experience decreases with age starting in adolescence.[116] If we are sleep-deprived, or we do something that reduces the amount of REM sleep we get on a given night—using cannabis, for instance—the next night we experience REM rebound by entering REM sleep sooner in the sleep cycle, and experiencing more REM overall. Chronic cannabis users who stop using cannabis often report vivid dreams in the first weeks and months after quitting.[117]

Alcohol and many prescription drugs reduce the fraction of our sleep that is REM as well. Once someone stops using these, they also experience an REM rebound.[118]

REM sleep is fascinating. As stated before, it is characterized by more brain activity than we ever experience in our waking life, and yet we are paralyzed while our brain is in that hyperactive state. And there's more. REM sleep is also the only time in our lives when our locus coeruleus—the brainstem region that releases norepinephrine and increases our focus and alertness—goes largely dormant. Also, we don't readily release adrenaline from our adrenals during REM.

Researchers believe that this paradoxical state, during which our brain is highly active but our body is paralyzed, our locus coeruleus is almost silent, and our body can't easily release adrenaline, serves as a sort of naturally occurring therapy, unloading the emotional burdens from our daytime experiences. Indeed, this general set of conditions parallels many established trauma therapies, in which patients recount a traumatic event while in an intentionally or progressively lowered state of anxiety, so as to detach the body's and brain's emotional responses from the details of the memory. People selectively deprived of REM sleep have a harder time unloading emotional burdens from past experiences, including traumas.[119]

REM, like some of the other sleep stages, is also a key time for the consolidation of new skills and information that are of a nonemotional nature. We will cover more on that in chapter 6.

Health risks of sleep deprivation

Given all this, it becomes clearer and clearer how lack of sleep, but also altered sleep architecture, affects our mind and body in a variety of ways. Sleep deprivation is associated with diminished response time, alertness, attention, memory, and executive functioning.[120]

Additionally, as described at the chapter outset, lack of sleep can bring about longer-term problems as well. Insufficient REM sleep may increase the risk of dementia. In 2017, a group of researchers published their investigation of links between dementia and sleep architecture.[121] They looked at three years of data on thirty-two adults over age sixty with dementia and found that the likelihood of cognitive decline fell in line with a reduction in REM sleep. In fact, with every 1 percent reduction in REM sleep, the risk of dementia rose by about 9 percent.

(Non-REM sleep deprivation did not share this connection.) The role of REM in building and consolidating neural connections, thereby protecting against cognitive decline, may also explain why truncating this stage would raise the risk of dementia, but direct evidence for this mechanism in humans is still lacking.

Getting sufficient REM sleep is also connected to overall longevity. In 2020, a group of researchers from multiple institutions reported that less REM sleep is associated with an increased mortality risk. Using data from 4,050 people, they found that for every 5 percent decrease in REM sleep, the mortality rate increased by 13 percent.[122] That held true for most causes of death, including cardiovascular disease.

Ask any sleep researcher "How can I get more REM sleep?" and they will tell you "Sleep in an extra hour or two." But most people can't afford to sleep in an extra hour or two past their usual wake-up time. The good news is that *when* we sleep is almost as important as getting enough of it. If we get to bed and wake up at a time that is in sync with our chronotype, we end up getting more growth hormone release, and we spend less time in light sleep and more time in deep sleep and REM sleep. As a consequence, we tend to need less sleep overall. Our sleep can become more efficient and restorative.[123]

Studies of shift workers tell us what happens if we sleep enough, but at the wrong times of the twenty-four-hour cycle. The short answer is: Bad things happen. Working at nighttime and sleeping in the daytime is associated with greatly elevated risk of type 2 diabetes, cardiovascular disease, depression, and suicide.[124] Shift workers are also susceptible to neurocognitive impairment and at greater risk for substance abuse.[125] One large survey from Canada found that executive function is significantly worse among people whose jobs take place outside normal work hours.[126] One study found the level of performance impairment to be equal to a blood alcohol concentration of 0.10, which exceeds the legal limit for driving in many places.[127]

To be clear: Being a night owl is not the same thing as forcing yourself to be nocturnal, so if that's your chronotype, don't worry. The health detriments of shift work are likely to be multifactorial—the lack of sunlight, the altered social interactions associated with an inverted schedule, and more. We know that one of the worst types of shift work for one's health is the swing shift, where people switch back and forth from daytime to nighttime work each week or even within the same week.

How long we sleep, when we sleep, and how consistent we are with our sleep-wake schedule affect our physical and mental health. That's why I hope you try the approach outlined here. Figure out what is best for you and then stick with it.

COMMON QUESTIONS:

Does changing time zones for travel or moving the clock for daylight saving time affect our sleep-wake cycle?

Yes. When we turn the clocks forward an hour to move from standard time to daylight saving time, or back an hour to return to standard time, or when we change time zones during travel, our circadian clock has to shift.

Changing our clocks forward or back means we have collectively decided that 7:00 a.m. is now 8:00 a.m., or 8:00 a.m. is now 7:00 a.m., but our SCN really doesn't care about clock time, it only knows time according to the entrainment cues it receives. You already know the most powerful entrainment cue and that's viewing morning sunlight. Even if we move the clocks just by one hour, the SCN needs a few days to shift its patterns of gene expression and communication with all the cells of the body to get them on schedule. In the meantime, we are groggy at times in the morning when we were perfectly chipper the day before. And a whole host of other systems in our body and brain have to shift before we feel like ourselves again. The dangers of such shifts extend beyond mere irritability. Traffic accidents increase in the days immediately following seasonal clock changes.[128] So do heart attacks.[129] It also makes people more susceptible to depression.[130]

Jet lag occurs when our sleep-wake cycle no longer matches the solar cycle of our location. Our internal timekeeper may be telling us it's time for bed when the locals are just eating dinner. Many people find that traveling east, into a later time, is harder than traveling west, into an earlier time, because we have to move our circadian clocks forward. It's often easier to stay up a few hours longer, or even take a brief nap, than to force ourselves to go to bed before we're ready.

Some people don't suffer much from jet lag. Others suffer tremendously. For those of you in the latter group, Sleep Protocol 15 offers a technique that can help avoid jet lag or at least dampen its impact.

Is it bad to sleep in on weekends or to stay up late now and again?

We should all strive to keep a consistent sleep-wake schedule, for the reasons discussed above. That means we should try to get to bed at the same time, plus or minus thirty minutes, on most nights. Same goes for waking up; try to wake up at roughly the same time each day, plus or minus thirty minutes. Larger changes in sleep or wake times every once in a while won't be too disruptive, because the entrainment of your SCN reflects the weighted average of inputs from multiple factors, as discussed. So by all means, enjoy that birthday or wedding or New Year's celebration and don't despair about arriving home late. One late night is not something to worry about.

Many people wonder whether wake times should be later after that occasional late night. If you usually go to sleep somewhere between 8:30 and 11:00 p.m. and have a night where you're up until 1:00 or 2:00 a.m., should you sleep late or wake up at your usual time? In general, it's best to get enough sleep to feel rested but not to sleep more than one or two hours past your usual wake time. So on those "I stayed up too late last night" mornings, get an extra hour in bed asleep if you can, and try to take a twenty-minute nap, or practice non-sleep deep rest (NSDR) in the afternoon (more on that soon), and then get to bed around your usual time that night. Your SCN—and thus you—thrive on consistency. If you go to bed much later than usual and sleep in much later, too, be sure not to shift your whole schedule forward. It's still fine (and encouraged) to view sunlight, exercise, and so on, but be especially mindful not to drink caffeine much later in the day than usual, or you will soon find yourself off your usual rhythm and it will take three to four or more days to get back to it.

What about children and teenagers?

The advice is a little different for young children and teenagers. Babies need to sleep A LOT and enter REM far more frequently and for longer than any other age group. Toddlers and young children should also sleep as much or as often as necessary, or desired, to support their extraordinarily fast brain and bodily growth rates. The amount of neuroplasticity in infants and children, all the way up to adolescence and beyond, is incredible—and sleep is a key part of that process. Limiting their sleep is never recommended but of course once kids are in school, setting a regular schedule (and keeping devices out of their rooms near bedtime and throughout the night) becomes important.

Sleep needs are somewhat different for teenagers. Bedtimes shift during puberty for at least two known reasons. First is what researchers call the homeostatic sleep drive. This term refers to a brain and bodily pressure to sleep that builds up gradually throughout the day, mainly due to adenosine accumulation.[131] The longer we are awake, the more adenosine in our bodies, and the greater the pressure to sleep. Adenosine levels drop while we sleep and begin to mount again when we wake up for the new day. This pressure to sleep is separate from the circadian clock mechanisms we have discussed a lot thus far. Teenagers (good rebels that they are) resist this pressure and force themselves to stay up late, building up more adenosine and, therefore, the desire to sleep in the next morning.[132]

And they often don't need to force themselves to stay up late; it just happens naturally, as the hormonal testosterone, estrogen, and progesterone surges of puberty shift their circadian clock to a later phase.[133] Melatonin production begins later in the teenage brain than in the brains of either adults or younger children.

All of these changes leave the typical sixteen-year-old awake until about 11:00 p.m.[134] And this age group should be sleeping about nine hours per night, making 8:00 a.m. the preferred wake-up time. Studies have found that moving school start times to 8:30 a.m. or later leads to better grades and other measures of academic performance. There is even evidence suggesting that this shift also reduces car crashes among teen drivers.[135] It's beneficial for teenagers to have days when they can sleep as long as they want, even if that means staying in bed until noon. That doesn't mean they should never be woken up earlier on a Saturday or Sunday, but parents and caregivers do not need to worry about prolonged sleeping on the weekends. Teenagers, yes, reference this book if you need leverage to sleep in and parents, yes, you still want to encourage them to get sunlight in their eyes once they get up, even though it is midday, and not low-solar-angle sun.

Current data indicate that teenagers in the US are in the midst of an epidemic of sleep deprivation that is likely having serious consequences for their health. Ideally, young people between the ages of six and twelve years should sleep at least nine hours per night, and thirteen-to-eighteen-year-olds should sleep at least eight hours per night. More than 70 percent of young people do not sleep enough, according to one large survey from the CDC.[136] Anxiety, mood disorders, obesity, high-risk behavior, poor academic performance, and substance use have all been tied to sleep deprivation among adolescents.[137] Good practices for teenagers include shutting off screens at least an hour before bedtime, keeping the phone (and the laptop, the tablet, etc.) out of the bedroom at night and the room cool and dark, having a consistent bedtime, and, ideally, sleeping for those eight to nine hours per night.

Do sleep patterns change for older adults?

Parsing the changes in sleep that arise in older adults is tricky. Ailments and medications of various kinds impact sleep in many ways. Absent any such interferences, sleep can vary in our later years, but not to a great extent. Older adults sleep a bit less than middle-aged adults by about an hour or so, on average.[138] It can take longer to fall asleep as we move past age fifty, but again, not in a dramatic way. And older adults are able to doze back off to sleep after a middle of the night waking, just as well as teenagers and younger adults can.

The stages of sleep also shift a bit as we age. The percentage of time we spend in deep sleep and REM decreases, although studies have shown a surge in REM in people between the ages of seventy-five and eighty-five years.[139] Older people also tend to nap more.

Does counting sheep help with falling asleep?

Counting sheep has long been recommended for calming a busy brain before bed. The idea is that by giving ourselves a task, we stop ruminating on the day and going over our to-do lists for tomorrow. It turns out that counting sheep isn't such a great nighttime activity. Allison Harvey, a psychologist at UC Berkeley, found that counting sheep actually made it more difficult for people to fall asleep.[140] She concluded that this basic mental imagery was not engaging enough to hold the attention of people lying in bed trying to keep anxieties at bay. Without that focus to help calm our brain, we're back to ruminating and reviewing to-do lists. A subsequent study in which Harvey instructed participants to deliberately suppress whatever thought was most likely to intrude into their mind before sleep found this didn't help—predictably, the thought they were supposed to be suppressing just became more preoccupying.[141]

Instead, try these somewhat weird tricks:

***Take a mental walk:* Imagine walking from your bed to your mailbox and then down the street and to a nearby location, then home again by the same or different familiar route.** Occupying a busy brain with an easy and engaging task can help stop ruminating thoughts. Mental walks like these are occupying but not stimulating. And they have the tendency to lull people off to sleep.

***Move your eyes following the pattern described below:* Warning: This is going to sound a bit out there, but it works well for many people, and studies are indirectly starting to suggest why.**

Lie down in bed and close your eyes. Keep your eyes closed and move your eyes slowly to the right then to the left, then up, then down, then counterclockwise and then clockwise. Then cross them somewhat by directing them gently toward your nose. Finally, do a big inhale and long exhale. Repeat one to three times as needed.

Told you this would sound a bit out there! This trick often helps people fall asleep, because to do so we need to stop thinking about our limb position, or proprioception. Our visual and vestibular systems, or balance, and proprioception systems interact, and the eye movements just described "confuse" those systems. A similar mechanism partially explains why gentle slow rocking and pacing can help babies, and slow rocking of a bed (yes, such beds exist) can help adults improve their sleep metrics.[142] We need more data to understand the mechanism behind this pattern, which is why it's not its own protocol, but it is reasonable to assume it is related to the eye-to-vestibular circuits involved in, among other things, proprioception and sleep. New eye mask and rocking-bed technologies that trigger this eye movement pattern are designed to cause similar eye movements. I have tried a few of these nascent technologies and confess I fell asleep in less than two minutes! Meanwhile, this technique is free and easy to try. "Next thing I knew it was morning!" is not an uncommon refrain from people with whom I have shared this trick.

SLEEP PROTOCOL

5

Lower Your Core Body Temperature at Night

WHAT TO DO:

- **Lower the temperature of the room you sleep in at night.** Cooler ambient temperatures facilitate sleep. Keep your bedroom between 65 and 68 degrees Fahrenheit, and a maximum of 70 degrees.
- **Warm your extremities before bed.** A hot shower, hot bath, sauna, or even washing your face with very warm water can help induce drowsiness by warming hands and feet and by triggering a drop in core body temperature in compensation for this heating.
- **Make sure your feet and hands can be easily exposed from underneath your covers.** The skin of these areas is a primary way we shed heat from our body. Exposing them to cool air is one of the most effective ways to decrease core body temperature. So untuck your sheets at the foot and sides of the bed.
- **Avoid wearing socks while you sleep, especially if you tend to wake in the middle of the night.** Socks can stop the natural cooling process that happens through the feet. (People who tend to run very cold at night may want to skip this recommendation.)

HOW IT WORKS:

Socks or no socks? Window open or closed? Blanket or just sheets? Feet exposed? We all have our sleep habits and a lot of them revolve around temperature. That makes sense. Thermoregulation—the maintenance of our core body temperature—and the management of our sleep environment to control our body temperature is crucial for a great night's sleep, both falling and staying asleep. Indeed, changes in our core body temperature both reflect and influence our circadian rhythm, how much melatonin and other hormones we release, and even the amount of deep and REM sleep we get in a given night.

As I mentioned earlier in this chapter, our core body temperature declines as the day goes on, eventually reaching its lowest point at a specific time—we call this temperature minimum time.[143] A decline in body temperature precedes us falling asleep. The rate of temperature reduction, and not just the absolute core temperature value, seems to matter. In one experiment, researchers made the case that people tended to head off to bed at exactly the time that their temperature was declining fastest.[144] Body temperature starts to increase shortly before we wake up. The relationship between core body temperature and our level of autonomic arousal—which is what sleepiness and alertness reflect—is causal but is best thought of as "necessary but not sufficient," meaning we need the change in temperature, but other factors are key too.[145]

Research has found that the ideal ambient temperature while we sleep is between approximately 66 and 70 degrees Fahrenheit, which typically brings the microclimate immediately around our skin down to somewhere between 88 and 95 degrees Fahrenheit.[146] To fall asleep our core body temperature needs to decrease by about 1 to 2 degrees.

A lower core body temperature facilitates various sleep-related biological processes you are now familiar with. First, research indicates that this reduction may help initiate non-REM sleep,[147] and our lowest body temperature is associated with deep sleep. Melatonin, a hormone that facilitates falling asleep, is released in sync with the nightly drop in body temperature. In one small study of twelve women who were entrained to the solar cycle, the secretion of natural melatonin at night occurred with a simultaneous decline in core body temperature.[148] Other studies have observed a similar coupling.[149]

The stillness of our body during early sleep also plays a role in further dropping our core body temperature. In sleep, our autonomic nervous system shifts from more sympathetic activity (or tone, as it's often referred to), which is related to being alert and able to generate movement, to a far more parasympathetic tone, which is associated with calmness, lower heart rate, and less or no bodily movement.[150] All that combined causes our blood to flow more to our periphery, to our hands and feet, where it "dumps heat," which in turn leads to a lower core body temperature.

This means that warming up our hands and feet a bit before getting into bed could facilitate falling asleep. That may seem paradoxical: Why would warming up your periphery help at a time when cooling down your core body temperature is the goal? Because heating your periphery acts as a trigger. A hot shower or bath, or a sauna, warms the surface of your body. That causes the preoptic area of your hypothalamus—a brain area that works sort of like a thermostat—to trigger a compensatory response, lowering the core temperature in your body.[151] This process makes it easier to fall asleep, a phenomenon known colloquially as the *warm bath effect*.[152]

Once you get in bed, having your sleeping environment cool is also helpful. Many people sleep best in a cool room but with their whole body under loads of warm blankets. Other people run hot and like to sleep under just a sheet or a light blanket. Try out a few of these recommendations and pick what suits you best.

In My Experience

I prefer a comforter and a weighted blanket, but stick my bare feet out from underneath them, which we know helps cool core body temperature. And I keep the room about 68 degrees Fahrenheit. Closer to morning, I find that I often bring my feet under the blankets (in my sleep!), which we know can increase the amount of time spent in REM in the final few hours before waking.[153] Temperature-controlled mattress covers like Eight Sleep make controlling your bed temperature across the night easy, and I use one. (They are a podcast sponsor, and I am a scientific advisor to Eight Sleep). But with or without Eight Sleep, it is a good idea to use programmable room temperature controls to help create that cooler-at-start and warmer-toward-morning sleep environment. Experiment and find what works for you.

COMMON QUESTIONS:

Do daytime temperature changes affect nighttime sleep?

Some data from animal studies suggest that a slightly elevated body temperature for a few hours in the afternoon may lead to more time spent in N3 sleep at night, when waste products from the brain and spinal cord are cleared away (among other processes).[154] That's one reason why many people find that doing some moderate to intense exercise in the early or midafternoon improves their sleep, provided they don't consume a lot of caffeine before their workout.

So should I avoid exercising at night?

It's best to avoid intense exercise late at night, within three to four hours of sleep. High-intensity exercise raises our core body temperature, which is counterproductive to falling asleep. That said, some people can only exercise at this time, and many learn how to down-shift afterward with a hot bath or shower, and by using some of the tools covered in chapter 3, like deliberate long-exhale breathing.

If you consistently find it difficult to fall and stay asleep after exercising hard at night, consider moving your more intense workouts to mornings and doing something lighter in the evening. A review of several randomized clinical trials found that meditative movement like tai chi and qigong improved sleep quality.[155]

However, if night is the only time of day you can exercise, then it's more important to get the workout in than to skip it just because it's late in the day (more on that in chapter 2). In this case, it may help to take some additional steps for ensuring a solid night of sleep: no caffeine after 1:00 or 2:00 p.m., a nighttime wind-down routine, a hot shower, some breathing exercises to reduce stress, no screens, and dim lighting will all help counteract the energizing effects of late evening exercise.

SLEEP PROTOCOL

6

Increase Your Core Body Temperature in the Final One to Two Hours of Sleep Before You Wake Up

WHAT TO DO:

- **Program your heating system for the room you sleep in at night.** If you have one that can be set to different times, program it to rise one to three degrees above your room temperature, starting one to two hours before your wake-up time.
- **Keep clothing by your bed.** If you wake up one to two hours before your preferred wake-up time or in the middle of the night to use the bathroom, try putting on some socks, sweats, or even a knit cap and go back to sleep until your preferred wake-up time. This can increase your core body temperature, which increases the amount of REM sleep you get and will help you wake up feeling energized.

HOW IT WORKS:

We touched on this in the previous protocol but given the importance of getting sufficient REM sleep for mental and physical health, and for performance, it's worth delving into this topic as its own protocol. So here it goes: Just as cooling our core body temperature facilitates falling and staying asleep, warming our core body temperature starting about one to two hours before we wake up can lead us to feel far more refreshed and ready to lean into the day.

Hot temperatures are disruptive to falling and staying asleep.[156] Interestingly the body tends not to adapt; even after several days of trying to sleep well in hot temperatures, sleep remains disrupted.[157] One theory holds that wakefulness itself is triggered by the need for thermoregulation; in other words, waking up is a way to bring our body temperature back to normal.[158]

We have less data on the use of temperature in this part of the sleep cycle than we do for the previous protocol. However, we know that our lowest body temperature, or temperature minimum time, occurs at about two hours before we wake up and begins to rise after that.[159] A return to our normal core body temperature accompanies our return to wakefulness, so it stands to reason that supporting the general process of warming up after we reach our temperature minimum helps us wake up feeling energized.[160] (It likely reflects having had at least two REM-enriched sleep cycles.)

Admittedly, there's a small problem here. It's hard to get out of a warm bed into a cold room. Heating the room you sleep in on a timer that increases the temperature one to two hours prior to waking solves that problem. Otherwise you just have to get up and get to the thermostat. As mentioned before, devices such as Eight Sleep mattress covers that can cool at first and then heat your sleep environment in the final hours of sleep are very effective. These can also measure your deep and REM sleep, and use AI to make real-time adjustments to your sleep temperature to help you get the best possible sleep. But these carry a cost that for many could be prohibitive, and most versions don't travel easily. Anyone can adjust their bedroom temperature and/or use clothes to try to achieve some of the ideal temperature ranges described here.

SLEEP PROTOCOL

7

Nap (Correctly) to Offset Minor Sleep Deficits

WHAT TO DO:

- **If you need a nap, make it short.** Keep the duration to no more than about twenty minutes, and avoid naps longer than ninety minutes.
- **Avoid late-day naps that interfere with your nighttime sleep.** Each person can determine what time constitutes "too late" with a bit of experimentation. See how groggy you are in the hours following your nap. Most importantly, note if you can still easily fall asleep at your regular bedtime afterward.
- **Know your goal.** Nap strategies depend on what you are trying to accomplish.
    - **If you need an energy boost to sustain your focus and drive for the rest of the day:** Aim for a fifteen-to-twenty-minute nap. Five to ten minutes will give you a mild energy boost and help your focus but it doesn't last long. After a fifteen to twenty minute nap, concentration, mood, and energy will improve in a way that will sustain you for the remainder of the day.
    - **If you are dealing with heavy emotions, say from a loss or a rejection or an argument:** Aim for a longer nap, but no longer than ninety minutes. You'll recall from Sleep Protocol 4 that the REM stage is when emotions are processed, and that stage arrives about sixty to seventy minutes into the sleep cycle. So know you might

feel groggy after a nap of forty-five minutes or so because sleep is cut off before the REM cycle is completed. And know too that when people's nighttime sleep is altered due to heavy emotions, and they nap in the day, they often go into REM more quickly; that's the REM rebound effect discussed in that same protocol.

- **If you are sleep-deprived for any reason:** It is fine to nap for thirty, sixty, or even ninety minutes but avoid longer naps as these can alter your circadian rhythm. It can often "split" your circadian rhythm so that you're asleep from 10:00 p.m. to 2:00 a.m., then awake for a few hours, then asleep again.

- **Consider other forms of daytime rest besides sleep to replenish mental and physical vigor.** Particularly if you have trouble falling asleep at night, napping may not be ideal. Sleep Protocol 8 describes non-sleep deep rest (NSDR), a highly effective alternative to napping that can help you feel refreshed without grogginess or impairment to your nighttime sleep. It has other benefits as well.

HOW IT WORKS:

There are conflicting views on napping among sleep experts.[161] Some say if you are sleepy enough to nap in the daytime, you must be getting less than optimal sleep at night, and you should focus on improving that instead. Others take the stance that napping is fine, beneficial even, and not always reflective of a sleep deficit. Provided you adhere to a few simple constraints, napping is great. But if you don't crave naps, there is no need to nap.

And yes, there is a proper way to nap.

First off, it's normal to feel a bit sleepy in the afternoon as your body temperature shifts from rising to falling—remember that the rate of core temperature dropping is what initiates the feeling of drowsiness. For people on a conventional schedule of being asleep at night and being awake in the daytime, this dip in early afternoon energy passes. I fall asleep at about 10:30 p.m.

most nights and wake up at 6:30 a.m., and I always get a bit sleepy between 2:00 and 3:00 p.m. irrespective of what I eat, how much caffeine I drink, and so on. After 3:30 p.m. or so, I feel wide awake and energetic again. The point is, you might get a bit tired in the afternoon, but the feeling is temporary. Not everyone experiences this dip. Some people just barge right through the day, morning until night.

We know that napping can increase our ability to focus and learn. Matthew Walker, a professor of neuroscience and biomedical engineering at the University of Texas in Dallas, conducted a study in which a group of participants learned a new set of facts at midday.[162] Half of them napped for ninety minutes afterward; half of them relaxed without sleeping. At 5:00 p.m., they learned a second new set of facts. The group that did not nap experienced a decline in learning capacity. The nap group sustained or even improved their capacity to learn. The difference reached about 25 percent, which is meaningful.

The finding goes back to the role of sleep spindles, which we covered in Sleep Protocol 4. These are the types of brain waves present during N2 sleep, which happens early in the sleep cycle. Even a brief snooze of twenty minutes takes us into N2.[163] Sleep spindles help us process new learning, but also prepare our brain for more learning after we wake up.

Napping also influences our mood. In another study, Walker and his group asked participants to rate the level of emotion they observed in a photograph.[164] How angry were the angry faces? How happy were the happy faces? Again, half the subjects napped for about an hour and half did not. Toward the end of the day, the non-nappers were rating the emotions as more extreme; angry people were angrier, and so on. The napping group was more likely to rate faces as happy; the rest time seemed to blunt the normal increase in anger sensitivity across the day. As Walker sometimes puts it, sleep gives us a "rose tint" to our worldview. In this study, the naps were ninety minutes, long enough to get some REM sleep, so the benefit is likely due to that, which as we discussed, is when we unload the emotional burdens from our daytime experiences. Although, in this case, it wasn't about the nappers' emotions; it was about how they perceived the emotions of others.

Finally, there is the simple benefit of restoring energy. Many people experience what sleep researchers call a postprandial drop, a dip in energy after eating, especially large meals rich in starchy carbohydrates. Aside from modifying your dietary pattern, naps can help get you to the other side of a postprandial drop if and when you do experience the phenomenon. That said, for anyone who feels tired in the middle of the day and would do better without that sleepiness, I suggest making sure you don't overeat, and possibly even reduce starchy carbohydrate intake, at lunch. Take a short ten-minute walk afterward; that can help for reasons related to blood sugar, or glucose, regulation (covered in chapter 2). Many people find that just reducing the amount of starchy carbs they eat at lunch allows them to go straight through the rest of their day feeling energized and focused. I'll talk more about the relationship between food and brain states in chapter 4.

When Not to Nap (and Why)

A short midday sleep isn't a good idea for everyone. To understand why, we need to return to adenosine. As you recall, adenosine acts as a neurotransmitter that inhibits neural activity in brain regions involved in strategic planning.[165] Sleep actually results from two processes: the circadian clock and sleep pressure from adenosine. Most of the protocols thus far depend on the former. This one has to do with the latter, which you might remember from Sleep Protocol 4. Adenosine is so vital to this process that we ought to explore it a bit further, so here goes.

ATP, or adenosine triphosphate, is the basic unit of energy for all our cellular processes. It is generated during the early stages of sleep. Adenosine is the downstream product of the burning of ATP.[166] It's a product of metabolism that accrues as we engage in activity over the course of a day. As we move from morning to afternoon to evening, more energy has been spent and therefore more adenosine builds up in our brains, gathering in the space between our cells. As it does, we register a need to sleep. This is, again, called homeostatic sleep drive.

The longer we are awake and the more physical activity and mental activity we engage in over the course of a day, the higher the levels of adenosine we accumulate. On days when we get more exercise, for example, our brains accrue more adenosine. And the more they do, the easier it is to fall and stay asleep. Additionally, greater amounts of adenosine are associated with an increase in deeper slow-wave sleep and a decrease in shallower sleep.

Napping—which is, after all, a form of sleep—reduces the amount of adenosine in our brains.[167] It won't zero it out like a solid eight hours of sleep will, but a forty-five-to-ninety-minute nap will clear away a substantial amount of adenosine. For this reason, people who have trouble falling asleep at night should not nap. You want the buildup of adenosine to create enough sleep pressure so that you easily fall and stay asleep at night.

How to Nap

Research at NASA back in 1995 found that napping for twenty-six minutes maximizes the benefits for alertness, focus, and motivation.[168] These became known as *power naps*, and are frequently used to improve memory, reduce blood pressure, and increase concentration. I don't believe there is anything magic about twenty-six minutes except that it is less than forty-five minutes and more than ten, so set your alarm for a fifteen-to-twenty-minute nap and perhaps hit the five-minute snooze button if you don't feel refreshed the first time your alarm goes off. Just don't hit it a second time!

A twenty-minute nap shouldn't make you groggy. That feeling, known as sleep inertia, happens when we wake up in the middle of the deeper stages of non-REM sleep. By keeping the nap to about twenty minutes, you get the benefits of N1 and N2 sleep without suffering from sleep inertia.

Perhaps surprisingly, some people find that resting without sleeping is sufficient to restore mental and physical energy. When you do, you can enter a liminal state in which you are still awake but some parts of your brain are in a sleeplike state. Many people find that even if they just lie down, elevate their feet on a few pillows or a chair, close their eyes, and rest for ten to fifteen minutes, they get some of the restorative effects of a real nap. Elevating your legs and feet slightly in this way promotes a parasympathetic response, increases venous blood flow to the heart, may lower blood pressure slightly, and—provided you don't ruminate on stressful topics—can shift your brain's state toward one of more "relaxation." No, it's not a good idea to spend this time tapping or scrolling on your phone, as it will offset the brain state shift you're seeking. You need to get your mind into a sort of idling mode. *Idling* is clearly not neuroscientific language. But it's a good way to describe how our brains shift to a very different pattern of activity under these resting conditions, moving from higher frequency beta waves (13–30 Hz) to lower frequency alpha waves (8–13 Hz). Napping, on the other hand, lets our brain enter N1 and N2 sleep, allowing even lower frequency theta waves (4–8 Hz) to emerge.[169] Experienced meditators can get themselves into a state where theta waves emerge quickly, although that takes practice. Relaxation techniques like those offered in the very next protocol can help you rest during the day without interfering with your ability to fall asleep at night.

COMMON QUESTIONS:

I'm not a napper but I don't have trouble falling asleep at night. Should I nap?

If you are not tired in the daytime, don't force yourself to nap. Some people get through a day just fine without naps.

Can naps help with insomnia?

People with insomnia should generally avoid naps.[170] The temptation to sleep during the day can be powerful when coping with poor sleep at night. But all evidence points to the idea that resisting the urge to nap is the way to go for insomniacs. If you are suffering from chronic insomnia, try the protocols in this book, and if those don't solve the issue then talk to a doctor who specializes in sleep medicine.

For older adults, is there an added health benefit to napping?

Studies of napping among older adults have shown mixed results.[171] A concern with prolonged midday rests among older adults is that the need to nap may be indicative of a problem with nighttime sleep. Older adults who always feel tired during the day should consider changes that can benefit sleep, such as making sure to get plenty of natural daylight in their eyes in the morning and dimming indoor lighting at night before relying on naps (Sleep Protocols 1–6 all have useful tools for this situation).

SLEEP PROTOCOL

8

Use Non-Sleep Deep Rest (NSDR) to Offset Sleep Deficits (and to Get Better at Falling and Staying Asleep at Night)

WHAT TO DO:

- **Do non-sleep deep rest (NSDR) if you feel tired and need to restore your mental and physical vigor.** NSDR is fast, safe, effective, and costs nothing. It has both immediate and long-term benefits for your brain state, and there is evidence it can improve focus and learning. It takes as little as ten minutes, although longer versions of twenty, thirty, or even sixty minutes can be even more effective. It's nearly impossible to do NSDR incorrectly (unless you are texting in the middle of a session).
    - Do NSDR first thing in the morning if you failed to get enough sleep the night before and want to feel more rested as you enter your day. If you don't have time just then, I suggest you do NSDR in the midmorning or afternoon. It will still help.
    - Do NSDR at night if you have trouble falling asleep, or if you wake up in the middle of the night and can't fall back asleep. NSDR is a far better option than tossing and turning and worrying about the sleep you're not getting.
    - There is a link below that will take you to a list of NSDR recordings available at zero cost in downloadable formats (no sign-up required)

done by me, and some by Kelly Boys—an expert in NSDR—if you prefer a female voice.

https://www.hubermanlab.com/nsdr

https://www.youtube.com/@kellyboys5313

https://www.kellyboys.org

HOW IT WORKS:

First off, it's important to emphasize that NSDR is not anything like traditional meditation. NSDR is not breathwork either. Rather, NSDR belongs to a category of techniques that can be broadly thought of as self-directed relaxation. NSDR is also not anything like a nap. A central feature of NSDR is to stay awake (but not focused on planning or action), while simultaneously bringing the body into an extremely relaxed state. It puts you in a unique brain state.[172] Meditation often involves holding one's attention on a specific location inside or near one's body (such as the spot just behind our forehead), or on an external object (a candle flame, for example), or even on a sensory experience (e.g., the taste of a single almond). These kinds of directed perceptual focus exercises have been shown to improve concentration, reduce stress, strengthen memory and improve mental health.[173] When done consistently, meditation techniques can lead to profound shifts in our awareness of our internal thought patterns. And over time, meditation can provide a rich understanding of how our minds work and can even change our temperament.

Self-directed relaxation protocols like NSDR are different. NSDR involves shifting our autonomic nervous system into a more parasympathetic, or relaxed, state by breathing in a manner in which the duration of our exhales is deliberately emphasized.[174] NSDR also involves deliberately and systematically moving our focus of attention from one part of our body to another, then to locations far from our body, then closer to us, then away again. The focusing, then defocusing, and moving and resetting of attention over and over keeps the mind active. And because it is done while the body is deeply relaxed, it brings about a somewhat dreamlike state, and yet you are completely aware and alert.

NSDR is a modification of an ancient practice known as yoga nidra, which roughly translates to "yoga sleep."[175] Yoga nidra has been described as creating the experience of moving our mind away "from thinking and doing toward a state of being and feeling"—which is an admittedly vague statement. There is a small but growing body of modern science on the brain and bodily states that yoga nidra and NSDR bring about and their ability to restore mental and physical vigor, improve consolidation of newly learned information, offset sleep loss, and more.

When I first tried yoga nidra in 2017, I found it to be incredibly restorative. Doing this technique for twenty to thirty minutes first thing in the morning after a restless or less-than-full night's sleep left me feeling fully rested, like I'd had the best sleep of my life. I also noticed that incorporating this practice in the morning improved my ability to fall back asleep quickly if I happened to wake up in the middle of the night. That's right—even though NSDR stands for non-sleep deep rest, and even though it is typically done in the morning or afternoon, something about doing it at that time significantly improved my ability to self-direct my brain and body into a relaxed state and drift back to sleep at night if ever I needed to. What's more, if I ever woke up in the middle of the night, listening to a guided NSDR recording beat tossing and turning, and often sent me back to sleep. Challenges with falling asleep and staying asleep are very common, so I was intrigued. I also noticed that replacing an afternoon nap with an NSDR session left me feeling especially reinvigorated and did not alter my nighttime sleep in any negative way.

I wondered how this simple practice really worked. So I dove into the literature and found there wasn't much known. But the few studies I did find were interesting. A 2002 study from Denmark found that doing yoga nidra dramatically increases levels of dopamine in a brain region called the basal ganglia, which are involved in taking, and withholding, action.[176] Yoga nidra also reduced people's blood pressure and heart rate. Although this and other studies of yoga nidra were small in terms of the number of subjects studied, other investigations indicated that this practice could improve various measures of mental health and help consolidate certain forms of learning.[177]

At one point, I decided to devote a portion of my lab to studying yoga nidra as a tool for stress reduction. To do so we needed to keep its core elements—breathing that emphasizes long exhales to slow the heart rate and place us into a more parasympathetic state, the deliberate and systematic movement of one's perceptual attention to the surface and then the interior of the body, then away from the body, and so on—but we opted to remove the "intentions" and any language pertaining to more spiritual aspects of yoga nidra.[178] This parsing was not an attempt at cultural appropriation of an ancient tradition. Rather, it was a way to examine this powerful tool within the context of Western science, where we seek to understand what works and why, and to then use this knowledge to build more efficient and effective tools. Any aspect of the practice that couldn't be reliably measured was discarded.

Later, as I moved into public education and spoke about stress mitigation tools, I coined the term *non-sleep deep rest*, which keeps the key elements related to the physiology of yoga nidra, but removes the subjective aspects that are hard to keep constant from one person to the next.

And eventually, given the wide interest in stress mitigation tools, my podcast team produced various NSDR scripts of short (ten minute), medium (twenty minute), and long (thirty minute) durations and made them freely available online.[179]

Public feedback has confirmed the positive effects of NSDR, but of course it just follows the thousands of years of people across the world doing this time-tested practice. (Later in chapter 3, I'll get back to what my lab's studies on stress discovered about the benefits of NSDR).

Among all the protocols that I have shared on the *Huberman Lab* podcast, NSDR is in the top ten of those that people tell me have changed their lives, especially individuals who struggle to sleep enough, to maintain high levels of daytime energy and focus, and also among those struggling with excessive work, school, or other demands. I am the last person in the world to suggest people sleep less than they need to at night, but I will be the first to acknowledge how challenging it can often be to get a full seven to nine hours of sleep, especially for parents of young children and those working very long hours. NSDR is a remarkable tool for anyone who simply can't get enough sleep because they have to wake up and meet the demands of the day. Or for those who don't like naps or who can't nap for whatever reason. We will revisit NSDR several times in this book, but in the meantime, if you're seeking tools for improving sleep, or even replacing missed sleep, I highly suggest doing NSDR.

COMMON QUESTIONS:

What if I fall asleep during NSDR?

That's just fine. Chances are, if done during the daytime, the sleep will be relatively shallow and won't create much, if any, sleep inertia. On many occasions, I have fallen asleep during a morning or afternoon NSDR session and then woken up at the last instruction to move my limbs, which meant I wasn't in a deep sleep. If you are using NSDR to reset during the day, or first thing in the morning to offset the effects of not getting enough sleep, just be sure you set an alarm in case you fall asleep.

How long should my NSDR session be?

That's up to you. A ten-minute NSDR is often enough for a quick afternoon reset, but I suggest doing a twenty- to thirty-minute NSDR if you have time. If you slept poorly the night before, you may find that a longer session in the morning or afternoon leaves you feeling more rested, compensating for the sleep you missed in the night. Find what works for you.

Can NSDR truly replace sleep or reduce the amount of time I need to sleep?

Claims that "thirty minutes of yoga nidra is worth two hours of sleep" abound. I've also heard that "twenty minutes of meditation twice daily reduces your nighttime sleep needs by several hours." I am not aware of much laboratory data supporting those statements. It can be hard to get enough sleep, and most of us would love to need less of it to feel fully rested. NSDR won't necessarily reduce the amount of nighttime sleep you need, but it may very well improve the quality of the sleep you get. Combined with proper placement of your nighttime sleep in the twenty-four-hour cycle (see Sleep Protocol 4 for more), and other protocols in this chapter, it may, however, reduce your total sleep needs by improving your sleep architecture, as we discussed earlier in this chapter.

In one study, researchers randomized forty-one people with chronic insomnia to participate in either cognitive behavioral therapy for insomnia or twice-daily yoga nidra for twenty minutes per session.[180] In both groups, participants slept a few minutes longer during the study than at the start of it. However, the yoga nidra group fell asleep faster, fell back asleep faster after night wakings, and had a more efficient sleep (an increase in the number of times they went through N1, N2, N3, and REM) compared to their sleep prior to the study. So while they weren't sleeping less, the sleep they were getting was better than before.

The study also found a significant reduction in cortisol following yoga nidra.[181] That may be one factor that reduces the total amount of sleep you need because, in theory, lowering your evening cortisol should improve sleep. If you practice relaxation techniques during the day and happen to need less sleep that night, that's an added bonus.[182]

SLEEP PROTOCOL

9

Consider Supplements to Support Sleep

WHAT TO DO:

- **Find a combination of supplements that support you in getting the best possible sleep.** Learn a bit about how each of these works. Consider your specific needs and consult with your physician to ensure that any supplements you take are safe for you and will not interfere with any medications you are currently taking. As stated in the introduction, supplements can have their place but ideally, try behavioral tools first. There is simply no pill to replace poor sleep habits, or "sleep hygiene." Below is a list of common supplements sold over the counter that can assist in getting the best possible night's sleep:
    - **Magnesium L-threonate or magnesium bisglycinate.** Dosage: 145–250 mg
      These two forms of magnesium are interchangeable for improving sleep.
    - **Apigenin,** a derivative of chamomile. Dosage: 50 mg
    - **Theanine.** Dosage: 100–200 mg
    - **GABA.** Dosage: 250–500 mg
    - **Glycine.** Dosage: 1–2 g (1,000–2,000 mg)
    - **Myoinositol.** Dosage: 900 mg
    - **Kiwi extract.** Dosage: 500–1,000 mg
    - **Tart cherry extract.** Dosage: 500 mg

    - **Saffron.** Dosage: 30 mg
    - **Valerian.** Dosage: 50–75 mg.
    - **Melatonin.** Dosage: 0.5–1.5 mg of rapid release; 0.5–1.5 mg of sustained release (Note the decimal points here; these are not typos. These are MUCH lower doses of melatonin than you commonly see recommended.)

- **Build a sleep stack.** The best approach is to experiment with one compound at a time in order to become familiar with the effects of each individually. Start with the lowest amount listed and adjust the dosage if necessary until you find the lowest dose that works for you. The dosages provided here are averages. All the compounds are considered safe for healthy individuals but results vary, so I suggest taking one at a time for a few nights each and then adding an additional supplement. That will be the most cost-effective and safest approach, and it will help you understand what works for you.

  That said, if you want to start with a small stack of two to three sleep supplements right out of the gate, here is one that has worked for a lot of people. Take it about thirty minutes before going to sleep.

    - 145–250 mg **magnesium L-threonate** (or **magnesium bisglycinate**)
    - 50 mg **apigenin**
    - 100–200 mg **theanine.** (Don't take theanine if you tend to have intense dreams or nightmares, or if you sleepwalk, as it can enhance the vividness of your dreams.)

- **Pay attention to potential side effects.** The supplements listed above are generally very safe but not all of them will sit well for all people. Here's what to watch for:

    - *Gut discomfort:* A small percentage of people (about 5 percent in my experience) who take magnesium threonate as a sleep aid experience digestive issues or other gut discomfort. Magnesium L-threonate and bisglycinate are far less likely to do this than other

forms of magnesium like citrate or malate, et cetera. Still, discontinue use of magnesium L-threonate or bisglycinate if gut discomfort persists. The dosage listed above for magnesium is already pretty low so you don't have a much lower limit to work with.
- *Vivid or disturbing dreams:* A small percentage (about 5 percent) of people who take theanine report having vivid dreams that wake them at night.

- **Proceed with caution.** Again, it is important to consult with a physician before you take supplements. You need to be sure that you are not risking a dangerous interaction, and that a medical professional has information about your sleep issues that may be symptoms of an underlying health problem. And always check that any product you decide to use is reliable.

HOW IT WORKS:

When it comes to getting optimal sleep, it's always best to start with behavioral tools and changes to your sleep environment. (Sun)light exposure, adjusting your core body temperature, and NSDR can all be employed to improve sleep. So, too, can exercise and proper nutrition (more on both later). These carry no cost, cause no side effects, and quite often resolve persistent issues.

Many people turn to supplements to help improve their sleep. Parsing the scientific literature on the efficacy of over-the-counter, supplement-based sleep aids can be difficult. The studies are often small, they have conflicting results, and they are too few to provide a significant body of evidence.[183] That being said, enough data exist to indicate that some supplements may be beneficial and carry a very low risk of harm for most people trying them. In my opinion, these are much safer than the majority of prescription sleep medications.

A major issue when it comes to supplements is that the dose of the pills inside the bottle often does not match the dosage stated on the label.[184] In addition, just because a supplement contains a "natural" ingredient does not mean it is safe. And these ingredients may react badly with a prescribed medication.

So a reminder here, again, to talk to your doctor before proceeding, and to only buy supplements from reputable brands. I discuss a few things to look for on the packaging to ensure this below.

- **Magnesium L-threonate:** Increasing brain magnesium with this compound may improve learning and memory.[185] A randomized study of magnesium L-threonate versus placebo found that this supplement improved the quality of sleep and also cognitive performance during the day.[186] There are more data on magnesium bisglycinate than threonate for sleep but these seem to work interchangeably for this purpose.
- **Apigenin:** This compound is among the most widely studied flavonoids (chemicals found in plants) and is present in chamomile, parsley, oranges, celery, and thyme, among herbs and vegetables.[187] A growing body of evidence supports apigenin as a sleep aid.[188] Animal studies have found a mild sedative effect from apigenin.[189] Studies in humans also indicate a sleep benefit. In one investigation, apigenin mildly improved daytime function among people with insomnia.[190] Among a group of new mothers suffering from poor sleep and depression, apigenin was found to improve both.
- **Theanine:** Evidence suggests that theanine increases levels of GABA, an amino acid that, when broadly increased in the brain, may reduce anxiety.[191]
- **Glycine:** Research suggests glycine works by elevating serotonin, which helps regulate sleep, and activating NMDA receptors in the SCN, where the circadian clock is headquartered.[192]
- **GABA:** As noted earlier, GABA is an amino acid associated with reducing brain activity. It promotes relaxation and is therefore conducive to sleep.[193]
- **Melatonin:** As discussed in Sleep Protocol 3, we produce natural melatonin, a hormone that causes us to feel sleepy. This production surges at night, leading to feelings of sleepiness. This hormone works well all on its own. However, melatonin supplements have been a staple of vitamin stores for years.

  Clinical trials and meta-analyses of multiple studies indicate that melatonin supplements may benefit older adults, who experience a lower level of natural melatonin production.[194] It may also be beneficial in combination with morning light exposure for people with Alzheimer's disease,[195] which tends to disrupt sleep patterns. However, there is no clear evidence of benefit for all other populations.

Once again, be aware of the dosages listed here. The amount of melatonin contained in the typical single, over-the-counter pill is far greater than what our bodies produce. I often see dosages of 3 milligrams, 5 milligrams, or even 8 to 10 milligrams of melatonin, which are incredibly high and not advised. That's a problem, because melatonin does more than make us sleepy; it can also interact with other hormones and biological pathways in the brain and body unrelated to sleep. Therefore, taking melatonin chronically can be problematic, especially in children and adolescents who are still growing.

If you decide to take melatonin, make sure that you are choosing a reputable brand with third-party certification and use the minimal effective dose. I would suggest taking no more than the amounts listed above (0.5–1.5 mg of rapid or sustained release, although it's fine, and useful, to take both).

- **Tart cherry extract:** A small, randomized, double-blind, placebo-controlled study found elevated natural melatonin levels and improved sleep quality among ten people who drank tart cherry juice for seven days.[196] This preliminary evidence suggests a potential benefit, with larger and longer-term studies needed. Tart cherry juice is safe to try as a sleep aid taken shortly before bedtime. Tart cherry extract capsules are preferable if you don't want the added calories from the juice.
- **Kiwi extract:** A small study of twenty-five people who self-reported their sleep patterns concluded that kiwi may modestly improve sleep duration and efficiency.[197] Consuming kiwi fruit with the skin on an hour before bed may be a mild sleep aid. More evidence is needed to be certain of this benefit, but kiwi is safe to try. Kiwi extract is a good noncaloric, capsule-based approach to get the same effect. (And you don't have to eat kiwi skins!)

COMMON QUESTIONS:

When should I take supplements for sleep?

It's best to take any sleep aid supplements about thirty minutes before you intend to be asleep. Magnesium supplementation during the daytime can be useful for other reasons, but if you're taking it specifically for sleep, best to take it before bed. The one exception is theanine, which some people like to take when they drink caffeine, in order to offset the jitters that they experience from caffeine. In fact, that is one reason energy drink manufacturers often include theanine in energy drinks.

I take AGZ, a powdered sleep supplement that you mix with water and drink. (Note: I helped design AGZ.) It contains many of the compounds listed above. It remains the best sleep supplement I have ever taken, and yes, I am incentivized to say that, but I am measuring my sleep stats most nights. I am able to take half a packet (one full packet is the recommended dose). It has outperformed all the other sleep pill/powder combinations I have tried over the years and even the "sleep peptide" I have tried called pinealon. There are, of course, other great sleep supplements with multiple compounds out there too. Compare and contrast ingredient lists and costs, and once again: Only by trying individual single-ingredient supplements can you really determine what does or doesn't work for you.

What brand of supplements should I use?

Always look for third-party testing. The NSF (founded as the National Sanitation Foundation) or US Pharmacopeia (USP) offer rigorous testing for supplements.[198] "NSF Certified for Sport" indicates that a product met the review standards of the NSF.

SLEEP PROTOCOL

10

Approach Prescription Sleep Drugs with Caution

WHAT TO DO:

- **Talk to your doctor.** If you're still struggling with sleep after working through the prior sleep protocols, and you have tried the stress-management protocols, too, talk to your doctor. There may be an underlying health condition that needs addressing. Or it may be that your sleep issues warrant more intensive treatment. Cognitive behavioral therapy has shown efficacy for sustained sleep disturbance.
- **Stay away from prescription sleep aids if you can.** These are best avoided, unless your physician prescribes them as a last resort. Most can carry side effects, like confusion and daytime drowsiness. Some, like Ambien, may harm sleep architecture and glymphatic function.[199] That means even if you have more time in bed, sleep might not be doing the "cleaning" job it's designed to do. Some, like trazodone, and the DORAs (dual orexin receptor antagonists), appear safer than the others, yet it is easy to become dependent on them for sleep once you begin. None are without side effects, and withdrawal then carries its own set of side effects.

HOW IT WORKS:

Below I've described the different and more common classes of sleep aids, so you can understand how each works, as well as the potential risks:

- **Benzodiazepines:** These drugs belong to a class often referred to as hypnotics or sedatives, although they have other effects too. They are often prescribed to treat insomnia. They work by increasing the effects of GABA.[200] They are older medications that can be addictive, and can have other serious side effects including confusion, memory problems, unsteadiness, and slurred speech.[201] The withdrawal from benzodiazepines is notoriously hard.
- **Non-benzodiazepine hypnotics:** These short-term insomnia medications tend to be less disruptive than benzodiazepines.[202] The most well-known is Ambien. However, the FDA has issued a "black box" warning for non-benzodiazepines following reports of rare but dangerous behavior during sleep, including wandering, driving, and using a stove, and amnesia and other forms of memory alterations after the drug has worn off.[203] And again, Ambien may harm sleep architecture and glymphatic function, the clearance of waste products from the brain at night.[204]
- **Antidepressants:** Drowsiness is a common side effect of certain antidepressants, leading to their use as a sleep aid. The American Academy of Sleep Medicine has recommended the use of certain antidepressants as a treatment for insomnia among people with depression, but clinical evidence for this benefit is limited.[205] Trazodone, a serotonin receptor agonist and reuptake inhibitor (SARI) seems to preserve sleep architecture better than other antidepressants when taken specifically for sleep.[206] Please note that many people who take selective serotonin reuptake inhibitors (SSRIs) like Prozac, SARIs like trazodone, or norepinephrine-dopamine reuptake inhibitors (NDRIs) like Wellbutrin/bupropion during the daytime for depression, anxiety, or other reasons do not experience altered sleep, and some of these, like bupropion, when taken early in the daytime, can indirectly improve sleep later that night.[207] Psychiatrists now will prescribe antidepressants specifically for sleep because some can improve sleep.

- **Melatonin receptor agonists:** This category of medications mimics the action of melatonin and may help with falling asleep faster and improving sleep quality. They do not appear to cause dependency or serious side effects.[208] However, the efficacy of melatonin receptor agonists is somewhat unclear.
- **Anticonvulsants and dopamine agonist drugs:** These may be prescribed to treat restless legs syndrome and other conditions involving nighttime limb movement that can make it difficult to fall and stay asleep,[209] as well as to treat pain. Examples include gabapentin and cabergoline.
- **Dual orexin receptor antagonists (DORAs):** Insomnia is characterized by abnormal wakefulness, and orexin, a neuropeptide that helps regulate the sleep-wake cycle and that is altered in narcolepsy, has been found to cause a state of arousal.[210] Thus it makes sense to investigate orexin as a potential target for insomnia drugs. That led to the development of the DORAs, which work by reducing the action of orexin and thus wakefulness circuits in the brain rather than by direct sedation.[211] Early evidence of such drugs shows that they do effectively block orexin, and indicate a potential role for them in safely treating insomnia.[212] A meta-analysis of ten randomized clinical trials that combined a sample of 7,086 individuals with insomnia found these drugs to be generally safe, with a comparably lower incidence of mild side effects and with improved sleep compared to a placebo.[213] These new medications are expensive, typically costing about $300 or more per month.[214] Generic lower-cost versions are not yet available.

SLEEP PROTOCOL

11

Adjust Your Caffeine Schedule to Improve Your Sleep

WHAT TO DO:

- **Avoid caffeine in the eight to ten hours before bed.** As it's a stimulant with a long half-life, caffeine should be avoided late in the day, especially if you have trouble falling asleep. Some people who are especially caffeine sensitive may have to avoid caffeine in the twelve hours before bedtime. Even those who can "fall asleep after drinking coffee" are likely not getting the best sleep they could. As someone who loves caffeine, I relate to anyone reluctant to stop drinking caffeine in the afternoon. As painful as it can be, I personally avoid it after 2:00 p.m. most days.
- **If you tend to experience an energy crash in the afternoon despite sleeping well, consider delaying drinking caffeine until thirty to ninety minutes after waking up.** This slight adjustment to your caffeine schedule may help you have more sustained energy levels throughout the day and may help you avoid the need to drink caffeine after 2:00 p.m.

HOW IT WORKS:

Remember adenosine, from Sleep Protocol 7? It's a chemical that builds up in our brains as we go throughout our day, eventually making us want to sleep through a process called homeostatic sleep drive.[215]

Our scientific understanding of adenosine is deeply intertwined with that of caffeine.[216] The research history dates back to 1911, when Coca-Cola asked a psychologist named Harry Levi Hollingworth to investigate the effects of caffeine on human behavior because the US government was suing the company for including what it considered to be a drug with a "poisonous tendency" in the soda. (The cocaine that had once been a major ingredient of Coca-Cola had been removed years earlier.)[217] The company wanted reliable evidence on exactly how caffeine altered human behavior. Hollingworth agreed as long as the company did not include his study results in its advertisements. He also insisted that the results be published regardless of what they revealed.

Hollingworth's investigation is often cited as the first time that the double-blind, placebo-controlled study design entered psychological research.[218] Although some may argue whether it was indeed a double-blind study, it is considered a landmark for its introduction of rigor into the process, and for its findings. Sixteen participants consumed caffeine daily at a range of doses (at amounts reflecting drinking a daily soda) or a placebo. They then completed various tasks that examined their alertness, coordination, and other mental skills. Caffeine undeniably improved their capacity in all these domains. The findings were favorable toward Coca-Cola because the chemical in question seemed to only help people, not hurt them, at least in the context of what was measured. But Coca-Cola wasn't interested in sleep. (If you were wondering, the US government's case was dismissed on a technicality when the company argued that caffeine wasn't added to the beverage but rather was naturally occurring.)

According to Hollingworth's report, published in the *American Journal of Psychology* in 1912, a few grains of caffeine taken on successive days were enough to impair sleep.[219] The connection relied on self-reporting and each individual recording their impression about the quality of their sleep following each study day. But the findings were consistent.

Decades later we know how that happens: Caffeine leads to longer sleep latency (that is, the time it takes to fall asleep) and more nighttime waking, thus leading to reduced wakefulness the next day.[220] We also now know that caffeine can alter sleep architecture, including less time spent in REM.[221]

Hollingworth's study was the first of many to come. Today we understand a great deal about how caffeine stimulates brain activity. It's a psychoactive stimulant that increases the actions of epinephrine and dopamine, in part by increasing the availability of dopamine receptors, the sites on cells where it can attach and thereby initiate its effects.[222] Caffeine also increases the activity of certain neural circuits and brain areas associated with alertness, such as the locus coeruleus, which we discussed earlier in this chapter.[223] We also understand now how it interferes with sleep. That brings us back to adenosine.

Caffeine is what is called an adenosine antagonist.[224] It parks in adenosine receptors, which prevents adenosine from exerting its normal fatigue-inducing activity in the brain. As sleep expert Matthew Walker describes it, "Caffeine keeps pulling out the chairs from under adenosine."[225] So even though adenosine is building up with each hour we are awake and increasingly so when we are very alert or active, our brains don't register that fatigue or the number of hours we've been awake accurately.[226] Caffeine dampens the communication between adenosine and the brain.

This process explains the phenomenon many of us know of as the caffeine crash. Once caffeine's actions on those receptors wear off, which our metabolism accomplishes in a few hours, the non-receptor-bound adenosine that has accumulated suddenly can bind and fatigue hits us. In addition, caffeine makes our brain more active and increases our capacity for physical effort, and that generates more adenosine as a by-product, which in turn means the crash is harder than it would be without caffeine.

This all sounds rough, but I want to reiterate: I love caffeine and I have no plans to give it up. The data say caffeine in moderation is fine . . . and may even be good for us. A recent large-scale study involving over 100,000 subjects found that daily intake of approximately two to three cups of caffeinated coffee or tea can reduce risks of stroke and dementia.[227]

"What is moderation?" you may be wondering. One or two cups of strong coffee, a few twelve-ounce diet sodas (we can debate artificial sweeteners later, in chapter 4, but we should all probably avoid the sugar in regular soda), or my favorite source of caffeine: hot brewed or cold brew yerba maté, which will deliver 100 to 300 milligrams of caffeine depending on the source.

The ramifications of caffeine on sleep depend on the dose of caffeine and the time of day you consume it. The closer to your to-sleep time you drink a caffeinated beverage, and the more sensitive you are to caffeine, the greater the impact it will have on sleep.

So now you may be wondering: How close is too close to your to-sleep time? This may seem somewhat obvious but most people don't realize just how long the effects of caffeine last, and that's what I hope to help with in this protocol.

People who are very caffeine sensitive have probably already learned by experience not to drink caffeine past a certain time of day if they hope to sleep later that night. For the rest of us who enjoy caffeine in both the morning and in the afternoon—yes, there are many of us—a bit more understanding of caffeine's effects can go a long way toward consuming it while still experiencing great sleep.

Caffeine is hard to study. Would-be study participants who consume caffeine daily (and that includes about 85 percent of American adults, for example) would need to quit prior to joining a well-controlled investigation of the effects of caffeine, and many people just won't abstain, even for a short while, just to be in a study. Also, researchers don't always know when a person who is in caffeine withdrawal is back to a baseline state of sleep.[228] And, as I've mentioned, people's sensitivity to caffeine varies.[229] That being said, the evidence shows that our sleep patterns tend to adapt to a daily dose of caffeine. Regular caffeine consumers are able to fall asleep, stay asleep, and cycle through the stages of sleep.[230] It appears that chronic caffeine users develop a sort of sleep-tolerance for the stimulant. This is good and bad. Good, because it means folks like me can enjoy a morning yerba maté and a 2:00 p.m. espresso and still fall asleep easily at 10:00 p.m. Bad, because there is a chance that anyone drinking caffeine past noon is getting less than optimal sleep. Not everything in life is about getting the best possible sleep of course, but if you are struggling to feel rested enough in the daytime or are waking after seven to eight hours of sleep and still not feeling alert, you may try avoiding caffeine in the eight to ten or even twelve hours prior to sleep. Note how you feel. Those tracking their sleep with Eight Sleep, WHOOP, Oura rings, or other devices can see how this impacts their REM and non-REM sleep.

The recommendation to delay caffeine by sixty to ninety minutes after waking is just a suggestion. Indeed, this suggestion—when I first made it on the internet—made a lot of people VERY upset. (People don't like it when you try to take away their morning coffee). To be clear: You don't have to do it.

It is also not supported by a clinical trial. It is, however, supported by ample mechanistic evidence of how caffeine adjusts adenosine, and how adenosine continually reduces in the first one to two hours of the day if we don't ingest caffeine. If you are someone who tends to experience energy crashes in the afternoon and you rely on caffeine to overcome them, I suggest at least trying to delay your morning caffeine by sixty to ninety minutes for a few days. It can be a bit painful at first, so maybe start with a thirty-minute delay, then sixty minutes, then ninety minutes, and see if you still need the afternoon caffeine kick. Then try NSDR, as described in Sleep Protocol 8, if you're having trouble making it through the afternoon without it.

One key thing: If you like to exercise soon after you wake up and need caffeine to do so—as I and many others do—then by all means, drink it upon waking and do your workout. Just be sure to hydrate well too. Caffeine can be a mild diuretic. It's much less of a diuretic than once thought but we tend to wake up slightly dehydrated as it is.[231] Before you slam back two coffees, it's probably best to hydrate first thing.

In My Experience

For my first caffeine of the day, I usually drink yerba maté, a Paraguayan (and Uruguayan and Argentine) tea that is traditionally sipped from a small gourd through a metal straw but that can also be brewed and consumed like any other tea. I'll drink it hot or a cold-brewed canned version. Mateina is my favorite. (Note: I am a partial owner of Mateina, but I love it without bias. Also, it is a good idea to avoid drinking smoked varieties of yerba. Mateina is air-dried, not smoked.) I find that the alertness effect from yerba maté is more gradual and causes fewer jitters, and results in a milder, if any, "crash" as it wears off. Sometimes I have coffee or espresso later in the morning. My absolute favorite time for coffee is in the early afternoon, after a twenty-to-thirty-minute NSDR session. Talk about a reset. My best work sessions seem to follow this protocol. However, my sleep suffers if I drink coffee after about 3:00 p.m. I can fall asleep perfectly fine, but my sleep is not as deep (I use a sleep tracker, and it confirms that I get much less REM sleep after late-day caffeine). So I try to limit coffee and other sources of caffeine after 3:00 p.m. That's not a hard-and-fast rule; sometimes I drink coffee late in the day, but that's rare and I always regret it when I'm still awake at midnight.

I like to exercise first thing in the morning, within an hour or two of waking up, so on workout days my target regimen is to drink water and caffeine soon after waking, view sunlight, and then exercise. On days when I cannot exercise early, I tend to delay caffeine intake until midmorning, which I find keeps my energy levels steadier into and throughout the afternoon. On these days, I often skip afternoon caffeine because I don't need it.

COMMON QUESTIONS:

Does the source of caffeine matter?

No. Different drinks contain different amounts of caffeine, and chocolate has small amounts too.[232] But the caffeine molecule works pretty much the same regardless of where it comes from. Some drinks like yerba maté and guayusa tea also contain non-caffeine stimulants in them like theobromine—a plant alkaloid also with antioxidant properties. And of course nowadays there are hundreds of different energy drinks available that combine caffeine, neuromodulator precursors like L-tyrosine (the amino acid from which dopamine is made), taurine, and on and on. I will drink a zero-sugar energy drink now and again. I discuss these and other stimulants more in chapter 6.

Is caffeine unhealthy?

Studies have consistently shown a health benefit from coffee, particularly when consumed before noon, up to a certain amount.[233] Generally, beyond four cups per day of coffee, or the equivalent of 400 milligrams, there are diminishing returns or possibly negative consequences, although larger individuals may be able to handle more than that with no problem.[234] Many of the benefits from coffee and tea are not from caffeine but from antioxidants contained in coffee beans and certain teas. That finding is supported by the fact that decaffeinated coffee confers the same benefit as caffeinated coffee, which includes a potential reduction in the risk of heart disease, prostate cancer, melanoma, endometrial cancer, liver conditions, type 2 diabetes, and neurodegenerative diseases.[235] In the case of yerba maté, research suggests that it may facilitate weight loss by reducing appetite and perhaps by its effects on digestion as well as the microbiome, a critical aspect of health we will address in chapter 4.[236]

SLEEP PROTOCOL

12

Avoid Alcohol Within Eight Hours Before Sleep

WHAT NOT TO DO:

- **Alcohol should not be used as a sleep aid.** Alcohol severely disrupts the elegantly sequential architecture of sleep, and reduces both the total amount of deep sleep and REM sleep, so even if it helps you drift off and you sleep for seven to eight hours, it will negatively affect the quality of your sleep.
- **If you drink, avoid alcohol within eight hours of the time you plan to be asleep.** This timing reduces the amount of alcohol in your body by the time you go to bed.

The "What Alcohol Does to Your Body, Brain & Health" episode of the *Huberman Lab* podcast remains one of the top downloaded and shared podcast episodes of all time, across all podcasts. It makes clear that the data show zero to two drinks per week is fine for nonalcoholic adults without confounding medical issues. However, zero is better than any, and there is growing data on the increased risk of cancer associated with alcohol consumption.[237]

I am not anti-alcohol! I know some people enjoy a drink now and again and that is my motivation for the inclusion of this protocol. I subscribe to a "do as you like, but know what you're doing" philosophy. I personally don't drink but I have never liked the taste or effects of alcohol.

But there's a key question for everyone that has not been addressed: Are many of the negative effects of alcohol the consequence of the negative effects of alcohol on sleep? This has not been systematically studied, but for those that like a drink now and again (and also for those who abstain), keep that question in the back of your mind as you read the section below.

HOW IT WORKS:

Alcohol is a sedative that affects the neural pathways associated with sleep in multiple ways. Alcohol decreases the amount of time it takes us to fall asleep.[238] But what happens next is not good. During the first half of the night, the presence of alcohol in the body suppresses REM sleep and it takes longer for us to reach whatever REM sleep we do manage to achieve.[239] Remember that each sleep stage is like a gate to the next, so the reduced REM means less deep sleep, and less REM in the next cycle. As discussed earlier in this chapter, REM sleep is critical to our cognitive functioning, to consolidating new information, and to daytime emotional regulation. So missing out on any amount of REM is a problem. And alcohol is a potent REM suppressor.

Alcohol has also been found to decrease the amount of growth hormone and testosterone released during the night—hormones critical for vitality and metabolism for both men and women.[240] Normally, growth hormone is released relatively soon after falling asleep, and testosterone is released before and during REM sleep.[241] The negative effects of alcohol on REM and these hormones happen acutely, meaning after even just a single night of drinking or for those who are alcohol sensitive, even one drink. Only if we metabolize the alcohol prior to bedtime do we avoid some of these consequences, which is why this protocol recommends a specific timing.

Chronic drinking is even more problematic for sleep. Insomnia and alcohol dependency frequently coexist, for example.[242] The cycle is self-perpetuating in that poor sleep leads to increased caffeine and other stimulant use during the day and into the afternoon and evening, which leads to difficulty sleeping at night, which leads to alcohol intake as a sleep aid. Beyond the changes one or two drinks can make on REM sleep, people with alcohol dependency tend to have decreased amounts of both N2 and N3 sleep, the non-REM period when we sink into a deep sleep.[243] These alterations in sleep architecture can persist for some time even after a person stops drinking. Frequent drinking also interferes with our circadian rhythm, disrupting or even decreasing the amount of melatonin our brains produce.[244]

Adolescents are at particular risk of turning to alcohol intake as a sleep aid. In 2008, public health researchers at the University of Texas Health Science Center reported their findings from a large, yearlong study of insomnia among youth between the ages of eleven and seventeen years. They collected data on 3,134 people in this age range from a baseline date and then twelve months later and found that chronic insomnia heightened the risk of alcohol use.[245] That's concerning because insomnia is the most common sleep disorder among young people, and because nighttime phone use, which is very common in this age group, also interferes with sleep quality and duration.[246] Phone use at night has been linked to insomnia.[247]

That means there are two major risks to this age group when it comes to good sleep, not to mention the chronic stress that kids at that age face. We'll discuss phone use in Sleep Protocol 14.

COMMON QUESTIONS:

It's not practical to avoid alcohol within eight hours of sleep because any drinking I do happens at night. How can I compensate for the negative effects of consuming alcohol close to bedtime?

For most people, social drinking happens well within eight hours of going to sleep. What's important here is that drinking this way every night, multiple times per week, or even once per week will disrupt sleep, and thereby health, in detrimental ways. Occasional alcohol use closer to bedtime, say once a month or less, is very unlikely to cause long-term problems, unless it's excessive during that once-a-month night out.

If you drink in the eight hours before sleep, make sure you also consume sufficient water before going to sleep and after waking. Take electrolytes too if you can, and emphasize other behaviors that support great sleep, as well as a healthy microbiome, to try to offset the effects of alcohol.

To be clear, it's good to enjoy life. If having a few drinks during a celebration or a night out now and again is how you do, you're not alone. The important considerations are that this isn't happening too often, that you're not driving, that you're not experiencing any kind of dependency, and that you're not too young to drink (the negative effects of alcohol are much worse for the developing brain compared to the adult brain).[248]

Does the type of alcohol matter?

Not with respect to the negative effects on sleep and the microbiome. As mentioned above, no alcohol is better than any alcohol. Although many studies have been done on the potential benefits of red wine, conclusive evidence of this link does not exist.[249] The amount of red wine you would need to drink to get benefits from grape skin, for example, would require consumption of enough alcohol to far outweigh any benefits. Put simply, the interaction between alcohol and our sleep processes is the same regardless of the drink.

SLEEP PROTOCOL

13

Avoid Cannabis as a Sleep Aid

WHAT TO DO:

- **Do not use cannabis specifically for sleep.** Cannabis should not be used to facilitate falling asleep or returning to sleep after night wakings. It potently reduces REM sleep.
- **Understand CBD's impact on sleep.** Some evidence exists on the benefit of CBD for sleep but those effects are mainly due to the reduced anxiety it causes.[250] At higher dosages (e.g., 160 mg or more), CBD is more of a sedative. The dosage of CBD that makes it an effective sleep aid varies depending on weight and other factors.[251]

HOW IT WORKS:

Cannabis is a psychoactive drug that comes from the cannabis plant. The main chemical behind its psychoactive effects is THC (delta-9-tetrahydro-cannabinol).[252] CBD, or cannabidiol, is another well-known component of the cannabis plant; this chemical technically is psychoactive, too, because it impacts the brain, but it's not responsible for the "high" that people are usually seeking when they use cannabis. THC can impair cognitive or behavioral functioning; CBD doesn't appear to do so.[253] When present with THC in the cannabis plant or in an edible, CBD can modify the way that THC works in the brain, so their ratios can determine the subjective effects of the drug.[254]

THC potently reduces the amount of REM sleep even at low doses.[255]

THC is often used as an aid for falling asleep, as its psychoactive properties are often accompanied by, or followed by, drowsiness. As with alcohol, people often come to depend on THC to fall asleep, which disrupts the sleep-wake cycle, and can put them at risk for the physical and mental health issues associated with a deficiency in REM sleep, including depression and cardiovascular disease, among other issues.[256] Not everyone who uses cannabis experiences these challenges of course but the link between REM sleep and health is solid: THC reduces REM. Ask people who have used cannabis regularly and then stopped and you'll often hear about the wild dreams they experience afterward. That is the REM-rebound compensation for the lack of REM they experienced while using cannabis.[257]

A multidisciplinary team at McMaster University, in Canada, conducted a review of the scientific literature on the link between cannabinoids and sleep.[258] One of their most noteworthy findings was that the direct effects of both THC and CBD on sleep are lacking data because most clinical studies of cannabis have focused on various health conditions, such as pain, post-traumatic stress disorder, or glaucoma. The researchers did identify data showing that cannabinoids could have a positive impact on sleep. But the small size of these studies and the fact that examining this connection was not the main objective of the investigations somewhat limits the usefulness of the findings. Furthermore, THC and CBD are vastly different, which makes any reference to *cannabinoids* confusing and unhelpful.

A survey of 4,637 ninth through twelfth graders in Colorado found that those who consumed cannabis through edibles or vaping tended to sleep fewer than seven hours per night.[259] Another study of adolescents found that the sedative effects of THC were followed by increased wakefulness at night and impaired memory the next day, which could have been directly due to the THC, which is known to impair memory, lack of sleep, or both.[260]

Researchers have also found a potential link between use of cannabis among pregnant mothers and poor sleep habits among their children during adolescence.[261] You might be asking, "How many pregnant women use cannabis?" A recent report said that anywhere from 4 to 12 percent of pregnant mothers in the US said they'd used cannabis during pregnancy, usually by edible and usually in the first trimester prior to learning they were pregnant.[262] Cannabis use during pregnancy has reportedly increased in recent years, from 3.4 percent in 2002 to 7 percent in 2017.[263] Smoking or ingesting cannabis during pregnancy has been tied to lower birth weight, possibly due to THC-induced changes to the placenta.[264] Rates of neonatal and infant death are higher with cannabis use during pregnancy compared to no such use (and combining cannabis with nicotine raises this risk even higher).[265]

Many people use CBD to try to induce sleep, but rigorous evidence of a direct benefit to sleep is currently insufficient. Chances are any positive effects of CBD on sleep are due to its anxiety-lowering effects. CBD may help people to stop ruminating—a prerequisite to falling asleep. As such, there are populations for whom CBD may be useful. In one study, fifty-seven of seventy-two adults with anxiety reported improved sleep with the use of CBD, although this study was retrospective, meaning the participants were reporting their recall of possible effects from memory rather than measuring them directly.[266] A 2025 review of twenty-nine studies identified a potential for CBD to reduce sleep disruptions but emphasized that research on this link has suffered from a lack of standardization.[267] There certainly is enough evidence to warrant continued study of CBD in this context and no known negative effects of CBD that would preclude trying it for sleep if you feel stressed at night. That said, in January 2024, a team from Australia published the results of a small, randomized, placebo-controlled study in which fifteen people received 150 milligrams of CBD and fifteen people received a placebo as a sleep aid to combat insomnia.[268] The investigators observed no difference between the two groups in the time it took to fall asleep, the efficiency of their sleep, the duration of sleep, or overall severity of insomnia. There were some signs of an improved mood upon waking among the CBD group, and that group had fewer night wakings after two weeks of treatment.

One more thing: An increasing number of studies report a potential for THC (but not CBD) to induce psychosis in certain individuals.[269]

If your goal is to improve your sleep, there are better tools covered in the other protocols of this chapter. The same goes for stress management—more reliable tools exist (and these can improve sleep too), which I'll explain in a later chapter.

SLEEP PROTOCOL

14

Avoid Screens Within an Hour or More Before Bedtime

WHAT TO DO:

- **Avoid screens in the bedroom at night.** This includes phones, laptops, tablets, and TV screens.
- **Avoid consuming information on an electronic device within an hour (at least) of bedtime.** Light from phones and other screens can disrupt your circadian clock.
- **If you opt to read or watch content on a screen in the hour before sleep, dim the screen.** I suggest lowering the brightness and/or activating the "red" screen function. You can also wear blue and green (short wavelength) blocking glasses.

HOW IT WORKS:

In 2011, the National Sleep Foundation conducted a poll.[270] They asked 1,508 Americans about their sleep habits, whether any technology was around them in the hour before bed, and if so, what it was and how they used it. Ninety percent of respondents said they used some kind of screen device at this time; for those under thirty, that percentage climbed to 96! Adolescent and young adult respondents were more likely to use cell phones or play video games before bed compared to adults over thirty, and the same went for computers and digital music players. I strongly suspect those percentages have either held constant or increased in the last decade and a half. In 2011, watching television was the most common activity among the entire sample. Others included doing homework, using social media, using a smartphone, sending work emails, and other activities. The researchers also asked about reading printed books and magazines before bed, which about half of respondents reported doing.

More than half the respondents—63 percent, to be exact—said they didn't get enough sleep on weeknights. And nearly all the people who reported insufficient sleep said it negatively affected both their personal and professional lives. The high rates of late-night technology use and insufficient sleep seen in the survey responses didn't automatically mean the two were related, so the researchers conducted some statistical analyses to check for such a link. They found that difficulty falling asleep rose in keeping with the amount of technology people used in the hour before bed. More passive devices like e-readers were less problematic than interactive devices like game consoles, cell phones, and laptops.

These screens are illuminated by LEDs, and as we've discussed in this chapter, this type of lighting is disruptive to our circadian rhythm. Evidence suggests that LED screens can interrupt melatonin production, which, as you now know, is essential for sleep. In 2014, a group of sleep researchers at Harvard Medical School reported that people who read on an e-book at night with a dim bedside light took longer to fall asleep, were less sleepy, had lower levels of melatonin, and were less alert the next morning compared to people who read a printed book with a dim bedside light before bed.[271]

And there's more. In 2018, a team of researchers, including UCLA psychiatrist Peter Whybrow, reviewed the data on the potential link between LED lighting and mental health.[272] They concluded that exposure to blue light, in particular, posed a risk to sleep and other processes governed by the circadian system. There is also evidence suggesting that the way in which artificial lighting at night interferes with this system may lead to depression.[273]

The problem with devices at bedtime is not solely due to the type of lighting. Technology, particularly interactive technology, stimulates our brains in a way that counters the calm that we need in order to fall asleep. For example, the devices in the 2018 study were most strongly linked to difficulty falling asleep and to poor sleep quality. Also, people who sleep with their phones in their rooms with the ringer on contributed to the numbers reported in the study, indicating that the problem isn't just about late-night scrolling.

We have known since at least the 1970s that the bedroom should be reserved for sleep and intimacy.[274] The evidence linking various stimuli to insomnia is well established. Yet decades later, here we are, with about 1,350 out of 1,508 randomly selected Americans ignoring this basic practice.

Believe it or not (believe it!), this protocol is one of the most potent in this chapter. It's also one of the most difficult to stick to for many people. Sleep-based apps and the use of smartphones as alarm clocks don't make it any easier. Still: I highly suggest you try it.

COMMON QUESTIONS:

Do blue-blocking glasses counter the negative effects of screens at night?

Yes, somewhat. Better, however, would be glasses that block both blue and green light, aka short wavelengths of visible light, at that time—especially if you use screens at night. (See Sleep Protocol 3 for more information.)

SLEEP PROTOCOL

15

A Tip Sheet for Avoiding Jet Lag

Some people experience terrible jet lag, others far less so. This changes as we age. And it depends on where we fly—which direction and if we need to push ourselves to wake earlier or stay awake later than usual. The latter is always easier for people.

Five factors allow you to shift your circadian clock. Knowing these can help you switch to a new time zone quickly, which allows you to be more effective on work trips and enjoy vacations more fully. The factors you use to entrain your SCN to a new local light-dark cycle are, in descending order of influence:

- **Light**
- **Temperature**
- **Meal times**
- **Exercise**
- **Social factors**

You might think: Can't I just hop on the local schedule? Alas, that's hard because your SCN is entrained to wherever you have been for the prior week or so before your trip. So for instance if you fly from California to London and arrive at 5:00 p.m. and you view the sunset, your SCN thinks it's morning sunlight and it wakes you up. But there is a way to overcome this. I'll explain.

WHAT TO DO:

BEFORE YOU TRAVEL EAST

Eastward travel is typically more challenging for the body. Why? Most people find it easier to stay awake later than to fall asleep earlier. But you can prepare for your trip and partially adjust your circadian rhythm before you leave:

- **Get early bright light exposure, but be careful when.** When traveling east, you need to shift to waking up earlier than you normally would. Starting two days before you leave, try waking up thirty to forty-five minutes prior to your usual wake-up time and view bright sunlight or bright artificial light as soon as you wake up.
- **Drink caffeine early.** This will help promote alertness early in the day and make it much easier to shift to your new time zone when you travel.
- **Get moving.** Within sixty minutes of your new, earlier wake-up time, exercise. Even just some light jogging will help if you can't do a full workout.

These three levers—light, caffeine, and exercise—will help adjust your circadian clock to your new eastward-of-typical location, fast.

BEFORE YOU TRAVEL WEST

As mentioned earlier, westward travel tends to be easier for most people. That said, it can still help to adjust your circadian rhythm before you leave by using light, exercise, and caffeine. In this case, however, you'll want to shift everything thirty to forty-five minutes later in the day as opposed to earlier. A slightly later wake-up time, a slightly later caffeine intake in the morning and early afternoon (but still avoid caffeine in the eight to ten hours prior to bedtime), and a slightly later workout—even just by forty-five minutes—will all help.

You'll also want to make sure that you view bright light from artificial lights one to two hours after sunset. Remember, you're trying to prepare to stay up later as you soon fly westward.

WHEN YOU ARRIVE AT YOUR NEW DESTINATION (REGARDLESS OF WHETHER YOU FLEW EAST OR WEST)

- **Eat like a local.** Adopting the local meal schedule when you arrive—eating breakfast, lunch, and dinner more or less at the same times as the locals, even if you're not hungry—will help you shift your circadian clock to the new time zone. Personally, I hate to eat when I'm not hungry (and love to eat when I am!), so I opt out of this protocol. If it works for you, go for it. The sooner you can get on the local meal schedule, the better. Many find it effective to fast for a period of fourteen to sixteen hours before the local breakfast time so they are very hungry when that time arrives.
- **Time your light exposure correctly by knowing your temperature minimum.** This is the real power tool to shift your circadian clock fast, but it involves learning your *temperature minimum* first. See Sleep Protocol 3 and Sleep Protocol 5 for more on that topic. For now, know that it occurs approximately two hours before your usual wake-up time. If you typically wake up at 7:00 a.m., your temperature minimum is very likely to be between 4:30 a.m. and 5:30 a.m. Here's the key: If you get bright light exposure in the one to two hours after your temperature minimum, you will adjust your circadian clock such that it will make you want to go to sleep earlier on the subsequent nights and wake up earlier on the subsequent mornings. Perfect for traveling east. Conversely, if you get bright light exposure in the one to two hours before your temperature minimum, you will shift your circadian clock such that it will make you want to go to sleep later on the subsequent nights and wake up later on the subsequent mornings. Perfect for traveling west.

But remember we are referring to the time of your temperature minimum before you leave! This is vital to understand. Get it right and you'll shift fast across time zones. Get it wrong and it can be a mess.

Why? Well, think about this. Imagine you fly from San Francisco to London (+8 hours). You land in the morning London time and the sun is out. I said get morning sunlight in your eyes, right? Yes, but for the first two to three days in London before you adjust your clock, viewing that London morning sunlight is the same to your brain's clock as getting a giant blast of light in your eyes at midnight San Francisco time. So you just made your body want to go to bed much later and wake up later. You got it backward. Many people sleep well their first night after flying east, wake up, see sunlight, and the second night is a mess. They can't sleep! It would be better to wear dark sunglasses during the two to three hours before your temperature minimum for the first two days in London. After those first two or three days, just view sunlight per the recommendations earlier in this chapter.

Obviously, I am just using London as an example. You must figure it out based on your own travel destination. I know it sounds complicated, but if you know the time of your temperature minimum back home, and follow the instructions above, you'll nail this protocol easily.

- **Use artificial light and blue and green (short wavelength) blocking glasses as tools.** Of course, it's often very cloudy, or you may land at night, and we can't control the time of sunrise and sunset—though if you can, please contact me.

What you can do, however, is travel with a portable bright light device (you'll want one with 5,000- to 10,000-lux brightness) to shift your circadian clock. Several are the size of a book and thin enough to fit in a carry-on bag. I have no affiliation with any companies that make these, but I use the Verilux Happy Light when I travel. They cost about $50. At home I use a larger countertop unit, the Carex Daylight (also no affiliation) and Ra Optics or Bon Charge full-spectrum LED bulbs in the daytime, as discussed earlier. Remember that even when it is cloudy, sunlight through cloud cover is still almost always far brighter than artificial lighting. Get outside and view that sunlight at the correct times and you'll shift your circadian clock fast. Then, you can return to the standard protocols to stay on the local schedule.

One more thing we can all control is the brightness of our evening and nighttime environment. As you get ready for bed, reduce exposure to bright lights—especially blue and green, or short-wavelength, light. Alas, as you now know, all LED lights are rich in blue and green wavelengths. For that reason, I wear blue and green (short wavelength) blocking glasses after sundown to help adjust to the local schedule. This protocol is known to protect against the melatonin-reducing effects of bright light and to prevent the cortisol-increasing effects of bright light.

- **Maintain a regular exercise schedule.** While traveling, try to maintain a consistent early-in-the-day exercise routine (adjusted to the local schedule). That, too, helps shift your circadian clock.
- **A final tip.** For trips that last fewer than two days, staying on (or near) your home sleep-wake, eating, and exercise schedule can be beneficial to minimize disruptions to your circadian rhythm.

These tips will help you quickly overcome any jet lag in your future travels—they've certainly helped me over the years, as well as people in the military, medical professions working night shifts, and more.

CHAPTER 2

PROTOCOLS for EXERCISE

I got really lucky with learning about exercise, and enjoying exercise—but only because I got unlucky first.

Like most kids in my town, I swam and played soccer, but unlike most I got really into skateboarding. I was decent enough at those other activities, but I loved skateboarding best. It felt the most liberating because I could do it any time of day or night, and I loved that there was no official court or playing field—city streets, curbs, benches, and stairs were as varied as they come. And it was transportation too, so it offered all sorts of possibilities for adventure. I could do it alone or with others, and I loved that you could innovate by making up new tricks. The sport was still relatively small at the time (this was the late 1980s and early 1990s) and, as I mentioned in the introduction to this book, several of my friends turned professional just out of high school. Not me. I kept getting hurt. By the time I was a sophomore, I had broken the same foot twice and messed up the arches of my feet.

And that's how exercise came into my life. Luckily, a supportive physical education teacher named Bob Peters noticed how often I arrived to class on crutches and pointed me toward a small weight room near the pool. No one really used it except the football team, and that was only during the summer months. So in many ways, it was a perfect situation. I could go in there and use the equipment whenever I wanted and I didn't have to compare my (lack of) strength to anyone else because I was mostly alone. Although I didn't realize it at the time, the dearth of other people weight training also saved me from the terrible, often dangerous advice people tend to give others in gyms.

The only problem was that I had absolutely no idea what I was doing. There were anatomy charts of muscles and bones and tendons on the walls, and a few diagrams of exercises that were easy enough to follow, but nothing else. That drove me to the library and local bookstore, where I read about weight training. Which left me even more confused. The recommendations were all over the place. "Do one set per body part but super slow." "Do twenty sets per body part." "Train for thirty minutes maximum, three times a week." "Train for two hours, twice a day, six days per week," and on and on. It was dizzying. I completely empathize with people who experience immense confusion when they try to figure out how best to exercise, because I felt that too.

Luckily (again), one of the books I stumbled upon was by Arthur Jones, the inventor of Nautilus exercise machines. Jones was a proponent of doing short, intense workouts two to three times per week, or even less. While that didn't sound like enough to get results, I liked that he had a rationale for his suggestions and I liked that his general training philosophy was based on science—in particular the work of physiologist Hans Selye, who studied stress and adaptations to stress.[1] (More about Selye in the next chapter . . .)

Exercise, Jones pointed out, is a form of stress that the body adjusts to with both specific adaptations, which reflect the type of stress that had been imposed to create them, and general adaptations, which come from pretty much any physical activity, to varying degrees.[2] Jones believed the goal of resistance training—or running, or any deliberate exercise for that matter—is the specific adaptations. The general adaptations that also occurred were a welcome bonus. Jones felt that when it came to resistance training, it didn't take much of the correct type of workout to stimulate the specific adaptations that would lead to, say, getting stronger or increasing the size of a muscle. And those two ideas formed the basis of his program.

I didn't know if Jones was wrong or right—after all, I had minimal experience with resistance training at that point. I also didn't have anyone to ask. Besides bodybuilders and football players—of which I was neither—not many people practiced resistance training back then, and most who did either looked big and puffy or veiny and really unnatural, neither of which was my goal. I wanted to get stronger and, at 6′1″ and about 150 pounds, I would not have minded having a bit more muscle too. The photos in Jones's books featured men and women who looked strong as well as lean. Some were younger, some were older. All that was a stark and welcome contrast to the extreme physiques highlighted in other weight training books and magazines.

And there was more: Jones emphasized that a good exercise program is one that doesn't take so much time that it disrupts one's school, work, and relationships. I liked the sound of that too. Hungry to learn more, I tracked down the phone number for one of Jones's protégés, Mike Mentzer, a legendary bodybuilder turned trainer from the late 1970s and early 1980s.[3] I called and left a message, and Mike called me back. I was sixteen at the time, and my mother was understandably worried. She wondered: Who was this grown man calling her teenage son at home? Apparently, Mike appreciated that when I called him, I rattled off a quick list of questions onto his answering machine that made it clear I had read Jones's books. We ended up speaking for several hours over the course of a few months about weight training, fitness more generally, and science—both actual science and scientists. It wasn't as if he gently took me under his wing though. Mike was super intense. He would sort of bark at me when he spoke, but there was always a hint of kindness in his delivery. And he did charge me $150 for the calls, which was most of my savings at the time but it was well worth it.

I'm telling you this story because what I learned from those calls with Mike has stayed with me and I credit much of my regular progress with resistance training over the last thirty years to him. Here are ten counsels Mike gave me that I never forgot and always strive to implement with respect to resistance training.

1 After warming up, do not train for much more than sixty to seventy-five minutes at a time . . . you'll progress much faster that way. Occasionally your training may go longer if you are waiting for equipment at a gym, but that's just about the only reason to extend a session much beyond seventy-five minutes.

2 Always strive to use good form, meaning use a full range of motion for every repetition of every set, and control the weight from start to finish.

3 Learn to use resistance as a tool to stress the muscles you're trying to train. Focus as you do the lift to feel the muscles you're trying to train working.

   Mike added: If you can't feel the muscle you're trying to target you'll want to use "pre-exhaustion" techniques when you train. I explain what pre-exhaustion is later, but as the name suggests, it involves doing an isolation exercise (where only one joint moves) immediately before you do a compound exercise (where multiple joints move) for the same muscle. Mike knew most people hate doing pre-exhaustion exercises because they require using less weight on the compound movement. But for getting results with otherwise hard-to-feel and slow-to-progress muscles, he was spot on.

4 If you're new to resistance training, you'll benefit greatly by taking one to three weeks to find the right movements that collectively allow you to target all the major muscles of your body and that work best for your body mechanics. Learn to execute those movements correctly using relatively light (for you) weights, meaning an amount of resistance where you can do ten to twelve repetitions, even though you could easily do five more.

This one-to-three-week "break-in" period is about learning how to train before you start the real work. If you've been regularly training with weights for a while, I suggest you take a full week off. Stay out of the gym completely for seven, or even up to ten, days. You may feel like you're standing still during this period but it's critical to your long-term progress, and you'll thank me later.

Once you start your real workouts, it doesn't take many sets per muscle group to get the results you want, IF you do them with proper form . . . and intensity.

5 Intensity is defined as working with a weight that is heavy enough (for you) that it limits you to completing six to twelve repetitions maximum in good form. There are times to deliberately use heavier weights that limit you to three to five repetitions maximum, or lighter weights that permit you to do thirteen to twenty repetitions maximum. When and where to do that comes later.

If you're not familiar with any of these terms, don't worry. I'll get into all this as the chapter unfolds. But what struck me looking back on these notes as I wrote this chapter is how many sets and exercises to do, and how often to train, was debated like crazy back then and it still is now. Mike was a bit extreme; he favored doing very few actual work sets of an exercise—meaning effortful sets, not warm-ups. In fact, he suggested doing even just one work set per exercise, and one to two exercises per muscle group. I will address the science-supported and practical reasons for doing a bit more than that later. But for now, let's take in Mike's points about a relatively low number of work sets, or what is referred to as a volume of sets. Because one thing most everyone agrees on now that Mike extolled is this: If done properly, you don't need a high volume of sets per exercise or muscle group, and that more is often counterproductive.

And so we continue, with more from Mike.

6 Train three times per week but know that your body gets stronger on the rest days in between training sessions, and mostly while you sleep.

Hard training taxes your whole nervous system, too, not just the muscles and tendons and ligaments you trained, so to make the best progress, every twelve to sixteen weeks, or even every ten to twelve weeks, take one complete week off from resistance training to allow your muscles and nervous system to recover. You'll likely make much more progress in the long run.

7 Your body adapts to training. Making progress requires continually stressing your muscles by increasing the amount of weight you use for exercise over time. You can also do more repetitions with the same amount of weight, but once you can do ten to twelve repetitions with a given weight on a given exercise, using proper form, you need to increase the amount of weight in order to continue to make progress. That is because to grow in strength and size, a muscle must be stressed to its limit. This is known as progressive overload. To ensure you're doing this, take notes on the number of sets and repetitions you're doing for each workout, along with the weights you're using. This is the best way to make sure you're progressively overloading your muscles from one workout to the next.

8 Take each work set to failure, the point where you can't move the weight anymore in good form despite your absolute greatest effort. And sometimes you have to push past failure by getting assistance from a training partner who nudges the weight just a bit, or by immediately reducing the weight and doing two to three more repetitions until you hit failure again.

9 Learn to enjoy training hard. Don't socialize in the gym. Warm up, train, and get out!

And undoubtedly the best and most classic Mentzer-ism of all:

10 "DO NOT LISTEN TO WHAT ANYONE ELSE TELLS YOU AS MOST PEOPLE WHO LIFT WEIGHTS ARE MORONS AND MOST OF WHAT THEY DO AND SAY IS TOTAL BS!"

(Mike literally yelled number 10 into the phone so loud that I winced and had to move the receiver away from my ear. Later I understood what words of wisdom and care those were. To be fair, there are many folks in the fitness education and training community who offer great advice, but Mike wasn't terribly off with this one.)

However coarse the delivery, those ten points were (and remain) gems that we can all benefit from. Again, as I said, I got lucky. We now have tons of peer-reviewed science to support the general logic of Mike's advice, although at the time, much of it ran countercurrent to the dominant views about resistance training, most notably the popular idea at the time that "more volume is better." As it turns out, quality reps and sets are what count, and it does not take much high-quality resistance training to trigger the specific adaptations Jones outlined in his book. (Note: *Quality* has many meanings, which we will cover repeatedly below.)

Of course, those ten points do not exhaustively cover all one needs to know about resistance training, and considering the results of studies that have been done since, there are some important caveats that I'll address. What I can say, however, is that I took Mike's general advice to heart.

After our first call, I took a full week off from any resistance training and then, even though I had been lifting for about six months, I devoted a few weeks to finding the free-weight, weight-machine, and body-weight-only exercises that worked best for me—meaning the ones I could do for full range of motion, pain free, and that allowed me to stress each of the major muscle groups. I found the right combination of compound (multi-joint) exercises and isolation (single-joint) exercises for each muscle group, like the shoulders, biceps, quadriceps, et cetera.

Then I started doing resistance training three times per week, training different muscles on each of those three days: calves and legs one day, then a day or two off, then chest, back, and abdominals (and neck), then a day off, then shoulders and arms, another day off, and then back to calves and legs day. So again, three days total in the gym per week. I've done that body part–split pretty much consistently for thirty-five years now. Even if I am traveling, I find a gym to do these workouts. And if I go to a location where I can't find a gym, I'll do body-weight-only exercises, or I take the week off and stay active in other ways. While general activity is no substitute for resistance training, I have found that a week off approximately every four months can be beneficial. I can arrange it to happen during a vacation or other travel, or if I get sick—fortunately a rarity for me—I don't train. I rest up and stay out of the gym (and thus avoid getting others sick too!) and that becomes the week off. Approaching resistance training this way has allowed me to make consistent progress with about three hours per week of resistance training while still fully enjoying other aspects of life and avoiding injuries.

Before going any further I want to acknowledge something that Mike got somewhat wrong and that is important to highlight here. There is not *one* best way to resistance train! You won't find too many effective programs that recommend fewer than three days of resistance training per week, but there are some good ones that involve more days. Some programs, like the one described in this book, are based on a body part split in which you train different body parts on different days. And even those splits can vary. For instance some people like to train all their pushing muscles of the upper body (chest, shoulders, triceps) on one day, and pulling muscles (back and biceps) on another day, and then legs a different day. Other programs have you train your whole body in every workout; others still alternate between upper and lower body workouts. All these can work. Below I explain the rationale for the split I use and suggest—because it offers some not-so-obvious benefits. The point stands, nonetheless, that there are a lot of ways to resistance train.

Yet there is a core set of principles upon which all people—women, men, inexperienced, experienced, young, old—must rely on to build an effective program. I define an "effective program" as one that people are likely to stick to over many years, and that works well for those also doing cardiovascular exercise, which we know is also vital to our health and provides distinct benefits from resistance training. Many people want to grow certain muscles and leave others as they are. Others want to grow all their muscles. An effective program should offer all those options too.

It also means a program that does not sap your energy but instead gives you more energy. After all, what good is a program that leaves you tired and hungry to an extent that inhibits your work and relationships? While it is normal (and reflective of an effective workout) to be tired after a training session, that fatigue should be somewhat transient, even that day. Your workout shouldn't leave you dragging. During your work sets, you work *hard*—both mentally and physically—and you'll sweat and perhaps get a bit sore, but those are not the goal. Those are the by-products of quality workouts. You also want to still be able to think and walk (!) in the hours and days that follow.

I've come up with a template to help everyone. It's part of why I call it a foundational fitness program—so named because it's grounded in research, the ideas above and that follow below, and the core physiological principles that undergird all effective programs. These principles will never change because they reflect the mechanisms by which muscles, bones, and connective tissues get stronger and, if desired, grow larger. If you make sure that your resistance training follows this template, you can still tailor it to your goals, body type, schedule, and the phase of life you are in. That's what I mean by a foundational fitness program.

You might be thinking, "What about cardiovascular training?" There too I got really lucky. By the time I was seventeen, I was doing resistance training three times per week per Mike's instructions. I got great results in terms of strength and muscle size increases. And I enjoyed it. But I quickly found that

I missed outdoor activities. Mike subscribed to the common idea back then that you couldn't make meaningful progress with resistance training while also doing endurance-type activities, like running or biking. The reverse was also thought to be true. Nonetheless, I disobeyed Mike and what all other training books at the time said and I started running on the days that I didn't resistance train. I had an excellent reason to. My girlfriend lived about fifteen minutes away by car, I didn't have my own car yet, there was no bus to her house, and Uber didn't exist back then. So, much of the time I would just run to her house, which took me about forty-five to sixty minutes, thanks to all the hills. Sometimes I would bike there instead, which took about thirty minutes. Once again, I had no idea what I was doing. I would just set out and go. Ah, the joys of being young and naïve. And in love.

Here's where I got lucky: I was surprised at what happened. Instead of getting weaker, which is what everyone said would happen, I got stronger. And instead of resistance training making me slower at running and biking, which is what our school's cross-country coach told me would happen, I found I could run and bike faster and farther, and without any pain.

I also noticed that I always felt better mentally when I did a mix of cardiovascular and resistance training across the week, as opposed to just one or the other. I thought perhaps it was the fresh air . . . but I noticed this even if it was raining and I was forced to run on a treadmill.

I should mention that this was the early 1990s, and the ideologies within different sports and sectors of the fitness world were still very siloed. Today, we believe that being stronger helps in pretty much every sport and physical activity. Back then people also thought that if you did resistance training and then stopped, your muscles would turn to fat. Today we know that is false—in fact, it's impossible. Nowadays, most every serious athlete resistance trains during both the main and the offseason. And we now know that even if you don't play a sport, if your goal is to be healthy and fit, and to stay uninjured, and live as long as possible, and to do so with vigor, you're best off doing a combination of both resistance training and cardiovascular training. This is true for women and for men. We also know that what defines an effective resistance training program is the same for women and men, such as the need for intensity—training to failure on work sets (or close to failure)—as well as proper form, allowing sufficient rest between workouts for specific adaptations to occur, and more. As Lauren Colenso-Semple, a PhD in integrative physiology and a strength and conditioning coach, and one of the world's leading experts in strength and hypertrophy training, stated so clearly (and adamantly) when she was a guest on my podcast, all the data point to the fact that when it comes to resistance training to improve strength and/or muscle size, the same principles and techniques apply to women and to men—including the need to train to failure or very close to it.[4] Looking back, for me it was thanks to those repeated foot injuries from skateboarding, the generosity of a physical education teacher, a few good books, some formative calls with one of the world's experts in resistance training, and being a naïve, lovestruck teenager that I learned early on how to get in and stay in great all-around shape. Lucky indeed.

And I promise you: If you follow the template here and add in cardiovascular training, too, you can get into and stay in great all-around shape at any age. Yes, nutrition matters but making exercise part of your life will absolutely make you a much healthier person, mentally and physically.

In this chapter I teach you how to do that. And if you already have a fitness program, I'm confident you'll still glean a ton of new knowledge that you can use from these pages.

Most people exercise because they want to feel and look good in their body. They also want longevity—not just to live as long as possible, but to be capable of doing any number of practical things without pain and, ideally, with relative ease. For example, having enough endurance for a long hike with a backpack. Being strong enough to lift boxes of books or help move furniture. Fast enough to sprint for (and catch) a plane or train without tearing a muscle. Able to open a jar when asked. The protocols here will enable you to do all that. They will also help you achieve the body composition (i.e., lean tissue-to-fat ratio) you want, while still allowing you to eat well, and feel more vital. Exercise is extremely potent medicine and, as with sleep, it's one of the best investments you can make toward your mental and physical health. The benefits start from the minute you begin each workout.

If all this gives the impression I love exercise . . . I do, on some days. Training is definitely a pleasure for me, especially if I've slept well, I'm hydrated, I'm caffeinated, and if there's no big stressor weighing on me. That's a lot of ifs, so it won't surprise you that those conditions are often hard to achieve because, well, life happens. I too sometimes get less-than-optimal sleep. I too have a full schedule. I too experience stress. I've had lapses due to the occasional cold. It happens to all of us.

That said, really understanding how exercise works and how much good can come from a few hours a week of focused training can keep us on the journey to get and stay fit when we are not feeling motivated. I look forward to workouts because I know that the way I'm training works. That is priceless. Especially for people who don't like exercise, but like the feeling of having done it, knowing your time was well spent—that it *will* get you results—is a game changer. In fact, a really good program of the sort I describe here can allow you to make progress most every single week.

I mentioned earlier in this introduction that I empathize with people who experience immense confusion when they try to figure out how best to exercise, because I felt that too. So perhaps you're wondering: Why not just discuss "the best way to exercise" here? Maybe you're sensing a pattern: Just like there's no "best" way to resistance train, there's no best way to exercise. We know that resistance training is key. So is doing cardiovascular training. And we need mobility and some degree of flexibility too. There are literally thousands of different programs for each of these. But, if you understand the *principles* by which different types of exercise benefit us in different ways, you can come up with the truly best exercise program for you. As Andy Galpin, PhD, an expert in exercise physiology, shared with me on my podcast, "The methods are many, the principles are few."[5] Meaning there are many different ways to go about generating specific adaptations like strength and muscle size increases, or improved heart stroke volume, which is the amount of blood your heart pumps. That's the power of understanding how the brain and body work, and that's why I explain the mechanisms behind each protocol.

I should say, too, that these principles are broad—I don't talk about specific demographics here. These are written to help the widest possible audience of women and men of any age. Know that I don't lump those two groups together casually. As mentioned above, the science shows that the principles of an effective exercise program are the same for men and for women. Of course, if ever the science points to key differences, I highlight them. But again, if you understand the mechanisms behind a protocol, you can personalize it for your specific needs. Likewise, if you are training for performance in a sport, you might adjust these, again, as you see fit.

What is exercise?

Peering into the history of exercise turns out to be both interesting and informative. And helpful, when it comes to our health goals.[6] An Indian physician named Susruta, who lived around 600 BCE, was one of the first known practitioners to prescribe exercise. "It should be taken every day," he wrote. "Diseases fly from the presence of a person habituated to regular physical exercise." Susruta's words are as relevant today as they were during his lifetime.

The problem is how to implement the prescription. Many people don't do it, or they do it wrong and end up discouraged, injured, or both. So many times I hear people say, "I used to work out every day," or "I used to be so fit," or "I don't have the time or energy to exercise anymore." What is rarely discussed is that exercise, done correctly, gives you energy. It extends your life (i.e., gives you more time). It also increases your level of focus for many hours afterward, which also saves you time. And there's more. Research shows that regular exercise can be as or even more effective for improving mood and lowering anxiety than prescription antidepressants or talk therapy.[7] On, and on, and on. Exercise is not a cure-all, but it is often a way to address many of the physical and mental health issues people struggle with. It's just that, as a species, we have not quite come to understand how potent a medicine exercise really is.

Then there are those who exercise consistently but overdo one type or just focus on their favorite sport, like running or tennis, Pilates or spin class, and miss out on the very real health benefits that come from variety.

In my experience, very few people know how to get in great all-around shape properly. Even fewer stay there. The good news is that doing so is pretty simple, again, once you know how.

It comes in three basic varieties: resistance training, cardiovascular exercise, and mobility and/or flexibility. Resistance exercise is where you use some weight—your body weight, weight machines, or free weights—to challenge your neuromuscular system and connective tissues. Resistance training also strengthens your bones. The hallmark of classic cardiovascular exercise is an increased heart rate for at least twelve minutes and up to seventy-five minutes—or in some cases even longer. There are arguments to be made that one can get effective cardiovascular workouts in shorter bouts of activity, through what's often called high-intensity interval training (HIIT). But we will return to that nuance later. Finally, mobility and flexibility challenges our ability to stably shift between different bodily positions, and to have access to a full range of functional motion if we need it for athletics or simply in everyday life. If you're now thinking "So I have to do three types of exercise? I barely have time for one!" don't despair. Although it can be great to have mobility and flexibility practice, as I describe later in this chapter, you can see meaningful benefits from protocols that take very little time to complete, in one case just five minutes. And the resistance and cardiovascular sessions I describe below are aimed to give you the maximum benefits for time spent.

What is the goal of exercise?

Believe it or not, the most important thing to understand about exercise is why you're doing it. I don't mean your psychology here. I am referring to what you are trying to achieve with each workout; why you are doing specifically what you are doing. It ensures every workout leads you to achieve your goals. For all that has been written and said about exercise, it often misses this crucial point. All effective forms of exercise share a common purpose: to trigger a set of specific and general adaptations in your body and brain.

Exercise is the stimulus, and the general and specific adaptations are your body's response to the stimulus. Exercise can also drive aesthetic changes, like fat loss, or improve sports performance, but those are secondary. "Wait!" I hear you saying, "I exercise to stay fit. Just tell me how to do that." I will, but I promise you will accomplish your goals much faster, and you will make consistent progress, if you understand exercise in this stimulus-adaptation context.

Here's an example of how specific adaptations work. Let's say you run or cycle at a moderate pace for thirty minutes. I'm talking about a pace where you can barely hold a conversation without gasping for air. While you do this your heart rate and blood pressure will rise substantially, you'll breathe more rapidly, you'll sweat, your muscles probably will burn a bit, and your immune system will release a bunch of pro-inflammatory molecules such as interleukin-6 into your blood.[8] Sounds terrible, right? Wrong. This constellation of responses—what we call the exercise-induced stress response—will lead to a set of adaptations that directly reflect the stress you just experienced but in the opposite direction. Thousands of coordinated, metabolic, molecular and even genetic changes occur when we exercise—a "molecular choreography," as one group of researchers has put it.[9]

After doing this for some time, your resting heart rate, blood pressure, and circulating levels of inflammatory molecules will be lower than they were before you set out on that run.

When most people think about what they accomplished by exercising, they tend to think about the calories burned or the mood enhancement it provides in the hours that follow. That's all well and good, but the real magic of exercise resides in the specific and general adaptations it produces. Those are the real "gains" of exercise. They last for days and they compound over time. They literally change your body and brain, and do so in ways that reflect the stress you experienced during the workout. That makes you a physiologically different person—capable of more in every area of life related to the exercise-induced adaptations—stronger, and faster, with more vigor and endurance, and more capable all around. Once you understand and experience the stimulus-adaptation process, you come to understand what effective effort is and when to rest to glean the adaptations you worked to trigger. It can make you wiser too. In fact, as we will cover later in chapter 6—neuroplasticity, or your ability to learn and rewire your brain—follows the same general contour of "failures" (from genuine efforts to do something!) prompted by specific adaptations that will help you overcome those "failures" in the near future.

The effects of quality exercise on your ability to learn extend way beyond just metaphor. Exercise can directly facilitate neuroplasticity by allowing it to occur.[10] Like heat makes metal pliable, so too exercise brings the brain into a state where new neural connections in the brain and body can be forged.[11] Take for instance a 2011 study by a group of psychologists at the University of Pittsburgh. They randomized 120 older adults (average age sixty-seven) into two groups: one to cardiovascular exercise, the other to stretching only. The cardiovascular exercise group walked for increasing durations of time, reaching a maximum of forty minutes per session by week seven. By that point, the walking was brisk enough to get the participants' heart rates up to 50 to 60 percent of their maximum. And they did three sessions per week. The participants continued with that regimen for a year. According to the results, the hippocampus—a brain region associated with learning and memory—increased in volume by about 2 percent among the cardiovascular group, whereas it shrank by about 1.4 percent among the stretching-only group. While that might not seem like a lot, these findings are noteworthy because a shrinking hippocampus is linked to memory impairments during the later decades of life. A rather simple low-intensity exercise intervention seems to not only prevent brain deterioration but also trigger brain growth. Other studies, including those exploring higher-intensity exercise and resistance training show similar—and in some cases greater—neuroplasticity brought about by exercise.[12]

It perhaps shouldn't surprise us that exercise can open the gates for learning in the brain. A disproportionate amount of our brain's volume is devoted to generating our movements. Rodolfo Llinás, MD, PhD, a neuroscientist at NYU School of Medicine, cites an odd but telling example of the sea squirt, a spineless marine creature.[13] Young sea squirts swim freely until they are fully grown. The adults then stick themselves onto a rock and become filter feeders, catching whatever happens to float by. When this transition from swimming to sedentary occurs, sea squirts eat their own brains, leaving only what is necessary for their new passive style of feeding. Llinás's story about a distantly related animal is relevant to us for two reasons. First, it provides a warning to humans with an overly sedentary lifestyle. As humans age and become less mobile, their brains degenerate too, albeit not as dramatically as does the sea squirt brain.[14] Second, people who continue to exercise—in particular those who do exercise that is challenging (but safe) for them, offset much of typical age-related brain loss that is otherwise observed. This has real implications, allowing them to maintain youthful cognitive function well into their later years, possibly through neurogenesis, the addition of new brain neurons.[15] Deliberate, repetitive, effortful movements that elicit the short-term stress responses (discussed throughout this chapter) trigger a battery of chemical and neural feedback signals to the brain, which both supports the existing brain cells and the connections we would otherwise lose over time, as well as releases signals that cause neurons to grow new connections. This makes sense if you think about the sea squirt anecdote once more. Our brain is the most metabolically demanding organ in our body. Much of that organ is devoted to our ability to generate movement.[16] If we don't move, much of our brain is less active too. Am I telling you that we must exercise just to maintain the brain capacity we have? Indeed I am. Exercise—provided it is of sufficient intensity—makes us cognitively resilient.

The benefits of exercise to brain health and neuroplasticity turn out to be robust at every age, for women, for men, for people vulnerable to age-related cognitive decline, and for both neurologically healthy and unhealthy people alike. Resistance training and cardiovascular training both impart huge benefits, but their combination (typically in separate workouts) turns out to be the most effective stimulus for brain health and neuroplasticity.[17] And when mobility and flexibility, and walking, are added in, the positive results increase significantly.

Some of the effects of exercise on brain health and neuroplasticity are the result of something called brain-derived neurotrophic factor, or BDNF, a protein our brain makes that can exert a powerful role on learning and memory by virtue of its ability to sculpt and reinforce new neural circuit connections.[18] Numerous studies have found that exercise leads to elevated levels of BDNF in the brain.[19] These elevations are temporary,[20] but enough to open the window for neuroplasticity for several hours after the exercise has ceased. Exercise also increases the release of catecholamines:[21] that dopamine, epinephrine, norepinephrine trio that we discussed in the chapter on sleep and that we will revisit throughout this book. When that trio is deployed in the body and brain, our levels of alertness and focus are increased, allowing us to access the memories, skills, and cognitive abilities we harbor in our neural circuits. As neuromodulators, the catecholamines also can open the opportunity for neuroplasticity. (I explain this process in more detail in chapter 6.)

The way to think about the effects of exercise on brain health and neuroplasticity, therefore, is that moderate-to-intense exercise reinforces and maintains the brain functions we already have and lets us access the best of our attentional systems for focus and memory. It also opens the window for you to learn at an accelerated rate after the exercise session. Exercise alone won't make you smarter, but it opens the door for you to become smarter, should you decide to put in the effort to do so. (Chapter 6 explains the best and fastest way to do that.)

It's important to remember that any learning facilitated by elevated levels of BDNF is not confined to the neural circuits involved in the exercise that triggered it. Rather, BDNF will facilitate whatever learning we pursue while its levels are elevated. As one of many examples, just six minutes of intense running improved the ability of twenty-seven healthy adults to learn new words.[22] The improvements in learning and retention were tied to elevated levels of BDNF, along with elevated catecholamines: dopamine and epinephrine. Moderate-to-high-intensity exercise is arguably the best type of workout to trigger this process. People will debate whether resistance training is as effective at increasing neuroplasticity as cardiovascular training is. The key variable seems to be the intensity of training; it has to be sufficiently high. When done correctly, resistance training can be at least as taxing as intense cardiovascular training when viewed through the lens of neurological demand, and perhaps more.[23]

Another way that exercise supports our brain and body is that it markedly improves sleep quality and duration.[24] Remember from chapter 1: Morning workouts appear to shorten the amount of time it takes to fall asleep at night, and regular exercise has been found to improve the overall quality of sleep for adults. In a study including forty-eight adults with insomnia, moderate aerobic exercise improved sleep, and helped the participants feel less stressed.[25]

One caveat. If exercise is very intense and done too close to your desired bedtime, it can be detrimental to sleep. (We cover this more in chapter 1 and chapter

3.) It's best to either avoid intense exercise in the hours prior to sleep, or if you can't, to make sure you engage in some deliberate downregulation practices, such as a few minutes of long-exhale breathing or a hot shower, so that it does not negatively impact your sleep.

There are many reasons why appropriately timed exercise improves sleep. As discussed in chapter 1, the chemical adenosine, which not only builds up in the brain and body throughout the day but is also further increased with exercise, creates an increasing pressure to sleep.[26] So exercise helps promote great sleep and reduces factors that lead to poor sleep. Regular physical activity also appears to increase the amount of time we spend in restorative slow-wave deep sleep, regardless of what time of day we exercise, and that translates to us feeling more rested when we wake.[27]

Then there is the benefit of moderate to intense exercise on our subjective waking experience, specifically on our feelings of well-being. Although "well-being" might sound nonscientific, for a lot of people it's an important barometer they use to gauge their quality of life. People who don't like exercise often look at me askance when I say that exercise improves mood, and not just because it helps us sleep better. But it's true: Exercise makes us happy.[28] And relaxed.[29] A moderate to intense workout is a proven, excellent way to snap ourselves out of a slump.[30] Exercise reduces our baseline levels of stress,[31] increases our capacity to show resilience in a wide range of circumstances,[32] and reduces anger.[33] These mood enhancements of exercise come from several different chemicals: dopamine, which increases motivation, focus, energy, and cognitive function;[34] and serotonin, which does many things, including help make us more resistant to challenges.

And here's a fun fact: The lactate your body produces during high-intensity exercise can physically modify—or lactylate—proteins in the brain, altering how neurons communicate. A recent study found that lactate production spurred by exercise reduced anxiety-related behaviors in mice, apparently by supporting the molecular machinery present at synapses between neurons in the prefrontal cortex.[35] The prefrontal cortex has many parts and functions, but will come up repeatedly in this book in the context of reducing impulsivity, decreasing anxiety, and learning new information and skills.[36]

There's more. Exercise has a surprising effect on our energy levels. The relationship between exercise and energy is key to understand, especially for those who feel they don't have the energy to exercise. After all, exercise requires energy, right? Right. For those who don't enjoy it or who have a ton of demands on their schedule and may not be sleeping well or enough, that's especially true. Add in a bit of low-level or major depression, anxiety about finances or the state of the world, or challenges with relationships in your life and, voila: You have a person who quite understandably does not want to exercise, and very likely won't exercise, no matter how many studies about its benefits or inspirational tales they see and hear. If this is you or someone you know, I hope what I'm about to share will help.

Yes, exercise requires energy to initiate and to complete, but it also gives us energy. I'm not just referring to energy in the psychological sense. I mean it gives us *actual chemical energy* and it does so by changing the electrical state of your nervous system. Work from neuroscientist Peter Strick's laboratory, at the University of Pittsburgh, identified three sets of brain areas that, when activated, communicate with our adrenal glands to cause them to release adrenaline.[37] In turn, this adrenaline activates receptors on our vagus nerve, which is a dense neural pathway that bidirectionally connects our body and brain. Our vagus nerve then triggers the release of norepinephrine from the locus coeruleus, which in turn can increase release of dopamine, acetylcholine, and other neuromodulators in other brain centers.[38] Other research found that exercise enhances a group of neurons in the hypothalamus—known as VMH SF1 neurons—whose activity is required in order for endurance-specific adaptations to occur.[39] Meaning, the brain is what actually coordinates the specific bodily adaptations that effective exercise triggers. Put differently, your body changes because your brain tells it to.

While the abilities of our brain to energize and change our body are incredible, the key practical questions are: "What are the magical brain areas that, when made active, flick the first domino in this brain–adrenals–vagus–locus coeruleus/basal ganglia circuit? And how do we activate those brain areas?" The answer, Strick found, is a set of brain regions that control voluntary movement of the major muscles of the limbs—and the core muscles; yes, your abdominals, or abs, but also the sheets of muscles below and all around them, such as the rectus abdominis and obliques. Translation: Deliberate movement of your limbs and your core muscles creates chemical energy that activates your brain to *want* to further move your body, and gives you heightened levels of motivation to continue doing so.

We can use that exercise-induced energy not just to exercise more or harder. It can be directed toward cognitive activities in the hours after you exercise or simply to go about the tasks of your day with more motivation and focus. Provided we don't exercise to the point of exhaustion, exercise markedly improves our brain function, psychological state, and overall energy levels. Yes, it involves hormones. Yes, it involves endorphins (everyone seems to know this based on the notion of a "runner's high"). But it also involves a shift in brain state.

And exercise affects more than just our brain. There's perhaps the most familiar benefit: our heart health. In 1986 researchers from Stanford and Harvard reported their findings from sixteen years of tracking physical activity and the causes of death of nearly seventeen thousand people between the ages of thirty-five and seventy-four.[40] They found that the more a person walked, climbed stairs, or played sports, the less likely they were to die of heart disease. And the correlation was linear: The more physically active someone was, the lower the risk. This connection existed regardless of smoking status, weight, or having a parent who'd died young (a potential indicator of an inherited condition). The report, led by noted epidemiologist Ralph Paffenbarger, MD, and published in the *New England Journal of Medicine*, was considered a landmark—proof that exercise improved longevity, largely by preventing cardiovascular illnesses.

Research since confirms this finding. In one study, researchers followed 3,307 people with heart disease from 1985 to 2014.[41] Everyone in the study had been encouraged to exercise and lose weight. After thirty years, the researchers could see that while weight loss alone did not reduce the risk of death, exercise did. Other data confirm exercise's significance, even when people have other risk factors. One group of researchers described this link starkly, back in 1996.[42] "Low fitness is an important precursor of mortality," they wrote. To put that in plain language: People who aren't active are more likely to die young.

One mechanism behind this link is increased insulin sensitivity.[43] Insulin is a hormone made and released from your pancreas that is essential for keeping your blood sugar, or glucose, levels within a particular range. Almost every cell in the body, including our neurons, requires glucose to function. Glucose comes from the food we eat and stored sources of energy, such as glycogen in our muscles and liver and adipose tissue, what is commonly referred to as body fat. Resistance to insulin leads to a buildup of glucose in our blood, which damages the endothelial cells that make up our capillaries, veins, and arteries, and deprives all cells of the glucose they need, impairing their functioning. It thus can cause cardiovascular disease and cerebrovascular diseases such as stroke and dementia. Exercise increases insulin sensitivity and can even improve the expression of genes that regulate insulin and glucose over long time spans which means more stable energy levels and reduced cellular inflammation and other symptoms of metabolic disorders.[44] People with diabetes are more sensitive to insulin after exercising,[45] too, and nondiabetics derive additional benefits from exercise-induced insulin sensitivity. Such benefits can be seen even after just one moderate workout.

What's more, exercise can make your muscles become much better at pulling glucose out of the bloodstream, which ultimately helps your body handle carbohydrates more efficiently.[46]

Finally (although I could go on!), there's this: As you now know from everything you've just read, exercise can make you healthier and happier, and it can allow you to get smarter too. It will also extend your life.

One analysis examined data from thirteen studies that directly compared life expectancy among active and inactive people.[47] Eight of those studies included both men and women, and the results showed an average increase of 3.7 years of life among people who exercised regularly compared to those who did not. While it's great to have a physically active job or lifestyle, the benefits of structured exercise are independent. You need both of these in your life.

And you don't need to have been a longtime fitness devotee either. A Swedish study of 2,205 middle-aged men found that people who started to exercise between the ages of fifty and sixty experienced the same life-extending benefit as men who'd been working out all their lives and continued to do so as they got older.[48] There are also now studies of people who started resistance training in their mid-sixties, seventies, and even eighties, and all made excellent progress in strength and derived many other general health and lifestyle benefits. In fact, the group in their eighties made the same degree of progress in muscle mass and strength compared to people who had been exercising regularly for decades![49]

There is a lot more to say about exercise and longevity, but the effects are multifaceted. Some of them arrive via improved metabolic health and fuel utilization. Some via improved sleep, and improved immune system functioning—again, assuming we don't chronically exhaust ourselves with over-exercising. The point is: Exercise gives us life—literally.

So by now I hope you're on board with the "why." We can move on to the "how."

How should I exercise?

As I've mentioned, there is no one best way to exercise but there is, I believe, a best way to structure an effective exercise program. It starts with setting a foundation that you can build on—not necessarily by adding more sessions but by changing the type and amount of exercise, and the sequence in which you do them each week. Let me show you how.

The data point to everyone—men and women, young and old—needing sessions specifically to maintain or build muscle and strength, as well as sessions to keep or improve cardiovascular fitness. Also, mobility and flexibility aren't just nice to have, they are crucial to ensure we can exercise for the rest of our lives relatively pain free, and just as importantly, to live full lives by virtue of the number and types of activities we can partake in. Sports, recreation, playing with our kids or grandkids, and even household chores require some degree of mobility and flexibility.

The five protocols that follow have everything you need to build an effective exercise program that can be customized for your age, fitness and aesthetic goals, and schedule. It makes the puzzle pieces I've outlined above fit together. They include the foundational fitness program I discussed: three days of resistance training—all relatively brief but intense workouts—and three days of cardio—each of different duration and intensity, and done on non-resistance training days. Plus daily walking that can be worked into your existing daily activities and some mobility and flexibility exercises that are fast, yet also effective. It is designed to be compatible with your life.

Yes, maintaining a consistent routine will require some commitment, even when a workout is the last thing you want to do. But remember: You will never feel worse for having exercised. And completing a workout is much easier than you might think, if you keep in mind that all effective exercise is stress designed to create specific and general adaptations. Collectively, these are certain to make you more fit and healthy and capable than you ever imagined.

EXERCISE PROTOCOL

1

Walk as Much as Possible Each Day

WHAT TO DO:

- **Incorporate walking into your daily life.** Also, in these instances in particular, if you can:
    - Walk for five to ten minutes after meals, when health benefits of this activity are amplified.
    - Walk or pace for at least five minutes for every thirty minutes of sitting or standing.
- **Consider a walk-and-work desk.** If you need to be at a desk for work for long stretches of time, a sit-stand desk may be a good investment. Even better is a walk-and-work desk, with a treadmill that fits below.
- **Seven thousand steps per day is a good goal, and ten thousand is even better.** Accelerometers, step counters, or even your phone can help you keep track, but are not necessary.

HOW IT WORKS:

This isn't that foundational fitness program I discussed; it's something even more essential. While walking isn't the only exercise we need to do, it's listed as the first protocol in this section because it should not be thought of as an add-on. Rather, it is at the bedrock of a healthy lifestyle, just as viewing morning sunlight is the basis of a good sleep routine. Simply walking for at least an hour a day (total, not even all at once) is one of the best things you can do to protect yourself against illness and improve your overall health. The data show us why.

A group of researchers from across the US recruited 2,110 people between the ages of thirty-eight and fifty years to wear an accelerometer, or a step counter, for one year.[50] The researchers then collected health data on these individuals for the next ten years (on average). Their analysis, published in *JAMA Network Open* in 2021, showed that people who took at least seven thousand steps per day during the decade of the study had a significantly lower mortality risk compared to people who took fewer steps.

In 2023, researchers from Kyoto University, in Japan, and UCLA published their study of 3,101 adults who took eight thousand steps three to seven days per week, eight thousand steps one to two days per week, or fewer than eight thousand steps on any one day in their week.[51] Health data were collected over the ten years following study enrollment. Like the earlier report, this one found that taking eight thousand steps or more correlated with a significantly lower risk of death from all causes, including heart disease. The benefit appeared to plateau at three to four days per week of eight thousand steps.

And walking protects against more than heart disease. Researchers from Denmark and Australia investigated the link between walking and dementia risk.[52] They monitored 78,340 adults for an average of seven years and, like the studies above, saw a link between walking and a lower risk for dementia. They noted that the optimal "dose" of walking to reduce the risk of dementia was just shy of 10,000 steps per day. Walking has also been tied to reduced risks of depression,[53] diabetes,[54] cardiovascular disease,[55] and the incidence of some cancers,[56] as well as increased survival after certain cancer diagnoses.

A paper published in *Nature Medicine* in 2022 found that walking 8,200 steps or more per day had a preventive effect against obesity, sleep apnea, gastroesophageal reflux disease, and major depressive disorder.[57] That is a remarkable set of benefits for such a simple, zero-equipment, zero-cost activity.

In other words: We should all be walking. A lot. If not every day, then almost every day.

A primary reason why walking is so beneficial is that it requires repeated muscular contractions. This activates an enzyme called AMPK. A 2018 paper by researchers at the Salk Institute for Biological Studies called AMPK the "guardian of metabolism," and with good reason.[58] This enzyme has multiple roles. It is involved in the process of stimulating glucose uptake into muscle cells. Animal research indicates that AMPK is also involved in generating more mitochondria through its interactions with PGC-1alpha, helps counter inflammation and improves vasodilation to help lower blood pressure and deliver more nutrients to cells, and under some conditions, can remove debris from them.[59] Taking enough steps each day is therefore beneficial for health in numerous ways that extend way beyond just the calories burned by walking.

Data also support the value of interrupting long bouts of sitting with short bouts of walking. A large review from 2022 gathered data from seven studies that examined the health benefits of interrupting long bouts of sitting with either standing or walking.[60] According to the analysis, standing between long stretches of sitting helps gradually lower glucose levels, but walking is far more effective.

Specifically, those researchers wanted to see which change is better at lowering glucose levels after meals. Walking is particularly effective right after a meal because glucose levels tend to increase at this time and preventing that rapid rise can help lower the risk of diabetes and heart disease.[61] (High glucose levels are linked to both.) A review of eight randomized studies examining thirty different interventions in 116 people found that walking within thirty minutes after a meal lowers glucose levels more effectively than walking before a meal or after a break.[62] That's because we use glucose as energy . . . to walk. Moving therefore helps clear glucose out of the bloodstream, which is both protective to our vascular cells—our arteries, veins, and capillaries—and is beneficial for all the cells of our body by making them more effective energy utilizing machines, as described above. There is no need to rest right after eating. Just head straight out for that walk, even for just five minutes, although ten to twenty or even thirty minutes would be better.

We are talking about walking, not a workout. Just low-level, repeated muscle contractions. In fact, these contractions don't even have to be created by walking: A 2022 study from the University of Houston found that repeated contractions of the soleus muscle, the deep muscle of our calf, significantly improve glucose regulation.[63] Remarkably, this was found to be the case even if people remained seated and repeatedly raised their heel off the floor. It seems that even though the soleus is only about 1 percent of our total musculature, it has an outsized (positive) effect in regulating our glucose levels when it is repeatedly contracted by walking or "soleus pushups." Of course, doing repeated soleus contractions while seated throughout the day, while possible, is not terribly compatible with daily life. Most people would not be able to concentrate on that while doing their work. But I include this recent finding here to emphasize just how powerful low-impact-repetitive muscle contractions can be. And of course, people who spend hours in meetings all day may want to consider doing calf raises while they're confined to a desk. It's not a replacement for walking, but it is certainly better than sitting still for long amounts of time.

What about standing still for long stretches of time? The study just described tells us that standing breaks are beneficial. Maybe you have a standing desk at your office, and that can be a great way to stretch your legs throughout the day. But walking is definitely better. A walk-and-work desk—where a treadmill fits underneath—can be a great way for some people to walk more.[64]

Curiosity about the health benefits of walking has generated a tremendous amount of data. As mentioned above, we now have studies showing that walking reduces the risk of heart disease, hypertension, type 2 diabetes, cancer, cognitive impairment, death by pneumonia, poor sleep, mental health issues, stress, hormonal imbalances tied to aging, and more.[65] Glucose regulation is certainly a part of it, but a deep dive into the molecular mechanisms behind all these effects is beyond the scope of this book. For those who are interested, a multidisciplinary team of researchers published a comprehensive review of the cellular mechanisms behind this wide range of effects.

There's one more useful but nonobvious benefit to walking that I'd like to mention here. Walking induces optic flow, the state of having the visual image of the world slide past us. We are usually unaware of what this does to our nervous system. When we ambulate—nerd-speak for "walk"—a stream of visual input flows past us, an effect called global motion.[66] Human and animal studies have found that forward ambulation causes reflexive lateral and repetitive (right-left-right . . .) eye movements that serve to stabilize the visual image on the eyes. Perhaps surprisingly, such eye movements significantly reduce neural activity in the amygdala, a region of our brain involved in threat detection.[67] In fact repetitive lateralized eye movements are the cornerstone of trauma therapies such as EMDR (eye movement desensitization and reprocessing), which pairs left-right-left-right repetitive eye movements with the recounting of challenging experiences to uncouple their memory from the anxiety response.[68] EMDR is done in a therapist's office but was developed by psychologist Francine Shapiro, PhD, after she noticed that recounting traumatic experiences was made less stressful when the recounting took place on a walk.[69] EMDR is still considered somewhat controversial in the therapy community. Some believe EMDR's benefits come from the hypnosis-like state it can cause—and clinical hypnosis has well-established effects on mental health and brain rewiring.[70] Others believe EMDR has its own direct effects on relief from trauma and depression.[71] We need more data to parse all that. For now, however, it is interesting to note that walking makes the amygdala less active, thereby reducing stress and anxiety.[72]

Alas, this benefit of walking won't happen if you're staring at your phone while doing it. That prevents the forward-ambulation-induced eye movements discussed here. The suppression of amygdala activity only occurs if we're looking forward and around. I believe this phenomenon is one reason why spending time simply walking or hiking in nature is so tied to well-being.[73] And also why walking or running on a treadmill—while better than not exercising—is less stress reducing than doing the same activity outdoors. The link between optic flow and stress reduction is an understudied area. However, walking outdoors is a zero-risk, zero-cost intervention that seems to translate to powerful results for your body and mental state.

In My Experience

I have a step tracker on both my phone and my WHOOP band (I'm an advisor for WHOOP). I track my steps every day but I don't look at the data every day. I check it every few days to make sure I'm "hitting my numbers." I know I get about seven thousand to ten thousand steps on average. More importantly, I am always seeking ways to take more steps. I make a point to pace indoors or walk outdoors whenever I take a phone call that doesn't require me to be in front of my computer. I take stairs rather than escalators or elevators whenever I can. I see stairs as an opportunity, not a task, especially on travel days when I am going to be sitting a lot on the plane. I always strive to take two short walks of twenty to thirty minutes each during the day, usually one in the morning and one in the evening. If I miss the first one, I make the evening walk longer. I often take work calls, check in with friends or family, or listen to books or podcasts while I do. Every time we finish recording a podcast with a guest, our whole team takes a walk together (in the direction of the sun of course). If I have to sit a lot on a given day, I make it a point to walk a lot more the next day. I have an indoor treadmill for days when I can't get outside to walk much due to work or weather.

I almost always use my standing desk to work at home. When I travel, I simply put my laptop on a box or stack of books on the desk or coffee table in the hotel room. It's low-tech but it works, and I can rotate it toward the window to get more natural light. You need to find what works for you, of course.

COMMON QUESTIONS

How fast should I walk to get the health benefits of this activity?

Any walking is better than no walking and brisk walking is better than slow walking.[74] Taking all studies discussed above into account, walking briskly for at least thirty minutes per day and ideally forty to sixty minutes should be the goal. Walking at least five days a week and making an effort to take stairs, et cetera, appears to be sufficient activity to meet current recommended guidelines.[75]

Again, walking is not "working out," but it is the basis of any good exercise program. Think of it as necessary for your health. We were made to move. Getting steps each day is essential and should be part of your life. You can weave it into time in the yard, time with friends, time on the phone, and so on. And when you are stuck in a meeting or on a plane and can't walk, try the calf raises discussed above. It's discreet enough that you're unlikely to get any strange looks.

Seven thousand steps are roughly an hour of walking, as I recommend, though obviously this will differ somewhat depending on the length of a person's stride, the terrain, and walking speed. And, again, these steps do not need to be done all at once but rather can be spread throughout the day.

Aim to speed up as you incorporate walking more into your life. If you already walk often, then try to walk a little faster. Faster walking obtains health benefits in less time.

Are other types of low-impact movement, such as tai chi or slow swimming, as beneficial as walking?

Yes and no. All movement is good movement, provided you don't get injured. Doing ten air squats—going from standing to a seated position with your thighs parallel to the ground, then standing up again, and repeating that ten times—every forty-five minutes throughout the day for an 8.5-hour period has been shown to have even better glucose-lowering effects than thirty minutes of walking, which makes it a decent alternative when you can't walk, like on really stormy days or on a long (or even a short) flight.[76] The ten-air-squats-every-forty-five-minutes approach obviously does not provide all the benefits that walking outside does (like optic flow, fresh air, sunlight, etc.).

There are other types of low-impact, continuous physical activity to explore. Tai chi is great for balance and is often done near sunrise and outdoors, adding to the benefit for reasons discussed in both chapter 1 and chapter 5, and it's typically done in groups, which has a positive social component. And tai chi certainly improves lower leg strength, balance, and coordination.[77] That's just one idea, but of course there are many others.

Everyone needs to find a low-impact, continuous physical activity that works for them in terms of enjoyment, and compatibility with lifestyle.

That being said, I'll come back to walking. Walking is a movement that draws on many different aspects of our anatomy: It puts weight on our skeletal structure, which is good for helping maintain our bone density and strength; it engages the soleus, which as mentioned before has a positive effect on glucose regulation; and it has the added bonus of optic flow for mental health. Add walking into your life wherever and whenever possible. Again, don't think of it as *exercise*, think of it as nonnegotiable movement that is foundational to a healthy day. Does that mean walking is the only thing we need to do? Of course not. In the context of physical activity, and to use scientific jargon, it is "necessary but not sufficient" for your health. So let's now discuss the things to do in addition to walking, starting with three times per week resistance training. Done properly.

EXERCISE PROTOCOL

2

Resistance Train Three Times per Week

WHAT TO DO:

- **Adhere to a program, starting with this foundational template that features three resistance training sessions every seven days.**

Day 1: Cardiovascular training (explained in Exercise Protocol 3)
Day 2: Resistance training of major lower body muscles: quadriceps, hamstrings, calves

Your glutes, core, and lower back are indirectly trained this day given the nature of the exercises involved, but direct glute training can be added.

Day 3: Rest day
Day 4: Resistance training of major torso muscles: chest, back, abdominals, and core (optional neck)
Day 5: Cardiovascular training (explained in Exercise Protocol 3)
Day 6: Cardiovascular training (explained in Exercise Protocol 3)
Day 7: Resistance training of shoulders, biceps, triceps, abdominals/ core (optional forearms and neck)

HOW IT WORKS:

This template is, in my experience, the best place to start and in many cases stay to achieve all-around fitness: strength, endurance, speed, and power. And it can be tailored to deliver the aesthetic changes you want.

It is grounded in the fundamental principles of effective resistance training,[78] and I strongly believe it offers the best time-and-effort to results ratio. It can also be easily modified when your schedule gets busy or you need a week off. I have seen it work for everyone I've suggested it to.

This program consists of three sessions of resistance training every seven days. It also includes three cardiovascular training sessions, done on non-resistance training days. (These are detailed in the next protocol. I include them in the template overview for clarity.) Together, these sessions provide the right amount of directed stress and recovery.

If you are already familiar with resistance training, you may think you need more sets to gain muscle or more training days for certain target areas than what this protocol suggests. Keep in mind that *each session works in the larger context of the program*. They synergize. For example, you'll train your legs but four days later, you'll sprint or row or cycle at an intensity that also taxes your legs (just enough, not too much). You won't lose ground.

For those new to resistance training, I highly suggest you do the "break-in" period, like the one detailed in Mike Mentzer's point number four in the introduction to this chapter. This will help you develop proper form with the exercises you select. For those experienced with resistance training, or novices who have completed the "break-in" period, you should design the specifics of each resistance training session with these variables as guidelines:

WORKOUT DURATION: ABOUT 60 +/– 20 MINUTES

- Brief whole-body warm-up: About 5 minutes
- Total number of warm-up sets: 1–3 per exercise
- Total number of work sets per muscle group: 4–9
- Total number of exercises per muscle group: 2–3
- For each major muscle group: Do at least one exercise that is a compound (multi-joint) exercise and one that is an isolation (one-joint) exercise. A third compound movement can be added, if needed.

- Total number of work sets per exercise: 2–3 sets (usually just 2)
- Repetition ("reps") range per set: As a general guideline, aim to use enough resistance so you reach "failure" after doing 6–10 reps of a given compound exercise, or in the case of an isolation exercise, after 8–15 reps. But if you can only get 5 reps, do that. Or if you can continue past 10 or 15 reps (reps in good form, that is!), keep going until you reach failure. Don't stop simply because you've reached a given number of reps. Remember, too, that you must use progressive overload to get results. Once you can perform 10 reps of a compound exercise, or 10–15 of an isolation exercise, in perfect form, you'll want to increase the amount of weight for work sets of that exercise in the next workout, which will very likely reduce the number of reps you can do until you progress further, and so on. This is absolutely key!

Note: *The rep ranges discussed here and throughout this protocol are just guidelines; venturing into heavier 3–5 reps or lighter 15–25 repetition ranges makes good sense for some exercises. So does systematically varying between very specific rep ranges for four to eight weeks at a time.*

- Rest duration between warm-up sets: 1–2 minutes
- Rest duration between work sets: 2–5 minutes, depending on repetition range. Typically people rest longer (3–5 minutes) between work sets of compound exercises than between work sets of isolation exercises (90 seconds–3 minutes), and I suggest you do the same.

On reading the above list I imagine novices might already be confused and experienced resistance trainers already might be furrowing their brows, but let's consider each of these points so the rationale is clear.

WORKOUT DURATION: ABOUT 60 +/– 20 MINUTES

You're in the gym to resistance train, and you're resistance training to trigger specific neural, muscular, and connective tissue adaptations. For most people the specific adaptations they seek are increased strength and perhaps also hypertrophy, or increased muscle size. Many want to also lose body fat.

It may surprise you to learn that body fat loss isn't a specific adaptation from doing a certain type of training. Why not? Because body fat loss is mostly the consequence of being in a caloric deficit. In chapter 4, I explain how certain foods and food combinations often make us want to eat more or less, but it's caloric intake that determines if we maintain, lose, or gain weight.

Some people say they want to get toned, and others say they want to get jacked, or ripped. For the record: Toned is not an actual exercise adaptation either, but instead refers to a defined-yet-still-slender aesthetic. And while we're talking nonscientific but commonly heard fitness terms: Jacked means larger, rounded muscles and relatively lean, and ripped means still muscular and extra lean. Leanness comes from a combination of training and nutrition, but mostly nutrition. The program here is great for gaining muscle, maintaining muscle while losing body fat, or for gaining muscle and losing body fat, depending on how you adjust your caloric intake.

Many people of course also resistance train for the general adaptation benefits discussed earlier in this chapter, including improved brain and body health and longevity, elevated mood, better sleep, and so on.

Unless you're socializing or texting or taking endless selfies, or the gym is packed, your resistance training sessions should rarely last longer than about 60 +/– 20 minutes. After a five-minute whole-body warm-up, and then two to three warm-up sets for your first exercise, sixty to eighty minutes of effortful, highly focused "work sets" is more than enough to stimulate the specific and general adaptations you're seeking. And that includes the rest periods between work sets too.

Why not longer? Because after eighty minutes of hard resistance training, the fatigue and stress on your body and nervous system is typically greater than is conducive for recovery before your next workout. Also, after eighty minutes, it can be hard to generate the focus and effort needed to continue to stimulate specific adaptations safely. While you might have the energy to train longer, it's good to finish your workout with some vigor left to devote to other aspects of life. Most people will find they won't progress much faster by training for longer sessions, or even more frequent sessions (and in many cases, they stop getting results altogether or even start regressing!). Especially when trying to incorporate the necessary cardiovascular training session discussed in Exercise Protocol 3. By resistance training three times a week for an hour or so, you're far more likely to be consistent over the long-term, which is ultimately what matters to both results now and in the future. There are times when because of long rest periods needed between sets in a crowded gym, workouts can take ninety minutes. Don't fret about it, but don't make that the norm. In fact, if you can get a great workout done in fewer than sixty minutes, even better.

Here are a few more nonobvious things that make a big difference to increase your efficiency in the gym:

A note about "intensity" and soreness

People sometimes think that being really sore in the days after a workout is the goal, but it's not. Delayed onset muscle soreness is not a requirement to make progress. Your goal is to effectively stress your muscles and nervous system across the training session, while still being able to recover before your next training session. This is how you continue to progressively overload your muscles each time you resistance train . . . and that's how you make progress.

Remember, done right, resistance training is a very potent stressor. Usually stress has a negative connotation, but in the context of exercise, just the right amount of local and systemic stress is what will bring you results quickly and consistently. That's why I designed this template with plenty of time for your muscles and connective tissues, and also your nervous system, to recover. Your goal is to trigger the proper adaptations by training really hard, then get out of the gym and recover while you live your life.

Don't think "workout," think "training"

First, training is, as the definition of the word implies, *practicing*. As Pavel Tsatsouline, world-renowned strength coach, explained on my podcast, it's best to view and engage in resistance training as if it were a self-taught class wherein you practice the skill of triggering specific adaptations.[79] The huge advantage of this approach is that it keeps you from adopting the "working out" mindset, which has most people merely going through the motions, thinking about burning more calories or the pump, or just getting through the workout. That mindset confuses effort with *directed effort*. And this template is all about directed effort designed to trigger specific adaptations. Calling it training carries a different level of seriousness that, in my experience, translates to higher quality effort and results. If someone asks "Training for what?" you can tell them, "to get stronger" or simply "life!"

Track your progress

Treating your resistance training as a self-taught class means you should track your progress. This helps you remember what you did last session so that you can make sure you're properly using progressive overload. I believe that whether you are a novice or highly experienced, you should take your training seriously—it's your body and your health after all.

Some people will track their sets and reps and the amount of weight they use on each exercise on their phone, others in a training notebook, others using an app. It doesn't really matter, although the phone offers so many chances for distraction whereas a good ol' pen and some paper have far fewer.

I usually put my phone on airplane mode when I start my workouts and only use it for music, or I simply train without it. Some people like to listen to a podcast or book while they train. You decide what is best for you but, again, take your training seriously. Avoid texting and scrolling social media while you're training. Your workouts will likely be much more effective, and I can guarantee you they will be more efficient. I use a paper notebook to write down every set and number of reps I do in order to track my progress, as described above. This makes a tremendous difference because it gives you a specific goal to beat every exercise and set. It also makes it fun. You can strive for and see objective progress in almost every workout.

Many people are haphazard about their training. Thus, they get some results when they start, but their progress quickly evaporates. It takes the same amount of time (or even potentially less) to do a truly effective workout as it does to do a half-baked one. So make sure you do the former. The great news is that as you practice resistance training, you get better at it.

BRIEF WHOLE-BODY WARM-UP: ABOUT 5 MINUTES

You'll get better results and avoid injury by including a brief five-minute whole-body warm-up at the start of each resistance training session. The goal is simply to increase your core body temperature a few degrees, to loosen up (a nontechnical term) your joints and to prepare for the sets to follow. I like to pedal on a stationary bike or walk briskly on a treadmill for five minutes until I break a light sweat. Alternatively, you can do jumping jacks, windmills, or get on the elliptical or stair climber. It doesn't really matter as long as you warm up. Physical therapist Kelly Starrett, PhD—famous for his work on mobility and all-around fitness—offered a great warm-up when he was a guest on my podcast, especially for when you're feeling less-than-motivated to train:

Just play for a few minutes. Shoot some layups and free throws on a basketball court, or shadow box, skip rope, or complete a simple circuit of body-weight-only exercises: first twenty-five air squats, followed by five lunges per side with just your body weight, and then jog in place for a minute before repeating, until five minutes have elapsed.[80]

You may recall that bodily movement activates two circuits: one in the body and the other in the brain. These trigger the release of adrenaline and norepinephrine, respectively, which in turn makes you more physically energized and mentally alert.[81] That's the other reason to do a brief whole-body warm-up. Many people find they are dragging themselves to the gym, and, after warming up, they feel like a new person. Some of that is psychological, but there is a physiological component too—the way that whole body movement stimulates adrenaline (via the body-to-brain connection) "wakes up" your brain, as we discussed at the start of this chapter.[82]

TOTAL NUMBER OF WARM-UP SETS: 1–3 SETS

Warm-up sets ensure that you are performing an exercise correctly across a full range of motion, and they prepare your nervous system, muscles, and connective tissues for the work sets that follow.

Most people do relatively high reps for their warm-up sets: For instance, they will do fifteen to twenty reps on the first warm-up set, add some resistance and do ten to fifteen reps more, then add a bit more resistance and do six to ten reps for the last warm-up set. Most people also tend to rest briefly between their warm-up sets, usually no more than thirty seconds.

I suggest doing warm-up sets differently, so you can get more out of your work sets that follow. Regardless of the repetition range you have planned for your subsequent work sets, make your first warm-up set only six to ten reps. Use a moderately light weight for you, around 40 percent of the amount of resistance you will use for your first work set. Lift and lower the weight under control throughout every set to make sure that you mentally engage the muscles you are trying to train. Then rest one to two minutes, and do a second warm-up set, but this time perform only four to eight reps using about 65 percent of the weight you'll use for your first work set. For some people that's enough warm-up before the first work set. If your work sets are going to be heavy on a given exercise, meaning they will have you reaching failure (that is, again, the inability to continue moving the weight in good form) after completing just five to seven reps, then I suggest you rest an additional one to two minutes after your second warm-up set and do a third and final warm-up set. For that third warm-up, use about 75 percent of the weight you'll use on your first work set. And for that third warm-up set, keep the reps low, to only two to four. Yes, you could do more, but that's not the goal. You're not trying to stimulate any adaptations with your warm-up sets. Rather, think of them—and especially that third warm-up set—as rehearsals for the real deal: the work sets to follow. Warm-up sets are about preparing your body and mind for the work sets.

Note the percentages above are approximate percentages of the weight you plan to use for your first work set, not a percentage of your one-repetition maximum (1RM), or the maximum you can lift once in good form. Most importantly, your warm-up set should never come close to failure.

TOTAL NUMBER OF WORK SETS PER MUSCLE GROUP: 4–9 SETS

To be clear: When I say muscle group I'm referring, for example, to your shoulders, or biceps, or hamstrings, or triceps, or quadriceps. "Arms" are not a muscle group. Nor are "legs." At least not in the context of resistance-training jargon. Quadriceps are called a "muscle group" because they are made up of several muscles. The same applies to your biceps and all the rest. Later in the chapter I provide links to exercise videos that will clarify any confusion about this and what exercises to select when training. Doing four to nine work sets per muscle group (divided across two to three different exercises) is more than enough to effectively trigger the specific adaptations you want, if you focus and work hard to control the resistance throughout every rep of every work set until you can't move the weight any more, aka failure.

So should you do four or eight, or five, or seven sets?

You decide, but be logical about it based on your goals and needs. One thing that is rarely discussed but important in designing the best program for you is that many people have muscle groups that, for a variety of reasons related to their genetics, the sports they played as youth, or their resistance training history, respond much faster to resistance training than other muscle groups. It makes sense to do fewer total work sets for those muscle groups. You heard me. Do fewer work sets for your quicker-to-respond muscle groups. That will ensure you don't throw off your proportions and create strength imbalances that eventually will lead to injuries. Women seem to be much better about training for aesthetic balance than men. We have all seen "that guy"—the one with the big chest and arms but disproportionately much smaller legs, or the one whose shoulders and back are as wide as barn doors, but with a tiny neck that makes it look like his head is on the wrong body. It's not just about aesthetics; muscle strength and size imbalances set you up for injuries in and out of the gym.

Aim for strength and aesthetic balance. If you have a muscle group that responds easily, limit yourself to doing four to five or even just three work sets total for that muscle group in a given workout. You should still focus on training to failure and in great form during those sets. For all other muscle groups, I suggest you do four to eight total work sets.

One last point regarding the total number of work sets to do. The better you focus and contract a given muscle group, the fewer work sets it will take to stimulate the specific adaptations you're after. Think about it this way: If you've ever hammered a nail into wood, you know that one to two clean, well-placed strikes of the hammer drives the nail in flush. If you don't hit the nail squarely on the head, however, you need many more swings. When you do four to eight work sets per muscle group, and just two to three work sets per exercise, focusing from start to finish as you lift and lower the resistance, your task of triggering specific adaptations in that muscle group is complete. Additional sets are not needed and might do more damage than good—just as continuing to pound on a nail that is already hammered in simply damages the wood.

How do you measure your neuromuscular control? Jeff Cavaliere, a physical therapist and strength and conditioning coach who worked with the New York Mets before founding his own online exercise platform, AthleanX, has a cool trick that translates to more effective (adaptation-stimulating) workouts too. Can you contract a muscle, let's say your bicep or calf or quadricep hard enough to make it almost feel like a cramp but with no added resistance, just by "flexing" the target muscle? If so, that is good news because when you train using isolation exercises, that's effectively what you are trying to do. You're just adding resistance to contract the muscle even harder, throughout the entire movement. This one takes some time for people to wrap their heads around because everyone thinks about "lifting weights," but effective resistance training aimed at generating hypertrophy and strength improvements is about challenging muscles, and the weight or resistance is just a tool to allow you to do that more effectively.

Compound exercises challenge specific groups of muscles and also train the coordinated action of those muscles as they work together to perform certain movements. A squat, for instance, calls on the muscles of the quadriceps, hamstrings (somewhat), glutes and lower back, and numerous stabilizer muscles. "Feeling" your quadriceps during a squat is crucial but the expectation is not that you completely isolate them; in fact, that's impossible. That is why in this program I suggest doing both compound and isolation exercises.

And if you can't feel the muscle you're trying to target when doing compound exercises, consider doing the isolation exercise for that muscle group first, then the compound exercise for that muscle group. For example, if you are having a hard time feeling your chest (pectoralis) muscles during your bench presses, do some sort of chest-isolation exercise first, then move to your bench presses. You don't have to move immediately from one to the other in classic "pre-exhaustion" format. You can simply do your one to three work sets of a chest-isolation movement and then do your one to three work sets of bench presses or other compound movement for the chest.

By the way, if you're feeling lost with these mentions of exercise names or anything else, do not worry! I provide numerous examples of isolation and compound exercises at protocolsbook.com/videos. You'll of course have to use less weight on the compound movement if you do an isolation movement for the same muscle group first, but remember why you are there in the first place: to trigger specific adaptations in specific muscle groups. And you can always reverse the order and proceed with the compound movement a few months later, once you have established a strong mind-muscle-connection with that formerly hard-to-feel and hard-to-improve muscle group.

Is it possible to do too few sets? Yes.[83] Or I should say, most trainers would say yes. Arthur Jones and Mike Mentzer were famous for taking the low-volume–high-intensity logic to the extreme, arguing that people should do just one to two work sets per muscle group per week. That was their suggestion: not *per exercise* but *across the entire workout*! Most everyone agrees nowadays (and the science does too) that you need more work sets. Studies over the last two decades reinforce the idea that somewhere more in the range of four to eight work sets per muscle group is both necessary and sufficient to trigger near maximal strength and/or hypertrophy adaptations.[84]

Many people try to train each muscle group twice per week, with twelve to twenty work sets per group at each session, believing that this is the "optimal" frequency for stimulating muscle growth. But believe me: Doing fewer sets with more intensity, with the focus described here, three times per week, allows for a more sustainable practice and thus better results over time. I will die on this hill! And again, the goal is to do cardiovascular workouts three times a week, too, some of which are intense. That mix is essential for health and is covered in Exercise Protocol 3.

And the great part about this program is that you still end up targeting each muscle group twice per week, just not the way you might think. Let me explain.

As I mentioned above, with regard to frequency of training, you can find studies that argue training each muscle group two or even three times per week is best for these results.[85] I suggest resistance training for each major muscle group directly only once per week. This is not by accident. By scheduling this way along with specific types of cardiovascular training sessions on particular days, you actually end up training each muscle group *twice* per week: once directly, and once indirectly. On chest and back day, your shoulders and arms get some indirect training. On shoulders and arms day, your chest and back get some indirect training too—because you are doing compound movements like overhead presses and dips and perhaps also some palms-facing-you pull-ups for your biceps. On "sprint" cardio day (covered in Protocol 3), your legs get indirect stimulation, and if you do your sprints on an assault bike, those stationary bikes with a fan and handles that you pump forward and back while you pedal, your back and arms get some additional indirect training too. Of course, these indirect training sessions are not enough to stimulate maximal strength or hypertrophy increases on their own, but they synergize beautifully with the direct resistance training that you're already doing for a total of three days a week with weights. A sprint four days after a proper leg workout for calves, quadriceps, hamstrings, and glutes, with multiple sets taken to failure . . . you'll be able to do that, I promise, but it's right as your legs start to feel fresh again . . . and a few days later you're back to your leg workout. You won't lose ground. In fact, you'll come out ahead on both. Try it.

In my experience, the overall program in this chapter provides a well-rounded combination of strength, hypertrophy, endurance, and flexibility and is the best time investment to achieve the results most people are seeking. It also keeps your motivation level for each workout high, which is crucial for anyone leading a busy life. Going to the gym for hard workouts five days a week is difficult for most to maintain. Pretty soon, people are downing two energy drinks and a coffee just to get going, not sleeping well, and getting sick. But three days a week, with just two to three hard work sets per exercise and two to three exercises per muscle group and three or four muscle groups? That's something I'm confident you can do for the rest of your life—and that's how to think of both getting and staying in great shape. It's for all these reasons that I strongly believe in this program. Let me put it this way: I've given this program to men and women of a wide range of ages, athletic backgrounds, and health histories, and I've never seen it not work for them to reach their fitness (and aesthetic) goals.

TOTAL NUMBER OF EXERCISES PER MUSCLE GROUP: 2–3 EXERCISES

TOTAL NUMBER OF WORK SETS PER EXERCISE: 2–3 SETS (USUALLY JUST 2)

In most cases, doing two exercises that target each muscle group is plenty, but in some cases you may want to do a third exercise if it's a muscle group of particular focus. Once again and so that we're clear on terms: Legs are not one muscle group. Quadriceps are. Hamstrings are another muscle group. Your legs have quadriceps, hamstrings, glutes, and calves—each of which has its own subdivisions. You do two to three exercises for each of these groups.

It's crucial that at least one of the two to three exercises for a muscle group be a compound (multi-joint) exercise. In most cases you'll also want to do one isolation (single joint) exercise for the same muscle group. Doing two to three exercises (with two to three work sets for each exercise) brings you to four to nine work sets per muscle group. (I recommend not going above nine work sets total for a single muscle group in a workout, given that you are training multiple muscle groups in each workout. Indeed, aiming for six hard work sets per muscle group per workout is often better, provided that at least three of those sets are from a compound exercise and you take those work sets to failure.)

Time constraints will often dictate exactly how much you do. So will how well you slept (I suggest aiming for the lower end of the number of sets on days when you are a bit sleep-deprived, but still doing the compound movements). So will nutrition. And stress. If you're well rested, fed, and you have the time, do the full three exercises for two to three work sets each, for six to nine total work sets. Or just do four to six work sets per muscle group total and pour every bit of focus and energy into those. With time, you'll learn when enough is enough for that muscle group on a given day and according to the context of the rest of your life.

Specific exercise selection:

As mentioned earlier, target a muscle group with at least one compound exercise and one isolation exercise for that same muscle group. (I provide a set of video tutorials and options to select from at protocolsbook.com/videos).

The rationale for including one of each is that compound exercises target a given muscle in conjunction with other muscles that it normally works with in various everyday movements. That also means compound movements allow you to use heavier weights, which provide not just a direct effect on the muscles you're training but also a positive "systemic effect" on various hormones and neurotransmitter systems of the brain and body.[86] And because they mimic a lot of pushing, pulling, kneeling, and lunging movements we do in everyday life, compound movements carry over to "real world" strength. The ones done standing, like squats and dead lifts, overhead presses, and even bicep curls or overhead extensions, help in developing more core stability and strength too. Taken to failure for two to three well-controlled, focused sets per muscle group, compound exercises are great . . . but they are pretty taxing on your nervous system. This is especially important considering you are doing at least one such movement, and perhaps even two, per muscle group, and training multiple muscle groups per workout.

Follow with an isolation exercise for each major muscle group. It lets you intensely target a specific muscle, it reinforces the mind-muscle connection to that muscle, and, because of the mechanics of the movement (the position and range of motion, etc.), isolation exercises tend to develop aspects of the target muscle that compound movements may not target as thoroughly.

And they don't create quite as much overall stress on your nervous system. Yes, exercise-induced stress is good (!) but it adds up and, as stated earlier, you have just one nervous system for both your workouts and for the other aspects of your life. You don't want to overtax it. That does not mean go easy on isolation exercises. You still need to use progressive overload and to take those isolation exercise sets to failure. By the way, once you do two work sets of leg extensions or side lateral raises (an isolation movement for the shoulders) for twelve to fifteen well-controlled reps to true failure, you'll realize that isolation movements done properly are their own special kind of intense!

To illustrate the importance of exercise and complementarity, let's return to that earlier example and talk about training your quadriceps. You're choosing two exercises. The compound exercise could be a barbell back (or front) squat (your hip and knee joints both move in a squat; hence, multi-joint), and the isolation exercise could be the leg extension machine (only your knee joint moves and your hips stay locked). If you have the energy that day, you might also do another two to three work sets of a compound exercise for your quadriceps, such as leg presses or hack squats.

As you likely realize by now, the exercises you can select from are nearly endless. And they can be free weight or you can use weight machines, or even just your body weight for some of them, like pull-ups or barbell dips. What's important is that you can do a movement safely, without pain, and while still pushing yourself to failure. And that you can safely add more and more resistance to the movement over time as you get stronger. People debate exercise selection a lot. Assuming you include both compound and isolation movements, you have to find what is best for you. What equipment you have access to is of course also a factor. Again, the video links I provide give you lots of options. In the meantime, let's discuss the "best exercise" myth.

The "best exercise/movement" myth

Barbell squats (where the bar is on your shoulders as you squat down and stand up again) are a terrific compound exercise many people can and should use to target their quadriceps, glutes, and other leg muscles. They challenge your lower back and core muscles too. Some trainers will say that you absolutely must do them, but that's simply not true. Some people have hip, leg, or shoulder mechanics that prevent them from doing barbell back squats without joint pain during the exercise or in the days after. You could work with a trainer to overcome those issues, but you could also substitute front squats, where the bar is held on the front of your shoulders, or hack machine squats, which have your back on an angled sled for support, or even leg presses for your quadriceps instead. There are Zercher squats, rear-leg-elevated squats, and goblet squats. There are also a near-endless number of lunge variations that target the quadriceps, glutes, and other muscles emphasized in the barbell back squat. The internet is filled with exercise clips showing all of these exercises. Again, I provide video tutorials of many to choose from at protocolsbook.com/videos.

Find the exercises you can really push yourself in, without joint pain. You'll enjoy it more, and your results will be greater . . . which will lead you to enjoy it even more. You'll experience a whole different relationship to resistance training if you make yourself the CEO of the process. Only do exercises that really work for your body. Just don't only do isolation movements. Compound movements are necessary to get the full benefits of resistance training.

A few quick notes about safety and pain

Safety: I'll be direct about this. Be careful as you train. Done correctly (warm up, don't add more weight than you can handle with control, and so on) and with caution to avoid a few potentially perilous mistakes, resistance training as described in this protocol is a very safe activity.

What sort of perilous mistakes am I referring to? Well, people have died barbell bench-pressing.[87] They couldn't push the bar up from their chest and they asphyxiated. It's rare, but it happens. Have a spotter who knows how to spot you correctly—which means they have to be strong enough to pull the loaded bar up off your chest or neck if need be. If you don't have someone who can do that, an easy solution is to use dumbbells if you're bench-pressing alone—those can be set down to your knees and dropped to your sides if you hit failure. A few dents in the floor are far better than the alternative. Or use a rack with safety pins (sturdy bars that can support a loaded bar) to set the weight on if you hit failure mid-repetition. Same goes for barbell squats. Yes, you can "dump" the bar behind you if you hit failure, but far better to have a knowledgeable spotter. If no such person is around, again use a rack with pins so you can set the bar down and crawl out. Many people opt for machines like the leg press or hack squat for compound quadriceps movements for just this reason: It's easier to hit failure without doing what I described. And they usually have "stops" you can engage when you hit failure. No, these movements do not engage the same muscles to the same degree as free weight compound exercises. Yes, they are safer. You decide your risk tolerance, but be safe regardless.

Also, think about your posture every time you are picking up or putting down weights, even if you're just replacing them on the rack or getting in position to start your set. A lot of resistance training injuries are the consequence of people not being mindful as they do the in-between work sets stuff because their mind is someplace else.

I'm proud of the fact that I have been training hard, and heavy (for me) for nearly thirty-five years and have never had a serious injury from resistance training. (Knock on wood!) Sure, I've had a few minor strains here and there but nothing that floored me or kept me from training or daily activities for more than a few days. I attribute that to staying mentally focused from start to finish in the gym, and to only making relatively small incremental increases (5 to 10 percent) in the amount of weight I add to any given movement from week to week, and only once I can do at least eight to twelve reps of that movement in good form.

Pain: We have all heard the mantra "no pain, no gain." News flash (!): That does not refer to joint or connective tissue pain. It refers to the burning sensation in muscles caused primarily by the accumulation of hydrogen ions inside muscle cells, brought on by the fact that the muscle cells need energy faster than oxygen can be delivered to them. (No, not lactic acid as was once believed. Lactate is created, but we know now it is not the cause of the burning.)[88] If an exercise causes sharp or dull joint pain—not post exercise soreness but, again, pain—either your form or the exercise itself is not right. Don't persist with that exercise. At least not that day. Find an alternative.

REPETITION ("REPS") RANGE PER SET

When it comes to selecting the number of reps to do for your work sets, you have options. After decades of debate about "optimal rep ranges," research from Brad Schoenfeld's lab, at Lehman College, found that using repetition ranges of anywhere from five all the way up to thirty on work sets stimulates essentially the same amount of hypertrophy. That is, if (and only if!) those sets are taken to failure.[89] Generally speaking, this is great news because it means that if you select a weight that you think you'll do eight reps with (and fail on rep nine) but somehow you are able to do eleven reps (and fail on rep twelve), you'll still make progress. It removes the need to stay in a narrow rep range, at least for hypertrophy.

At face value, these findings suggest you don't ever need to train with low reps and heavy weights to get results; you simply need to push until the final reps of your work set are very hard to complete. In some sense, yes, you can use moderate or even light weights (for you) that limit you to twelve to thirty reps before reaching failure. But you should also regularly use heavy (for you) weights, which means weights that limit you to just five to eight reps and no more, despite your maximum effort to complete more. Turns out using a mix of weights stimulates different muscle fiber types and ensures you activate different forms of cellular stress and thus adaptations.[90]

More on that below but in the meantime, if you don't want to have to think much about rep range selection, here's a good guide:

For compound exercises, use the amount of weight on your work sets that has you reaching failure between five and twelve reps.

- Occasionally use heavier loads that limit you to just 3–5 reps before you reach failure.
- Experiment with lighter loads that allow you to complete higher repetition compound exercises, especially for quadriceps and calves. Many people find that 12–20 repetition squats (or its variations) are very effective for hypertrophy.
- Warning: High-repetition quadriceps work sets taken to failure are brutal. The loads you use will be lighter than you would use for 5–10 reps taken to failure, but the pain tolerance level on the final reps (and mental fortitude) required for 15–25 reps of a compound leg movement, like squats or even one of its machine variations, like a hack squat, taken to failure is no joke.

For isolation exercises, use an amount of weight on your work sets that has you reaching failure between eight and fifteen reps.

- Doing isolation exercises for heavier 5-8 repetition sets (to failure) is not bad per se, but most people find that doing higher (8–15, or as many as 25) reps on isolation movements like leg extensions, shoulder lateral raises, preacher curls for biceps, and so on, is more effective. But feel free to experiment. You may find, for instance, that your hamstrings respond best to heavier sets of lying leg curls (an isolation exercise) that limit you to 5-7 reps.

Just remember, no matter what the repetition range you use for a movement, go to failure on work sets, even if it has you exceeding your target repetition range for that day and exercise.

Now before you say, "I heard leaving one to three 'reps in reserve' (RIR) is just as good as training to failure," we need to get honest: If you use heavy (for you) weights that would make you reach failure somewhere between five and ten reps, but you stop a rep or two before failure, you probably will still stimulate some strength and hypertrophy adaptations. That is because heavier loads generate levels of mechanical tension that readily stimulate muscle and nerve-to-muscle adaptations.[91] However, given that this program has you doing relatively fewer work sets (four to nine), and directly targeting each major muscle group only once per week (and a second time per week, indirectly, as described above), you really should take all your work sets to failure.

Still not convinced? Well, consider this reality: We all like to think we are training our absolute hardest, but what most people consider taking a set to failure almost always leaves one to two more repetitions in reserve. How can I be so sure? Well, if you hit failure on the eighth rep of a set but were told that getting a ninth rep would save someone's life, I am willing to bet that ninth rep would happen. So failure is somewhat subjective. Thankfully lives are not on the line according to when we reach failure on our lifts. But that momentary muscular failure is the closest thing you have to an objective measure of intensity of effort. So seek it out.

Here's a bit more information so you can make the best-informed decisions about whether to train heavy, moderate, or light (for you). Hypertrophy adaptations are thought to be stimulated by at least three things:[92]

1. Microdamage caused to the muscles using heavier loads. (Here, we can define "heavier loads" as sets that have you fail after completing three to six reps.) The extent to which this contributes to hypertrophy is a matter of emerging debate, but it still has some solid evidence in its favor.
2. Mechanical tension (from moderate to heavy loads and/or the contraction or stretching of the target muscle).
3. Metabolic stress (including the pump and cellular swelling, all brought on by enhanced blood flow, along with the release and delivery of various cellular factors to the muscles you are training).

Muscle size and strength are correlated so if you make a muscle bigger it will get stronger, but training specifically to maximize strength is typically done by using loads that limit you to three to five reps (or fewer) and doing a large number of sets for each muscle across the week and not training to failure on any one set. Getting strong is great but the vast majority of people who resistance train do so to get stronger and for aesthetic changes that are best brought about by the rep and load ranges discussed above.

That is why I suggest you mainly use five to twelve reps on your compound work sets, and occasionally venture into using heavier loads that limit you to just three to five reps before you fail. In reality there will be times when you can do ten reps of a movement with a given weight, so you increase the amount of weight the next time you're training that body part and somehow you can only do three or four reps before you reach failure. Don't worry about it. Just keep striving to add more reps or weight each workout in great form. If you want to obsess over something useful, obsess over the amount of focused effort you put into your work sets and using great form!

About ten years ago, I decided to train exclusively with heavy weights that limited me to three to five reps on compound exercises and six to ten reps on isolation exercises—which is called periodization. I did that for three months and I got a lot stronger, such that when I went back to doing five to twelve reps, I was stronger on every movement. Later I ran a similar experiment using lighter weights and more reps (12–25) for a few months . . . all still to failure on work sets of course. I made considerable progress in terms of hypertrophy, but when I went back to using heavier weights for lower reps, I found I had lost a lot of ground. So I learned something. Nowadays I almost always train with weights that limit me to five to twelve reps and only venture up to fifteen to twenty for an especially intense leg workout or on certain upper body isolation exercises. That's what is best for me and my goals. You should experiment and find what is best for you.

Progressive overload is key!

I know that the requirement for progressive overload is a giant "duh" to many of you out there, but others may need this reminder. If you do the same workout every week, using the same weights, reps, and sets, take note. You might sweat, work hard, and feel the mood enhancements of exercise but your progress will halt. Because we're keeping the work sets to just two or three, you must challenge your muscles by either increasing the amount of weight or the number of reps, or both, while keeping your form excellent.

"More weight or more reps, perfect form, and pushing to failure." That should be your resistance training mantra!

Be aware that it's unreasonable to expect to add weight while maintaining the same rep count you performed the previous week, but it will happen. Those are great workouts. However, there will be weeks when, for whatever reason, you are not able to hit your target weight and rep goals in the gym. Consider the reasons: Are you sleep-deprived? Underfed, under caffeinated? Unfocused? Life happens, so don't obsess about it. Just do your absolute best for that day. If you find you're not making progress for two weeks in a row, you may need to reduce the set volume. Yes, I said it: Try doing *fewer* work sets and see if that budges you forward. Or maybe it's time for a week off to rest, so you can come back stronger.

Finally, while 1RM lifts and even 2RM lifts are great for building strength (and allow you to answer the "How much can you bench?" question you'll invariably get at some point), I recommend most people avoid doing 1RMs. They come with too much risk of injury. If you really want to do them, fine, but use a spotter, please! And understand that 1RM lifts are what you train for in powerlifting—which is a specific sport. If that's what you're interested in, there are great programs out there for powerlifting. But most people are lifting weights for other reasons. They want the variety of benefits that come from the resistance training I've described here. If someone ever asks me how much I can bench, I usually just tell them what I did for five to eight reps the preceding week because that's all I know for certain!

An important note about training to, and past, failure

As I've said about a hundred times now (but still a hundred fewer than Mentzer would have in the same time frame!): Do the first work set of an exercise to failure, using perfect form. Pour everything you have into that set, on every repetition. That means, as the final reps approach, think: "This is what stimulates the adaptations I'm here for." Strive to keep your form stricter, and stress the targeted muscles more, not less as failure approaches. Then, when the weight won't move any more, try HARD to continue to move it for an additional three to five seconds, then re-rack the weight.

Then rest two to three minutes, or perhaps even four to five minutes on compound exercises for legs or back or other large muscles. Then do a second set of that exercise, also to failure, but don't fight to push the weight once you've hit failure, like I described for the first work set above. This is not a back-off set. You're just stopping when you can't move the weight anymore.

Should you do a third set of that exercise? Maybe. But usually not. Two sets done the way I just described should trigger the specific adaptations you're seeking. And you still have another exercise or two to complete next for that muscle group. Am I like Mentzer and think that if you do a third set, it's going to be counterproductive? No. I don't know if it will help your progress, but I don't think it will hurt you if done in good form and with intense effort. You decide. One thing's for sure: If you can't make the set a highly focused, max effort work set, move on.

Once you hit failure, should you do assisted (sometimes called "forced") reps? Or a drop set, where you reach failure then quickly lower the amount of weight and grind out one to three more reps before hitting failure again? These techniques can be helpful, but they stress your nervous system a lot. I would suggest pushing beyond failure for two to three sets maximum across the entire workout. On days where you're feeling a bit stressed, don't push past failure. And if you have someone assisting you with forced reps, make sure they don't jump in before you reach failure. Make sure they force you to do the work. It's a fine line between spotting someone to ensure they don't get stuck in a dangerous position during a lift and getting someone to help you with forced reps.

Spotting someone in the weight room is a skill—it's not brain surgery but there is a right and a wrong way to do it. On social media, you often come across videos of gym disasters, where people get stuck under the bench press or squat bar because they were too shy to ask for a spot. There are, however, a nearly equal number of gym disaster videos of young kids who were not able to pull the bar off their dad's chest because they are too weak. Avoid all of this by making sure anyone you ask to help you is (1) strong enough to help with the amount of weight you're using and (2) understands that you need to do the majority of the work. They are there to help keep you safe (again, especially on bench presses or squats where getting stuck can be dangerous), but not hinder your progress. Tell them: "I'll let you know when to help but don't touch the weight until I say." And if they check their phone during your work sets, find a new training partner!

REST DURATION BETWEEN SETS

Just as I listed above, take one to two minutes off between warm-up sets, and two to five minutes between work sets, depending on repetition range. Typically, people rest longer (3–5 minutes) between work sets of compound exercises than between work sets of isolation exercises (90 seconds to 3 minutes). Some people adhere to the clock for between set rest, others go by feel. You decide. I use the clock to get a sense of how my subjective "Okay, I'm ready for another set" sense matches up with various time ranges. Just don't talk, text, or scroll too much between sets. Stay focused, get the training done and get out.

Recovery tips

Then there's the rest that comes after your resistance training session.

Great things happen for your health during your resistance training sessions but the really big benefits—the actual changes in your muscles, connective tissues, and brain—occur during the two to four days afterward, mostly while you sleep.[93] The protocols provided elsewhere in this book will help you get your sleep right and your nutrition and stress control right—all of which support recovery from, and adaptation to, exercise. You do not need to overhaul your sleep schedule or diet just because you resistance train. It is true that if you do a particularly hard workout, you may find you need a bit more sleep on subsequent nights, but in general, resistance training has the effect of improving the quality of your sleep, not increasing your sleep duration needs.

Same with nutrition. Resistance training doesn't massively change your nutritional needs. Assuming you are already eating in the manner I describe in chapter 4—meaning you strive to eat about 1 gram of quality protein per pound of lean body weight daily, as well as plenty of vegetables, some fruit, unprocessed starches, and healthy fats.

It is true that if you are actively seeking to gain muscle, you'll need to eat more calories than you burn each day, but not by much—200 to 400 calories more than your maintenance calories is fine.[94] The old-school practice of bulking up by eating many more calories than you need is just not healthy—and brings with it a lot of body fat that you'll be trying to lose later.[95] I suggest you don't go that route. Provided you are not undernourished in calories or protein, you'll make progress with resistance training. Keep in mind as you gain more muscle and/or lose fat, your caloric needs change—fortunately in a way that lets you eat the same or more while staying lean or even getting leaner. Muscle tissue is metabolically demanding, which means it burns more calories than fat tissue, which is just one of the many benefits of resistance training.

There is a formula for determining your maintenance calorie needs per day, or what is called your basal metabolic rate (BMR). That's how many calories you should eat each day to maintain your current body weight if you did no physical activity whatsoever.

The formula is called the Katch-McArdle formula.[96] It takes about five minutes to figure out, and it's very easy to do. It requires a few other simple calculations first, which I'll walk you through.

Determine your body weight (BW) in kilograms:

- The formula uses kilograms so if you're used to thinking about weight in pounds and not kilograms, first divide your body weight (BW) in pounds by 2.2 to get your weight in kilograms.
- For example, I weigh 220 pounds, so 220/2.2 = 100 kilograms.

Calculate your lean body mass (LBM):

- Multiply your BW in kilograms by 1 minus your body fat percentage as a decimal.
- For example, I weigh 220 pounds (100 kg) and am about 10% body fat, so my LBM is approximately 100 × (1 – 0.10) = 90 kilograms.

- To estimate your body fat percentage, these online resources can help you figure that out:
  - Men: https://athleanx.com/articles/body-fat-percentage-men
  - Women: https://ultimateperformance.com/your-goal/fat-loss/female-fat-loss/womens-body-fat-percentage-in-pictures/
- There are more precise methods to measure body fat percentage, but they can be costly. This works pretty well, and is available at no cost.

Calculate your basal metabolic rate (BMR):

- **Katch-McArdle equation:** BMR = 370 + (21.6 × LBM in kilograms).
- So for me: BMR = 370 + (21.6 × 90) = 370 + (1944) = 2,314 calories per day, my BMR.

Multiply your BMR by an activity multiplier to account for how active you are throughout the day:

- **Sedentary (no exercise at all):** BMR × 1.2
- **Lightly active (e.g., walking 7,000–10,000 steps):** BMR × 1.375
- **Moderately active (e.g., same as lightly active, plus yoga, "easy" cardio):** BMR × 1.55
- **Very active (e.g., walking 7K–10K steps, effortful resistance training or cardio):** BMR × 1.725
- **Extremely active (e.g., same as very active but two-a-day-workouts):** BMR × 1.9

I'll add one comment on estimating your activity levels from sports performance expert Andy Galpin. Based on his experience training hundreds of clients in reaching their fitness goals, Andy notes that people are typically far less active than they think. For example, most who rate themselves "very active" are actually moderately active. He recommends that people select the activity category below the one they think they fall into if they're interested in losing weight.

I don't do resistance training and cardio on the same days, but I try to get seven thousand to ten thousand steps in every day, and I resistance train three times a week and do some form of cardio three days a week.

Occasionally, I will resistance train or run, and then also go for a hike. That constitutes extremely active but it's too rare an occurrence. Also, given Andy's recommendation, I'll consider myself "very active" and therefore multiply my basal metabolic maintenance calories (2,314 calories) by 1.725 = 3,991.65 calories . . . and I round that up to 4,000 calories per day.

I naturally tend to eat less on days I don't exercise, so for that day, I multiply 2,314 by 1.375 = 3,181.75 calories.

Voila! I need about 4,000 calories per day on my training days and about 3,000 calories per day on my non-training days. Do I neurotically count every calorie? No. Truth be told, I probably eat about 3,500 calories on training days, and about 3,000 calories on days I don't train.

Should you count calories? Maybe, but not every day and certainly not forever. I suggest figuring out your basal metabolic maintenance calories, what you're consuming now, and what changes you need to make, and then stick to that revised plan most of the time.

After you've completed the simple formula above, a great tool to track what you're eating is the Carbon app developed by Layne Norton, PhD, who is an expert in training and nutrition. (Carbon is a sponsor of my podcast because I believe it to be a terrific product.) Another option is the Cal AI app. Both make it very easy to enter what you eat and the apps then do all the calculations of calories, as well as macronutrients like protein, fats, and carbohydrates. Each carries a nominal cost, but it is very easy to use. Personally, I don't like to count calories every day, but I use the Carbon app for periods of time to see how I'm doing.

If you want to lose weight, eating 300 to 500 fewer calories than you burn daily is the best way to go. By resistance training while in this caloric deficit, you're better able to spare lean muscle and preferentially lose fat.[97] This is further helped by making sure you're eating a protein-rich diet, despite eating 300 to 500 fewer calories. In short, resistance training and a good diet are two of the most effective and durable paths to body recomposition—a fancy term for "gaining muscle and losing fat," as opposed to simply losing weight.

Pre-training and post-training nutrition:

I prefer to resistance train early in the morning or midafternoon, and I consistently have my best workouts when I have not eaten anything in the hours before I begin. I like to wake up, get sunlight, hydrate, caffeinate, then train, and then eat afterward, but some people just can't do that. They feel weak, tired, hungry, or nauseous if they train on an empty stomach. But I know myself well. If 10:00 or 11:00 a.m. rolls around and I haven't eaten, I need to ingest some calories before training. That's usually a few scoops of whey protein, a small bowl of oatmeal, a piece of fruit, and some nuts. Nothing fancy. Or two to three eggs, instead of the whey. You'll have to experiment to see what works best for you. If you eat before you train, ideally give yourself at least an hour to digest your food before you begin.

After resistance training, your body is primed to convert any food you consume into energy to burn at a very high rate, so it can replace glycogen you used during the workout.[98] That does not mean you should gorge on pastries or pizza after training. Unless you're deliberately low-carb or keto, the meal following a resistance training workout ideally should include both natural sugars (a few pieces of fruit) and starchy complex carbohydrates (such as rice, potatoes, bread, pasta, or oatmeal) to replenish glycogen stores in your liver and muscles. It should also include some quality protein (such as whey, beef, chicken, fish, turkey, or eggs).

This meal doesn't have to be complicated. The enzymes that facilitate restocking of glycogen are upregulated after resistance training,[99] and you direct more of the amino acids coming from the protein you eat into your muscle tissue after resistance training too,[100] so it's a good idea to eat within the three hours after training.[101] BUT, contrary to the lore in the 1990s, if you don't eat in this window, it's not the end of the world! As long as you don't eat far too few calories, you'll still make progress. You'll likely recover faster if you do eat in this window, but follow your hunger cues. There is a lot more to say about nutrition and training. Far more than can be covered here, but I provide a few more tips below, and even more in chapter 4.

Hydration:

Drink water before, during, and after a workout, especially on hot days or if you tend to sweat a lot. I cover hydration later in chapter 4 as well. Yes, there is a protocol for how to hydrate properly, as this is one of the most undervalued tools for mental and physical performance.

Supplements:

You do not need supplements to make progress with your resistance training. What's most important is that you train hard, get enough sleep, and eat right. If you want to explore supplements, however, there are two that have been shown to increase strength and hypertrophy: creatine monohydrate and whey protein.

Creatine brings more water into your muscles, enhancing training capacity and recovery ability, which thus makes you stronger. It also can have some positive effects on brain function,[102] especially after mild sleep deprivation.[103] I take five to ten grams of creatine monohydrate daily, as a powder dissolved in water. You can take it any time of day, with or without food. Any reputable brand with third-party testing and that is "Certified for Sport" is fine. I have seen no evidence that creatine harms your kidneys[104] or makes your hair fall out,[105] which is what some online claims say. It's normal to gain a few pounds of water-in-the-muscles weight with regular creatine use. If you stop taking it, you urinate out that extra fluid.

Whey protein is simply a high-quality, easily digested protein. It's convenient and cost-effective when compared to other quality proteins. It doesn't have many other micronutrients like meat or eggs do, however, so I wouldn't make whey protein your only quality protein source. I drink one to two scoops of whey protein mixed with water once or twice a day, which equates to 20 to 80 grams of protein (it's about 20 g of protein per scoop). Along with the foods I eat, this helps me meet my daily protein goal. Without whey protein I find it challenging to eat about 1 gram per pound of lean body weight each day.

The other supplement worth mentioning in the context of resistance training is caffeine, which has been shown to improve exercise performance when 100 to 400 milligrams is consumed about thirty minutes prior to and even during exercise.[106] That's about one to four cups of coffee, depending on the brew strength and size of the serving. Not everyone can or should consume caffeine, however. It makes some people anxious. I personally love caffeine and tolerate it very well, so I drink a cup or two of black coffee and/or a yerba maté about thirty minutes before resistance workouts.

A lot of people are into energy drinks these days as pre- and intra-workout energy sources. I will occasionally drink an energy drink (Jocko Go or Gorilla Mind—I know, wild names!—are the ones I like best for taste and effect) before and during a workout, but not every time. If I am facing a particularly challenging leg workout I tend to make my own pre-workout by drinking (or taking) 200 milligrams of caffeine and alpha-GPC (300–900 mg). I discuss alpha-GPC and other compounds more in chapter 6. Just remember, if you're working out in the evening, drinking caffeine beforehand will really disrupt your sleep.

There are a few other supplements which have been shown to improve exercise performance—like *Rhodiola rosea*, which can reduce fatigue during training,[107] but I consider it a distant fourth place to the three mentioned already.

But I want to reiterate: You do not need supplements to make progress resistance training. Focus on training properly! Then focus on recovery, meaning letting the adaptations you stimulated in the gym actually occur by getting proper sleep and nutrition. That is what really moves the needle.

A week off every twelve to sixteen (or even ten to twelve) weeks:

I attribute taking a week off from resistance training every three to four months or so as one of the main reasons I have been able to make regular progress in resistance training over the last thirty-five years. I know that sounds crazy, and that it runs counter to much of the "no days off" advice seen online, but I am convinced it's the way to go, for three reasons.

First, it gives your joints and your mind a chance to reset. Any nagging aches or residual muscle soreness tend to go away during that week off, and you come back feeling reset.

Second, most people make actual progress during the week off. Training-induced stress is cumulative; when we train and recover between workouts, we get stronger and can manage more reps and/or more weight in perfect form from week to week, but not all our bodily tissues adapt at the same rate. By the time we are eight, nine, or even fourteen weeks into training since our last week off, we tend to have a harder time recovering from workouts. Taking a week off lets everything catch up, and lets you come back stronger.

Third, it's common that after twelve to sixteen weeks of training we feel less motivated to keep training hard. The relatively low frequency of resistance training I recommend in this program—just three times per week—usually staves off boredom but some people do start to lose steam after ten or more weeks of training. If you find yourself dragging yourself to the gym, and you're more interested in texting than training once you're there, take a week off, and come back. That usually does the trick. You'll be more energetic when you do.

Keep in mind, too, that sometimes we are just forced to take a week off because life says we have to! I don't think training when you're sick is a good idea, and it gets others sick, too, so please stay out of the gym until you're better! Other times we are forced to take a week off because we have a major deadline or a family vacation or other demands. I personally like to train on vacations because it helps me get over jet lag when I travel, but you may feel like it's a waste of time. It's a matter of choice, and how you view vacation.

Regardless of whether your week off is due to a cold or pre-planned for the end of a twelve to sixteen week stretch of training, or simply because a work deadline hits, don't worry about it causing a setback. It's part of the process. Just get back to training (properly) after that week off.

COMMON QUESTIONS:

Does it matter what day I begin this sequence?

No. Start it on Sunday or Tuesday or whenever you like. What's important is to follow the sequence.

You listed abdominals/core as "required" but neck and forearms as optional. Why? And am I supposed to train neck and abdominals/core and forearms the same way I train other muscles, with progressive overload, to failure, et cetera?

Some people need to work on their forearms—and their grip strength—and others don't, for a variety of reasons. It could be genetics, or because that second group targets their forearms and grip strength with plenty of work from deadlifts, pull-ups, rows, and similar movements. Grip strength is a correlate of longevity but not a cause. It's also one of the things that starts to wane as we age. I like training forearms when I train shoulders and arms, and just for three to four sets of flexor and/or extensor movements (see protocolsbook.com/videos for examples). Use higher rep ranges, say twelve to thirty reps—

no need to train forearms with lower reps and heavy weight. You'll get that indirectly from your heavier pulling movements when you train your back, such as chin-ups or rows.

Abdominals are a specific set of muscles in your midsection and your "core" includes a lot more than just these. I suggest you train your abs and core one to two times per week. Endless crunches are not the way to go. There are better options to train these muscles. And some let you train your forearms and strengthen your grip, and let you get in a great stretch too, all at once. Like hanging from a bar and doing knee raises, then progressing over time to hanging chair sits and L-sits, where you hold your legs straight out, parallel to the floor, and eventually hanging pikes, where you bring your shins up to the bar. You don't just leap into pikes, by the way; you work toward these with the exercises above, and everyone—yes, everyone (men and women)—I have taken through this progression has eventually been able to do multiple sets of three to five reps of hanging pikes! They were surprised, but I was not. Your body is amazing in how it will adapt if you give it the right stimulus, and the right recovery. (Oh, and I know three to five reps is not ten, but when you reach that number you will have a very strong core and grip!)

Other reasons to train your core: It's vital for posture and back health, and it will help your resistance and other fitness training. Six-pack abs are the consequence of having low enough body fat to see the contour of the abdominals. You don't get that from training alone. But abs and other muscles of your core react to progressive overload just like any other muscle (here too, see protocolsbook.com/videos for examples).

Neck exercises are the least performed of any exercises in any gym, but they are so important! Your neck is your upper spine, and a strong neck is crucial for posture. It also helps to keep your shoulders uninjured. Also, done right they won't give you a huge neck—or (oxymoronically) the "no-neck" look. Women and men who train their neck properly can avoid that look if they want to, and yet can still enjoy the better posture and facial tone that work can bring, as the neck and face muscles both activate during these exercises. For wide-shouldered men, balanced neck development is crucial to avoid appearing as if your head is too small for your body! This will be of great aesthetic and structural benefit. Neck training is simple to do safely and effectively once you know how, and requires little or no equipment. I include several examples also at protocolsbook.com/videos.

Everyone should be sure to train their rear deltoid muscles—small muscles on the back of the shoulders that, when made sufficiently strong, greatly improve posture and shoulder stability. There is a way to train this muscle along with other muscles of the middle back that will also help make your default posture more upright. The exercise is called a "face pull," and no, it does not involve attaching weights to your face or jaw. You do them during your "shoulders and arms" resistance training day, using exercise bands or a cable machine. I have a video of the person who popularized these, Jeff Cavaliere from AthleanX, teaching me the proper form at protocolsbook.com/videos.

What if something comes up and I have to miss a workout, what then?

I address this in Exercise Protocol 3, because the resistance training outlined here is part of a larger program. In the meantime, know that you have a fair degree of flexibility, and you can move a workout forward or back a day if needed.

Can I still play sports and do other activities?

Of course. You'll be stronger for it. And the relatively low volume of sets in this program means you won't be sore all the time. (Again, soreness is zero indication of an effective workout—it does not mean you effectively stimulated specific hypertrophy or strength adaptations.) Please don't add additional resistance training work or CrossFit workouts and the like until you've tried this program, but tennis, Pilates, hiking, yoga, archery, golf, soccer, et cetera, and being active with house and yard work is encouraged. Most people nowadays are too sedentary. More movement is nearly always better than less. And of course, cardiovascular training is key. I discuss that next.

EXERCISE PROTOCOL

3

Do Cardiovascular Training Three Times per Week

WHAT TO DO:

- **Elevate your heart rate for anywhere from six to seventy-five minutes, three times per week.** Plan three sessions, each focused on stimulating a different specific adaptation: a long, a medium, and a brief cardiovascular workout, scaling the intensity inversely with the duration of each session. That means the long cardio workout should be of low intensity, the brief cardio workout should be of high intensity. Here is how to incorporate cardio into the overall program:

  Day 1: Cardiovascular training, 45–75 minutes (low intensity/long duration)
  Day 2: Resistance training (legs: calves, quadriceps, hamstrings, glutes)
  Day 3: Rest day
  Day 4: Resistance training (torso: chest, back, abdominals/core; optional neck)
  Day 5: Cardiovascular training, 25–30 minutes (moderate intensity/moderate duration)
  Day 6: Cardiovascular training, 6–17 minutes (high intensity/brief duration)
  Day 7: Resistance training (shoulders, biceps, triceps, abdominals/core; optional forearms and/or neck)

The first cardio workout each week marks the first day of the foundational fitness program schedule. It should be relatively low intensity, and long duration. And it should be continuous. Your goal is to sustain a steady output of effort for forty-five to seventy-five minutes without any pauses except perhaps to drink some water or wait for a stoplight to change so you can cross the street. This falls into the category of classic endurance work. The primary adaptation you're stimulating with this workout is to increase your heart's *stroke volume*, which is the amount of blood your heart pumps with each beat. This means the heart can pump more blood per beat, and thus does not have to beat as fast to deliver the same amount of oxygen. The consequences of that for your health are manifold, including a lower resting heart rate when not exercising.[108] This workout also stimulates a number of metabolic pathways related to utilizing fat for fuel and for vascular growth and even lymphatic health.[109] It indirectly improves mood and sleep too.[110]

The challenge of this workout resides in its duration, not its intensity, and for many people the most challenging aspect is refraining from going faster and harder as they complete it. The forty-five to seventy-five minute duration is intentionally broad. In fact, if you're out of shape when starting this program, I suggest you begin with just fifteen to twenty minutes, and add a few minutes to that each week, until you're doing forty-five to seventy-five minutes of continuous movement. In my observation, most people find that sixty minutes is about the upper limit of their psychological tolerance for this sort of exercise, unless they really love the activity or it's made social, like a hike or bike ride with family or friends. In any case, your goal pace throughout should be such that you can just barely hold a conversation. It's quite all right if you must pause your speech here and there to catch your breath, but the idea is to exert yourself at a level that, were you to push yourself any faster or harder, holding a conversation would be impossible.

Another way to calibrate to that goal pace is to push as hard as you can while still breathing in and out only through your nose. No mouth breathing whatsoever, unless you are talking. As soon as you feel you have to gasp to get air through your mouth, you know you're pushing too hard.

In the language of percentage of maximum heart rate this cardio session is done at 60 to 70 percent of your maximum heart rate (HR), but ideally closer to 70 percent. Your max HR can be estimated by this formula: 220 – your age = your approximate max HR. That's not a perfect measurement but it's close, and for most it's more than sufficient to use here. If you want to be more precise about it, max HR is better approximated by the following formula: for men, you take 208 beats per minute – (0.7 × your age in years); and for women, it's 206 beats per minute – (0.88 × your age in years).[111] Once you have determined your approximate max HR, multiply that by 0.6 and 0.7 to get the lower and upper range, respectively, of your target heart rate for this cardio session. I've shared this formula because some people like to use an HR monitor while training to be sure they stay in that target HR zone. I prefer to use the "upper limit of effort while maintaining nasal breathing" approach, because whenever I have measured my HR while running and restricting myself to nasal breathing, it lands at about 70 percent (+/–5 percent) of my max HR. I have nothing against HR monitors. I just prefer not to use one when doing this workout. I like to let my mind wander or to listen to a book or podcast or music but if you like tracking your HR in real time, go for it.

A few other things to consider for this workout: Some people refer to this as Zone 2 cardio, which is a term that describes the intensity of the exercise with regard to heart rate training zones. But on that scale, I consider it more Zone 2/3 because it's done at the high end of Zone 2 and the low end of Zone 3.[112]

Ideally you would get outside to do this workout so that you're getting all the benefits that come with being outdoors. This raises the issue of what type of exercise is best for this. That's an easy one to answer. Select any activity you can do for the specified duration and intensity without getting hurt. That means do what is safe for your joints, works for your skill level, doesn't stress any of your injuries, and can be completed in safe conditions. I love running and much prefer doing it outside on a trail or city streets to all other forms of cardio, but many people loathe running, or it hurts their knees, or it's not safe for them to run in a given area. You don't have to run! You can opt for cycling, or use the elliptical machine or a stair climber, or hike with a weight vest or a rucksack or, heck, even a backpack with a one-gallon jug of water in it. The possibilities are nearly infinite, and many of these cost very little. If I don't run, I'll sometimes swim laps in a pool or swim parallel to shore in the ocean. If the weather is bad, I'll occasionally run on a treadmill or use a stationary bike.

Pick your poison and deliver it slow and steady for forty-five to seventy-five minutes. Many people find this workout meditative and learn to enjoy it. While you can of course go longer than seventy-five minutes, remember you're training your legs the next day.

The second cardio workout each week is done three days after your leg workout (day five of the program). By then, your legs should be feeling mostly or completely recovered. This second cardio workout should be moderately fast-paced. It should have you breathing fairly hard but not gasping for air or needing to stop to recover. I suggest you start with five minutes of low-intensity movement to warm up and then shift to twenty-five to thirty minutes of "work" where your heart rate is kept between about 75 and 85 percent of your maximum heart rate.

Using the heart rate training zones, this workout falls in the high Zone 3 and low Zone 4 range.

Notably, although this workout is more intense than the first cardio session, it generally leaves you feeling energized and focused for many hours afterward. The key is to not push overly hard at any one time of that approximately twenty-five to thirty minutes. You want to stay roughly in that "75 to 85 percent of max HR" range. That said, it's perfectly all right to move between high and low within this range by pushing harder at times, and pulling back at times. Say, for example, you're climbing a hill or you're just feeling strong on your bike for a stretch and want to push yourself. Your pace and your heart rate don't have to be perfectly constant throughout. Remember: It's not a sprint! You don't want to overly tax your body. The third cardio workout is the one that is intense. Luckily, it's brief too.

The third cardio workout each week lands four days following your leg workout. If you still have a bit of residual leg soreness, no big deal: Proceed anyway. Some people refer to this type of workout as Zone 5 training or HIIT (high-intensity interval training), but I like to refer to it as "max heart rate training" or simply "intense cardio" because there are non-interval ways to do it, and—for reasons that will become clear in a minute—getting your heart pumping near your maximum heart rate is highly beneficial.

There are a few variations in the "classic" versions of this workout. All begin with five to ten minutes of warming up at an easy to moderate pace. HIIT has you modulating between near-all-out efforts that put you at 90 to 95 percent of your max HR, interspersed with bouts of lower intensity effort where you let your HR fall a bit before repeating the sequence.[113] Another approach is to start at an easy effort and build in a continuous and progressive manner—for example, increasing the level of resistance to your effort (think: increasing treadmill speed and incline)—until your effort plateaus, or starts to drop. (That actually mirrors how a VO_2 max test, a measure of fitness and endurance, is conducted.) There are many ways to do max heart rate training but the total time spent at near-all-out effort is always pretty brief: as short as about six minutes, and up to about sixteen minutes. Either works for this third cardio session.

What form of exercise you choose can vary. For example, you could hop on an assault bike—those stationary bikes with a fan and handles that you pump forward and back while you pedal. You'll soon realize that the fan is there to increase the resistance, not just to cool you down. Or you could use a stationary bike that lets you adjust the resistance of the pedals. You could also go sprint at a track or on a trail, or swim in a pool. The important thing is to do something in which you can really exert yourself without getting injured.

A "fun" HIIT session is this: brief five- to ten-minute warm-up, then pedal (or run, row, or swim, etc.) as hard and fast as you can for thirty seconds, then rest or slow down for sixty seconds, then another thirty seconds of all-out effort, then back again to sixty seconds of rest or low effort, and so on, for a total of six to twelve rounds of alternations. I do this on the assault bike once a week. I love-hate it.

You will quickly realize that with each round of all-out effort it gets tougher and tougher to recover, such that by rounds six to twelve, those sixty seconds of rest will seem to go by *extremely* fast. There is actually a neuroscientific basis for the warping of time perception we experience under stress that I discuss in the next chapter. The good news is, even though this workout is intense, the whole thing, including the warm-up, only takes about twenty-five minutes. At the end, you will feel fatigued, but remarkably, within five to ten minutes after stopping you will likely feel extra energized from all the adrenaline and norepinephrine you generated in your body and brain.[114] You will also have provided a great stimulus to improve your VO_2 max, and max HR, the importance of which I cover below.

Other options for this workout include the Cooper test, where you see how far you can go (run, swim, cycle, etc.) in twelve minutes of steady, hard effort.[115] That is a "fun" one too.

Or you can try to run your best mile time. This is something performance coach, author, and former elite runner Steve Magness has emphasized as being a terrific correlate of VO_2 max.[116] It's one of my favorite workouts. Here is how to do it properly:

First find a 400-meter track. Start by warming up with an easy jog of four to six laps slowly interspersing the occasional faster-paced 100 meters—not all out but just quickening your pace to about 60 to 70 percent of your subjective "run for your life" speed. Perhaps do that on one straight-track segment between turns on each warm-up lap. Once you feel properly warmed up, run four laps (which is 1,600 meters—about 9 meters shy of 1 mile). It's a skill to run the mile and pace everything just right for your best time. But you're not aiming to be a competitive miler here. So set out at a pace you can maintain for three laps—about 85 percent of "running for your life" speed, then push it harder on the last lap, or 95 percent of "running for your life" speed. The key is to pace yourself so you're not sprinting laps one to three and then forced to walk or jog the remainder. It can take a bit of practice but within a few weeks you'll know the pace to take for each lap. Almost everyone likes to really push the final 200 meters or so.

I test my approximate best mile time about once every two months lately. I'm not training to be a competitive miler but it's nice to have one version of the short intense cardio workout where I can track my progress across the year. I doubt I'll beat my best time from high school ever again, but it's fun to have an "a bit faster than last month" run. My goal is to maintain or reduce my mile time each time I run it.

And there is the Norwegian 4×4, if you want to try it.[117] That's where you warm up, and then run, bike, or row hard for four minutes, then rest or slow down for four minutes. Repeat this cycle for a total of four work-rest rounds.

As you can see with all these examples, the exact work-to-rest ratio and total time can vary dramatically, and yet all can be effective. What's key is that during the work periods, you're truly working hard. That is because, during the rest periods, you're allowing enough time for recovery so that you can again come back to a truly hard effort. Don't be overly caught up in the exact protocols. You can alter them if you like and still get the same results.

I'm recommending three different types of cardio training sessions every week because this variation is typically what delivers the best results over time for improving your VO_2 max. We're trying to balance duration and intensity in this program. It's best to emphasize both. You want longer moderate efforts and you want brief and very intense efforts. And while the shorter, intense efforts are extremely effective (and time efficient), they take longer to recover from compared to the longer, moderate efforts. Given that you're also balancing this cardio training with the resistance training, a blend of longer/lower, moderate, and brief/high intensity cardio training sessions is what works best for results across the board.

HOW IT WORKS:

The cardio workouts described above each help trigger beneficial adaptations. They all increase your heart's efficiency in delivering blood (and thus oxygen and vital nutrients) to the rest of the body.[118] They trigger capillary growth in your muscles, which allows more oxygen to move through these vessels during all activities.[119] They stimulate an increase in the number, size, and efficiency of your mitochondria, the energy producing organelles in our cells known to be critical for preventing chronic disease and premature aging. Further, they all acutely elevate levels of the catecholamines: dopamine, epinephrine, and norepinephrine.[120] Also, because they rely on a mixture of aerobic (oxygen dependent) and anaerobic (oxygen independent) processes, cardio of the types in this program increases metabolic flexibility, or your body's ability to rely on different fuel sources for energy. And that's just a small sampling of the many beneficial adaptations.[121]

The extent to which brief, high-intensity or longer, lower-intensity cardio triggers these different adaptations varies, but there is also synergy between them.[122] Those brief, intense cardio training sessions will allow you to move faster but with less effort on your long and medium cardio days, not unlike how getting stronger with low repetition heavy sets in the gym equates to you being able to move more weight on your higher repetition sets once you get stronger.

So, while people often debate which form of cardiovascular exercise is best for overall health and longevity, that's not the lens through which to look at it. I suggest a practical lens. (And you know by now, I don't believe in any best type of exercise; only the best way to structure an effective exercise program.) For instance, consider that your one-mile time is a good reflection of your VO_2

max.[123] Does that mean you should only do one mile distances for cardio? No. In fact, whether you're a competitive miler or simply using the one-mile time test as a fun workout and barometer of your VO_2 max, doing some longer/lower, moderate, and brief/high intensity cardio workouts across the week is how to get faster at the mile.

In science we love to isolate variables, so people have done the "which cardio exercise is best?" experiment. That research made clear that if you have to choose one type, you want to opt for brief/high intensity cardio rather than, say, three thirty- to forty-five-minute Zone 2/3 sessions.[124] But doing a mix of durations and intensities is recommended, and for the reasons mentioned above, it meshes well with your resistance training. A Zone 2/3 jog or hike for an hour the day before you train your legs with weights is no problem. Sprinting the day after leg training to failure? Not a good idea. The injury risk is too high.

Doing these three cardio training sessions also means you're logging a total of about two hours per week of cardio. Considering the immediate and long-term health benefits, that's a great return on investment.

We hear all the time about "fitness" and it reflects many things. But from a health perspective consider that two studies—one published in 2018 and another in 2022—both showed essentially the same thing, which is that as you move from the lowest to the higher tiers of cardiorespiratory fitness (one measure of that is your VO_2 max), your mortality risk drops.[125] These are meaningful shifts in life expectancy too. One of the studies states, "Those with the highest fitness had roughly five times lower mortality than the least fit."

Resistance training is less about cardiorespiratory fitness, but its effects in maintaining (or increasing) muscle mass and bone density, promoting cognitive function and healthy body recomposition, make a combination of resistance training and cardio training two of the three vital interlocking puzzle pieces for excellent physical health.

COMMON QUESTIONS:

Does doing three cardio training sessions per week prevent you from building muscle? And does resistance training harm my cardio efforts?

To be clear: If your goal is purely to put on as much muscle as possible, or to do an endurance event like a half marathon or marathon as fast as possible, there are better training programs for those specific goals. When splitting your time across both building muscle and building endurance, there's going to be a performance trade-off. You can't *maximize* for both at the same time because of so-called interference effects.[126]

That said, for vitality, health, longevity, aesthetics, and all-around fitness, you want to do both resistance training and cardio training. Research indicates that the interference effects are minimal when done on separate days at the duration and intensities similar to those in this foundational program.[127]

What if I play a sport?

If you're training for a competition or a race, or you play a sport like soccer or tennis or basketball, and you play hard for an hour or more one to two times per week, the program here is still great. You may want to do the lower number of work sets, and you'll really need to tend to your recovery and nutrition by making sure you get enough hours of quality sleep and calories—including, yes, enough quality protein, but also starches and fats.

Again, the program here will get you the most all-around fit as possible at any age. That does not mean you won't gain strength and muscle—you will. You will also burn fat. You'll increase your endurance too. And once you learn how different exercises impact your body, you can emphasize some and reduce others, per the suggestions I describe in this protocol. Exercise done correctly is very potent in that way. Assuming you pay attention to the points

I make about recovery too—that is, eat well and sleep well—I'm certain you'll achieve remarkable results with this program.

What if I haven't slept well, should I train or not?

If you are healthy, and you happen to have had a bad night's sleep—by which I mean only one to two hours less sleep than usual—then try to stick with your workout. There is a growing amount of data that say it can help offset some of the short-term cognitive disturbances from sleep loss.[128]

Just be careful not to push too hard in the gym (or in life) after a poor night's sleep as injuries happen more often when people have not slept enough.[129] And don't make it a regular thing to get less than enough sleep, and expect to remedy that with exercise. You'll end up sick, injured, or both. Maybe do some non-sleep deep rest (NSDR) (see Sleep Protocol 8) and then push through the workout. If you have had a really bad night's sleep for two or more nights in a row, for whatever reason, I suggest you get back on track with your sleep before exercising again. Consider some deliberate heat exposure (sauna or a hot bath, for example), and if you feel you *must* exercise, try a restorative activity, like stretching, light yoga, or just walking.

Is it better to eat before or after training?

There is no clear rule here. Personally, I prefer to train in the morning on an empty stomach. Figure out what works for you. It may be best to eat prior to training if you wake up hungry and you know that hunger will distract you during your workout, or you get dizzy or nauseous training on an empty stomach. Some people may find that eating about sixty to ninety minutes prior to exercise gives them an energy boost without the discomfort of feeling full. It's highly individual. Experiment with your timing of your workouts and meals.

If I miss a day of cardio or resistance training, should I change the weekly schedule?

It's hard to answer this one because . . . it depends. However, I would not change the order of your resistance or cardio training sessions across the week because the schedule starts to fall like dominoes, and it's hard to get back on track. But maybe something comes up and you can't do the long, slow cardio day as planned. I would not recommend moving that workout to the same day you train legs. I would simply skip the long cardio day and train your legs on schedule. Skipping leg day is a bad idea. You do three days of cardio per week, so having to miss one every now and again is not a huge deal. But you only train your legs directly once a week, and done correctly as outlined above it creates major positive systemic shifts in your brain and body. So when people say, "Don't skip leg day," it's not just about aesthetics. In fact, if I could only train once per week in the gym and do one cardio training session—not what I recommend, but if I *had* to—I would do leg day and I would do some sprints followed by light jogging four or five days later. That's just to illustrate a point about the potency of those two workouts. I recommend the full program described in this chapter.

Let's say you can't do the moderate cardio training session for whatever reason. You could, in theory, shift it to immediately after your arms workout that same day. But remember, you're scheduled to do the long, slow cardio session the very next day, and you don't want your legs to feel like noodles when you wake up the following morning for leg day! So think ahead a bit about your recovery.

I suggest you stick to the schedule as best you can, missing days here and there or doubling up when there is no other option. Plan your workouts, follow through, and if people get curious about how you're getting such great results, teach them the principles, or even better, share the program. No one owns this or any exercise program; they are all derivatives of each other anyway, and based on what science says works.

EXERCISE PROTOCOL

4

Incorporate Brief Mobility and Flexibility Work Two to Four Times per Week

WHAT TO DO:

- **Do four specific movements to improve your mobility, two to four times a week.**
- **Refer to the instructions below to target areas susceptible to injury as you do these movements.** Wrist, back, knee, hip, and shoulder injuries are common. The movements described here will ensure mobility in these areas. They aren't a guarantee against injuries, but they can help tremendously.

HOW IT WORKS:

First, I'm not giving you yet another workout to do. The current program—about three hours a week of resistance training, about two hours of cardio—is not terribly time-consuming, considering the years (literally!) it can add to your life. Still, I acknowledge that people's time is limited. That is why I suggest incorporating just a few minutes of mobility exercise two to four times per week. It can be done at the end of one of your other workouts, or any time of day really. It does not take long at all, only about ten minutes per session.

That might seem woefully inadequate to the mobility experts out there. I get it. I would love to add two thirty-minute mobility workouts to my own schedule but alas "my dance card is full," as they say. I'm assuming yours is too.

The good news is that some aspects of the training suggested in the earlier protocols in this chapter are pro-mobility and pro-flexibility too. Remember the emphasis on using a full range of motion for resistance training sets, as described in Exercise Protocol 2? Doing that will not only build your strength and muscles but can also enhance your flexibility and mobility. In fact, some studies find that full-range resistance training can be as effective as static stretching, a type of stretching in which you hold a muscle in a stretched, or elongated, position and gradually deepen the stretch using body weight. Controlling the eccentric, or lowering, phase in full-range resistance training may be critical for this effect, which makes sense as that is when the muscle is elongating.[130]

There are easy ways to get even more flexibility from resistance training too. In the resistance training video tutorials at protocolsbook.com/videos, I also emphasize some exercises that are hardest for a given muscle when the muscle is in the elongated, stretched position, as well as exercises where the tension is greatest when the muscle is in its shortened, contracted position. Consider a stiff-legged deadlift or similar variation for your hamstrings, glutes, and lower back—the so-called posterior chain. It involves holding a barbell or dumbbells and moving from standing to something resembling a toe-touch (or an attempt to) by lowering the weight under control toward the ground, and then standing up again. You can imagine the stretch to your hamstrings and lower back that movement provides if you use a full range of motion. Including some movements that are most challenging for a given muscle group when it is in the elongated position can help build flexibility and can help you remain "strong in any position," which assists mobility too.[131] Again, if any of this is confusing, I provide a gallery of movements to choose from at protocolsbook.com/videos.

I also hope you'll include the direct mobility exercises that I describe below in your weekly routine but even if you don't, by training the way I describe above, most people will improve their mobility, and flexibility too. We're talking about the ability to touch your toes while keeping your legs straight or just slightly bent, to hang from a bar with no pain, to twist around to look behind you while seated in a chair, to sit in a deep squat for one to two minutes (and be able to stand up at the end!), and so on. You can develop those basic abilities through resistance training with a full range of motion, and focusing on the relevant muscles at all positions in each rep.

There are many great ways to improve mobility. Here I have created what I believe is the minimal effective dose of it. And if you want to do more mobility work, please do!

At least two to four times a week, take ten minutes and do the following four movements. You can do these most any place and at any time.

1 Deep sumo squat, torso twist, point, and look up

Set your feet a few inches wider than your shoulders, then squat down as far as you can.

Put your elbows against the insides of your knees and your palms and fingers together in "prayer" position, and push out gently with your elbows until you feel a stretch in your hips and inner thighs. Then raise one arm and, with your index finger, point directly up at the ceiling (or as high overhead as you can) while keeping your other elbow against the inside of your knee. Let your gaze follow your finger, which will naturally have you twist your torso and turn your neck to raise that arm. Look directly up at your index finger for three to ten seconds. Inhale and exhale.

Then put your arm down, reset to the first squat position with both elbows against the insides of your knees. Place your hands in prayer position for three to ten seconds, and then raise your other arm up to point at the ceiling. Twist your torso and look up at your index finger for three to ten seconds. Repeat three times for each side. You may have to stand up between sets. That is fine.

This is a great movement because it gets you squatting deep, it improves your thoracic spine and neck mobility, and you'll also feel a decent stretch in your inner thighs and hips. It will also reveal if you have any asymmetries in your mobility (perhaps one side versus the other) which is common.

I demonstrate this movement here: protocolsbook.com/videos.

Note: *If you can't point and/or look all the way up to directly overhead, start by pointing and looking up at a lower angle. Gradually progress to pointing and looking directly overhead.*

2 Get your knees behind your glutes, one at a time

This is one I learned from mobility expert Kelly Starrett whom I mentioned earlier in this chapter. Since it may not be easy for most people to envision, try this: Start in a standing lunge by placing one foot in front of you and the other foot behind you. Bend your front knee and keep your rear leg straight or a bit bent. Now nudge the foot in front of you slightly farther out. Bend that front knee more and focus on stretching the hip flexors at the top of your back leg. You may need to lean your torso back a bit to really feel the hip flexor stretch. Okay, notice the knee of your back leg is now behind your glutes? That is what I mean by "get your knee behind your glutes." Slowly ease into this hip flexor stretch for ten to thirty seconds while exhaling. It's fine to reach up and look overhead while doing this, as that will help extend the hip flexor, but keep your attention on the back leg. Your front leg is there for stability and you can bend it to provide more rear-placed-leg hip stretch. Repeat for each side three times. I demonstrate this movement here: protocolsbook.com/videos.

Next, you're going to kneel on both knees. Then put one knee up in front of you (the foot of that same leg is thus flat on the ground). The shin of your rear leg is parallel to the ground. That means your back foot will be sole-facing-up. Place your hand on that raised front knee for stability and gently extend the back leg until you feel a stretch in your hip flexor. Again, think "I need to get my knee behind my glutes." Keep your torso upright, your eyes forward or up, and even lean slightly back at the waist. Hold the stretch for ten to thirty seconds. Repeat three to four times. Don't forget to breathe.

I demonstrate these movements here: protocolsbook.com/videos.

The reason to do this: Your hip flexors are located where your leg meets your pelvis. When you sit, your hip flexors are partially flexing. When you run, bike, or walk up a set of stairs, your hip flexors are repeatedly flexing as you bring your knee up and forward. Modern life has us flexing our hip flexors all the time. A key step toward good mobility is to make sure you can extend your hips. Hip extension is the opposite of hip flexion—it moves your knee away from the front of your pelvis, to a location *behind* you. Hence the directive here. Once you experience how good it feels during (and after!) this stretch, you'll be looking for ways to do it more often.

3 Get into a reverse tabletop position

Sit on the floor with your feet in front of you, the soles of your feet and butt on the ground, and with your knees bent. Place your hands at your sides a few inches away from your hips, with your palms down. Turn your hands so your fingers point away from you out to each side.

See if you can slowly push your pelvis up so that the tops of your legs and torso are parallel to the floor, and your knees are at a 90 degree right angle. Many people find they can't get into this "reverse tabletop" position for very long, if at all, but some can. See if you can hold that position for ten seconds.

If you can't do this, practice doing this each week for three sets of however long you can hold it until you can easily remain in this position for ten seconds. Once you can do that, move to the following progression:

Sit on the floor with your feet in front of you, with the soles of your feet and butt on the ground, and your knees bent. Place your hands just behind your hips, with your palms down. Turn your hands so your fingers point backward.

See if you can *slowly* push your pelvis up so that the tops of your legs and torso are parallel to the floor, and your knees are at a 90 degree right angle.

Once again, the goal is to get into the flat reverse tabletop position and hold for ten seconds. For some people this will take a while to achieve. For others it will be easy depending on your level of shoulder mobility. These movements are also great for wrist mobility, too, by the way.

Once that final "reverse tabletop" variation is achievable, then you can start to experiment SLOWLY with this next movement. Sit on the floor with your legs straight in front of you, heels on the ground and the soles of your feet facing forward. Place your hands flat on the ground just behind you, with your fingers pointed backward. Keep them there as you gently and slowly scoot your glutes forward. Remember, your hands stay flat on the ground and fixed in place. Keep scooting forward until you feel a stretch in your biceps and shoulders. Exhale, and see if you can ease into it another centimeter or so. Once you can extend your shoulders back behind you with the edges of your hands touching, you are getting to quite mobile shoulder status.

The reason to do this: Tight shoulders can arise from many sources, but often there will be people who can raise their arms to the front or to the side without issue but who don't have the mobility to raise their arms up behind them, meaning they don't have much shoulder *extension* mobility. This is made worse by desk work, and the chin-down/forward-leaning posture that is nearly ubiquitous nowadays, thanks to excessive amounts of time texting and scrolling on our phones. Shoulder tightness and neck and back pain are often linked too. Improving your shoulder extension mobility is straightforward. It just requires a willingness to work through these progressions.

Wrist, back, knee, hip, and shoulder injuries are super common and many can be avoided by a quality strength training program and by including some basic mobility exercises like the ones in this protocol. Some quick movements you can incorporate in your routine are the "face pulls," which strengthen these and other areas, as well as neck training a few times a week, as described in Exercise Protocol 2 and shown at protocolsbook.com/videos. You will be amazed at how strong, mobile, and stable your shoulders, neck, and upper back will be if you do.

Do not push too fast when it comes to mobility work! Work through the progressions listed above over the course of months or more. Make it painless but deliberate, and you will build and maintain much greater shoulder, hip, knee, back, and wrist mobility.

4 Practice the Founder pose

The final mobility exercise is the Founder pose, made popular by chiropractor Eric Goodman, who has served as a conditioning coach for numerous top athletes in sports ranging from cycling to surfing to water polo. I was referred to his work by friends who previously had back pain and shoulder pain, and who sit a lot of the day. "You have to try this thing called Founder pose," I kept hearing. Mind you, in my role, I hear that about a thousand times per day about a variety of things, so I'm not easily moved to try them. But I heard this decompresses the spine and trains your musculature to work properly as a functional unit.

I tried Eric's Founder pose and, wow, it's great. Not just because it feels good while you do it but your posture improves. And it definitely made me more flexible.

So what is it? It's similar to the "chair pose" in yoga but while that mainly emphasizes the musculature of the front of the body, the Founder pose emphasizes mobility of your posterior and lateral chains: your hamstrings, glutes, lower and upper back, and thoracic muscles.

Here is how you do it: Stand with your feet a bit wider than your shoulders, toes pointing slightly out.

Stand as tall as you can by pressing your heels down and lifting your head up, as if a string were tied to the top of your head but your heels were fastened down to the ground.

Hinge your hips so you lean slightly forward at the waist—almost as though you're about to sit in a chair but freeze only about a third of the way down into the movement. Your hips and glutes are back behind your heels, and your knees are just slightly bent. Keep your head as far away from your glutes as possible. You should feel a stretch in your lower back and hamstrings. If not, lean farther forward at the waist until you do.

Raise your chest, and with your arms at your sides, turn your thumbs out and away from the midline of your body (away from your belly button).

Keeping your thumbs rotated out, start to slowly lift your arms. Stop when you feel more stretching in your lower back and/or the backs of your legs.

Now move your hips back a few inches more. And raise your chest and head, aka "make your spine long," still pressing your heels down.

Raise your arms a bit more if you can (thumbs still pointed away from your navel in external rotation), all the while pushing your heels down.

Hold this position for five more seconds then stand up straight.

Repeat that one to two times, as often as every day or even just a few times a week.

Thank me later. No, thank Eric Goodman!

I demonstrate this movement here: protocolsbook.com/videos.

CHAPTER 3

PROTOCOLS

for STRESS CONTROL

I, like everyone else, don't like the feeling of being stressed, but I have grown accustomed to the idea that life inevitably involves stress. Whether it was my high school classmates (most of whom were very driven), the athletes I've met, or the students, professors, and people in tech or creative fields around me, I have always found that stress accompanies ambition, and that for many of the top achievers, it's a constant.

The weird thing is that many of the unambitious people I have known often said they were stressed out too. Lack of direction, lack of money, the feeling they were slipping behind in life, health issues, and more . . . Eventually I had to conclude that this was indeed part of life—like breathing, sleeping, or eating. That meant there had to be a good way to address it.

The problem was that when I looked to see what the science said about stress, it was uniformly negative. It made clear that stress wasn't just uncomfortable, it was damaging to the brain and body. And that only made stress more stressful. Moreover, the whole framing of stress seemed wrong, or at least rather one-sided.

For instance, "fight or flight" is one of the most common phrases we hear when the topic of stress comes up. It's easy to remember and it seems science-y—because it sounds like it *could* describe how the brain and body respond to stress. Unfortunately, it's more misleading than informative. We also often hear that the stress response is an inconvenient holdover from our evolutionary past. Meaning, the uncomfortable state of arousal we call stress was helpful for us long ago, propelling us to escape from saber-toothed tigers and other large predators, but it's no longer useful.

I always appreciate when science shows up in a conversation, but I confess phrases like "fight or flight" make me shake my head. It's not just that they are misleading; they also don't provide any valuable information about how to navigate the stress response. And actually, the stress response is no holdover. And research has shown that the beliefs we hold about stress can change how stress impacts our health, for better or for worse, so we need to be careful what we tell ourselves about it.[1]

Stress is an area I've thought a lot about from a neuroscience perspective. My lab has studied it in animals and humans. Decades into my career, I now know that there is, in fact, a good way to address it. There are excellent stress management tools based in science. So, given how pervasive stress is, I am especially excited to share the information in this chapter.

First let's begin with the facts. Forget saber-toothed tigers. Many of the same situations that stress us out now have been stressing out humans for thousands of years. An argument with a loved one, a persistent pain of unknown cause, a worry about a child, a looming payment, and on and on. Scenarios like these are not unique to modern times.

A good way to think about stress is this: Stress is nature's attempt to create a single solution to all matters that might be, or actually are, urgent. I'll say that again. Stress is nature's attempt to create a single solution to all matters that might be, or actually are, urgent.

So no matter what the stressor (and there are an infinite number of them out there), the basic architecture of the stress response—that is, what happens to our brain and body when we perceive a stressor—is the same. Cortisol and other hormones, including the catecholamine neuromodulators adrenaline and norepinephrine, flood our system. Adrenaline, or epinephrine, as well as cortisol are released from our adrenal glands. Norepinephrine is released from specific locations in the brain including the locus coeruleus, which we discussed in chapter 1 and chapter 2. Dopamine is released in the brain and in the body too. All of these chemicals change the activity level of specific neuronal circuits and, in doing so, initiate a coordinated shift in the ways our organs function, and thus in our overall state of mind and body. We often hear about the increase in heart rate, breathing, and blood pressure that stress brings about. Less discussed, however, are the perceptual changes. Stress changes our visual field and narrows our mental attention.[2] We become fixated on the events related to the stressor: "How did this happen? How can I undo this?!" Stress causes our perception of time to slow down. Seconds start to feel like minutes, minutes like hours, hours like days . . . Meanwhile, our rate of thinking—the sheer number of thoughts we have per second—seems to speed up. And yet, our cognitive flexibility is reduced. We default to simple black-and-white thinking. Nuance evaporates. Mild-to-moderate stress makes us feel jittery whereas intense stress can cause us to freeze. At its extreme, it can make people feel as if they have left their body, as if they are viewing themselves from above.[3]

While that all sounds dreadful, we must remember that the stress response is adaptive. The purpose of it is to put our brain and body into a state that gives us the best chance of addressing the problem at hand. A single solution. In an ideal world, the degree of stress response would perfectly match the stressor we face. Running late? A little bit more arousal to help us focus on the key items we need to get out the door with grace would be perfect. See our toddler running toward the traffic? A huge surge in energy to quickly grab them is what we want! In fact, the parts of our nervous system that govern stress—called the autonomic nervous system—can be calibrated to generally match our stress level to the stressor we face, from mild to severe, from brief to ongoing.[4] But nowadays, the many comforts most people enjoy thanks to technology—indoor heating and air conditioning, abundant food and shelter, and all in all our general lack of actual survival stressors—have our autonomic nervous systems uncalibrated. We are far more labile under the constant barrage of minor psychological stressors all day and night, and a lot of people are in a constant state of stress related to things they simply cannot control or influence even slightly. Put simply, the frequency and/or magnitude of the stress response is far too high relative to the stressors many people face. The occasional bout of stress lasting a few hours or less is no big deal, and even a few days is something our bodies can handle without long-term consequences. Once we experience a few weeks to a month or more of daily (which usually also means nightly) stress, that's when we start to suffer. Chronically elevated resting blood pressure and heart rate, not sleeping well or enough due to rumination or feeling "tired but wired," and other shifts to our internal state become detrimental to our immediate and long-term health. We've all heard the laundry list of things that stress harms: our hormones, memory, mood, and decision-making ability, as well as the many diseases it makes worse or can bring about to our heart, brain, gut, and liver. The body of evidence that chronic stress is bad for us is vast and robust.

Yet some stress is good for us. In fact, the occasional spike in our stress hormones can increase testosterone[5] and improve our immune system functioning during the hours that follow.[6] In the short term, it can improve our memory.[7] The problems arise when the intensity or the duration of the stress response is too great.

Eliminating stress from our lives is unrealistic. So our goal with stress should be twofold. First, we need to be able to adjust the intensity and the duration of our stress response so we can better handle stress in the moment. Second, many of us need to increase our stress threshold—that is, the subjective point at which events and thoughts trigger large amounts of adrenaline release in our body—so our stress response is calibrated to any stressors we may encounter.

Ahem, I mean, that we *will* encounter. When adrenaline release occurs as the consequence of tiny things, that is not good. It negatively affects our physical health and relationships, including our relationship with ourselves. Do you like being around you when you're stressed? Didn't think so. We can change our relationship to stress through cognitive reframing, but an effective approach is to learn to quickly control our stress response once it hits, and to periodically reset our stress threshold to a level that best serves us. We can't always control what life throws at us, but we can indeed control our stress response, and we can raise our stress threshold. That's what this chapter is all about.

I first became interested in investigating the neuroscientific mechanisms behind stress back in 2015. At the time, grit, resilience, and mental toughness were popular themes in books and media. And those are great qualities. The examples—both historical and contemporary—of people being gritty and resilient and mentally tough are there to remind us that humans harbor within them an enormous capacity to manage and even channel their stress.

While there is a lot known about the neural circuits and hormones that control the stress response, I specifically wanted to understand the mechanisms that determine its intensity and duration. I wanted to know which features of the stress response, like heart rate, blood pressure, attentional narrowing, and so on, were amenable to adjustment in real time. I also wanted to know whether there are levers for adjusting the duration, the intensity, and maybe even the probability of the stress response getting triggered in the first place.

I was able to find some data about stress inoculation,[8] including some studies supporting the idea that certain forms of early-life stress can set the stage for resilience later in life by virtue of how they tune the physiology of the stress response to better match the intensity of a stressor.[9] But it was hard to find evidence for specific tools that kids or adults could reliably apply to recalibrate the stress response across different circumstances. I wanted to find mechanistic data that could be translated broadly and that were accessible for the average person.

I continued my search. I found studies on the benefits of positive self-talk[10] but just as many studies on its lack of effectiveness.[11] Despite the fact that we are all born with the same biological stuff—adrenals that release adrenaline, locus coeruleus neurons that release norepinephrine, and prefrontal cortices that can exert top-down control over our impulses and feeling states—I just couldn't find any really convincing studies in humans that pointed to tools people could use to improve their capacity to manage stress. Meanwhile, we know that slogans like "Just do it" and mantras like "Embrace the suck," or telling ourselves "You got this," can be good for pushing us through a stressor we have chosen to face—a long run, the final reps of a hard set in the gym, a study session or big exam—but most people would agree that self-talk fails the vast majority of the time when the stressor isn't one we've chosen, or when our efforts have us falling short of our goals. And at some point, real life brings the sorts of stressors we simply cannot control, like a medical emergency or the loss of a beloved friend or family member. In those circumstances, "Just do it" just doesn't do it.

Of course, much has been researched and written about what I call offline practices to manage stress. Meditation, massages, vacations, hot baths, deep breaths, talk therapy. Great! Who doesn't love a massage at the end of a hard day? Meditation is powerful as a tool to buffer against the stress response; a randomized clinical trial conducted by researchers at Georgetown University found that people with generalized anxiety disorder who meditated experienced a noteworthy reduction in pro-inflammatory cytokines—chemical messengers essential to our immune system but that can also trigger a stress response—compared to those who didn't meditate.[12] Other studies, including one done by my lab at Stanford in collaboration with my colleague David Spiegel's lab, also at Stanford, have shown clear benefits of meditation practices as short as five minutes per day on stress, mood, and sleep.[13] That might seem like a trivial level of time commitment, especially given the many benefits of meditation.[14]

But I wanted to know how people can navigate stress while they are in the throes of the stress response. When their pulse is racing, their vision is blurry, their hands are shaking, and all they can think about is the stressor and the potential bad outcomes from it. That's when the capacity to manage stress matters most. Not offline, but in the moment.

As I pointed out above, the stress response is universal. Whatever the specific stressor might be, the stress response is the same. It varies in degree, not kind. This suggests that if we have reliable tools to reduce the stress response in one context, we ought to be able to reduce it in another. The problem? No one had dissected the universal features of stress control, only the stress response.

One valuable thing everyone should know about the stress response, though, is that it is asymmetric: It starts extremely fast and turns off relatively slowly. The adrenaline release that is the first domino of the stress response happens in seconds or less and can continue for several minutes after we perceive a stressor.[15] Think of a time when you were groggy from just waking up and you picked up your phone to see a disturbing text. BOOM! You are wide awake and ready to move in an instant. That's the speed of adrenaline in action.

Then, even after the stressor is resolved, the stress response persists. Imagine getting a text that says, "I think Mom was on the flight that just crashed," and ten minutes later, "I just spoke to her, she wasn't on there. She's fine." Your feeling of relief will no doubt outpace how quickly your body settles down. That's an extreme example, but the same thing applies when someone almost sideswipes you while driving, and you swerve just in time to avoid a collision. A shot of adrenaline wicks out through your body in an instant, and almost as fast, norepinephrine is released to ramp up attentional circuits in your brain. Cognitively, you realize you're safe almost as quickly as you thought you were about to get hit, but your body and mind don't relax immediately. More often than not, we plummet into the stress response and it takes time to return to baseline. And that's when everything turns out okay. When stressors persist, you experience wave after wave of adrenaline. And while the basic circuits for stress are the same in everyone, seldom discussed is that not everyone has the same threshold, or trigger point, for a stress response to kick off. For some people it's as if that first domino is fixed in cement. Such people are rare. For most people, however, the domino falls too easily. I wanted to understand this aspect of stress too, in order to develop tools anyone can use to raise their stress threshold, to allow them to calibrate their autonomic set point. That is, the balance point that our nervous system works to maintain—so that the stress response happens when it's needed and not when it isn't. Even better would be to find ways such that when stress does happen, it occurs in proportion to the stressor. I wanted these tools to be mechanistic and behavioral, not pharmacological, because pharmacological tools—while they can be helpful—don't allow for real-time adjustments. You swallow a pill and that's that. And they have to be taken before stress arrives, which is problematic because we don't always know when stressors are coming. I also wanted to develop tools that do not rely on practice, like cognitive behavioral therapy, which is great but can take a fair amount of time to master[16] and doesn't always translate across stressors very well; there is evidence both for and against generalizability.[17] Like all protocols in this book, I wanted tools for stress management that could be effective the first time and every time because they are anchored in hardwired circuits and processes we all possess. So I dove into the research on the physiology of stress to come up with a different way to frame the whole concept of stress. And stress control. That led to . . .

The Seesaw Model

Think about the stress response as existing somewhere along a spectrum of arousal, with very low arousal at one end of the spectrum and very high arousal at the other. At the extremely low arousal end is a comatose state. Slightly more aroused than that would be deep sleep, then light sleep. Then toward the middle of the spectrum is a state in which we are alert but calm (which incidentally is the ideal state for most of our waking activities). As we progress further along toward the highest arousal end of the spectrum, we enter mild stress, then severe stress, and finally, full-blown panic. When we think about stress on a spectrum of low-to-high arousal, we realize that arousal—and what increases or decreases arousal—is the thing to focus on if we wish to deliberately lessen the stress response.

Where we happen to be on the spectrum of arousal at any given moment reflects the level of activity in our autonomic nervous system. Our autonomic nervous system regulates involuntary functions like our heart rate, digestion, blood pressure, and breathing. It also controls our level of alertness, and thus our ability to focus. It is comprised of two sets (sometimes called "arms") of neural circuits: the parasympathetic nervous system (PNS) and the sympathetic nervous system (SNS). These function more or less independently of one another, but their balance of activities combines to determine our arousal level, and thus our overall brain and bodily state.[18]

But what sets the balance between these two systems? Or, to put it another way, what regulates our autonomic nervous system? There are three main categories of autonomic regulators. The first is our twenty-four-hour circadian rhythm.[19] If you follow a typical diurnal schedule—awake in the daytime and asleep for a major portion of the night—then your SNS activity levels will dominate in the daylight hours and your PNS will dominate at night. In fact, the incredible impact your circadian rhythm has on your ability to reason,[20] exert physical effort,[21] and resist infections[22] stems from how it controls the balance of SNS versus PNS activity. In the morning and early daytime, elevated SNS activity (sometimes called "sympathetic tone") caused by a natural and healthy increase in our baseline levels of cortisol makes us physically stronger and better able to focus, whereas in the later evening and at night, when our baseline cortisol levels are markedly lower, our parasympathetic tone is elevated, and we become mentally and physically weaker, and our immune system becomes far less capable of warding off infections.[23] (Circadian variation in the expression of specific genes and the actions of various molecules—neuromodulators, hormones, peptides, etc.—are what underlie those dramatic morning-versus-nighttime variations in autonomic tone, as discussed in chapter 1.)

The second category of things that control our autonomic nervous system, and thus our level of arousal, are the sensory inputs—or stimuli, as neuroscientists call them—that we experience. For example, our level of physical comfort or pain, how well-fed or hungry we happen to be (not surprisingly, hunger makes us more alert), whether we are in a brightly lit or dim environment, the environment is quiet or loud, et cetera. And, of course, by the presence or absence of psychological stressors. In general, when we are hungry, thirsty, tired, or otherwise in need of basic sustenance, our arousal levels increase and, with that, our propensity to think and move increases. It should be obvious why that is adaptive. (It helps us seek out food, water, etc.)

The third category of things that control our autonomic nervous system is pharmacologic. Caffeine and other stimulants are sympathomimetic, meaning they stimulate the SNS and increase arousal.[24] Other drugs promote PNS activation, and thus decrease arousal levels. For example, alcohol and barbiturates indirectly increase PNS circuit activity,[25] as does the molecule apigenin, which is found in chamomile tea.[26] By the way, if you're wondering why alcohol initially makes people more talkative and alert before it makes them drowsy or has them pass out, it's because before it reduces central nervous system activity and lowers arousal, alcohol first transiently stimulates the SNS. "It lifts you up before it drops you," as they say.

Autonomic means "automatic" and indeed our sympathetic and parasympathetic nervous systems are, for the most part, not under our direct conscious control. We of course can adjust them indirectly. We just discussed three categories of ways to do that. The pathways and mechanisms by which different activities like exercise,[27] or mechanical inputs like massage or a warm bath,[28] or drugs like caffeine[29] elevate or lower arousal by adjusting the activity of our SNS or PNS are fairly well known, but again, it's crucial to note these are all indirect ways of adjusting autonomic arousal. As such, they tend to be slow and hard to titrate—meaning hard to get just right. Moreover, some, like barbiturates or prescription stimulants, have addictive potential and/or are costly.

There is, however, one major exception to all of this: one lever by which we can quickly, directly, and reliably change our level of autonomic arousal by shifting the balance of SNS versus PNS activity. That lever is our respiration pattern, aka our breathing.

Why? Because the neural circuits that control our breathing are part of our autonomic nervous system. In fact, they are the one (and only!) component of it that is both autonomic—breathing works just fine without us having to think about it—but that we can also consciously and directly control at any moment we choose. The same cannot be said about our heart rate, digestion, or immune system. As my colleague at Stanford, David Spiegel, MD, has described it to me, breathing and the neural centers that control breathing represent a bridge between our conscious and unconscious mind. We will return to this idea shortly, but to understand the specific patterns of breathing that allow us to consciously and directly control our stress response, and to understand the best tools for adjusting our stress threshold, we need to take the autonomic spectrum—that continuum spanning from deep states of calm to intense states of panic I described earlier—and turn it into a seesaw.

A seesaw? Correct. The simplest model for understanding how to control stress is a seesaw: parasympathetic at one end and sympathetic at the other. When the seesaw is tilted toward the parasympathetic end, we feel calm and relaxed. Tilt it further in that direction and we start drifting off to sleep. A flat, balanced seesaw represents when we are alert, but calm. Tilt it a bit in the other direction, toward the sympathetic end, and we feel more alert and energized. Tilt it further, and we feel stressed. At its steepest tilt, we are in full-blown panic. Reducing the intensity or duration of the stress response can be accomplished either by increasing the load on the parasympathetic side, by reducing the load on the sympathetic side, or both. How do you do that? We just need to understand a bit about the neural circuits and physiology of the SNS and PNS. And how breathing impacts each of these.

Because it turns out that inhales and exhales modulate the activity of our autonomic nervous system. Inhales reduce PNS activity, leading to relatively more SNS activity and thus, arousal. Exhales directly increase PNS activity. This means your heart rate is faster during inhales than during exhales—which incidentally is the basis of heart rate variability (HRV). Higher HRV in sleep and throughout your day is better than lower HRV, because it means PNS activity is periodically slowing your heart rate down. It's a good marker of your body controlling its own level of arousal, and keeping stress in check.[30] More on all that later but for now, it's going to be helpful to understand what "feeling stressed" is about at a neurochemical level. If you are stressed, that likely means that adrenaline and cortisol have been released and are circulating in your body at higher-than-typical levels, and that norepinephrine has been released at higher-than-typical levels.[31] You can't just make those molecules go away with positive self-talk. Also, when stress hits, your prefrontal cortex changes its pattern of electrical firing in a way that limits the range of solutions you can come up with to a problem.[32] It even changes your ability to link previous experiences in insightful ways.[33] Most of us are familiar with this stress-induced black-and-white thinking. These facts should help alleviate some of the frustration you may experience when someone tells you to "just relax," and you can't. Or when someone says, "Don't worry, this too shall pass." The first form of encouragement ignores that we must actively do something to our *physiology* to relax. You can't out-think adrenaline. The latter encouragement is spot on, as stress does indeed hinder our ability to see the big picture, but it's not particularly helpful in the moment. It's sort of like telling you that the splitting headache you're suffering from right now won't suck in the future. Fortunately, there is a way to get right to the physiology of the stress response. Rather than try to directly reduce sympathetic tone, you need to instead tilt the seesaw back toward the parasympathetic side by increasing the activity of your PNS. That is going to be the fastest way to calm down in real time whenever you are feeling stressed.

Resilience defined

If you think about it, this is a big part of what resilience is really about. It's not our ability to tolerate or eliminate the stress response but rather our ability to reduce its intensity quickly and in real time, when our arousal exceeds a useful level, so that we can move forward. Resilience is our ability to control stress. Sometimes that means going from extreme stress to very alert and energized, so we can perform a task and quickly problem-solve under intense pressure. Other times it means taking ourselves from endlessly looping thoughts to deep sleep. Resilience is also about an ability to deliberately increase our stress threshold, so life's minor stressors don't disproportionally hijack our mind and body. Once you learn how to do those two things, then you will truly be in the driver's seat.

Maybe that all sounds overly simplistic. Easy to say but harder to do. Well, it turns out there are science-supported tools to adjust your stress response in real time and to raise your stress threshold, and they work exceedingly well—and fast. They can also work the first time, and every time, because they are grounded in biological mechanisms and circuits that you already have inside you and can access. Some involve adopting a specific pattern of breathing, but they are not breathwork. After all, when we find ourselves in a high stress situation, we can't run off and do five minutes of box breathing! Other protocols don't involve breathing at all. I've been blessed to play a partial role in the discovery and application of several of these stress control protocols, although like so many other scientific "discoveries," aspects of them were known about and used by nonscientists in other contexts first. None of us gets the patent. The following pages explain what they are, how they work, and how to use them.

STRESS CONTROL PROTOCOL

1

Do One to Three Physiological Sighs to Reduce Stress Fast

WHAT TO DO:

- **Breathe in the pattern known as the *physiological sigh*.** Inhale deeply through your nose until your lungs are full (your belly should expand out while you inhale), then sharply inhale a second time, also through your nose, to maximally inflate your lungs. Then slowly exhale through your mouth until your lungs are empty of air. Repeat this in-in-out breathing pattern up to three times, in succession, as needed to reduce your stress level (meaning, your level of autonomic arousal) fast.

HOW IT WORKS:

Physiological sighs are, to my knowledge, the fastest and most effective way there is to deliberately calm yourself down. Often just one physiological sigh does the trick.

That's because our state of mind and body changes our breathing but our breathing also changes our state of mind and body.[34] Remember the locus coeruleus that releases norepinephrine to make us alert? Well, specific populations of neurons involved in specific patterns of breathing connect directly to and modulate this release from the locus coeruleus.[35]

The conversation between the neurons in your brainstem that control breathing also extends downward, into your spinal cord, which contains neurons that in turn control the muscles between your ribs (called the intercostals) and a dome-shaped muscle attached to the bottom of your rib cage called the diaphragm that actively inflates and deflates your lungs.[36]

When we inhale, oxygen enters our body, fills our lungs, then passes from our lungs into our bloodstream. That only happens because our lungs are not just two big, hollow bags; they contain hundreds of millions of tiny sacs called alveoli, which inflate with air as we inhale. The walls of the alveoli are extremely thin—about 1/2000th of a millimeter (!)—and yet rich with capillaries, the smallest diameter blood vessels. Together, they allow oxygen to move from the air-filled alveoli into the bloodstream. Having hundreds of millions of alveoli greatly increases the surface area through which oxygen can pass into our blood, and thus increases the amount of oxygen we absorb with each breath. (As wild as it sounds, you have approximately 70 to 100 square meters—about the size of a regulation tennis court—of alveolar surface area packed inside your lungs.) Big, deep breaths inflate more alveoli and the more alveoli that inflate, the more oxygen passes into your bloodstream to get delivered to your organs, including your brain.[37]

Carbon dioxide from the bloodstream passes into the alveoli—again through capillaries—and then is expelled from your body when you exhale. We need both oxygen and carbon dioxide, but we need them in the right balance. If we breathe too little, carbon dioxide builds up in our brain and bloodstream, leading to headaches and tiredness.[38] If we breathe too much—rapidly inhaling and exhaling, or what we typically call hyperventilation—we expel too much carbon dioxide, which is problematic because carbon dioxide is crucial for making sure oxygen gets to our brain cells. If you've ever wondered why it's advised to breathe into a paper bag if you're having a panic attack, it's to recapture some of the carbon dioxide that would otherwise be expelled. In this chapter you'll learn faster and better ways to calm down, but the logic is the same. Overbreathing causes anxiety, dizziness, confusion, poor sleep, and even muscle spasms.[39]

As mentioned in the introduction to this chapter, the neurons in our brainstem that control our breathing represent a bridge between our conscious and unconscious mind. They are equipped to sense the ratio of oxygen to carbon dioxide in our blood, which prompts any necessary alterations in our breathing pattern to keep us alive and well. That happens regardless of whether we are exercising hard or deeply relaxed—it even happens while we sleep.[40] Unlike other autonomic neural circuitry, however, we can take immediate conscious control of these neurons. We can decide "I'm going to extend my next exhale a bit" or "I'm going to take one more inhale before holding my breath" and—voila!—we can make that happen. We just don't have that level of conscious control over any other autonomic function. There are some reported examples of people who used biofeedback to learn to directly control their heart rate or the size of the pupils of their eyes, but that requires a fair amount of training.[41] Extended exhales and physiological sighs are something that anyone can do.

Certain internal states are associated with certain respiratory patterns. And by deliberately changing how we breathe, we can shift our internal state. That's a big deal and something I wish they had taught us in grade school. Alas, it wasn't until recently that Western science embraced controlled studies of respiration and, in doing so, revealed what had been known in Eastern traditions for thousands of years. We owe it to a small set of dedicated researchers, mostly neuroscientist Jack Feldman's lab at UCLA, for discovering how the brain controls breathing, both our unconscious reflexive breathing and deliberate breathing, and how they impact our emotional and cognitive states.[42] Before and during our discussion on the *Huberman Lab* podcast, Jack told me stories of setting out to study this topic in the early 2000s, and a luminary of neuroscience making fun of him at meetings. He would jab: "Why would you study something as boring as breathing? Why don't you study something important, like memory?"[43] (That guy studied memory.) Jack knew to ignore him and follow his intuition. His work ignited a field that is now positively impacting the mental and physical health of people of all ages. Detecting and modifying certain breathing patterns also turns out to be important for predicting heart attacks,[44] strokes,[45] and seizures,[46] and for preventing sudden infant death syndrome (SIDS).[47] Some of his recent work has also shed light on the fact that some opioid drugs can lead to death because of how they change the firing patterns of the neurons that control breathing.[48] It is fair to say that Jack's work has literally saved lives.

Breathing isn't just about getting oxygen into your lungs; it also helps control heart rate. While you can't directly control your heart rate, you can leverage the fact above and use your breathing to control it indirectly. Deliberately inhaling more vigorously or longer (or both) increases your heart rate, whereas deliberately exhaling more vigorously or for longer slows your heart rate down, through a process called respiratory sinus arrhythmia. Exhales also activate a specific branch of the vagus nerve, which is part of the PNS, which in turn reduces the rate of electrical activity in neurons of the sinoatrial node of the heart, your heart's natural pacemaker. So deliberately emphasizing the intensity and/or duration of your exhales for a few breathing cycles will caaaaalm youuuu dooooown. The breathing pattern described in this protocol does just that.

Once you learn the relationship between breathing and heart rate, and deploy the physiological sigh to reduce your heart rate on the spot, it gives you a significant feeling of confidence in dealing with stress, and uncertain circumstances too. You no longer have to be afraid you will get stuck in an anxiety response in a key moment, or any moment for that matter. You also realize that what most people say to themselves or others when stress hits—"Take a deep breath"—is the exact *opposite* of what we need to do! When stress hits we should do a big exhale. It is when we really draw out that exhale that our heart rate starts to slow down.

So why am I recommending "Do one to three physiological sighs to calm down fast" and not just "Do a big exhale"? And why aren't I suggesting box breathing, a popular breathing pattern that asks you to inhale-hold-exhale-hold, each in equal duration? Because some breathing techniques are far more potent and fast acting than others for stress reduction. And physiological sighs are particularly powerful for that purpose, because they capitalize on a hardwired set of neural circuits and neuromuscular pathways, which at once slow our heart rate down and adjust our oxygen-to-carbon-dioxide ratio in our brain and our bloodstream. The first two steps of the physiological sigh—the long inhale, followed by the quick inhale—are vital because of those hundreds of millions of alveoli we discussed. The insides of alveoli are a bit damp, not unlike a deflated balloon that once held water. And they tend to stick together due to surface tension. The long inhale inflates many alveoli, and the second quick inhale that immediately follows helps generate the force needed to reinflate alveoli that would otherwise stay deflated. This is especially effective when you inhale through your nose, because nasal breathing generates more resistance than mouth breathing and thus more force to reinflate those alveoli. Doing a physiological sigh also stimulates a collateral (meaning a branch of a neural pathway) that emerges from the brainstem area controlling your breathing and reaches other brain areas important for emotional and cognitive control.[49] Thus, physiological sighs, unlike just a big exhale or box breathing, are a three-pronged tool to quickly (1) slow your heart rate, (2) reestablish proper oxygen-to-carbon-dioxide ratios in your brain and bloodstream, and (3) engage brain areas that let you think logically about your situation. It's adaptive biological engineering at its best and works to calm you down.

Infants do physiological sighs reflexively.[50] Animals do too.[51] Observe a dog right before it goes down for a nap. You'll see that double inhale, long exhale pattern. Rats physiological sigh when placed into a claustrophobic environment.[52] People reflexively do physiological sighs about once every few minutes when working[53] and even in their sleep to reset their oxygen-to-carbon-dioxide ratio.[54]

In fact, you have dedicated sets of neurons in your brainstem for generating physiological sighs.[55] Nature just doesn't create discrete neural pathways by accident; that's how important this breathing pattern is. One respiratory region, the pre-Bötzinger complex, controls your rhythmic breathing, the regular alternation of inhales and exhales.[56] But a second region, the parafacial nucleus, controls breathing that involves double inhales, double exhales, or any combination of inhales and exhales in ratios other than the 1:1 inhale-exhale pattern.[57] The parafacial nucleus does things other than generate physiological sighs but that's one of its primary functions.

I'd like to clarify that physiological sighs are not breathwork. *Breathwork* refers to setting aside five to twenty minutes to do a specific breathing pattern (or designated sequence of patterns) to get you into a specific state of mind and body. Physiological sighs are a naturally occurring breathing cycle that we can deliberately recreate. And they are the fastest way to consciously tilt your seesaw to the parasympathetic side of your autonomic nervous system.

Do it before public speaking or a hard conversation. Do it when you're stuck in traffic or late to an important meeting and starting to feel your tension level rise. Do it to stop yourself from overreacting to an offhand comment. It won't guarantee that you'll always do the right thing in response, but it will put you in a better frame of body and mind, so that you have the best chance of navigating the stress that comes from these or similar situations.

There are data showing that doing physiological sighs outside of stressful moments can help buffer you against future stress too.[58] Several years ago, my lab collaborated with psychiatrist David Spiegel to investigate just that.[59] We conducted a study that randomized 108 participants to one of four groups. One group did five minutes per day of cyclic physiological sighing: Inhale, inhale, long exhale, repeat, and so on for five minutes. The second group did five minutes per day of box breathing, a breathing technique I've mentioned before, which follows a pattern of inhale-hold-exhale-hold-repeat, where each inhalation and exhalation, and the holds, are the same duration, until five minutes have elapsed. The third group did five minutes per day of cyclic hyperventilation: You take a big deep breath in through the nose and a shorter exhale through the mouth, putting more vigor into the inhalation than the exhalation. A fourth group did five minutes per day of meditation, seated with eyes closed, and focusing their attention on their breath but with no specific instructions about breathing pattern.

Most participants, regardless of their group, reported an improvement in mood and outlook. But cyclic physiological sighing had a notably bigger effect. We also observed improvements in resting heart rate, improved sleep, and other metrics of well-being related to autonomic function. In other words, doing one to three physiological sighs is a great tool for when stress hits and doing five minutes of physiological sighs on repeat can help buffer us further against the inevitable stress of life. Given what you now know about exhales slowing heart rate, oxygen and carbon dioxide levels, and the autonomic seesaw, it should make sense as to why this works. Your brain and body were literally built to do this.

STRESS CONTROL PROTOCOL

2

Use Deliberate Cold Exposure to Raise Your Stress Threshold

WHAT TO DO:

- **Put yourself in uncomfortably cold water three to seven times per week.** This can be as simple as a cold shower, or as involved as an ice bath. For the duration, choose one of these options:
    - **Timed protocol:** One to three minutes per session.
    - **Count "walls of adrenaline" protocol:** Rather than committing to a specific amount of time, try committing to a specific number of mental "walls" to climb over. When you feel the impulse to avoid or exit the cold but you stay, that's one wall you've scaled. Decide in advance how many times you will encounter this impulse and keep going. You do not have to always increase the number of walls. There are days when you will decide to "go over" five walls and other days where two walls will be enough.
- **The water should be uncomfortably cold.** This means it should immediately trigger your impulse to get out, but it should be warm enough that you can safely stay in the water for up to three minutes. Why do I suggest using such annoyingly subjective criteria? Because the specifics will differ by person, the time of day, the ambient temperature, how well rested you are, and on and on. It should be cold enough to require you to overcome some mental resistance to get in. And once you get in, it should be cold enough to cause your breathing to quicken. It should

make you want to raise your shoulders. If the water is so cold that it burns or gives you a headache, however, it's probably too cold. For most people, somewhere between 40 and 50 degrees Fahrenheit works great.

HOW IT WORKS:

The previous protocol will help reduce the intensity and the duration of your stress response. This one takes a different approach to stress control by increasing your stress threshold.

But let's first address some of the common myths about deliberate cold exposure. You may have heard that it can increase your metabolism. In my view, the data are not strong enough to support those claims, at least not by doing a typical one-to-three-minute cold shower or cold immersion (and staying in the cold much longer than that could be unsafe).

You also may have heard to avoid deliberate cold exposure after any resistance training session aimed at increasing muscle growth and/or strength. That counsel is legitimate. Deliberate cold exposure in the six to eight hours after resistance training can prevent some of the strength and hypertrophy adaptations that would otherwise occur. (Chapter 2 explains more about those adaptations, and how to achieve them.) That inhibition of muscle growth is likely due to the vasoconstriction the cold causes, which limits both nutrient delivery and waste removal from the recently trained muscles and also blunts protein synthesis.[60] Wait at least six hours after resistance training to do deliberate cold exposure, or do it before you train, or just save it for another day. Or do it any time relative to your resistance training, but be sure to end with a hot shower or bath to reestablish perfusion of the muscles to correct for this. One study argued that deliberate cold exposure done in the first six hours after resistance training does not prevent strength adaptations, but most of the work on this issue indicates that deliberate cold exposure done in the six hours or so after resistance training will significantly reduce any hypertrophy or strength increases that would otherwise occur.[61] So it is best to simply do it before resistance training, or on rest days. Or allow six or more hours to elapse after resistance training before deliberate cold exposure.

Another common myth is that deliberate cold exposure is harmful for people wishing to limit their cortisol levels. You often hear that people should avoid deliberate cold exposure to keep their cortisol levels low too. Yet the cortisol increases caused by deliberate cold exposure, while significant, are transient and small compared to the dramatic increase that a moderate intensity exercise session triggers.[62] You won't hear that people should avoid exercise to keep cortisol low because the cortisol increase caused by exercise is, again, transient and, what's more, beneficial. (Indeed, it is a key aspect of the specific and general adaptation triggers we discussed in chapter 2).

Many of the "cold exposure is bad for you" stories involve people going into the cold for very long periods of time at excruciatingly cold temperatures, or combining deliberate cold exposure with hyperventilation breathwork and/or jumping or diving under ice. All of which are dangerous and should be avoided.

Now that those points are out of the way, let's look at why deliberate cold exposure is beneficial. Done correctly, deliberate cold exposure is a powerful, safe, and reliable tool for rapidly adjusting your internal state and stress threshold. There are two key phases, each with distinct benefits. First, the state shift that occurs during the cold exposure itself. Second, the state shift that occurs for many hours afterward. Anyone who has done deliberate cold exposure consistently—that is, three to seven times per week—will tell you there is a third phase too, which is the change in your subjective experience of stress and your ability to navigate other forms of stress.

When you enter the cold, it sharply tilts your autonomic nervous system toward the sympathetic end of the seesaw. It does this the first time and every time, and it happens fast, within one to two seconds upon entering the cold. Then, once you get out of the cold, you tend to remain in a very "alert but calm" state—meaning (in the context of the model I described) with an evenly balanced autonomic seesaw—for many hours afterward.

Deliberate cold exposure increases the levels of circulating catecholamines in your brain and body: adrenaline, norepinephrine, and dopamine, and increases in the hormone cortisol too.[63] Some, including dopamine in particular, remain elevated long after you dry off and warm up.[64] These catecholamines increase mood, energy, and alertness. They also can increase your stress threshold; more on that below.[65] But first I want to pause for a moment because you may be asking this: Why would I want to trigger the release of these "stress" chemicals? Won't that make me feel more, not less, stressed? Yes, but that's what this protocol is all about.

We need to challenge the notion that stress is always bad for us.

In fact, when we have control over when, how much, and especially for what purpose we experience stress, the impact of that stress can switch from being health-perturbing to health-promoting, and this reshapes the body's response to all forms of stress.[66] This is not "mind over matter," it's leveraging the brain circuits that convert the arousal response we call stress into something called eustress—a term coined by Swiss physiologist Hans Selye.[67] (You may remember him from the previous chapter.) He was nominated for the Nobel Prize seventeen times for his work on this and related topics,[68] long before we knew what the underlying mechanisms were, but as those mechanisms have become elucidated, many of his theories have largely been deemed correct.

We now know that your prefrontal cortex—that patch of brain real estate involved in context-dependent decision-making (as well as "top-down" inhibition of impulsive actions) is also a key component of our limbic system, which is involved in different arousal-based responses.[69] Usually when people talk about the limbic system, they focus on the amygdala, a brain structure often touted as our fear center. They also talk about our reptilian brain, which is pop neuroscience language for structures like our hypothalamus, which contains dozens of subareas involved in regulating hunger, thirst, aggression, mating, and much more. The hypothalamus and amygdala are often placed conceptually opposite "more evolved" or "higher" brain centers like the prefrontal cortex. But alas, that framework is a gross misrepresentation of the way our brain actually works.

Human brains don't have one system for positive arousal and another entirely different system for negative arousal. We simply have a system for autonomic arousal that is linked to, and impacted by, areas of the brain that evaluate the context of our experiences and then help us make adaptive decisions. Think about it: There are an infinite number of different contexts in which arousal could be good, and just as many where it could be bad. Your prefrontal cortex carries out the basic analysis when arousal happens, asking questions like, "Did I choose this situation?" "Can I control how long and/or how intense this arousal is?" and most importantly, "Is this state of elevated autonomic arousal good or bad for me?" Of course, the answers to those questions depend on the context. And your prior experiences and knowledge.

In fact, our knowledge about stress—not just our memories of stressful circumstances we have been in before, but what we believe to be true about stress—affects how we respond to it. Work from Alia Crum's lab at Stanford shows that humans who learn about some of the (true) positive effects of stress-related arousal on physical health and mental performance experience those positive effects when they are subjected to stress.[70] Her lab also showed that if people learn a bunch of (also true) information about how stress can make us physically unhealthy and cognitively impaired, well, that's what happens to them when they get stressed![71] We can thank our prefrontal cortex for that ability to reframe stress in ways that change its actual effects on us. It's not just a decrease in its negative effect but an inversion from deleterious to beneficial. There's more that shapes our experience of stress as good or bad. Perhaps one of the most interesting things that determines the outcome is whether the stressor has a known end point and resolution that we control.[72] With that in mind, it should now make perfect sense why deliberate cold exposure meets all the criteria of eustress, and why I coined it *deliberate*. If you are the one who elected it, and you control its duration, and you understand how it is good for you, you can turn stress into eustress.

So how, exactly, is it good for you? Two ways. First, the stress of deliberate cold exposure helps us become better at handling other moments of stress. That's sometimes called cross adaptation. It's often studied in the context of physical stress, where exposure to one type of stress—say, exercising in extreme heat—prepares a person to tolerate another type of stress, such as thriving in environments with low oxygen levels.[73] The idea is that we can precondition ourselves to cope with challenges by seeking out situations that draw on similar aspects of our physiology. Cold water swimming has been proposed as a way to improve surgical outcomes,[74] for example, because the stress of the former helps patients better handle the stress of the latter.

Controlled studies showing that cross adaptation focused on physical stress can prepare us to face emotional stress are slowly accruing. In one study of eighty-six people, combining cold exposure with breathing techniques changed the participants' perception of stress in their everyday lives.[75] Participants rated statements such as "You feel calm" and "You enjoy yourself" following a few minutes of vigorous breathwork and a quick cold shower every morning for a period of two weeks. And participants who did both during that period reported a greater sense of control over irritations, and stronger feelings that life was going their way and that they were on top of things, compared to participants who did only the breathwork or the cold exposure, or neither.

Some data are more tangential in nature. For example, cold exposure appears to improve the body's response over time to hypoxia, or low oxygen levels in the blood, which is relevant because hypoxia can rapidly set in when we hit a state of anxiety or panic.[76] Some preliminary evidence has pointed to a possible role for cold exposure in the treatment of depression, not as a replacement for medication but as an accompaniment.[77] In 2018, a group of researchers from the UK reported that a twenty-four-year-old woman who had been treated for major depressive disorder and anxiety since the age of seventeen with little to no relief began weekly sessions of cold water swimming in an attempt to find something that could diminish, or negate, the need for medication after she became a mother. The intervention worked for her. Within four months, she no longer required drug treatment.[78] That was a case study of just one person, but interesting nonetheless.

A 2023 review of fourteen studies on the mental health benefits of outdoor cold-water swimming found this practice to be associated with stress reduction, mood improvement, and a positive outlook.[79] That result is not necessarily entirely tied to cold; being outdoors and part of a community (many people do winter swims in groups or with friends) certainly contributes, but cold exposure is responsible for at least some of this benefit. Other work has also shown a connection between winter swimming and well-being.[80] In one study, fifty-three people in the UK who participated in eight weekly sea swims reported a reduction in both depression and anxiety.[81] Interestingly, "confronting a challenge" was commonly reported as a reason why the experience was rewarding. In another investigation, forty-two undergraduates at the University of Chichester, in the UK, completed a mood profile questionnaire before and after cold immersion, with an additional twenty-two students completing the questionnaire twice but without cold immersion in between.[82] Energy and self-esteem increased significantly in the experimental group, which also experienced a decrease in tension, anger, and depression. No comparable changes were observed in the control group.

The overarching concept here is really about the intentional discomfort brought about from doing deliberate cold exposure. As Mike Tipton, a sports and exercise scientist who has studied cold exposure extensively at the University of Portsmouth, has noted, the kind of discomfort stemming from a cold bath was once a commonplace occurrence.[83] Humans have been exposed to cold for a very long time, and modern living has eliminated it. As a result, we are never forced to move out of homeostasis, which means our various systems are rarely challenged. "The dynamic equilibrium that underpins homeostasis needs to be perturbed," Tipton wrote in an editorial first published in 2018. Stanford University psychiatrist Anna Lembke, author of *Dopamine Nation*, has also spoken about the role of deliberate pain exposure to combat addictions. As she explained it, we are living in the midst of a "fire hose of dopamine," triggered by our phones, caffeine, sugar, and other aspects of modern life.[84] And part of the way out of this is to temporarily abstain from pleasure and to intentionally seek pain—not life-threatening pain, not anything dangerous, but discomfort.[85] We need to learn to cope with stress, not just eliminate it. Stress is a part of life, and we are capable of withstanding it. Cold immersion shows us how.

The second way deliberate cold exposure is good for us is the state it puts us in after it's over. And no, I'm not just talking about a state of relief—although it is fair to say that nearly everyone enjoys getting out of the cold plunge or cold shower more than getting into it. In all seriousness, very few people actually enjoy deliberate cold exposure while they are in the cold. It is a potent stressor and no amount of learning about eustress will change that. In fact, I often find myself cursing Selye when I'm in the cold. But once we get out, ahhh, that's when the real magic starts. The sharp increase in adrenaline, norepinephrine, and cortisol we just triggered also sets in motion a dramatic and prolonged increase in dopamine—the molecule that, as we will discuss more in chapter 6, induces a heightened sense of motivation and focus and, with the pain of the cold now gone, buzz. Dopamine doesn't act alone to create the post-deliberate-cold state, but it is a central player in that neuroendocrine cocktail. It's the perfect state for a work session, for exercising, socializing, pretty much any activity that requires us to be alert and focused.

If the way I'm describing the post-cold state sounds almost drug-like, it is. Only better. One study found that full-body (up to the neck) immersion in water at about 57 degrees Fahrenheit for one hour triggered a more than fivefold increase in norepinephrine levels compared to baseline.[86] It also produced a rise in dopamine levels in the body, raising them more than twofold for hours afterward. We call this peripheral dopamine, because it was measured from the body. We don't yet know the exact relationship between dopamine levels in the body and in the brain, but we do know they tend to increase and decrease in parallel. And there is emerging evidence that when peripheral dopamine is elevated, it increases dopamine in reward and motivation circuits in the brain in a dose-dependent manner.[87] When adrenaline is released in the body, it doesn't cross the blood-brain barrier but it does activate receptors in the vagus nerve that project from the body to the brain. In doing so, it causes the locus coeruleus to release norepinephrine, which increases alertness in the brain. So there is reason to assume that peripheral increases in catecholamines triggered by deliberate cold exposure are mirrored by similar increases in the brain.

It is worth noting that drugs known to sharply increase dopamine and epinephrine, such as amphetamines or cocaine, also produce fast, large increases in catecholamines but with the important caveat that they cause levels of the catecholamines to rise so fast and then drop so fast, that they plummet below pre-drug levels. That is part of what, as Anna Lembke, MD, explained in *Dopamine Nation*, puts people in a state of psychological and physical discomfort, and leaves them craving more of those drugs right away, which partially explains why they are addictive.[88]

Deliberate cold exposure then seems an almost perfect way to significantly increase and maintain elevated levels of catecholamines. You get the mental focus and mood benefits they provide, and you also raise your stress threshold.

Most of us don't have an hour available to spend sitting in chilly water, however. Fortunately, you can use colder temperatures for much shorter periods of time to get the same effect. Studies show that even thirty seconds can work.[89] Yet I suggest one to three minutes or two to ten "walls." As mentioned above, pinpointing an exact temperature for every reader isn't possible because it will vary according to differences in the amount of body fat, time of day, tolerance for cold, and other factors. That being said, adrenaline levels reliably increase when we expose our body surface to temperatures below 59 degrees Fahrenheit (15°C) and the colder the water, the faster and larger the resulting catecholamine response will be. This relationship isn't linear. We cannot say, "Sit in this temperature water for this long and you'll get this much more adrenaline and dopamine released." It doesn't work like that. We don't work like that. Nor can we say that x number of minutes in x degrees water will elevate our dopamine x amount for x number of hours after.

That's why, although I refer to deliberate cold exposure as a protocol, like resistance training or cardio, you will need to consider what number of sets, so to speak, works best for you. It is best thought of as a time to practice triggering specific types of adaptations to build resilience. Some people say you should try to relax and breathe slowly during deliberate cold exposure. Others suggest distracting yourself with mental arithmetic or singing a song. I disagree and view both those approaches as the loss of a valuable opportunity to focus on stress control. You can take this time to learn to steer your mind and body through the stress response.

Resilience, grit, and mental toughness are really about the ability to stay in control of your thoughts, words, and actions when you experience that stress response. When you get into the cold, your prefrontal cortex experiences a surge in norepinephrine input, which causes a disruption in its communication with subcortical areas.[90] This is true of any stressful circumstance, whether deliberate or involuntary. With your prefrontal cortex function essentially impaired for the first thirty seconds after you get in the cold, all your thoughts and actions initially will default to removing the stressor. It's where the immediate "I want out!" response comes from. The key is to remind yourself that it is normal to feel like that. You're in what I call "pure impulse" mode. Do this: Try to consciously watch your mind shift from "I want out!" to "I've got this," which will likely happen again and again very rapidly in that first thirty or so seconds. By observing that phase and not trying to grind your way through it, you are actively engaging your prefrontal cortex in a way that is not typical of someone going through a mild cold-shock response. That's an extremely valuable skill, to be able to observe your own mind during stress. It's not about passively observing or dissociating, nor is it about getting hijacked by stress. It's about learning adaptive self-control during stressful moments.

The first time you try this, it's hard, but most people find that within a few sessions the mind racing starts to lessen, and pretty soon, they feel in control of their thoughts and actions from the start. Few people have mastered this valuable skill in any domain of life, but anyone can learn it. Deliberate cold provides a safe way to practice.

I believe the walls approach mentioned above is the best way to practice this skill, whose benefits translate to other forms of stress. When we measure time elapsed in the cold, we focus, not surprisingly, on its passage. As you learned in the introduction to this chapter, high arousal states tend to slow our perception of that. We count, we wonder why time seems to be moving so slowly—a known function of stress—and we focus on it . . . 3, 2, 1, okay, done! Real-life stressors are very different. Some hit when we least expect it (e.g., an accident or crisis), others are stressful in large part because we know they are coming (e.g., a public talk we need to give, a medical appointment we would sooner avoid, etc.). The way to train for real-life stress in the cold is therefore to learn to sense the increases in adrenaline that occur as we approach, enter, stay in, and exit it. Each of these can be the walls you need to climb over. If you think like that, you'll notice something very useful: Stress is not constant. It's not, as we say, a step function. It oscillates, often very quickly and irregularly. The walls appear, and then disappear and reappear with unpredictable frequency.

If you dread the cold, remember that adrenaline is released merely from the anticipation of getting in. Congratulations! That's the first wall. And as we lower ourselves into the cold, that's another wall; next comes the first "I want out!" wall, then it passes . . . then comes the next wall, the next, and the next. Importantly, the time between walls is variable. This is also important to notice, as that is exactly how real-life stress feels. We often can't predict when the next stressful event is coming.

Basically I'm suggesting you approach deliberate cold exposure as resilience training. And by doing it you'll become mentally stronger in the face of nonvoluntary stress. Just be sure you don't stay in the cold longer than five minutes. Stick to the one to three minutes recommended here, or "go over" two to eight walls. Then get out and go about the rest of your day. Some people, myself included, like to take a hot shower after deliberate cold exposure. People debate whether it's better to end on cold or not. I don't care. I like a hot shower after and, in my experience, it does not seem to diminish any of the benefits. Find what works for you.

As a final point, you actually have more moment-to-moment control over the temperature of the water than you may think. While you can't quickly make the water temperature change, you can dynamically adjust your experience of it. If you hug your arms around your body, raise your shoulders toward your ears and bring your knees up toward your chest, you will feel slightly warmer. Conversely if you keep your arms and legs extended and move them around, you'll break up the thermal layer of heated water around your body, making the experience much colder. Want it even colder? Make sure to let the cold water reach as high as your armpits and keep your hands and feet under. You'll want to remind yourself that this is all very good for you now, and in the hours to come. Cursing Selye, as I do, or cursing me (feel free), is allowed and encouraged.

COMMON QUESTIONS:

Is deliberate cold exposure safe?

Cold exposure can be dangerous if the water is exceedingly cold. Exercise caution and prudence with this tool. If you are new to cold immersion, start off slowly, with short exposures in temperatures that are outside your comfort zone but not extremely so. Try a cold shower, which allows you to adjust the temperature higher or lower quickly. Alas, there is not much data on deliberate cold exposure for pregnant women so if you're concerned about potential negative outcomes, avoid this. Don't do it when sick with a cold, the flu, or other respiratory illnesses. Regardless of what you may see online, it's likely to make your illness worse. Here's a good set of guidelines for nonpregnant individuals with no serious health issues:

- Start with water around 50 degrees Fahrenheit the first time, maybe in the mid- to high 40s. Test the water temperature with your hand or foot before getting in; it should feel cold and make you think, "Whoa, that's cold!" but it should not "burn."
- If the water triggers a reflex to raise your shoulders and huddle your arms when you get in, then it's cold enough. If your breathing involuntarily quickens, it's cold enough.
- Get in up to your neck with your feet under. Put your hands under last.
- If you opt for a cold shower, back into the water until your whole body and head are underneath the stream.
- Expect your mind to start racing with thoughts like, "I want out! Why am I doing this?!" Congratulations, you have a functional autonomic nervous system.

Note: *Never, ever jump or dive into very cold water. Lower yourself in while holding something reliably stationary like a ladder or the sides of a cold plunge, or back into a cold shower. I recommend against deliberate cold exposure in cold or frozen outdoor bodies of water unless you have an expert with you, know the location well, and there are real safety measures in place. There is a video on the internet of a woman who drowned after jumping into an ice hole; unbeknownst to her, there was a rapid current under the ice and she was* *swept under. Her husband allegedly went in after her and also drowned. I have a professor friend who nearly drowned doing deliberate cold exposure in a river. He had done at-home cold plunges many times before but hadn't realized how cold the river was until he swam out a few feet from shore. He couldn't breathe properly in a shocked state and he was alone. Have someone with you and decide on a nonverbal signal for "Save me!" before you get in.*

*Never—never, ever!—combine immersion in cold water with any type of deliberate hyperventilation before or during. Your breathing will naturally quicken when you get in cold water, but what I am referring to is deliberate hyperventilation (*Wim Hof *or* Tummo *breathing, as it is sometimes called). This breathing method causes the lowering of carbon dioxide and will delay the gasp reflex, potentially leading you to black out and drown; sadly, people have died this way.*

Deliberate cold exposure is easy to do safely. Almost all deaths from it occur because people were reckless in some way or combined it with hyperventilation. Don't be reckless.

Are there additional benefits to deliberate cold exposure?

A study from metabolic scientist Susanna Søberg, at the University of Copenhagen, and colleagues showed that if people did eleven minutes total per week of deliberate cold exposure, divided into two to four sessions, they enhanced the amount of brown fat in their bodies, a healthy, mitochondria-rich fat that surrounds the heart, neck, and clavicles.[91] That additional brown fat allowed them to feel more comfortable in other cold environments, because when the sympathetic nervous system is active it causes brown fat to burn fatty acids and glucose, which generates heat in the process. In that way, brown fat is like an internal furnace. So if you're someone who is often cold, deliberate cold exposure can help shift your thermal set point. This is connected to the metabolic benefits of cold immersion, which are outside the scope of this protocol.

(Note that the participants didn't gain weight; they just added this special—and beneficial—type of fat.)

I hate the cold so much. Is there any alternative method?

Yes. As an alternative to deliberate cold exposure, you can do three to five minutes of cyclic hyperventilation *away from water*, which reliably raises adrenaline levels. Cyclic hyperventilation, as the name suggests, involves taking long, vigorous inhales through your nose and passively exhaling through your mouth—think of it as letting the air fall out rather than forcing it out—over and over. It's not easy to keep up this breathing for several minutes. You'll find it makes you quite agitated and a bit lightheaded.

Data suggest that cyclic hyperventilation works similarly to cold exposure.[92] Adrenaline rises. Your heart rate increases. Your limbs will feel like they want to move. And your brain will ask "Why am I doing this?!" It's normal to feel some light burning in your nostrils as well. It feels uncomfortable while you're doing it, but it can improve mood and sleep afterward. Also, you can back off the intensity and/or duration of the inhales and thereby modulate your stress response as you go, an advantage that cold exposure doesn't offer.

So if you really hate the cold or if you don't have access to it, cyclic hyperventilation is the next-best alternative. Just never do it in combination with deliberate cold exposure as, again, you can pass out and drown. People have died combining cyclic hyperventilation with cold immersion; that's why I'm repeating the warning here yet again. And of course never do cyclic hyperventilation while driving or operating machinery, or other activities that demand your attention. Just sit or lie down somewhere safe for a few minutes to use this tool.

STRESS CONTROL PROTOCOL

3

Do Non-Sleep Deep Rest (NSDR) to Buffer Against Stress

WHAT TO DO:

- **Do a non-sleep deep rest (NSDR) session for 10 to 30 minutes.** Sit or, ideally, lie down in a quiet place and listen to a scripted NSDR session. Guided NSDRs in different voices are available online (hubermanlab.com/nsdr) for zero cost and can be downloaded to use offline (also at no cost). NSDR is especially useful in high-stress times lasting weeks or longer, such as intense work or school periods, or when facing deadlines and life transitions, such as raising young kids or caring for an elder. Ideally you do NSDR once per day but it is beneficial to reduce stress at any point. I do it at least once a week, depending on my schedule.

HOW IT WORKS:

I talked about NSDR earlier in this book (remember Sleep Protocol 8?). It is impossible to overstate what an extraordinarily potent tool NSDR can be for mental and physical health. In chapter 1, I covered NSDR's ability to restore mental and physical energy without creating sleep inertia grogginess. But it is particularly potent when it comes to limiting unhealthy stress. I was first introduced to this tool nearly ten years ago. I often get asked "What is something you wish you had known when you were younger?" and my answer is always, "I wish I had known about yoga nidra (aka NSDR)."

NSDR has so many benefits. It replenishes your mental and physical energy,[93] it can offset many of the negative effects of sleep deprivation,[94] it improves the depth and continuity of your sleep at night,[95] and it buffers you against the harmful effects of both acute and chronic stress.[96] To get the most out of this practice, I'll make a few things clear. First, NSDR is not a nap. Nor is it hypnosis. Nor is it meditation, as I explained in chapter 1. Rather, NSDR belongs to a category of techniques that can be broadly thought of as self-directed relaxation. You shift your brain and bodily state from one of "alert and ready to move" to "alert yet deeply relaxed." It emphasizes parasympathetic nervous system (PNS) activity, or increases your parasympathetic tone, tilting you toward that calmer side of the autonomic seesaw that I described in the introduction to this chapter. Sounds like a shallow nap . . . but it's not. Because you deliberately stay awake during this practice, your sympathetic nervous system remains engaged too. It's a unique brain state that has important implications.

Research shows that during NSDR, parts of your brain enter sleeplike states, while other brain areas remain in a state of alertness.[97] We don't quite know what to call the overall brain state that NSDR creates, but we know that it's self-directed and has significant stress-reducing and energy-replenishing effects.[98] We also know that people typically emerge from NSDR in an alert-but-calm state of mind and body, that center of the seesaw. When one considers that it costs nothing but ten to thirty minutes of time, that is quite a return on investment!

As discussed in chapter 1, NSDR involves shifting one's focus throughout the session, which for some people makes it easier than meditations that demand you anchor your focus or "clear your mind." NSDR asks that you shift from thinking, doing, and planning, to being and feeling—I know, that sounds super New Agey. But the instruction is based in physiology, not mysticism. Here is why: Turning off our thoughts is really hard. In fact, we can't do it. Even in sleep, we dream. Even in REM sleep people can solve and respond to math problems.[99] (If you're wondering how the experimenters knew that, given people are paralyzed during REM, the subjects signaled correct answers to simple subtraction problems using eye movements.) So forget trying to destress by not thinking. It just won't happen.

We can, however, easily shift our immediate experience from planning and analyzing to just experiencing physical sensations. NSDR has us do that. We deliberately shift our attention from one aspect of our sensations in that moment—for instance from our toes to our fingers, then to a location away from our body such as to sounds in the room, then to sounds far away, then back to a specific location on our body, and so forth. This regular and deliberate shifting of our focus on different aspects of our perception both eliminates the strain of trying to continually focus on one thing, and the tendency of our mind to default to planning and analyzing. With NSDR, your mind drifts from one sensation to the next in an intentional but relaxed way. When you do that, your mind goes into an atypical, almost liminal state, the one described above—somewhere between that of deep sleep and being awake. Cortisol levels drop, discrete brain areas fall asleep while others remain active.[100] Because NSDR is done lying down with eyes closed, from the outside it appears you are napping but you're not. You're in self-directed reset mode.

If you've never done yoga nidra or NSDR before, this may all sound a bit abstract, but it's really very concrete. It is grounded in what we know about self-directed brain states. And it's very easy to do. One of the biggest advantages of NSDR is that, in contrast to mindfulness meditation—which is a skill you build up gradually over time and that requires daily (or near daily) practice to maintain the positive effects—NSDR can work the first time, and every time.

You lie down, listen to the instructions, and voila! Ten to thirty minutes later you emerge feeling renewed and rested. Most everyone who tries it marvels at the immediate positive effects. It's starting to be used in schools, by elite military operators, professional athletes, Fortune 500 CEOs, and many other men and women around the world as a tool for managing stress and even as a means to accelerate recovery from illness and injury, to offset some of the negative symptoms of menopause, sleep deprivation, trauma, and more.[101] I encourage everyone to try it a few times and experience the benefits for themselves.

COMMON QUESTIONS:

When should I do NSDR?

This is the most common question I get about NSDR. You can do it ANY time. In the morning if you wake up and don't feel fully rested and don't have time to get another hour or more of sleep. In the afternoon instead of a nap and if you know you'll be working harder or longer than usual that day. Before a workout if you're feeling less-than-motivated or lacking energy. In the evening if you get home and want to destress from the day. In the middle of the night if you wake up and can't fall back asleep. (In that case, get out of bed and do an NSDR then get back into bed; a return to sleep will arrive easier.)

The simple answer I default to whenever asked "When should I do NSDR?" is "First thing in the morning, or in the afternoon, or any time of night . . ." It is that versatile and that useful.

STRESS CONTROL PROTOCOL

4

Do a Micro Meditation Immediately After Waking Up

WHAT TO DO:

- **Incorporate a simple, five-minute daily meditation into your routine.** Any time of day can be beneficial, but doing it before getting out of bed each morning ensures you don't have to carve out time later and may offer distinct benefits as well.
- **If you feel an urgency to get out of bed before five minutes have elapsed, stay put.** Contrary to how it is usually framed, meditation is one of the best forms of resilience training. So see this as an opportunity to practice resilience. This meditation is not about clearing the mind. It's about building the capacity to sit with the stress that even micro meditation can trigger. This will help you better deal with real-life stressors once your day starts.

HOW IT WORKS:

Plenty of evidence exists that mindfulness-based meditation practices buffer us against stress, and even brief daily sessions reduce anxiety.[102] I mention both stress and anxiety here, because there's a difference. Some say stress has an identifiable cause, or a known stressor, whereas anxiety does not. That's a good working distinction. But the fact that meditation protects us against both highlights that each experience is based in the same thing: an elevated sympathetic tone that exceeds the demands of the stressor.

Meditation can adjust your autonomic seesaw, bringing you back to the center. But just how may surprise you.

Most everyone assumes the goal of a meditation practice is to quiet the mind and that it involves cultivating a sense of peace during the practice. In some sense that's true. One study found that four consecutive days of a meditation practice reduced anxiety and increased mindfulness, a broad term encompassing a sense of awareness, calm, and being in the present moment.[103] A 2019 report by New York University neuroscientist Wendy Suzuki and colleagues found that doing eight weeks of thirteen-minute daily meditation notably decreased anxiety.[104]

But data also show that meditation can make us more resilient by allowing us to observe stress when it hits without reacting to it. When psychologist Richard Davidson—one of the world's foremost experts on the science of meditation—appeared on my podcast, he described that his lab saw a statistically significant increase (!) in people's anxiety levels in the first week that they started doing a regular meditation practice.[105] Wait, what? Meditation increases anxiety? Yes. Because it can be maddening to force yourself to focus and refocus on your breathing over and over for five minutes when you wake up and you have to dive into your day. Your mind wants to shift to planning and doing. In that way, meditation can serve as a way to increase your stress threshold. Not unlike learning to stay in uncomfortably cold water.

This is as hard as it sounds, but well worth it. Regular meditation teaches us to observe, rather than act on, our autonomic arousal. It also reduces the likelihood that real-life stressors will hijack our mind. Just like Stress Control Protocol 2.

One study found that the intensity of the emotions people experienced while viewing potentially disturbing pictures was reduced when people did so from a "mindful" state, indicating that meditation promotes a kind of awareness that makes a person's autonomic nervous system less subject to outside stimuli.[106] Indeed, neuroimaging studies have confirmed that meditation consistently alters brain regions connected to both body awareness and mental awareness, as well as emotional regulation.[107] The underlying mechanism appears to be connected to the production of GABA, an inhibitory neurotransmitter—meaning a chemical that generally suppresses the firing of other neurons. People with panic disorders and anxiety tend to have decreased GABA activity in particular regions of the brain.[108] Researchers have theorized that the increased blood flow to the prefrontal cortex that seems to occur during certain types of meditation may, in turn, lead to increased GABA activity, along with improved top-down inhibition of brain areas that generate reflexive thoughts and actions, and this equates to a general sense of relaxation.[109]

A bit more on the format of the micro meditation: stay in bed or, if you must, get up and use the bathroom first, and then set a five-minute timer, sit or lie down, and stay as still as you can while you focus on your breathing. Observe where your mind goes. If it wanders—which is completely normal by the way—redirect your focus back to your breath. Slow nasal-only inhales and exhales are best. But the most important thing is to do it, and on days when you feel stressed, do it anyway. In fact, that's a bonus opportunity. The benefits to your ability to observe your stress rather than have it engulf you that come from a daily five-minute meditation are well worth it. And of course, if you want to do a longer meditation, go for it.

As simple as this protocol may sound, I and countless others can attest to the fact that it provides immediate benefits, and benefits that extend throughout the day. And one more thing: We don't yet understand the science of exactly how, but it also seems to create the ability to "see" when stress is coming your way. Perhaps it sensitizes the brain circuits that respond to autonomic arousal. Perhaps it leads to better recognition of adrenaline in our body rising, or our heart rate starting to increase. After all, a five-minute meditation will gradually have you feeling more anxious as you progress from start to finish; it's very different from getting into cold water, which causes a big spike in adrenaline right at the start. But that ability to sense approaching stress is a game changer, as it can reduce your reactivity and improve your ability to make decisions about what to do and say—and in many cases, what not to do and say—when the inevitable stressors of life appear.

STRESS CONTROL PROTOCOL

5

Boost Your Morning Cortisol and Catecholamine Peak

WHAT TO DO:

- **Stack three to four of the pro-cortisol and pro-catecholamine triggers below in the morning, and limit them at night.**
    - **Get bright light, ideally sunlight, in your eyes for about ten minutes, as soon as possible after waking.** If you wake before the sun is up, you'll either have to wait for the sun to rise or use a 10,000 lux light for this trigger. (I cover how in detail in **Sleep Protocol 1**.)
    - **Hydrate with 16 to 32 ounces of water and consume some caffeine in the first two hours of your day.** How much caffeine? 100–400 milligrams depending on your body weight and caffeine tolerance. A strong cup of coffee or yerba maté (my preferred caffeine source) has 150–200 milligrams of caffeine. Note: Chronic caffeine drinkers don't get as much of a cortisol increase from their usual amount of caffeine as those who aren't, but it still has a positive effect on other catecholamines for reasons covered in chapter 1.[110]
    - **Exercise in the morning.** If your schedule allows, do cardiovascular or resistance training within the first two to three hours of waking; the closer to waking the better. (The foundational fitness program in chapter 2 offers a sustainable weekly structure, but of course there are many others out there.) If you can't exercise in the

morning, take a brief walk, do some jumping jacks, skip rope, or do some light calisthenics, even for just five to ten minutes. While not a full-fledged workout, it will help stimulate the morning cortisol and catecholamine increase you're after.

- **Do one of the deliberate cold exposure protocols discussed in this chapter.** Remember, this takes only one to three minutes, and a cold shower works too. Just do it before resistance training, ideally not after (refer to Stress Control Protocol 2).

  As an ALTERNATIVE to deliberate cold exposure, try cyclic hyperventilation: Do a cycle of twenty-five to thirty deep, vigorous inhales through your nose, with each inhale followed by a passive exhale—meaning just let the air fall out of your lungs via your mouth. Afterward, you'll feel a bit lightheaded. That is a normal response. Exhale all your air and hold your breath for thirty to sixty seconds. You should no longer feel lightheaded. You can repeat this process for two to three more rounds. Note: NEVER do cyclic hyperventilation before or during deliberate cold exposure, anywhere near water, while driving, operating machinery, or performing other activities that demand your attention. You may recall from those protocols that deliberate cold exposure doesn't spike cortisol all that much, but it does significantly increase the other catecholamines. And that is beneficial here.

- **Consider occasional (once or twice per week) use of low-dose licorice root containing glycyrrhizin or consume grapefruit in the first one to three hours of your day.** Both have been shown to significantly increase cortisol and the duration of cortisol action. Subjectively, they can increase feelings of morning and daytime energy and focus. Warning: Despite licorice and grapefruit sounding natural (and they are), their effects can be very potent. They can increase blood pressure and/or fluid retention at high doses, so use the minimal effective dose and, as with all supplements discussed in this book, consult your doctor first.

HOW IT WORKS:

Cortisol and the catecholamines adrenaline and norepinephrine, but especially cortisol, are often thought of purely as stress chemicals. The third catecholamine—dopamine—escaped this reputation but is usually thought of (also incorrectly) as purely a pleasure chemical. And while cortisol is involved in the stress response, thinking about it as purely a stress chemical is wrong. I wish I could banner this across the sky: *Cortisol Is Not a Stress Hormone!*

In fact, if I could impart just one message about how to improve your health, it would be this: Strive to get your morning cortisol high (yes, high!) and your nighttime cortisol low.

The main function of cortisol is to ensure there is enough energy in the form of glucose, or blood sugar, for you to meet life's demands. Yes, that can include overcoming stressors, but it also includes simply waking up each morning with the physical and mental energy required for work, school, family, and exercise. Cortisol causes glucose (as well as fats) to get released into the bloodstream, and it also stimulates the liver to make more glucose.[111]

Cortisol and adrenaline play additional key roles in our body's everyday functioning. They improve our immune system's ability to ward off infections, they elevate our mood, they allow for our capacity to form new memories, and they increase metabolism . . . so just forget the idea that cortisol and adrenaline are only about stress.

A gradual rise in your cortisol levels starts three to four hours before you wake up each morning and its levels eventually hit a threshold level, at which point you wake up, open your eyes, and get out of bed. Keep in mind that cortisol doesn't act alone to rouse you from sleep; a parallel rise in body temperature and clearance of the sleepiness-inducing molecule adenosine follows a similar schedule. Nonetheless, scientists call this rise the "cortisol awakening response" or CAR. Now that makes it sound like a medical problem of some sort, but CAR is a normal and (provided it is timed correctly) health-promoting aspect of our biology.[112] And it helps buffer you against unhealthy stress.

Cortisol first starts to rise as a result of a signal from your SCN, your brain's master circadian clock that we discussed in chapter 1. For most people, that rise starts somewhere around five hours into their night's sleep and continues sharply over the subsequent two to three hours until it reaches a threshold level and bam! You wake up. Even if you use an alarm clock, you can be sure your cortisol levels were rising as you approached the start of your day. Now, once you're awake, cortisol *continues* to increase until it hits its peak for that twenty-four-hour cycle. For most people, that peak occurs anywhere from 0.5 to 1.5 hours after waking up.

Then cortisol levels slowly start to decline—a process that continues into the late afternoon and evening. Assuming you encounter no major stressors, your cortisol levels continue to drop in the hours before you fall asleep and reach their lowest level about three to four hours after you doze off, and then slowly start to rise again to eventually trigger the next morning's CAR, and so on. This is the ideal cortisol pattern for mental and physical health, energy, and resilience to stress.

Night shift workers deal with a very disrupted sleep-wake schedule, and their cortisol pattern gets fragmented, with multiple peaks and troughs throughout the day. For some, the pattern inverts to match their wake-sleep schedule. Although that might seem like not that big of a deal if they are still getting enough sleep, it's known to cause serious and long-lasting health issues. Indeed, many of the known health detriments of nocturnal schedules are due primarily to alterations in the pattern of cortisol release and its downstream effects. I cover what shift workers can do to partially offset those negative effects in chapter 1 and chapter 5.[113]

Most people, even night owls or those staying up too late on their phones, are not completely inverting their sleep-wake schedule, and yet there is reason to believe that they have less than ideal cortisol patterns. I say "most people" because the vast majority of questions I get are about wanting better sleep, more energy, improved focus, and less stress and anxiety. And when I inquire about the structure of their days, I learn that very few people are doing the few simple things to ensure high cortisol in the morning and low cortisol at night. This sets them up for health problems and lowered resilience to stress.

Numerous studies show that if your cortisol levels fall too slowly as you approach the later hours of your day—a so-called "flattening of the diurnal cortisol rhythm"—or if your cortisol is spiked by stress or bright light in the evening, you can experience that as increased anxiety, and sleep can suffer too.[114] If this happens once in a while, it's no big deal. Acute stressors—an argument, a small crisis at work, and so on—are part of life. They spike our cortisol and catecholamines. But these levels ordinarily return to baseline a few minutes or hours later. So don't freak out about a bit of stress here or there even late in the day! The stress management tools discussed elsewhere in this chapter will assist in helping you navigate those events.

If, however, your cortisol undergoes stress-induced peaks in the late evening or nighttime, or if your morning cortisol is too low or declines too slowly, that flattening of the cortisol curve is what puts you into a state of chronic stress.[115] This can cause a cascade of detrimental events in your body and brain. Diabetes, hypertension, depression, and weight gain can result, as can physical imbalance, leaving a person feeling unsteady on their feet.[116] Studies have also linked abnormally high cortisol levels later in the day and into the night to acne, irregular menstrual cycles, and digestion issues.[117] High cortisol at night has been linked to insomnia and reduced amounts of REM sleep.[118] Given this, everyone would do well to try to anchor and amplify their cortisol and catecholamine peak in the first hours after waking to start their day and limit their cortisol and catecholamine levels at night. That simple framework goes a long way toward limiting your chronic stress. And that's what this protocol is all about.

Let's start with what to do at night, because how you prepare for bed affects your cortisol and catecholamine levels the next day. Some of what you're about to read will be familiar to you from chapter 1. Before bed, implement a wind-down routine of dimming the lights, maybe taking a hot shower or bath or even washing your face with hot water. If you're feeling stressed from the day, take a few moments to do some physiological sighs to lower your heart rate, and/or do a ten- to thirty-minute NSDR session. Don't drink too many fluids or eat in the two to three hours before sleep, and definitely try to avoid caffeine in the eight to ten hours prior to bedtime. Viewing bright overhead LED lights (of the sort that are in many bathrooms) is a quick way to spike your cortisol and quash your melatonin, and checking your email or the news in the last hour before sleep is definitely a risky move if you want to keep your cortisol low at night (see chapter 1 for details). And to be clear: Low cortisol at night should be your goal!

If you happen to wake up in the middle of the night for whatever reason, avoid viewing bright lights or looking at your phone. Again, do some physiological sighs to help keep your heart rate low, and let yourself drift back to sleep. If you can't fall back asleep, listen to an NSDR session. Or try the weird eye-movement trick I shared in chapter 1.

By the way, if you exercise in the evening or at night, that does significantly increase late-day cortisol. It's better to exercise than not to, if you have a workout planned. To help keep your cortisol and catecholamine rhythms on a diurnal schedule, you can reduce the intensity of your evening training a bit and/or be sure to include a wind-down routine afterward. Andy Galpin, an exercise physiologist, encourages this after all workouts, but especially nighttime ones. Even moderate-intensity exercise can cause a large increase in cortisol (as discussed in chapter 2), especially if you consume caffeine first.[119] That is one more reason to drink caffeine before moderate to intense exercise in the morning, but also to avoid it before moderate to intense exercise at night.

I don't want to demonize late-day exercise. Better to do it than not do it. But just know that if you exercise intensely within four to six hours of bedtime, your next-day waking cortisol may be lower due to the negative feedback regulation of cortisol.[120] That's a mechanism you often see with hormones in the body, like cortisol or testosterone: When those hormones reach a certain high level, it signals specific brain areas and glands, such as the hypothalamus and pituitary and adrenals, to reduce their release of those hormones. Just another reason why spiking your morning cortisol is a good thing. It not only sets you up for the day, it helps keep cortisol levels low at night.[121] So if you exercise at night and wonder why you're dragging a bit the next morning, this may very well be why. Be diligent about using the tools in this protocol and you'll be A-OK.

What about spiking your cortisol and catecholamines in the morning—how best to do that? There too you have options: Viewing bright light can boost your morning cortisol peak by 50 percent, making it a very easy, effective and beneficial practice (see Sleep Protocol 1 for more). Sunlight is ideal, but a 10,000 lux light works too.[122] Hydration, caffeine, moderate to intense exercise, deliberate cold exposure, maybe cyclic hyperventilation (but never with deliberate cold exposure): Doing one of these is better than none, two is better than one, and so on. If I had to place them in order of effectiveness, I would say: sunlight viewing, exercise, and caffeine are the big levers here, but don't worry about the order. Let logic be your guide. Obviously hydrate before and during your exercise, drink caffeine for an energy boost, get the sunlight before or during exercise if you can, but if the sun isn't up and you're ready to train, train! Don't wait for the sun to rise, thinking that it has to come first because it's a big lever. The cortisol and catecholamine systems are primed for release in the early hours of your day and will synergize without the need to get the relative timing (of all the things that cause their release) perfect.

When people ask me, "Who has time for all this?" I respond that it takes mere seconds to drink 16 ounces of water, a few minutes to make a caffeinated beverage and step outside into the sun while you drink it, and then depending on your schedule, exercise. Do not obsess over the details of relative timing of these tools.

A number of people have asked me over the years: "Given the importance of ensuring elevated morning cortisol, is there anything I can take to boost it besides caffeine?"

In chapter 6, I cover the many prescription drugs and supplements that can increase dopamine and norepinephrine, but when it comes to things that boost cortisol there are two that are particularly useful. And they are inexpensive. And commonplace. You may even have one of them in your kitchen right now.

They are grapefruit and licorice root extract. Not licorice candy, but licorice plant root extract.[123]

Each can increase the size and duration of your morning cortisol peak and thereby increase your level of alertness and the other subjective effects associated with elevated sympathetic tone. How is this possible? Well . . .

Grapefruit impacts cortisol levels by two known mechanisms. First, it inhibits the enzyme (11β-HSD2) that blocks cortisol to cortisone conversion—cortisol being the chemical that imparts the functions we've been talking about so far in this protocol. Slower conversion means more active cortisol stays in our system for longer to impart its effects. Second, grapefruit inhibits the enzyme CYP3A4, which blocks the liver's metabolism of cortisol, the net effect of which is to increase cortisol's duration of action.

Licorice root extract contains something called glycyrrhizin (pronounced gly-cer-ry-zin) that potently inhibits the same abovementioned enzyme 11β-HSD2.

You may be thinking, *Grapefruit and licorice?! Is he serious?!* Yes, quite serious. There are human data to support the use of each to increase cortisol's duration of action including studies demonstrating dose-dependent effects. So much so that well-informed MDs will warn patients with Cushing's syndrome—which is a condition marked by pathologically elevated levels of cortisol—to avoid grapefruit, licorice root extracts, teas containing glycyrrhizin, and any licorice candy. (Note: Some traditional black licorice root candy, typically sold in Scandinavian countries but elsewhere too, contains glycyrrhizin, though versions without glycyrrhizin exist too.) I suggest most everyone avoid licorice root extract consumption late in the day and at night. If you want to experiment with taking licorice root extract that contains glycyrrhizin please talk to your doctor first. At high doses it can raise blood pressure, cause fluid retention, and even affect the metabolism of certain pharmaceutical drugs and potassium because of the many roles of the abovementioned enzymes in the liver.

I use licorice root extract with glycyrrhizin as a tool occasionally (once or twice a month). I find that 100 to 250 milligrams of licorice root in capsule form is enough to feel its effects. I make sure to use a version containing glycyrrhizin, and I take it with my morning caffeine usually before a hard workout that I need to start earlier than is typical for me. The energy-increasing effect is very noticeable. On very rare occasions I will take it around noon to try to extend my window of elevated cortisol to work for an especially long day, or to exercise hard midday. Again, I use it as a sometimes tool, not a regular tool, to boost cortisol in the morning.

Overall, grapefruit and grapefruit juice have a milder, but still meaningful, impact on cortisol's duration of action. Most people can consume these without an adverse effect. But they can interact with various medications, so be sure to consult your doctor before taking. If you'd like to try incorporating grapefruit as a cortisol-boosting tool in your routine, perhaps eat a grapefruit or drink a small glass of grapefruit juice in the morning (pink or conventional is fine; it doesn't matter). See how that affects your energy throughout the day. I would avoid these at night for obvious reasons.

One more thing to note here is that it is hard to find very-low-dose licorice root extract with glycyrrhizin. Most are 400 milligrams or more, and even at

200 milligrams it works very well to increase energy, so I empty half a 400 milligrams capsule into water or my coffee, and drink that. It tastes good. Remember: It raises blood pressure, and taking glycyrrhizin every day can lead to serious problems over time, so if you experiment with it, try a low dose—even if it means having to open up a capsule to remove a portion of the contents. Once more, talk to your doctor before you do. And if you have high blood pressure, don't take it!

I can't end this protocol without one more reminder about caffeine: If you consume caffeine in the late afternoon, too, don't overdo it. I get it; I love yerba maté in the morning, and I love, love, love the taste of coffee in the afternoon. But if you're an afternoon caffeine drinker and having sleep issues or trouble getting going in the mornings, you can bet it's at least partially because the caffeine levels in your bloodstream are still too high from your afternoon coffee or tea. Try to drink only decaf after 2:00 p.m., or limit yourself to roughly 60 milligrams of caffeine (that's about 3 to 4 ounces of regular coffee, or an espresso shot), and do your best to avoid it altogether within eight hours of bed (refer to Sleep Protocol 11 for more guidance). You could also opt to ditch the afternoon caffeine and instead to take 300 to 900 milligrams of alpha-GPC, which is a short-acting stimulant that can increase energy and focus and may actually improve REM sleep at night if taken six to ten hours before bedtime. I discuss this tool more in chapter 6.

This protocol includes several tools, so to recap: By increasing the slope and height of your morning cortisol and catecholamine peak, you buffer yourself against later-day stress in several ways. First, you're likely to experience improved energy and focus for many hours afterward. Viewing bright light,[124] consuming caffeine,[125] exercise,[126] and cold exposure[127] all increase cortisol and/or catecholamine release. This helps us keep our reactions proportional to any stressors we may encounter later. By starting your day in a state of focus and readiness, if a stressful situation arises you don't need to produce more cortisol to confront it effectively. Researchers who have examined the link between morning cortisol and stress call this connection the CAR anticipation hypothesis.[128] It suggests that a big cortisol peak in the morning isn't just to wake us up; it also prepares us for whatever stressors lie ahead.[129]

And just remember this: You *want* your cortisol and catecholamines relatively high in the morning and daytime, and you want them low in the evening and at night. Stack the tools described here to do just that.

STRESS CONTROL PROTOCOL

6

Consider Specific Supplements to Help Offset Excessive Stress

WHAT TO DO:

- **Find a combination of supplements that might help you combat severe or prolonged periods of stress.** Remember: Behavioral protocols are the foundation of mental and physical health and performance, and that is especially true when it comes to stress control. It's also true that if your sleep duration and quality are not sufficient, no amount of pharmacology will help, at least not for long. Refer to chapter 1 for more on that topic. With that said, below is a list of supplements that have shown some efficacy for reducing various aspects of the stress response:
    - **Ashwagandha:** 200–300 mg, 1 to 2 times per 24 hours, but taken only in the afternoon and/or evening.
    - **L-theanine:** 100 mg or 200 mg, 1 to 3 times per day; if you drink caffeine regularly or are in a period of unusually high stress, take theanine with your caffeine.
    - **Phosphatidylserine:** 400–800 mg, once per day anytime after 4:00 p.m.
    - ***Rhodiola rosea*:** 200 mg, once or twice per day
- **Proceed with caution.** As always when discussing supplements or medication, it is important to consult with a physician. You need to be sure that you are not risking a dangerous interaction, that the product is reliable,

and that a medical professional has information about what may be symptoms of an underlying health issue.

HOW IT WORKS:

Certain supplements can help in times of excessive stress, such as when you are dealing with two or three nights of poor sleep due to an emotionally challenging circumstance, or if you've made behavioral changes but are still finding it hard to balance that autonomic seesaw. Alternatively, changes that occur with age can cause hormone surges or other shifts that can make you more vulnerable to stress.

On these occasions, certain supplements, taken alone or in combination, can help. The supplements in this protocol can increase parasympathetic nervous system activation and reduce sympathetic nervous system activation, either directly or indirectly, helping you to tilt that seesaw in the direction that is most beneficial to you. The studies described below are selected from the body of research on each supplement. These summaries are not comprehensive but provide an overview of the evidence.

If you decide to explore supplements for limiting stress, I would suggest taking one of them and seeing how it works for you before adding another. That is going to be the most informative and cost-effective approach. (I am well aware that some people will opt to just dive in and take all four because they hate stress that much. Try to hold back.)

Ashwagandha:

Ashwagandha, also known as Indian ginseng or winter cherry, is used as an adaptogen—a term that broadly refers to substances that improve a person's resistance to stress. A large review published in 2021 that included forty-one total studies in humans included seven that focused on stress and anxiety, enrolling a total of 491 adults who either reported being under high stress or were diagnosed with an anxiety disorder.[130] Ashwagandha dosages varied from 240 milligrams per day to 1,250 milligrams per day for an extract and up to 6,000 milligrams when administered as a powdered root. (Most ashwagandha capsules sold over the counter in the US contain 200–600 mg per capsule.) Taken together, these studies showed that ashwagandha reduced stress and anxiety when compared to a placebo, and also reduced sleeplessness and fatigue. Cortisol levels in the blood were also lower among people taking this supplement, and it appeared that the cortisol-lowering effect of ashwagandha is likely the major basis of its effect on lowering stress and anxiety. A study of sixty adults found that those who took 225 milligrams or 400 milligrams per day of ashwagandha reported reductions in anxiety, depression, and food cravings compared to people randomized to a placebo.[131] One study found that men and women taking ashwagandha had a 22 percent and 25 percent reduction in cortisol, respectively, when they took ashwagandha for sixty days versus taking a placebo for sixty days.[132]

Research has identified several components that could contribute to the stress-reducing effects of ashwagandha. Most likely the effect is due to a "cocktail" of several different compounds in ashwagandha that work in parallel on various aspects of the hypothalamic-pituitary-adrenal axis, which, as you may remember from Sleep Protocol 1, is our main biological circuitry for mobilizing a physiological response to a stressor. The most potent of these mechanisms is the suppression of the signaling pathway for corticotropin (ACTH), a hormone that acts to stimulate the release of cortisol from your adrenals.[133] The ashwagandha-suppression of corticotropin (ACTH) happens through a multistep process that begins with compounds called withanolides (naturally occurring plant hormones). These compounds can lower corticotropin-releasing hormone (CRH) in the hypothalamus.[134] Limiting the amount of CRH in turn dampens the signaling that would normally trigger the release of cortisol. The fact that ashwagandha works "upstream" from the adrenal glands has a potential downside: Namely, it is likely to impact all the biology connected to CRH, which includes the gut and the immune system, among others. That's one of several reasons why I suggest not taking ashwagandha at dosages higher than 600 milligrams per day for more than a few weeks before taking at least a few weeks off. There is at least one report of someone taking a high dose (950 mg) of ashwagandha daily for a year and developing adrenal insufficiency.[135] People seem to vary quite a bit in their sensitivity to ashwagandha, so if you decide to try it in times of excess stress, I suggest starting with one dose per day, taken in the evening or an hour before bedtime at a dose of about 100 to 200 milligrams, and only increase the dosage, if needed, to find the minimal effective dose for you. Importantly, you don't want to suppress cortisol in the early part of your day. If you decide to take more, take ashwagandha in the afternoon around 3:00 to 4:00 p.m., and perhaps again an hour before bedtime in a dosage of 200 to 300 milligrams each.

As mentioned above, I suggest you do not take ashwagandha at doses exceeding 600 milligrams per day for periods of longer than a couple of weeks. While the reports are largely anecdotal, some people taking high doses of ashwagandha (700–1,200 mg) per day experience apathy, starting about three to four weeks after continuous intake. The reasons for this are not clear and may be similar to the case report mentioned above, but because efficacy has been shown at lower doses of 300 to 600 milligrams per day, I suggest people use it as a tool to augment stress reduction by taking about 300 milligrams on a regular basis as described above, or reserve its use to high-stress periods and take higher dosages (greater than 600 mg/day) only during those times. And don't let up on the behavioral practices for stress reduction.

A quick note about sourcing ashwagandha and other herbal adaptogens: The herbal supplement world is full of fake and contaminated products, perhaps even more so than for other types of supplements. Stick to major brands with third-party testing, especially ones that test for and remove metals from their products and ensure purity. Gaia Herbs has a good reputation for doing this and sells single-ingredient formulations. Barlow Herbals is another. I have no affiliation to either.

L-theanine:

L-theanine is an amino acid present in green tea and has been recognized as one of its active compounds, alongside caffeine, catechins, and other molecules.[136] Many studies of green tea have investigated a potential protective benefit against cancer and other chronic diseases,[137] with the evidence from laboratory and animal studies indicating that it may reduce the risk of obesity and type 2 diabetes, as well as heart disease[138] and breast cancer.[139]

Large-scale clinical trials exploring the efficacy of theanine in humans are still lacking. It's unlikely such studies will ever happen given their high cost and the fact that theanine is unlikely to be made into a pharmaceutical drug. That's just how it goes with most naturally occurring compounds.

The reason L-theanine is in this chapter is that it is widely used to reduce arousal. That's why nowadays L-theanine is sometimes added to energy drinks, and even to some coffee blends, to offset the jitters associated with drinking too much caffeine—presumably a clever trick on the part of the manufacturers that allows people to drink more of these beverages without feeling too strung out.

In one small, blinded, randomized study, thirty participants between the ages of thirty-six and sixty took L-theanine 200 milligrams per day or a placebo for four weeks.[140] The investigators, a team from Japan, used several standard measures to gauge depression, anxiety, and sleep quality. They reported that the group taking L-theanine had significantly fewer stress-related symptoms.

In another study, a group of researchers in Australia and the Netherlands enrolled thirty-four adults between the ages of eighteen and forty in a blinded study to measure stress response in reaction to a series of cognitive tests involving mental arithmetic, memory, and coordination.[141] Tasks like these can trigger stress because they challenge us. The tasks were presented following consumption of either a placebo or L-theanine as a nutrient drink. They found that the stress response, measured through the amount of salivary cortisol, was reduced compared to the placebo, an effect that appeared to last for several hours. In addition, the L-theanine group showed an increase in alpha brain waves, suggesting a more relaxed state of mind. That being said, cognitive performance was no different between the L-theanine and placebo groups. The reduced stress reaction may be beneficial for other reasons, but it's useful to know that theanine didn't make people better at the tasks they were given.

In terms of the underlying mechanisms, L-theanine research has found that this compound indirectly increases GABA—the major inhibitory neurotransmitter in the brain—and dopamine.[142]

Theanine taken in the hour before bedtime is part of the sleep stack I describe in chapter 1. There, I warned that people who have especially vivid dreams *not* take theanine. I suggest that people who want to try theanine to reduce their stress do so by taking about 200 milligrams of it in the early afternoon and perhaps another 100 to 200 milligrams again in the evening, especially if you had caffeine in the early afternoon.

Phosphatidylserine:

Phosphatidylserine is a type of phospholipid. It is naturally found in the membranes of neurons, and comprises about 10 to 20 percent of the total phospholipid content of the brain—an enormous percentage when one considers that much of the nonliquid content of the brain is phospholipids. Naturally occurring phosphatidylserine plays a role in cognitive function,[143] and the loss of phosphatidylserine in neurons known to occur in later adulthood may partially explain age-related (non-dementia) cognitive decline.

What's more, in its natural state in our brains, this compound is known to decrease the stress response.[144] As a supplement, phosphatidylserine has shown some benefit in older adults who experience chronic stress. There is some evidence phosphatidylserine taken late in the day may preferentially reduce evening and nighttime cortisol,[145] which may explain how it indirectly supports sleep.

In one investigation, from 2004, participants took a phosphatidylserine supplement at a dose of 400 milligrams, 600 milligrams, or 800 milligrams, or a placebo (twenty people per group) and then completed a type of social stress test that involves performing in front of an audience.[146] Data collected on biological indicators of the stress response revealed a significant decrease in these symptoms among the 400-milligram group, but not among those taking the higher doses (or the placebo). It's hard to interpret the effect of higher doses, but this is not uncommon in pharmacology studies. Many studies of stress and cognitive performance show an inverted U-shaped response, where low- and high-dose conditions yield similar or no effects, but mid-range dosages do. Such are the complexities of biology. Another study found no link between phosphatidylserine and measures of a stress response across all sixty participants, but the researchers did observe an effect among participants with high chronic stress levels.[147] Initially, this group had a diminished cortisol rise in response to a social stress test. That may sound like a good thing but it's not. A blunted cortisol response is often a sign of underlying issues, such as depression.[148] Treatment with phosphatidylserine appeared to restore the healthy rise in cortisol in response to the test, meaning it seemed to recalibrate the stress response rather than stop it. I say all this not to confuse you but to remind you that though the best model for your autonomic nervous system might be a seesaw, we need to consider the "hinge" of that seesaw (metaphorically speaking). How it bends, or sticks, matters. And compounds like phosphatidylserine may change people's stress response by adjusting mechanisms analogous to how you might treat a hinge, rather than merely increasing or decreasing cortisol or adrenaline. Finally, in a six-week study from

2014 of seventy-five men randomized to phosphatidylserine (at a dose of 200 or 400 mg per day) or a placebo, the higher dose of the supplement appeared to lower the stress response among participants with chronic high stress.[149]

If you opt to try phosphatidylserine for stress control, I recommend starting with a low dose of 100 to 200 milligrams, taken a few hours before bedtime, and increasing the dose only as needed. I know many people who like its effects on lowering stress late in the day, and for sleep.

Rhodiola rosea:

Rhodiola rosea is a yellow-flowered plant that grows in northern regions of Europe and Asia and on the Atlantic coast of North America. It's long been part of traditional medicine practices in Europe and Asia, used to address fatigue, mild anxiety, and symptoms of burnout.[150] It is considered an adaptogen, because it alters the subjective experience of effort, apparently by adjusting the threshold for perceived effort, and by increasing effort endurance in physical and mental exertion. Subjectively, people taking *Rhodiola rosea* report less post-physical-exertion-related fatigue and that mental stressors feel less stressful, meaning they can lean into sustained effort without feeling exhausted. Indeed, *Rhodiola rosea* has been shown to reduce the symptoms of burnout, which is a multidimensional feature of chronic stress that includes the "wired but tired" feeling that is a common consequence of prolonged periods (days, weeks, etc.) of stress and altered sleep-wake cycles. European medical authorities approved the use of *Rhodiola rosea* for short-term relief of stress in 2012[151] and data on this connection have been slowly accruing.

One study examined the effects of *Rhodiola rosea* among fifty-six physicians working night shifts for fourteen days.[152] Signs of mental fatigue were tested before and after the night shift for three two-week stretches. The investigators reported an improvement in tests examining memory, concentration, perception, and other aspects of brain function during the first two-week administration of *Rhodiola rosea*.

Another trial, from Russia, randomized 161 military cadets to one dose of *Rhodiola rosea* per day at either 370 milligrams or 555 milligrams, or placebo, and found a reduction in fatigue among both supplement groups.[153] And in another investigation, a phase 3 clinical trial at Uppsala University, in Sweden, sixty people were randomized to receive four daily doses of *Rhodiola rosea*, for a total of 576 milligrams per day, or four placebo tablets.[154] The participants completed several questionnaires gauging quality of life, depression, fatigue, and attention. Both groups experienced improvements in overall mental health and reduced feelings of burnout. But in the group taking *Rhodiola rosea*, the reduction in fatigue was more pronounced, and linked to improvements in performance and concentration.

Rhodiola rosea is among the better-studied supplements for stress control, and we have copious evidence pointing to its usefulness in this context. With regard to the underlying mechanism, *Rhodiola rosea* contains numerous phytochemicals (compounds made by plants) that could contribute to its benefits, including by interacting with cortisol pathways[155] and by activating heat-shock proteins,[156] which our cells make in response to stressful conditions such as the excessive heat or cold, the presence of heavy metals, or an infection. Researchers are still investigating the exact mechanisms tied to the stress-reducing effects, as well as its apparent contribution to physical strength and endurance.[157] The picture emerging is that *Rhodiola rosea* buffers against stress by calibrating the amount of adrenaline that is released in moments of high physical exertion and high emotional stress.

I recommend one of two approaches to trying *Rhodiola rosea*. The first is to take it thirty to sixty minutes before a known stressor, like a hard workout or big exam or study session or public speaking engagement—basically any event that you know will require an intense and prolonged effort. I take 120 to 240 milligrams of *Rhodiola rosea* before hard resistance training workouts, which is per the standard protocol used in most peer-reviewed studies of *Rhodiola rosea* for physical exertion. The second way to take *Rhodiola rosea* is during periods of chronic stress, when you can't get as much sleep as you would like and/or when your output is greater than usual. Think final exam week, the days of long work hours before a vacation, the vacation with your in-laws where you are coordinating everything, et cetera. In those times, I suggest taking 100 to 120 milligrams (the typical capsule dose of *Rhodiola rosea* in most supplements) three times daily (morning, afternoon, and evening). It can be taken with or without food. I would not suggest taking *Rhodiola rosea* multiple times throughout the day for more than three to four weeks without taking a break of at least two weeks, as all the biological pathways *Rhodiola rosea* is known to impact are subject to feedback loops and downregulation. Use 100-milligrams-plus daily dosages of *Rhodiola rosea* as a short-term tool to combat stress and burnout, not as a mainstay of your supplement regimen. And I know I sound like a broken record, but don't just pile on supplements for managing stress. You need—and now have—multiple behavioral tools to reduce stress. Use them!

CHAPTER 4

PROTOCOLS for NUTRITION

Nutrition advice is everywhere, and it's often conflicting. Eat meat. Don't eat meat. Eat breakfast. Fast until noon. Carbs are the enemy. Carbs help you burn fat. Fats are key. Fats are bad. Sugar is poison. Calories, not sugar, are what matters. Seed oils are good for you. Seed oils are bad for you . . . It's enough to make anyone dizzy.

And there are avid debates. While some get into nuanced biochemistry, others are surprisingly basic. For example, people still argue about whether the types of foods you eat are more important than how much you eat or whether protein guidelines are off by a factor of two. People also debate whether the timing of when you eat different types of food affects body composition—that is, your body fat to lean mass ratio. Worse, dietary fat and body fat share the same name: fat. That has millions of people avoiding certain dietary fats that, were they to eat them, would likely improve their health.

I'm old enough to remember the "low fat" trend of the early 1990s—when seemingly everything was labeled low-fat or nonfat, including things that never had fat in the first place, like soda and candy, but for which labeling as "no fat!" gave the false impression they would promote body fat loss.

I also remember the 40-30-30 carbohydrate-protein-fat ratio trend, too, which was good in principle, but difficult to adhere to because—at least in my opinion—it wasn't restrictive *enough* to make it easy to follow. That's right, it was too permissive to allow for easy decision-making about food choices. So people ate too much. They needed to be told what not to eat.

The point being: A clever way to start a diet trend is to demonize one type of food.

Which may partially explain why low-carbohydrate and ketogenic diets became popular in the early 2010s. Eating mostly just fat and protein requires some "no thank you" discipline but is otherwise pretty simple . . . until a few weeks in, when a person realizes that even a bowl of salad is off limits and that packaged "keto" snacks often contain a lot of calories . . . and that calories still matter.

The rise and somewhat-fall of keto seemed to usher in time-restricted eating, or intermittent fasting, which emphasizes extended periods each day (and night) with no food intake. This approach was attractive for people who find it hard to have "just a few bites" of a certain food yet find solace knowing they can eat that same food later, once they are in their "eating window." But this diet can challenge even the most disciplined, because while it has practical, psychological, and some health benefits, it doesn't work if people eat with abandon during that window.[1]

Oddly enough, a reptile from South America entered the picture and settled one major debate. Yes, a reptile.

Long story, made short:

The Gila monster doesn't need to eat very often. Just three to four times a year. A year!

A curious biologist asked why.

He discovered Gilas make a peptide called exendin-4 that potently suppresses appetite.

It was then discovered that humans make a peptide similar to exendin-4, called glucagon-like peptide (GLP-1).

Humans made drugs that mimic GLP-1, but a thousandfold.

People don't want to eat as much and . . .

They lose weight.

And a trillion-dollar weight loss drug industry was born.

More importantly for this chapter, GLP-1s really did settle that major debate about why people gain, maintain, or lose weight. They proved that sure, you can argue about which foods may indirectly impact satiety, or which foods are healthiest, but when it comes to body weight, how many calories we eat relative to how many we metabolize matters.

And yet there is a lot more to nutrition. A LOT more. For health. For brain health too. And not just neuron health, but also for mental health. Even for our focus and ability to learn.

There's a lot more to nutrition, in part because there are a lot of experts with different perspectives. True experts, who have done the research, observed what works or fails in the real world with women, men, kids, healthy and sick people, and with those who exercise and those who don't, or just won't.

I have had a closeup view of just how many perspectives are out there through my podcast. I've talked for hours with "pro-plant-based" scientists like Christopher Gardner, PhD, professor of medicine at Stanford University.[2] I've learned from nutritional scientist Layne Norton, PhD, and nutrition educator Alan Aragon, MS, who draw from both their academic training and their experience working with thousands of people.[3] I hosted osteopathic physician Gabrielle Lyon, DO, to discuss protein needs for both women and men, and endocrinologist Robert Lustig, MD, professor at University of California, San Francisco, about sugar.[4] (P.S. Robert is not a fan of sugar!) Justin Sonnenburg, PhD, a microbiologist at Stanford and perhaps the world expert on the human gut microbiome, spoke with me about how to support a healthy gut with specific foods.[5] Harvard Medical School psychiatrist Chris Palmer, MD, explained the now-demonstrated benefits of the ketogenic diet for depression and other mental health issues.[6] And Satchin Panda, PhD, who directs the Regulatory Biology Laboratory at the Salk Institute for Biological Studies, in San Diego, shared his extensive knowledge on the science of intermittent fasting.[7]

These experts disagree—sometimes vehemently—on many things . . . no surprise there. But they also agree about many things, and one foundational understanding in particular: that when it comes to body weight, how many calories we eat relative to how many we metabolize does matter.

In this chapter, you'll learn the consensus from nutrition experts that you likely have not heard anywhere else. I'll also share my own experience and observations, having tried many different approaches to nutrition. And I share one that is seldom discussed but that I, and many others, have used to great success. It builds on this consensus. It cuts through the noise. It puts you in the driver's seat so you can make satisfying food choices that don't sacrifice taste; that support your body composition goals; and that help ensure you get the macro- and micronutrients you need for brain and bodily health. And it can be done on a budget.

The Clean Omnivore Diet

I call the approach I'm suggesting here the "Clean Omnivore Diet." As you'll see in the pages that follow, this approach to nutrition is based in science. We begin, as we have for each of the topics in this book, with data. I provide an overview of nutrition to get everyone on the same page, and to help you navigate what follows. I do hope you'll read it, because I know it will empower you, but I'll understand if you'd like to jump to the protocols so you can learn what to eat and when for maximal health.

Body composition affects health and longevity. People with a higher ratio of lean mass to body fat tend to live longer than those with relatively higher percentages of body fat.[8]

More than 70 percent of Americans are overweight and more than a third are obese,[9] which basically means the majority of Americans are likely shortening their lifespan with their eating habits. The harshest messaging of this I've ever heard was from an MD colleague of mine who said, "You just don't meet many obese eighty-year-olds." Fill in the blanks on that.

Physicians are known for gallows humor, but this point matches the data. Body composition matters.

The advice for most people, given the above, might simply be "lose weight." But that is short sighted. I said body composition, not weight loss. If you lose weight and much of it is muscle mass, your metabolism drops, and then it's very easy to gain the weight back. (Muscle, if you recall from chapter 2, is very metabolically active, and plays a role in blood sugar management and therefore affects insulin sensitivity, which refers to how well your body responds to increases in blood sugar.) You need to maintain and/or increase muscle mass, along with bone mass, while you lose mostly body fat. And while bone is not as sexy sounding as muscle, having adequate bone mass and density is vitally important for your health and longevity too.[10]

The not-so-secret secret solution? Do resistance training, and eat at what we call maintenance calories, or slightly submaintenance calories (300–500 calories less than you need per day—more on that in a moment) . . . unless of course you are among those trying to gain weight, in which case you want to eat a bit more (300–500) each day. In the short run, this works. But in the long run, everyone—not just those seeking to lose or gain weight—needs to eat for health and longevity, but also for taste, and in a way that is compatible with their social life, schedule, and budget. That's a tall order.

The great news is that there's considerable overlap among diets that do just that—and that includes the Clean Omnivore Diet. They won't leave you avoiding restaurants, either. But they require understanding what food and nutrition are really about.

WHAT TO EAT

There are three macronutrients: proteins, carbohydrates, and fats. Each of these can be subdivided into categories according to how they are used by the body. Let's take a closer look at each, one at a time.

How to Think About Protein

Dietary proteins are foods rich in amino acids, compounds that our body needs to make its own proteins. All the cells and tissues of our body—hair, muscle, bone, et cetera—contain those proteins. So we need amino acids from food to keep our cells and tissues functional. Of the twenty amino acids found in the human body, there are nine that we cannot make on our own; they must come directly from outside sources—namely from dietary protein.[11] These nine amino acids are called the essential amino acids, and foods containing them are referred to as complete proteins. Many foods sourced from animals, such as red meat, poultry, fish, eggs, and shellfish, such as scallops and oysters, as well as many dairy products, contain all nine essential amino acids, and thus are considered complete proteins. Some plant-based foods such as quinoa, hemp seeds, and soy also contain all nine essential amino acids.

Most plant-based foods, however, do not have all nine essential amino acids and must be combined with each other to be considered complete proteins. Examples include beans with rice, or nuts with lentils. There is a lot of debate (of course) as to whether animal-based proteins are superior to plant-based proteins, but the debate is often misleading because it neglects a key feature of any protein. And that is what I will refer to as the complete-protein-to-calorie ratio (CP:C ratio). Even when comparing animal-based complete proteins to one another, it is important to consider their relative CP:C ratios. I'll illustrate this concept by comparing some examples of different foods: 150 calories of chicken versus 150 calories of lean beef versus 150 calories of whole eggs versus 150 calories of tofu versus 150 calories of beans and rice. All are considered complete proteins.

Now, importantly, while you would need to eat beans and rice (or nearly any legume and any grain combination) to get all nine essential amino acids, these do not need to be eaten in the same meal to be utilized effectively. As long as you get sufficient essential amino acids across your meals over the course of a day, it works.

150 calories of chicken has about 28 grams of complete protein
150 calories of lean beef has about 25 grams of complete protein
150 calories of whole eggs contains about 13 grams of complete protein
150 calories of tofu has about 15 grams of complete protein
150 calories of beans and rice has about 6 grams of complete protein
150 calories of peanut butter on a slice of wheat bread has about 6.5 grams of complete protein
And let's throw in 150 calories of scallops, which has about 29 grams of complete protein.

The reason different foods and food combinations yield different amounts of complete protein at the same caloric level is because none of these foods are 100 percent protein. They also contain some fat, or in the case of plant foods, carbohydrates and fats.

Most animal-based foods like meat, eggs, and shellfish contain zero (or close to zero) carbohydrates, and varying amounts of fat. Dairy products contain protein and fat (unless defatted, like skim milk, for example), and dairy includes carbohydrates to varying degrees.

So we need to ask: Does a given "protein" contain all nine essential amino acids? And: What is its CP:C ratio?

In other words: How many calories of a given "protein" food do we need to eat in order to get enough of those nine essential amino acids?

The answer to that question matters for body composition, health, and the pleasure you experience from eating, because getting those nine essential amino acids is crucial for satiety. That's because how much you eat at a meal is driven in part by your brain's and body's hunger for complete proteins. When you get enough complete protein, you tend to feel satisfied during, and for a long while after, the meal. When you don't, you tend to feel hungry again soon after eating.

The nine amino acids are not the only reason we eat, but they are a big part of it. Below I'll explain how, if we don't get enough complete protein per calorie, we start to run into problems. Luckily, those problems are easy to fix. I'll explain how to do that too.

I often hear: "But I eat protein! I eat beans, I eat peanut butter . . ." Well, neither of those are complete proteins, but if the beans are served with rice or if the peanut butter is spread on wheat bread, then they become complete proteins. Problem solved? Usually not. In fact, often it's problem *created*. Remember, beans and rice together provide 6 grams of protein for every 150 calories. That means you would need to eat more than four times as many calories of beans and rice (700 calories) to hit the same amount of protein (28 grams) found in 150 calories of chicken. Peanut butter on wheat bread is a similar story, given that in those 150 calories, you're only getting 6.5 grams of protein. That brings us back to CP:C ratio. Chicken has a high ratio; beans and rice or peanut butter on wheat bread has a low ratio.

To be fair, some animal-based foods also have a low CP:C ratio. Take most pork for instance. One hundred fifty calories of lean pork will give you about the same amount of protein as 150 calories of chicken or beef (about 25 grams). But most commercially sold pork products, such as bacon, ham, and pork chops, are not lean. Most contain a high percentage of fat, and often have sugar added to them too. One hundred fifty calories of low-sugar bacon has only about 10 grams of protein. Typical store-bought bacon with sugar added? About half that, at 5 grams. You would need to eat about 400 to 500 calories of bacon to get the protein found in 150 calories of chicken.

The takeaway here is that we need to prioritize eating complete protein foods, and we need to consider the CP:C ratio when selecting which to eat. While protein is not the whole story, the best nutrition plan typically places proteins with a high CP:C ratio at the center of the plate.

WHAT PROTEINS ARE BEST?

If you eat animal products, I suggest you prioritize lean cuts of beef, elk, venison, or bison, as well as fish and chicken. They have a high CP:C ratio. Many dairy products do, too, such as Greek and Bulgarian yogurt, and cottage cheese. Eggs are great as well, even though they do not technically meet the benchmark, given their ratio of protein to fat. That said, I still incorporate eggs into my diet most days. After years of public debate on whether eggs are healthy or unhealthy, the FDA consensus as of 2025 is that, yes, eggs are healthy. They appear on a list right next to salmon, 100 percent olive oil, fruits, and vegetables.[12] Our grandparents were right (again!).

Powdered proteins such as whey protein have a very high CP:C ratio and are a convenient way to get enough protein for perhaps a meal or snack per day, maybe two if you're on the go. But they should not be your only complete protein source because they lack a number of important vitamins and minerals and other micronutrients found in whole foods. You want to prioritize whole foods for that.

Plant-based sources of proteins, by contrast, tend to have a low CP:C ratio. So much so that it is best not to think of most plant-based foods as proteins at all. It's more accurate to think of grains, like rice and quinoa, and legumes, like beans, simply as carbohydrates, because that's mainly what they are. And think of the lipid-rich plant-based sources of proteins, like nuts, as fats, because that's mainly what they are. There are exceptions, but by and large the CP:C ratio of these foods is just too low to consider them otherwise. Unless you're burning significant calories through long-duration exercise or physical labor, relying on low CP:C ratio foods to try to get enough complete protein often leads to eating excess calories and putting on body fat. And for those trying to gain weight—yes, such people are out there—devote your additional calories to high CP:C ratio proteins, carbohydrates, and healthy fats.

And before you say "He's an anti-vegan, ketogenic carnivore!" I assure you that is not the case. None of this is leading up to me suggesting a purely animal-based diet. I think vegetables and fruits are fantastic. I eat them daily and some grains too. Vegans who are willing to put in the work to seek out or prepare dishes with a variety of ingredients—such as beans and other legumes, rice and other grains, and tofu and tempeh—can get adequate amounts of the nine essential amino acids across the day without eating animal products. They just need to be mindful not to eat too many calories relative to their overall energy needs. I have seen a vegan diet work great for some people, but admittedly they tend to be very diligent about the sourcing and combining of their plant-based foods to achieve complete proteins. Or they do a lot of cardiovascular exercise—they run marathons, triathlons, and distance races of that sort—which comes with very high caloric needs compared to that of most people.

One more consideration as you select a protein source is the bioavailability of that protein source—how much protein you can absorb as you digest it, and then how much your cells can make use of it. There is ongoing debate about this amount. Classic studies concluded that we can only absorb about 30 grams of protein per meal.[13] That amount became a sort of "law" of nutrition, especially in resistance training fitness circles that prioritize muscle protein synthesis—a process that is stimulated by weight lifting, but that is also involved in muscle maintenance for everyone, lifters and non-lifters alike. Later studies showed, however, that our bodies can use pretty much any amount of protein we ingest.[14] What changed? Mostly the conversation around protein absorption.

A portion of the protein that we consume at any given meal is used by our muscles. But there's a limit to the "dose" of protein our muscles can synthesize; that dose is around 30 to 50 grams at one time.[15] Whatever amount we consume beyond that will be absorbed by the gut and the liver, and used for things like neurotransmitter production, hair and collagen growth, immune system function, and much more. (Note that for kids still growing, and for those who resistance train regularly, the amount directed for protein synthesis is probably closer to 40 to 50 grams per meal, with the excess available for other tasks.)

Does this mean that you must consume 30 to 50 grams of protein at every meal if you want to maintain your current muscle mass? Nope. Research on intermittent fasting (a good setting to investigate this question because daily calories are consumed in a small window rather than as three meals spread across a day) found that lean muscle mass is preserved as long as enough total protein is consumed in a day.[16]

All of this explains why people versed in nutrition don't just talk about how much protein we can absorb, but the metabolic fate of the proteins we eat. In fact, there are times when assimilating 100 grams (!) per meal is possible.[17] Does that mean you should eat 100 grams of protein per meal? Not necessarily. First off, how many meals are you eating? And how much protein do you need? Again, we return to the data.

HOW MUCH PROTEIN DO YOU NEED?

Most people should aim to consume 1 gram of protein, ideally from high CP:C ratio protein sources, per pound of body weight each day. It's not crucial that you eat exactly that much every day. I suggest it as a target from which you experiment a bit to find your protein needs. If you find yourself too full or otherwise unable to hit it, that's okay. You should never feel like you're force-feeding yourself just to hit a protein goal. Strive to hit the 1 gram of protein per pound of body weight (or close to it) most days. And if you prefer to divide your protein into multiple meals and snacks per day, do that. If, however, you prefer to eat twice a day and ingest more protein at those meals, do that, even if you're resistance training specifically to gain muscle. While it's true that spreading out your protein across four to five meals and snacks per day can provide a marginal increase in muscle protein synthesis if you're resistance training and aiming to gain the maximum amount of new muscle, the difference it makes won't be meaningful for the majority of people. So figure out the timing of your meals and snacks that works best for your hunger, energy levels, sleep, and schedule. Be mindful of, but don't obsess about, that 1 gram of protein per pound of body weight target.

Some people worry that eating too much protein can cause kidney problems or gout, but the data show that only becomes an issue if people consume something in the vicinity of more than 3 grams of protein per pound of body weight—an absurdly high amount that most people would struggle to reach.[18] So don't fear eating high CP:C ratio foods. That's one more debate that's easy to settle.

Another debate: There is also talk that deliberately eating far less protein than we need can help us live longer. The theory is that eating protein stimulates a rise in the level of mTOR (which stands for mammalian target of rapamycin), a protein related to cell growth that, when suppressed, has been shown to extend lifespan in animals.[19] So far, however, the data point to "NOPE" on whether a low-protein-to-suppress-mTOR diet helps humans live longer.[20]

Entire books could be devoted to any of the topics above but for now, let's just keep the CP:C ratio in the back of our minds as an important metric to consider when making food choices. Prioritizing eating enough foods with a high CP:C ratio to reach that 1 gram per pound of body weight removes a lot of confusion in the "what to eat" debate.

How to Think About Carbohydrates

Carbohydrates, or carbs, as we often call them, have become appropriately controversial in the last few decades. I say that because carbs include both healthy and very unhealthy varieties. And no, that's not determined by just whether a carb is complex versus simple, a term that refers to their molecular structure (more on that later). Some carbs quell hunger. Others can make you eat with abandon. Sometimes it depends what those carbs are combined with. Carbs combined with fat and with sugar, for example, can make people with a sweet tooth feel like an addict who just scored: focused on getting more. It becomes very easy to overeat.

Should you just cut out all carbs? Well, cutting out carbs completely will make you lose weight fast, but mostly you lose water weight as carbs cause you to "hold" water.[21] For most people, I don't suggest suddenly cutting out carbs completely, though cutting back on certain types of carbs can be beneficial for many people. I've seen folks with autoimmune issues resolve them by moving to a carnivore (meat, salt only) or ketogenic (very low carb) diet. Then, most gradually reintroduce carbs over time, learning which carbs are problematic for them and which are not. I have also seen people who could not lose body fat do so on very low carb diets. Ketogenic diets have also been shown to be an effective treatment for some forms of drug-resistant epilepsy[22] and in some cases for schizophrenia[23] and depression.[24] Also, some people just "feel better," both mentally and physically, on a zero or near-zero carbohydrate diet. Incidentally, I am not one of those people. I love fruits and vegetables and I eat starches, but I am thoughtful about which and, to some extent, when.

I also know people who have done well on an "animal-based" diet, which recommends people eat only meat, fish, eggs, and dairy. It's actually a misnomer because the actual animal-based diet made popular by Paul Saladino, MD, includes not just meat, eggs, fish, and dairy, but also fruits such as dates, bananas, cucumbers, and tomatoes (yes, those last two are fruits).[25] This diet is much easier to adhere to, and arguably much healthier in the long run than a pure-meat carnivore diet. The controversial part is that it is ostensibly "anti-vegetables." In the last year, I have seen public messaging from Paul that asparagus now gets the green light. (No pun intended.)

The low starch, minimal-to-zero vegetables thing can be a real challenge. The vast majority of us are—and want to continue to be—omnivores, meaning we would like to eat meat but also fruits, vegetables, and, yes, other carbohydrates. So with that in mind, let's parse this category of macronutrients.

First, there is no such thing as an essential carbohydrate—you can survive by eating only proteins and fats. But all our cells run on glucose and, assuming we eat them, carbs readily get converted to glucose. That glucose is absorbed into our bloodstream—which leads to a rise in blood sugar, which in turn triggers the release of hormones like insulin that help manage this fuel. Typically, the breakdown of carbs into glucose is what our bodies prioritize for energy, then fats, and finally protein. That's an oversimplification, but all things being equal, that's the sequence.

To fully understand how carbs work, you need to know a bit more about how carbs are processed alone and in combination with other foods, and how they impact appetite. Carbohydrates can be broadly divided into complex carbohydrates and simple carbohydrates. Complex carbohydrates can be further (and still broadly) divided into starchy complex carbs and fibrous complex carbs. As a general rule, starchy complex carbohydrates, aka starches, are complex carbohydrates that completely or mostly dissolve in your mouth (after they are cooked or manufactured). Examples include rice, potatoes, beans, yams, pasta, lentils, bread, chips and crackers, and so on. When consumed with little or no added fats or sugars, non-processed starchy carbs are what some call clean starches. So if you're wondering—chips and crackers, while mostly starch, are not clean. Although fairly calorie dense, clean starches like oatmeal, potatoes, rice, beans, and lentils are terrific sources of energy because they are more slowly converted to glucose by the body. Breads made without excess sugar or preservatives such as rye bread, sourdough, and unbleached wheat bread can also be considered clean(ish) starches.

That being said, you can overconsume starchy carbs.[26] Four things tend to lead you there:

- If you don't eat enough high CP:C ratio protein along with them.
- If you add sugar to them including jams, honey, syrup, and more.
- If you add fat to them like butter, oil, or cheese.
- If you add both sugars and fats.

Starchy carbs are easy to overconsume, in no small part because they literally melt in your mouth. They are flavorful especially when combined with fat and salt (think bread alone versus bread and butter with salt or bread dipped in olive oil with salt, or french fries, or macaroni and cheese). And when starches are combined with fat and sugar and just enough salt to bring out the sweet taste (think cheesecake, doughnuts, chocolate cake, pie, ice cream, and most breakfast cereals nowadays) most people find them super tasty, and hard to not overeat. Processed starchy carbs, like chips, crackers, store-bought cookies, frozen pizza, burritos, et cetera, are basically starches with fats and/or sugar blended evenly throughout, so every bite tastes identical—identically scrumptious that is. Chips and crackers are especially easy to overconsume because they activate the "eat more of this!" circuit in your brain and body, without any of the usual satiety promoting features of whole foods. They tend to have a very low CP:C ratio, and they are incredibly calorie dense for their size. You can easily eat 800 calories of chips without feeling full . . . and in many cases doing that will tend to increase your appetite. By comparison, you would have to eat about 16 ounces (a pound!) of cooked steak to get to the same 800 calories. I'm betting by the tenth ounce of steak, you're going to feel very satiated, and would stay that way for many hours.

I don't want to demonize starches. I eat them. I love them. Rice and pasta dishes and a great thick-crusted rye, or sourdough bread with olive oil or butter and salt are some of my favorite foods. I also think most people can enjoy a slice of cake or pie, a scoop of ice cream, a hot dog, a slice or two of pizza, and other carb-fat-sugar combinations now and again without any issue. But even if they are homemade, or from a bakery or restaurant that uses quality ingredients, they should not be a staple of anyone's diet. And the packaged, processed versions are certainly damaging to our health. This is true for a variety of reasons, but their low micronutrient value and their tendency to make people overeat are just two.[27]

SO WHICH CARBS SHOULD WE EAT?

Most people, unless following a ketogenic, carnivore, or animal-based diet, should consume some clean carbs one to three times per day. How much? A simple solution is to scale your starchy carb intake with the amount and type of physical activity you're doing. Unless you are still growing, are very lean (less than 10 percent body fat for a man and less than 15 percent for a woman), or are doing a lot of cardio (1.5 hours or more per day on average) or hard manual labor (3-plus days a week), it is probably best to limit your starch intake to a third or less of your daily calories. Strive to make that from clean starches, and don't add more than one to two tablespoons of fat (butter or olive oil, etc.) to any one starch serving. And don't add sugar.

If you do intense cardio or hard resistance training three or more times a week (meaning you are doing compound multi-joint exercises and take your work sets to failure; see chapter 2 for details), then consider also consuming some clean starches in the meals that follow your training session. Ideally, eat some fruit too. Long, intense cardio and resistance training of the sort described in chapter 2 can deplete your glycogen reserves.[28] You would be wise to consume 30 to 75 grams of high CP:C ratio protein in that same meal. By the way, unless it's very intense, a yoga class or bodyweight workout won't meaningfully deplete your glycogen reserves. Nor will half an hour of Zone 2 running or easy laps in the swimming pool. That is not what I'm talking about. But if you push yourself running, swimming, or cycling or training with heavy (for you) weights for forty-five to seventy-five minutes, or do a truly hard Pilates workout, then you likely need to replenish your glycogen reserves. Eating some clean starches (and fruit and some high CP:C ratio protein) is a great way to do that. In fact, unless you're in ketosis and familiar with that state, failure to replenish your glycogen, or dropping your starches to zero for one to two days in a row, can lead to sleep challenges, headaches, and brain fog. Resistance training with any real intensity when you haven't eaten any starches in the preceding days can be extremely difficult. Most need those clean starches, just not in excess. And if you resistance train with intensity—taking sets to failure or close to it (as described in chapter 2)—you'll want to eat those clean starches to have the glycogen your muscles need to continue your workouts.

On that note, if you follow a ketogenic, animal-based, or carnivore diet, you'll have to make up for the lack of starch with calories from fat and/or protein, and be mindful of replenishing your glycogen in other ways after hard workouts. Protein can be converted to glucose by your liver through a process called gluconeogenesis. I know very few people who consistently follow a pure ketogenic or pure carnivore diet who also consistently resistance train with intensity, but they exist. Shawn Baker, MD, a popular public educator and proponent of the carnivore diet, is a good example of someone for whom this approach works. I've seen a fair number of low/no-carb folks who do pull-ups and push-ups and other body weight exercises as well as cardio. But for most people, if you train with weights in a manner similar to how I described in Exercise Protocol 2, you're going to want to eat starches, especially in the meal following training.

There's another type of carbohydrate to discuss: fibrous carbohydrates, which as their name suggests, are high-fiber-containing carbohydrates like broccoli, cucumbers, lettuce, kale, chard, asparagus, and so on. These tend not to dissolve in your mouth, even if they are cooked first. It's hard to overstate how great complex fibrous carbs are for us. Indeed, most of us should be trying to eat more of them. They are rich with vitamins, minerals, and other micronutrients and, as their name suggests, they contain a lot of fiber. We're told all the time that we need to eat more fiber, but trying to get fiber mainly from starches is a mistake. That tends to make people gain body fat, and I'm hearing from more and more people about allergy and gut issues due to eating too many grains. Look to get most of your fiber from vegetables. Though be mindful to chew your fibrous carbs well or they can be hard on your digestive tract. And it's good to note if any specific fibrous carbs do not agree with you (you'll know!). But as a general rule, ingesting more fiber from vegetables and from low-sugar fruits is associated with better health outcomes and longevity.[29] Fibrous carbs also slow the absorption of glucose into your bloodstream for a steadier rise in your glucose levels, and they make you feel full.[30] Our sense of satiety comes from a combination of having eaten enough essential amino acids and fatty acids, and from our glucose levels having risen (but not too high), but also from the mechano-sensation of the stretch sensors in our gut . . . which is nerd-speak for "feeling full."

There are even more benefits. As I mentioned, vegetables contain remarkably high levels of micronutrients, like vitamins, minerals, and more, and deliver those with very few calories. Whether they taste "yum," "yuck," or "meh" to you tends to be a function of age (know many kids under eight that love chard?), and how these foods are prepared. It should be obvious that adding a lot of oil or butter or sugary sauces can quickly make fibrous vegetables easy to overeat, and very calorie dense—especially if the vegetables are cooked—so add those sparingly.

And we should all avoid fried vegetables, fried starches, and fried meats. Fried foods are terrible for your cardiovascular health and longevity and even have been linked to poorer mental health.[31] They are high in calories, often high in sodium, and can contain trans fat, which has been linked to heart disease and other bad outcomes. If you're serious about your health, ditch them. If you indulge occasionally with a doughnut or French fries, no big deal. But if eating fried foods is a daily, or even a weekly habit, it will likely catch up to you.

There's one last carbohydrate relevant to this conversation. Simple carbohydrates are what are often referred to as sugars—although that can lead to a lot of confusion.

Unfortunately, when most people hear the word *sugar* they immediately think of white table sugar, or sucrose, but simple sugars exist in many forms. Naturally occurring simple sugars in foods that have fiber and fairly high water content, like fruits or vegetables, are absorbed more slowly. The simple sugars found in honey or maple syrup, which have very little fiber, and no fat, are absorbed very quickly. Lactose, the simple sugar found in full-fat milk, is absorbed slowly because of the presence of fat. The point is that sugars vary in type, and how fast they are absorbed depends on the other macronutrients (proteins, fats, and carbs) you eat with them.

Maybe you've heard that "sugar is poison." This is not true of the sugar in fruit and vegetables, or in many full-fat milk products. If your goal is to have stable blood sugar and energy levels, those sources of sugar should account for about 95 percent of your sugar intake. And while you must be careful not to overconsume maple syrup or honey and other natural liquid sweeteners—they are very dense with sugar and calories—they are not poison. So adding a small bit of pure honey or pure maple syrup to your food or drinks every so often is no big deal.

Refined sugars are another story. Refined sugars are simple sugars that have been stripped of their fiber or fat content and are often chemically modified to taste extremely sweet. Some are so sweet that consuming them may change your sweet taste threshold and make otherwise savory or sweet tasting foods taste more bland.[32] Luckily that effect is reversible if you cut out refined sugars even just for a few days.

Sucrose, which is refined from sugarcane, is the most basic example of a refined sugar. A bit of it here or there, like table sugar in dessert, is generally not a problem for most people. Keeping refined sugars to 5 percent or less of your sugar intake is a good idea. Or, if you loathe tracking that sort of thing, simply limit yourself to one serving—a scoop of ice cream or piece of cake—per week. To some of you that may seem spartan. To others, that may seem indulgent. Later we will discuss sugar cravings, and how to beat them. In the meantime, I can assure you that it is possible to stop craving sugar, and cutting out refined sugars entirely, or close to it, is the first step in that process.

Alas, these days, sucrose or high-fructose corn syrup are put into all sorts of foods that we think of as savory (e.g., soups, cereals, sauces, and salad dressings) in order to make them taste sweeter than they would otherwise. So be a bit more vigilant and read food labels if your goal is to avoid added sugars of any kind.

Sugar is immensely reinforcing—ingesting it makes you want to eat more. So while people debate if sugar is truly "addicting," most everyone agrees that consuming refined sugars is highly reinforcing, and is not healthy—or at least offers little, if any, nutritional benefit.[33]

So while I don't think that sugar is "poison," nor do I feel it meets the classic definition of addictive, which would mean its use is progressive and destructive to multiple areas of life, I do, however, think eating too many sugars, and especially refined sugars, is bad for us. It can lead to gaining body fat due to the overconsumption of calories with little nutritional value, as well as insulin sensitivity problems that, at the extreme, can cause diabetes and other metabolic issues.[34] It can even lead to mental health challenges, such as depression.[35]

And sugar is everywhere. Consider that complex starchy carbohydrates—like wheat, rice, potatoes—if refined to remove their fiber content become more like simple carbohydrates. Foods containing refined flours, such as bread, pasta, cereals, crackers, and most packaged snack foods, are good examples. And they often contain added sugar as well. Even if the packages show some amount of fiber, these foods almost always act more like sugars in the body—they get absorbed fast, and almost always lead to an overconsumption of calories with little nutritional value. While eating something fibrous (like a salad) or fatty (like almond butter) with these refined complex carbs will typically slow their absorption, the outcome is almost always the same: an overconsumption of calories with little nutritional value. I'm not out to demonize the packaged food industry but their goal is simple: to get you to buy and consume more of what they sell. And it's clear they've been successful in reaching that goal given the prevalence of these foods and the declining health of those who consume them. We have plenty of evidence now linking ultra-processed foods with serious health issues, including heart disease, type 2 diabetes, obesity, depression, and impaired sleep.[36] The more cryptically problematic foods, in my opinion, are refined carbohydrates with added sugars. We don't think of them as highly processed compared to, say, chips or microwave meals, but they are nearly as bad in terms of our propensity to overeat them. Luckily there is an easier and much more satisfying way to eat. One that is affordable too. But first, we have to understand fats.

How to Think About Fats

First off, it's a real shame this category of macronutrients is called *fats* because that immediately makes people think about body fat, which almost no one wants. But you do want fats in your diet. *Lipids* would have been a better choice in my opinion but alas, here we are.

Fats are lipids, and they are calorically dense: 9 calories per gram compared to 4 calories per gram for carbs or protein. And fats are vitally important. We can't live without them. In fact, a large part of each of our cells is made of fats, and thus consuming enough fats is crucial for cellular function and repair throughout the body. You need to eat fats, but the right kinds and the right amounts. So get it out of your mind that fats are bad. Remember, there are no essential carbohydrates, but you absolutely must eat protein and fat to survive.

Fats can be broadly divided into saturated fats and unsaturated fats.

The simplest way to recognize a saturated fat is that these are generally solid at room temperature. The saturated fat in cheeses and meats are good examples of this. While some non-animal sources such as coconuts and Brazil nuts contain saturated fat, most saturated fats come from meat, dairy, and eggs. People love to debate if saturated fats raise your cholesterol, and it's become a circular argument because yes, they do, but then the discussion turns to if cholesterol levels, HDL and LDL (classically referred to as the good and bad cholesterols, respectively), are truly meaningful in predicting heart disease and longevity, or if there are more important metrics. The whole thing can get rather confusing.[37] Some people who eat low saturated fat diets have high LDL, due to genetics or other factors like age; some people who eat high saturated fat diets don't have high LDL, but they also tend to eat a lot of fiber, and not much starch and sugar. Pretty soon, talk turns to how insulin from carbs and not just fats impacts LDL . . . and the debate rages on.

SO HOW MUCH FAT DO I NEED IN MY DIET?

If you are eating animal-based proteins daily, and that includes eggs, red meat, or full-fat dairy, chances are good that you are getting enough saturated fat. If you are vegetarian or entirely plant-based, you might consider incorporating eggs and dairy (if vegetarian), along with coconut or coconut oil, macadamia nuts, cashews, or other foods and oils that have saturated fat.

Although debated, the data show that you want only moderate amounts of saturated fats in your diet because high levels of saturated fat consumption can increase systemic inflammation—an effect that is only made worse if you also ingest sugar.[38] Some might argue that is a consequence of eating saturated fats and carbs, not the fats per se. Yet, even if you're following a strictly ketogenic diet, excess saturated fat consumption is not good for your immediate or long-term health.[39] So regardless of whether you are an omnivore, keto, or vegetarian, consuming leaner cuts of meat and emphasizing proteins with high CP:C ratios will help keep your saturated fat intake relatively low. It's worth noting that I regularly do blood work to keep an eye on my cholesterol levels and other blood biomarkers. I think this is a good practice to truly understand how diet is affecting your blood lipids. Function Health, a company I'm an advisor to, makes this type of testing quite affordable. There are other companies entering the space as well and helping to drive the cost of blood tests down.

WHAT ABOUT UNSATURATED FATS?

Unsaturated fats tend to be liquid at room temperature. There are two types: monounsaturated and polyunsaturated fats, both of which come mainly from fish, seeds, olives, and avocados. (More on the benefits of unsaturated fats in Nutrition Protocol 5.)

And for those of you following the ongoing debate about seed oils—canola, grapeseed, corn oils, et cetera—I give my take on them in Nutrition Protocol 5. Some evidence points to the idea that if seed oils are used to replace someone's saturated fat intake, their health improves.[40] Though that overlooks the fact that consuming seed oils often tends to correlate with eating more processed foods, and carb-fat combination foods. And some argue excessive heat during seed oil processing makes them potentially hazardous, which is why this topic is contentious. (Nutrition Protocol 5 gives you a fuller picture.)

My recommendation is to save yourself a giant headache and when given the choice between cooking with seed oils or other fats, go with pure olive oil or avocado oil, or perhaps some small amount of butter, tallow, or ghee. If you need to cook at high temperatures, avocado oil is your best bet given that it has a high smoke point. Smoke point is the temperature at which an oil starts to smoke under high heat—which can lead to it degrading as the fats oxidize, and that produces harmful compounds linked to inflammation. When it comes to seed oils, I personally avoid them, opting to cook and make salad dressing from olive oil and using small amounts of butter here and there. No one debates olive oil's health benefits.[41] And it's delicious.

THE BEST DIET FOR YOU

We have covered a lot here. But if you're realizing that the use of words like proteins, carbs, sugars, and fats requires distinguishing the different types of each and how they interact, then you're on track to devise the best diet for you. The good news: There are several different diet frameworks that allow for that, so you have options. Here they are:

Low Carb/Keto

Technically speaking, as discussed, we can get all we need to survive from consuming only proteins and fats, and can skip carbohydrates entirely. Done right, the ketogenic diet tends to raise energy levels and assist weight loss, because you excrete a lot of water that starches normally cause you to retain. Ketogenic diets have also been shown to help resolve symptoms of epilepsy, as mentioned already, as well as major depression, bipolar depression, even schizophrenia, in some people, and there is growing evidence it may help for people with gut and autoimmune issues.[42] But to do it right means eating mostly fat, some protein, and very, very little carbohydrates, along with all the vitamins and minerals you need—which takes a lot of discipline and attention to detail. Most people just won't do that for long because they can't imagine saying goodbye to bread, fruit, pasta, salads, et cetera, forever. Still, it might be the right choice for you. Ask yourself this: Are you willing to give up starches and fruit?

Pure Vegan

By pure vegan, I mean no animal products whatsoever. That's possible. A vegan friend of mine (yes, I have some vegan friends) is a "platinum star" vegan, meaning he's never knowingly eaten any animal products. The real challenge with this diet is getting enough high CP:C ratio proteins without eating too many calories, and to make sure you don't overconsume processed foods, just because many of them—such as French fries or coconut ice cream—are vegan (and convenient and delicious). I know people who have been vegans for many years and thrive. One thing all vegans must be careful of is muscle loss, especially as they age. Resistance training can help offset that, but getting those high CP:C ratio proteins is key, of course, too.

Animal-Based

This diet has a very misleading name, as, yes, it includes meat, eggs, and fish, but also fruit, honey, dates, tomatoes, avocados, coconut, hard cheeses, and other full-fat dairy. Sounds decadent, no? It is. But it also takes some discipline to follow because it's an omnivorous diet minus any starches or vegetables. That means no rice, no oatmeal, no bread, no broccoli, no lettuce, and on and on. Yes, it intentionally lacks vegetables. And the only processed food you'll eat on this diet is hard cheese like Parmesan. This diet is possible for pescatarians who want to eat fatty ocean fish such as salmon and sardines. It's also fine for people who don't like red meat but eat poultry. I have heard from many people who have achieved impressive body composition results and improved their health outcomes by following an animal-based diet. That said, because it includes a lot of calorie-dense foods, you still need to watch your total caloric and saturated fat intake. In my view, any dramatic effectiveness of this diet is likely to be multifactorial, including that it limits starch-fat and starch-sugar combinations, and that it makes no room for processed foods or refined sugars of any kind. It tends to quell hunger fairly well and contribute to stable blood sugar. That said, it can tend to lead to very high LDL levels in some individuals, which can be correlated with increased risk of heart disease and stroke, a result of fatty plaque building up in arteries.[43] If you opt to follow an animal based diet, I suggest getting a calcium CT scan of your heart before starting and again a year later to see if it causes you to add plaque to your arteries. I know people for whom it has made plaque worsen, and those for whom (independent of their LDL levels) it has not caused increased blockages. We still have a lot to learn about the relationship between LDL, markers like ApoB, diet, and cardiovascular diseases. Meanwhile, assess your current cardiovascular risk profile and how your diet—animal-based or otherwise—is impacting it.

Clean Omnivore

My diet of choice is what I call the Clean Omnivore Diet because it checks off all, not just a few, of the key pillars of effective, health-promoting, delicious, cost-effective, and practical nutrition, which makes it easy to stick to. If we take a step back from the debates, and ask what we need and want from a great overall diet, the answer that emerges is this:

- **Plenty of protein from high CP:C ratio sources:**
    - Aim for 1 gram per pound of body weight of high CP:C ratio proteins. Some days a bit more, some a bit less. If that feels excessive, and you find yourself dreading eating these foods, scale it back a bit.
- **Plenty of fiber, vitamins, and minerals and micronutrients, from vegetables:**
    - 35 grams of fiber recommended for men each day.
    - 25 grams of fiber for women each day.
- **Healthy fats:**
    - Like olive oil, avocados, and maybe a bit from dairy like Greek or (my favorite) Bulgarian yogurt or nuts. Small amounts of butter are fine. Nuts and nut butters are calorically dense, and most people tend to overeat them, but assuming they contain no added oils or sugars (including cane sugar) they are also fine. (Read the packaging; manufacturers seem to sneak those into everything nowadays!)
- **Fruit:**
    - Two to four pieces or servings per day depending on activity levels and caloric needs. Berries are a great choice, but expensive. Look for citrus, apples, peaches, and on and on. If you want to look up the sugar and fiber content of different fruit, do; opt for the lower sugar, higher fiber varieties if you can.

- **Clean starches:**
    - Think rice, oatmeal, potatoes, yams, sourdough or rye bread, beans, lentils. The goal is to eat enough of these to fuel your brain and bodily activities, including regular moderate to intense exercise four to six days per week.

That's what to seek out.

And not to sound like a broken record, but most people are best off limiting starch-fat combination foods and starch-fat-sugar combination foods. That means very little, if any, highly processed food like candy or cookies, boxed or frozen meals, or sugary drinks. Just cut them out. You'll feel so much better in every way—not just in appearance, but your cravings for sugar will be greatly reduced.

If you want a decadent homemade or real bakery-made dessert, homemade pasta, or a couple of slices of pizza or ice cream now and again—as in up to once a week—no big deal (especially if you're exercising as described in chapter 2).

Alas, there is no official name for this diet. While it's pretty straightforward, it's certainly not the Standard American Diet. Nor is it paleo or Mediterranean or animal-based. That's why I called it the Clean Omnivore Diet. It's clean, it's healthy, and it's satiating. It's also flexible, meaning it works both for your preferences and your goals. For instance, at the end of this section I offer a suggestion that explains how one slight modification of this diet can allow for meaningful fat loss that you can maintain over time.

So aim for 30 to 50 grams of high-quality protein at each meal. That's about one large chicken breast, a 6- to 8-ounce piece of salmon or other fish, or a 5- to 7-ounce steak. This will fill about a third of a standard dinner plate.

Fill another third of that plate with vegetables.

If you're having starch with that meal, the starch can fill the remaining third of the plate. This is approximate. Don't obsess. If you completed an intense resistance training session or a hard cardio training session lasting longer than forty-five minutes that day, feel free to increase the starch portion a bit. Otherwise, keep your starch intake moderate.[44]

HOW MUCH TO EAT: CALORIES IN, CALORIES OUT

Whatever diet you decide is best for you, you'll need to pay attention to how many calories you consume. Calorie is the unit we use to measure how much energy is in what we eat and drink. And the number of calories you consume versus the number of calories you burn determines whether you will gain weight, lose weight, or stay at your current weight. "Calories in, calories out" is the phrase to remember. Or, if you prefer acronyms, CICO. This is not a matter for debate; it's a matter of thermodynamics.

If you want to lose weight, then you must consume (and absorb) fewer calories than you burn. I say "absorb" because not every calorie you consume is absorbed. Complete proteins are 4 calories per gram as they head into your mouth, but the metabolic requirement of processing those proteins ends up making them closer to 3 calories per gram when all is said and done. And while it's not a dinner-table-appropriate topic, some of the calories in food pass through your digestive tract without being absorbed. For example, humans have engineered fats that improve the taste of a food, but that get eliminated from your digestive tract with no absorption of calories. Other calories fail to be absorbed because they have a rapid rate of passage through your digestive tract, or bind to fiber. But for the most part, calories eaten equals calories absorbed.

Which takes us to the calories-out part of CICO.

As covered in chapter 2, your basal metabolism is the number of calories you burn if you were to just lie in bed all day and night and do literally nothing. Contrary to what many people once believed, your basal, or resting, metabolism doesn't change a whole lot with age, at least not after age twenty-five or so.[45] Unless your muscle mass changes. If you lose muscle, your resting metabolic rate decreases. If you gain muscle, your resting metabolic rate will increase. This suggests that one reason people put on weight as they age is they lose muscle mass. Another is that as people get older in age, they tend to walk less and just generally move around less (even while seated!) and thus burn fewer calories each day. This kind of non-exercise movement, or non-exercise activity thermogenesis (NEAT) in nerd-speak, may not seem important, but it is. It can burn greater than 1,000 calories a day in some people . . . so knee bouncers and fidgeters rejoice.[46]

While NEAT is (amazingly) a key aspect to your daily caloric expenditure, you of course can't get away with just fidgeting and walking. As explained in detail in chapter 2, exercise—specifically resistance training and cardiovascular training—is critical to maintaining healthy body composition over time. Also, if you are choosing to be in a calorie deficit to lose weight, and you resistance train, more of the weight you lose will come from body fat and less will come from muscle. If you don't resistance train, you'll lose roughly equal amounts of body fat and muscle.

The reverse is also true. If you're in a calorie excess, you'll gain weight that is a mix of muscle and body fat, but probably more body fat. That is, unless you resistance train, in which case you'll gain more weight that is muscle, especially if many of the additional calories are from high CP:C ratio proteins.[47] And if you resistance train while eating at maintenance levels, you'll likely add muscle and reduce your overall body fat percentage.[48]

So viewed purely through the lens of thermodynamics, does it matter what you eat? If you are thinking about total weight on the scale, then technically no, it doesn't matter. A calorie is a calorie. But as you can see from everything we've discussed so far in the chapter, there's more to it than that.

Physiologically speaking, we eat for four main reasons:

- To provide our cells with the raw materials like amino acids and fatty acids that they need to rebuild themselves

- To provide our cells with glucose to fuel their activities, that is, to give them energy
- To get micronutrients (such as vitamins and minerals) for our cells
- To provide sustenance for the beneficial bacteria that live in our gut

(We also eat for psychological reasons, but those reasons are countless in number: because it's social, or it reminds us of home, or it reduces our anxiety, or it just tastes good, and on and on.)

That's why I believe, given most people are (and want to remain) omnivores, that the healthiest possible way to eat is to get enough high CP:C ratio proteins, plenty of fibrous vegetables and some fruit, healthy monounsaturated and polyunsaturated fats, and a bit of saturated fat, too, and enough clean starch to fuel our brains and bodies. And to do all that without eating more calories than we need. It hits each of these four reasons, while helping us stick to the requirements of CICO.

A Word About Weight Loss, or the Clean and Lean Omnivore Diet

One of the best ways to avoid eating too many calories is to avoid processed foods entirely, while also restricting starch-fat and starch-fat-sugar combinations, even if the ingredients are not processed.

There is even a case for dropping starches entirely—at least for a while. I know it seems crazy, but I have a dozen or more close friends who really struggled with their weight for years who switched to a diet consisting of meat, fish, eggs, vegetables, fruit, olive oil, coffee, tea, and water (there's an argument to be made that diet soda is fine to include too) and only used salt, pepper, and cinnamon for added flavoring.[49] Without any calorie counting, they have lost anywhere from twenty-five to sixty pounds in four to six months, and kept it off. These friends also made sure to consume some low-sugar fermented foods each day, too, such as sauerkraut or kimchi, which promote microbiome health. All of them exercised but no more than they were doing prior to eating this way. Each reported "cheating" two to three times a year, usually for a holiday meal or birthday. They simply got right back to the plan the next day. And after a year or so of eating this way, the ones exercising regularly and intensely were able to start adding moderate amounts of clean starches, like potatoes, beans, and rice, back into their regimen with no detriment.

Their results were remarkable, but not atypical. Again, since the laws of thermodynamics are immutable, we have to conclude this diet naturally puts active people into a caloric deficit. What is wild is how fast it works, and how easy it is to stick to, and how it stands in bold contrast to their many other failed attempts to lose body fat in a sustainable way. You might say "No bread?! No ice cream?! No pasta?!" All I know is that the people who elected to eat this way report feeling very sated, which I attribute to the fact that they were getting everything their body needed physiologically and psychologically, without counting calories. And their improved body composition and other indicators of health, including sleep, just further reinforced their decision. I guess if we had to name this diet we would call it the Clean Omnivore No Starch Diet but that's a mouthful so I've defaulted to calling it the Clean and Lean Omnivore Diet instead.

Calculating Your CICO

After you've decided on what to eat, you'll want to dial in to how much. That's where calculating your CICO comes in.

I actually think it's a good idea for people to calculate their CICO for a few days or so, at least one to two times a year, and update their food intake accordingly, the same way that I think it's a good idea to get your blood pressure checked one to two times a year, and update your stress control tools accordingly.

Luckily there is an easy, no-cost way to determine your caloric needs. It's called the Katch-McArdle formula. I discussed it in chapter 2, so please refer to page 174 to refresh your memory on how your daily caloric needs are calculated.

If you want additional support for body fat loss, muscle gain, et cetera, as I mentioned I highly recommend the Carbon App, created by Layne Norton, one of the world's foremost experts on nutrition, especially for health and body composition. (Note: Carbon is a sponsor of my podcast.) It allows you to determine what you need to eat and how much of each macronutrient and it makes it easy to enter your calorie and specific food intake. It also learns your nutrition patterns over time, and makes valuable suggestions. So it's not just a calorie and macronutrient counter; it's a nutrition coach. I have used it for years now and everyone I have recommended it to thanks me for the ease and results it's brought them around nutrition and body composition.

STRAIGHT TALK ABOUT HIGHLY PROCESSED FOODS

It is true that eating 3,000 calories of highly or "ultra" processed food will not cause any more or less weight gain than eating 3,000 calories of non-processed food, but the damage the former does is real. Let's acknowledge the one thing everyone in the nutrition field seems to agree on—the vegans, the carnivores, the keto enthusiasts, the vegetarians, and the omnivores: Highly processed foods are genuinely bad for us.

When we talk about highly processed foods, we're referring to multi-ingredient, packaged products that are either ready-to-eat or only need to be heated up to eat. We're not referring to single ingredient starches that just need to be baked or cooked in boiling water, like rice or potatoes or beans. That's not "processing"; it's "preparation": And those are healthy, non-processed foods. Highly processed foods are problematic for many reasons related to our short- and long-term health. These products—even the ones labeled "Heart Healthy"—are often high in sugar, as well as various preservatives and artificial dyes that, while perhaps not deadly on their own, seem to pose a risk to health.[50]

And recent studies suggest that eating a lot of processed foods can increase your risk of psychiatric illnesses, likely due to changes in brain metabolism.[51] In fact, that is one reason why, as mentioned above, ketogenic diets (which are very low in carbohydrates) are increasingly being prescribed as a tool to improve mental health. Whether that is due to the absence of carbohydrates, the reduced intake of processed foods, or a direct effect of improved insulin sensitivity remains unclear, but the results are nonetheless compelling. We also have reliable evidence that diets low in fiber and high in processed foods, or even simply just high in refined carbohydrates, such as white rice and white wheat flour, increase the risk of cancer[52] and cardiovascular disease.[53] As do deli meats, which are effectively highly processed meats.[54]

It's hard to tack the health-degrading effects of processed foods to one aspect of their makeup. A study published in 2017 reported that nearly half of all deaths due to cardiac or metabolic issues are rooted in poor diet.[55] The Center for Science in the Public Interest, a nonprofit organization, estimates that 678,000 US deaths each year are due to diseases stemming from an inadequate or otherwise poor diet.[56] Half! Personally, I view highly processed foods as destructive to health mostly because of the other actually healthy foods you could be eating in their place. You still have to obey CICO according to your goals, and make sure you get the right macro- and micronutrients, but avoiding processed foods will likely add years to your life.

WHEN TO EAT

Then there is the question of when we eat. Here again, people debate. In the 1990s it became popular to eat four to six small meals per day, following a 1989 study published in the *New England Journal of Medicine* on the subject of "nibbling versus gorging."[57] The idea was that grazing throughout the day would prevent overeating in any one sitting and stimulate metabolism. It fell out of favor because it's impractical. It also turned out to have a trivial impact on metabolism.[58]

Most people default to eating three to four times a day, with one to two of those instances as snacks and the others as meals. Job, school, and social constraints usually dictate when, exactly, people eat.

The practice of time-restricted eating, also called intermittent fasting, as discussed earlier in this chapter, became popular a few years back, and many people follow this practice either deliberately or by default because they are not hungry in the morning. They end up restricting their eating to a window of four to ten hours each day, and most typically seven to eight hours.[59] Some people limit themselves to one meal a day, which means their window is only one to two hours a day. There is now a fair bit of science—including clinical trials—on time-restricted eating. Intermittent fasting was made popular first as a way to lose weight and improve insulin sensitivity, meaning the extent to which our cells use glucose for energy (the more efficiently this happens, the less insulin we need to produce in order to regulate blood sugar levels). Soon it was studied and touted as a tool to live longer, to avoid cancer, and on and on.[60]

When it comes to losing weight, the data show that intermittent fasting does indeed help when compared to "unrestricted eating." However, it likely helps because people end up eating fewer calories when they limit their eating to a specific time window. So ultimately, it all comes back to CICO. When you put intermittent fasting head-to-head with a diet where people can eat whenever they want, but the two diets are matched for total calories consumed, the results end up being the same. A yearlong randomized study found that people with obesity who followed a calorie-restricted diet and ate only within an eight-hour window did not lose more weight or body fat compared to those who followed calorie restriction without the accompanying time-restriction plan.[61] That being said, many people find it easier to control the hours in which they eat than to control the portion of what they eat, and thus find intermittent fasting a very effective tool for eating fewer calories than they would otherwise.

Many people opt for intermittent fasting because they incorrectly think that means you don't have to think about the types or amount of food you eat, but if you care about your health you still do. Fasting doesn't change our need for micronutrients.

Debate continues about what it can do. Intermittent fasting has generated interest for its potential to extend life.[62] However, the only strong link between fasting and extended lifespan appears to be restricting calories, not meal timing.[63] That said, Satchin Panda's lab at the Salk Institute has shown that mice who eat across a twenty-four-hour window of time compared to an eight-to-twelve-hour window, even when calories are held constant, suffer negative health outcomes such as obesity, elevated glucose levels, insulin resistance, and fatty liver.[64] Studies from Satchin's lab have also shown similar adverse effects for humans.[65] Further studies show that not eating within two to three hours of bedtime does seem to improve sleep quality,[66] growth hormone release[67] in sleep, and next-morning glucose regulation,[68] all of which may indirectly impact lifespan. While restricting eating within two to three hours of bedtime does seem to be a best practice, there are some exceptions based on the type of meal. For instance, if you're hungry and need a snack, consuming 30 grams of casein, the protein found in dairy, can help reduce blood pressure and perhaps even aid in exercise recovery, especially for those doing resistance training.[69]

Some research suggests that time-restricted eating extends life because it increases autophagy, a process that removes damaged or used cells and cellular material from our bodies.[70] We also know that extended fasting, such as consuming only water and electrolytes for one to three days, is linked to increased autophagy.[71] But again here, it's not the timing that increases autophagy; it's the overall daily calorie deficit.[72] And whether autophagy truly extends human lifespan is still unclear.[73] Most evidence we have linking caloric restriction or intermittent fasting to lifespan is still largely from animal studies.[74] Prolonged fasting in humans will no doubt improve certain health metrics, like insulin sensitivity, but it risks reducing lean mass. Exercise—both resistance and cardio training—stimulate autophagy but improve lean mass with the added benefit of improving fitness.[75]

I reflexively do something similar to intermittent fasting. My first meal is typically around 11:00 a.m. or noon. I wake up at about 6:00 a.m. most days and I find it easy to wait to eat my first meal because I tend not to get hungry until 10:30 or so. Around 3:30 p.m. I usually get hungry again and I'll have a snack. I prefer to eat my last meal of the day around 7:00 p.m., but I stay somewhat flexible on that depending on my schedule.

Since I'm typically done eating around 8:00 p.m., my eating window is usually eight to nine hours, maybe a bit longer. I've found that this slightly restricted window allows me to feel at my best while also helping me to manage my daily caloric intake.

From a health standpoint, it's best to eat at fairly consistent times each day,[76] but you don't have to be neurotic about it. If someone sets a dinner time for an hour earlier or later than usual, or a bit outside your eating window, it's not a huge deal.

WHAT'S AHEAD

The following protocols are not yet another trend to follow. When I said I hoped you'd find the best diet for you, what I meant is one that you can stick to.

These protocols are not complicated, they are not expensive, and they do not involve searching out obscure ingredients or creating an elaborate schedule of meal prep. They follow directly from the ideas discussed in this introduction to the chapter. Each explores a key point here, then offers one simple tool. My hope is that they will provide you with the inspiration and rationale to make easy yet meaningful shifts in your nutrition, and therefore immediate and long-term health. Adopting any of these into your daily routine can improve your digestion, your energy levels, and your ability to focus and concentrate. For those of you seeking dramatic positive transformations in body composition, I offer a sustainable way to do that too. Of course, exercise—per the recommendations in chapter 2—is critical for getting sustainable and healthy body composition changes, and exercise has its own benefits altogether. Some of the suggestions that follow will be familiar. Others may sound a bit heretical. But I assure you they work.

NUTRITION PROTOCOL

1

90 Percent or More of the Food You Eat Should Be Unprocessed or Minimally Processed

WHAT TO DO:

- **Eat and cook with single-ingredient, non-processed foods.** These include meat, fish, eggs, poultry, fruit, vegetables, rice, lentils, beans, oatmeal, pasta, olive oil, avocado oil, and even butter (albeit in small portions). They can be consumed alone or combined in recipes, and of course you can use spices, seasonings, and salt as well.
- **Avoid ready-to-eat packed foods or packaged multi-ingredient foods.** Most pre-packaged sauces and condiments should be avoided; these typically contain a fair amount of added sugar. Read nutrition labels to check.
- **Consume nut butters in moderation.** These can be healthy, but some contain processed oils and even added sugar. Even when nuts and salt are the only ingredients, all have a very high calorie-to-protein ratio. If you're trying to lose body fat, then it's best to abstain from nut butters entirely.
- **Consume full-fat yogurt and cottage cheese and other forms of dairy, but in plain flavors only.** Here too added sugars should be avoided. Add fruit, a drizzle of honey, or a pinch of cinnamon for taste if you don't like these foods plain.

HOW IT WORKS:

Food is amazing. Despite the debates, I think we can all agree on that. We eat for the building blocks food supplies our brain and body, as described in the introduction to this chapter, and of course for the pleasure of it. For many people, food is one of their biggest joys. I count myself among people who love to eat.

But the type of food we eat is probably second only to sleep and exercise for its importance to our long-term health. Centering our meal and snack choices on whole (that is minimally or non-processed) foods has so many benefits—disease prevention, longevity, cognition, mood, energy, reduced inflammation, healthy weight management, and more. The increasing concerns about processed foods stem from the plethora of data linking them to obesity, high blood pressure, heart disease, gastrointestinal disorders, cancer, and other serious ailments.[77] Chemical additives used to color, preserve, texturize, and flavor these products have been linked to potential health hazards.[78] Processed foods also tend to contain high amounts of sugar, even in products that would seem to not require it. And excessive sugar consumption is tied to diabetes, heart disease, cancer, and an increased risk of early death.[79] All of which is to say, we need to make it a point to eliminate, or at least vastly reduce, processed foods.

The good news is that eating healthily is not complicated or expensive. We can all make incredible tasting meals and snacks using whole foods, if we learn just a bit about how to prepare them. Think: a perfectly cooked steak and carrots roasted with olive oil, salt, and some spices. In some cases, these foods need no preparation at all. Like a juicy orange or fresh berries. If these sound bland or overly simple, chances are your taste circuits in your brain and body need some recalibration.

If you have grown accustomed to eating processed foods, this recalibration can seem difficult. Processed foods alter our brain and gut to make us perceive other, more nutritious foods as less appetizing. It's because of how sugar, certain starch-sugar, and starch-sugar-fat combinations are metabolized in our gut, and how they change our brain's reward pathways. You'll be happy to know, however, that the cells in your gut and brain are perfectly happy to rewire to make healthy, unprocessed foods literally taste better. It doesn't take long, and it will make eating healthy most of the time reflexive.

This protocol looks at the gut-brain axis, the connection between the cells in our digestive tract and specific areas of our brain. That connection is the key to understanding how processed foods affect us.

Our gut talks to our brain via two main parallel pathways. The first involves the cells in our gut communicating with our brain using a neural pathway called the vagus nerve, a bidirectional superhighway linking the organs of our body and our brain. You may remember the vagus from chapter 3.

Our body and our brain are connected by a second pathway, through secreted hormones and small proteins called peptides (in general, the vagus pathway is the faster of the two). The hunger sensation arises, in part, because our stomach produces a hormone called ghrelin[80] in amounts proportional to how much time has elapsed since our last meal. Ghrelin travels to our hypothalamus, a marble-sized brain region located over the roof of our mouth, where it activates our drive to seek food.[81] Other hormones and peptides made by both our gut and our brain make us want to eat less; for example, the peptide GLP-1 gives us a feeling of fullness, which is why GLP-1 analogs are used as drugs to treat obesity. (The gut microbiome, the trillions of bacteria living in our digestive system, also influences hunger—more on that in Nutrition Protocol 6.)[82]

At the same time, specific nutrients in the foods we eat—most notably sugars, but also fatty acids and amino acids—activate cells in our gut called neuropod cells that communicate with the brain via the vagus nerve, leading to the release of dopamine.[83] And while dopamine does many different things in the brain and body, when it is stimulated in this context, it can drive the urge to consume more of that food. It's an elegant mechanism if you think about it, because the taste of food in our mouth is not a great indication of the actual nutrients in a given food. Taste is more of a guess, a correlate. The cells in our gut, on the other hand, are poised to respond to the broken-down components of food, letting the rest of our body and brain know what we ate and what to eat more (or less) of. Amazingly, all this happens below our conscious awareness.

Given how sugar drives the urge to consume more, it's no mystery why it's in so many foods. Processed food manufacturers add sugar to foods so we buy and consume more of these foods. That's why sugar can be found in everything from packaged mac-and-cheese to frozen pizza, and most everything else on the supermarket shelves. Even tortilla and potato chips can have added sugar. So does most store-bought pasta sauce. And salad dressings. And condiments. Which is why so many people crave sugary food all the time.

You get the idea. It's a clever, albeit diabolical, tactic.

As mentioned in the introduction to this chapter, sugar that gets added to food is considered a simple carbohydrate. Typically it is added as sucrose, but sometimes as high-fructose corn syrup, or something similar. The exact form doesn't really matter however. Our brains are hardwired to detect simple carbohydrates. Studies in both mice and humans show that even when we are unable to taste sweetness, we still show a strong preference for sugary foods and beverages, indicating that the brain can detect sugar by a pathway other than conscious taste.[84]

Here's a simple and fun experiment you can try; it's something that Anna Lembke, MD, a world expert in dopamine and its role in craving and addiction, taught me. Eat one small piece of chocolate or one spoonful of your favorite ice cream. Both have sugar and fat, a combination known to trigger a lot of dopamine compared to eating either one alone. Pay attention to how it tastes, but then also notice your thoughts as you swallow. You'll notice how quickly they move from "mmm, yum" to "I want more." The immediate sense of craving that overlaps with pleasure is the power of dopamine in action. Sugar, in particular, amplifies that response, even after the flavor experience has passed, by activating the gut-to-brain pathway.[85] It even works for sugary foods that don't taste that good! And it's why processed foods that we don't even think of as sweet often contain added sugar.

Again, I want to be clear that I do not subscribe to the view that all sugar is inherently bad. A homemade dessert, chocolate, or ice cream once in a while . . . all can definitely fit within a healthy diet. But I do think we should limit these foods and avoid, as much as possible, consuming non-dessert foods that have added sugar, as well as any highly processed foods, except on rare occasions or out of true necessity.

Maybe you're wondering about fruit, which as I mentioned contains a sugar called fructose. Fruit contains a lot of water, fiber, valuable nutrients, and polyphenols, compounds found in plants that have various beneficial properties. All these components contribute to the prevention of heart disease, cancer, and other serious health issues.[86] And the high fiber content of most fruits slows down the absorption of sugar, which makes them less stimulating than desserts, sweets, or highly processed foods. But there are a few fruits that contain more fructose than others—like grapes. Note, too, that dried fruits, without their water content, now contain concentrated amounts of sugar. Fruit juices, like orange juice, are generally best avoided. They are high in sugar and calories, too, and the absence of fiber means that the sugar contained there is easily absorbed into the body, which means it spikes blood sugar quickly. Because that spike leads to a subsequent crash in blood sugar,[87] consuming it often can lead, in the short run, to fatigue, sugar cravings,[88] and, in the long term, an increased risk of diabetes[89] and heart disease.[90]

Then there are artificial and low-calorie sweeteners. The data show that artificial and low-calorie sweeteners do not drive the same craving typical simple sugars do. Stevia for instance, is safe, and may even have some health benefits.[91] Aspartame appears to be safe too.[92] Saccharin and sucralose, though, may negatively impact the gut microbiome.[93] And there's interesting data on diet sodas. In a randomized controlled trial from 2024, people who consumed diet sodas lost more weight than people who drank equivalent amounts of water.[94] The underlying reasons include less hunger among soda drinkers and more cravings for sweetness among the water drinkers. At the same time, people who consume a lot of artificial sweeteners often experience increased overall appetite, perhaps due to glucose and insulin disruption.[95] There isn't a broad rule that applies to all artificial and low-calorie sweeteners. For some people, they seem to help with weight loss, whereas for other people, they stimulate hunger in ways that may make it harder to keep from overeating. You have to figure out which group you are in.

If a few diet sodas a day help quell your sugar cravings at a time when you're trying to lose weight, then great. If you don't like diet sodas, there is no reason to consume them. I drink beverages containing stevia and occasionally enjoy an aspartame-sweetened diet soda. When developing the zero-sugar cold brew yerba maté for Mateina (as noted, a company I partially own), I chose to include a small amount of stevia. I drink that for much of the early part of the day. I avoid sucralose and saccharin.

COMMON QUESTIONS:

Do you have any suggestions for beating sugar cravings?

Yes. Some are conventional; one is not (more on that in the last protocol of this chapter). As with many cravings, sugar can be hard to quit. If you think you're overdoing it with sugar, then try committing to having no sugar for a certain period. I suggest one week. I promise that soon you will stop craving it so much, though it takes a few days to "get over the bump" (the heightened cravings) as they say.

Focus on consuming high CP:C ratio proteins, at least three times per day. And dietary fiber, mostly from vegetables and lower sugar fruits like apples and berries. If you crave chocolate, try and slowly develop a taste for raw cacao beans (five or six per day), which are rich in polyphenols, which again have various beneficial properties. Similarly, you can try 100 percent chocolate (not baking chocolate!). You read right. That's no sugar, and no stevia either. It's an acquired taste, but once people develop a taste for it, they generally like it. If you really struggle with sugar cravings, cut sugar out entirely but consider drinking a half tablespoon (about 3–5 g) of l-glutamine powder dissolved in water two to three times a day; this powder may reduce cravings by regulating blood sugar levels and thereby quelling the need for sugar.[96] This is a somewhat unconventional tool—one for which we need more studies—but anecdotally speaking (about my own experience), it works.

NUTRITION PROTOCOL

2

Stay Hydrated

WHAT TO DO:

Regardless of what and when you choose to eat:

- **Consume 18 to 24 ounces of water upon waking.** Try to do this first thing in the morning before drinking or eating anything else, including coffee or other forms of caffeine.
- **Aim to consume about 80 ounces of water across the first ten hours of the day.** That's about 2.4 liters. It is not necessary to consume 8 ounces each hour, but try to spread it out in a way that works for you. The earlier in the day you drink it the better. It's typically best to avoid a lot of water in the hours before bedtime, since you want to wake as infrequently as possible to use the bathroom.
- **For optimal performance during exercise, consume water according to this equation: Your body weight in pounds divided by 30 equals the number of ounces to drink for every 15 to 20 minutes of your workout time.** This calculation originates with the work of human performance expert Andy Galpin, director of the Human Performance Center at Parker University, and is referred to below as the "Galpin Equation."

    Example: Total body weight of 150 pounds ÷ 30 = 5 ounces every 15 to 20 minutes, which means 15 to 20 ounces consumed during an hour-long workout. You can sip water throughout, drink at regular or non-regular intervals. Your pattern of consumption during exercise will of course be dictated by the type of exercise you're doing: running, cycling, swimming, et cetera.

HOW IT WORKS:

Your body is made mostly of water. By one estimate, obtained by sending a weak electric current through the body, an adult human is about 62 percent water, with that percentage starting to decrease around sixty years of age.[97] Water is essential for every biological process that we need in order to live and function.[98] If there is one protocol that is most overlooked and that can immediately and significantly improve your energy levels, focus, and general feeling of well-being, it is this: Hydrate properly. It is rarely discussed. When we do hear about hydration, the message is typically a warning against dehydration, not the great benefits of hydration.

So let's talk about what hydration is, and why it's so powerful.

Hydration is the process of providing the cells of our body with the water they need for all those biological processes. Some hydration is achieved by breathing, some is produced through metabolism, and some comes through the foods we eat. Most hydration comes from the liquids we consume. The water we take in through eating and drinking enters our gut and is absorbed into our bloodstream and finally our cells.

Proper hydration is crucial to both the body and the brain. Hydration helps prevent injuries, improves recovery, and is also important for maintaining body temperature during and following exercise.[99] It reduces the risk of kidney stones.[100] Drinking water stimulates the sympathetic branch of your autonomic nervous system, the circuitry that increases your alertness and focus. (See chapter 3 for more on this.) Research indicates that drinking water can trigger the release of norepinephrine, the hormone that helps keep us focused and alert.[101] In a study of fifteen children, proper hydration was tied to improved performance on tasks involving motor skills and memory.[102] Similar findings have been observed in adults.

Dehydration, on the other hand, quickly becomes problematic. It's also common. This is unfortunate because even slightly insufficient amounts of water in your body can diminish your concentration, alertness, short-term memory, visual perception, and other cognitive functions.[103] Mild dehydration can cause low-level confusion, fatigue, depression, and irritability.[104] One review found that a 2-percent decrease in body mass due to dehydration was enough to diminish mood, increase fatigue, and reduce alertness. That is remarkable because most people do not consume enough water to maintain hydration, and spend much of their day suffering the ill effects of mild dehydration . . . without even realizing it.

A mildly dehydrated state can reduce brain volume and alter the activity of neural pathways associated with motor output and cognition.[105] It also reduces blood flow, which in turn diminishes the supply of oxygen to the brain. What's more, it can cause headaches and lethargy, and of course a dry mouth and thirst.[106] It's important to note amidst all this that we can be dehydrated without registering thirst.

People engaging in intense exercise need to be especially vigilant about hydration, and not just in hot and/or dry environments either. In one study, eight trained cyclists rode for two hours on a stationary bike, consuming either 2.4 liters of an energy drink or 0.4 liters of water plus sports gel to equal the carbohydrates in the energy drink. The low-hydration riders became exhausted sooner and exerted less energy as they rode.[107] In a study of seven experienced resistance trainers (all male), insufficient hydration decreased performance during exercise.[108] These studies are small but are representative of what happens when we exercise.

The quantities provided in this protocol do not need to be followed to the precise ounce or milliliter. They are general guidelines to help ensure sufficient hydration.

One reason to focus on getting about 80 ounces of fluid in the first ten hours of the day is that this time is when our kidneys function at their best. Our kidneys filter fluid and produce hormones to regulate water and salt balance, among other things, and their efficiency at doing so is strongly governed by our circadian clock[109] (see Sleep Protocol 1 for more on the circadian clock). Our kidneys are simply much better at filtering water and other fluids we drink in the morning and daytime than at night; their function tends to peak in midafternoon and is slowest around midnight.[110] Focusing most of your water intake to the time of day when fluid filtration by the kidneys is at its most efficient will also help prevent, or at least reduce, having to get up in the middle of the night to use the bathroom, which is among the more common causes of sleep disturbance.

The quantity of 80 ounces across the first ten hours of the day gives us a solid metric to aim for. Simply make sure to drink 8 to 16 ounces of water (one to two glasses) upon waking, and again approximately every waking hour during the day. That will get you in the ballpark of 80 ounces in the first ten hours. Individuals living in hot environments tend to need more water. So do people who move around a lot, even if that's in a temperature-controlled office or home.

But if you're exercising, that's where the Galpin Equation enters the picture. If you want to improve your exercise performance, hydrate according to this calculation. You'll be amazed by the difference it makes. Again, anyone living in hot environments will tend to need a bit more water here too; so increase the amount from the equation by a few extra ounces every fifteen to twenty minutes.

Beyond these three points, just remember: Stay hydrated. Hydration sounds boring but it's actually really powerful when it comes to improving health and performance and again, it's one of the more overlooked tools out there. It's important for your brain, for your skin and appearance, for your digestion, and for your mood. You will notice the difference in all these areas after starting to follow this protocol.

COMMON QUESTIONS:

How do I know if I'm dehydrated?

There are so many myths around this. Among the more popular ones is that clear urine indicates sufficient hydration. Wrong. Many factors impact urine color besides hydration status. Your urine can be yellow and you can still be plenty hydrated. Another: If you pinch the skin on your hand, it should retract in less than two seconds. Wrong again. This response depends on age, skin thickness, and other factors. It's true that if you pinch the skin on the top of your hand and it does not return to its original state within three to five seconds, then there's a decent chance you're dehydrated. Same goes if your urine is *much* darker than usual. But that's not the best way to guide your hydration, nor is whether your ankles are swollen . . . all of these are myths.

The best way to be certain that you are hydrated is . . . to not wait for some less-than-reliable marker to tell you so. Simply drink enough water.

Do I follow both protocols at once when exercising? In other words, do I drink the recommended amount during general waking hours plus the amount recommended for hydration during exercise?

Yes. Drink the amount recommended for ten hours of waking, and add more using the Galpin Equation. If you don't want to bother with the calculation, then just aim to ingest 80 ounces of water across the first ten hours of the day and add an extra 15 to 20 ounces of water for every hour spent exercising—and drink it while exercising.

Should I drink more if I'm someone who sweats a lot?

People who tend to sweat a lot can increase the Galpin Equation by 50 to 100 percent during exercise. The same holds true if you are doing some kind of heat exposure that promotes sweating. For example, it would be appropriate to drink 8 to 16 ounces of fluid for every twenty to thirty minutes you spend in a hot sauna.

Electrolytes (particularly sodium, magnesium, and potassium) are also beneficial, especially if you are sweating. If you're working or you're exercising in a warm environment, or you're spending time in a hot sauna, add a pinch of sea salt to water (and add a little lemon juice to offset the salty taste). Or use a commercial source of electrolytes to help replace those lost through sweat. I'm a fan of LMNT, a sponsor of my podcast, which has more sodium than most electrolyte formulas. (It also has zero sugar, which is good since many hydration formulas have added sugar.) Many people worry about salt intake but if you eat clean—meaning limited or no processed foods—there is a good chance you need more, not less sodium.

Even if I slow down my water intake after the first ten hours of the day, I'm still concerned about frequent nighttime waking. Is there a way to reduce this?

It's normal to wake up once during the night to urinate. To avoid waking more than once, try this:

1. Hydrate sufficiently during the day to ensure you are not excessively thirsty in the evening.
2. Reduce fluid intake in the evening (obviously).
3. If you do drink fluids (of any kind) later in the day or in the evening, sip them slowly. The rate at which fluid moves from the gut to the bladder is determined partly by the rate at which we drink. Gulping water quickly leads to sooner urination; sipping slowly leads to more time between urination.[111]

That said, if you are still waking up often, that could reflect a bladder or prostate issue. Talk to your doctor.

I drink coffee, tea, diet soda, et cetera. Does that count toward my daily hydration needs?

Technically, yes, but drinking good ol' plain water is still important. Beverages containing caffeine act as diuretics; they stimulate urine production and therefore do not contribute to hydration to the same extent as non-caffeinated drinks. The amount of caffeine most people consume is usually not enough to cause significant dehydration, but anyone who drinks more than two cups of strong coffee per day—meaning more than 200 to 400 milligrams of caffeine—should make sure to drink at least those 80 ounces of water in addition, and perhaps as much as 100 ounces.

Keep in mind that many commercial coffee vendors brew their coffee strong, as in 300 milligrams or more of caffeine per serving. If you tend to feel shaky or lightheaded after drinking that coffee, you may be low on electrolytes, as caffeine causes excretion of sodium, a key electrolyte. I've known a lot of people who were able to eliminate caffeine-induced lightheadedness and shakes, and even the caffeine crash, by drinking a glass of water with a small pinch of salt dissolved in it, or by drinking water with a serving of electrolytes (sodium, magnesium, and potassium) alongside their coffee or other caffeine-containing drink. In fact, people who drink a lot of caffeinated beverages report that they feel much more energetic, and avoid the caffeine crash, when they are careful to also ingest some electrolytes before, alongside, or after their caffeine.

NUTRITION PROTOCOL

3

Eat High CP:C Ratio Protein at Each Full Meal

WHAT TO DO:

- **Aim to include 30 to 50 grams of high complete-protein-to-calorie ratio foods at each meal or snack.** Your daily goal should be around 1 gram per pound of body weight. This is the cornerstone of your diet.
- **The number of calories from those foods will depend on what you select.** Poultry, lean red meat, fish, and shellfish are the best high CP:C ratio sources of protein for those who eat animal-based products. Eggs are great as well, but they do have a relatively high calorie-to-protein ratio. Whey protein and plain full-fat Greek yogurt and cottage cheese too. Plant-based complete protein sources include beans and rice (together), lentils, soy, seitan, and some grains, such as quinoa. Just be aware that these have a less-than-favorable protein-to-calorie ratio.
- **Nuts, nut butters, and most cheeses are not high-quality protein sources.** And all of them are very calorie dense. Peanut, almond, and other nut butters are mostly fat, and most nut butters on the grocery shelf often also contain added sugar and/or seed oils. If you're going to eat nut butters, limit them to a few tablespoons a week and be sure they contain only nuts and salt. No sugar or added oils. It would be better to avoid nut butters and eat whole seeds and actual whole nuts. But these are mostly fats; they are not high CP:C ratio proteins.
- **If you are someone who tends to overeat, whichever foods you choose, eat your high CP:C ratio proteins first.** Then any starches, then

your fibrous vegetables. You'll enjoy more satiety, better appetite regulation, and better digestion because apparently the French have it right about "salad last."

HOW IT WORKS:

I know it's not much fun to see a delicious steak and think "amino acids," but that's what your body does. If you took apart any protein, you would find an array of amino acids.

As I explained in the introduction to this chapter, all living things need amino acids to make protein. The human body needs twenty different amino acids. Nine of these are impossible for our body to make on its own. We get them through the proteins we eat. The proteins that have all nine are considered complete proteins, and we want to consume these proteins, because the body uses them to maintain a healthy immune system, produce certain hormones, and maintain and increase muscle mass, among other functions.[112] You might be amazed to learn that most of your organs, not just your muscles, are made of proteins that are remade every few weeks to months. And it's these nine essential amino acids that allow for this to occur. Your spleen, your heart, your liver, your muscles—the protein we consume allows them to keep working as they should.

Your body is smart. While you might think you eat for pleasure, it's actually how your body keeps you seeking the food it needs to maintain these processes—that is, seeking those nine essential amino acids.

Whole grains, vegetables, seeds, and legumes do not contain all nine amino acids, but it is entirely possible to obtain all nine by consuming a variety of these plant-based proteins. Whether you eat meat or not, you are foraging for amino acids as you choose your proteins each day. That's why we feel so satisfied after we eat complete protein; it's because the feeling of satiety is strongly linked to obtaining enough essential amino acids.[113]

And there is one particular amino acid we prioritize in that foraging, even if we are not consciously aware of it. An expanding body of evidence indicates that leucine, one of those nine essential amino acids, is especially impactful.[114] Rising leucine levels in a cell launch a signaling pathway associated with the protein mTOR (I mentioned it in the introduction to this chapter), which in turn triggers the body to make muscle.[115] This amino acid also has several other known effects. Research has found links to improved immune function, for example,[116] as well as increased muscle mass among older individuals.[117]

As discussed earlier, mTOR has been linked with aging and cancer. One mutant strain of mice lived three times longer than usual after treatment with the drug that lowers mTOR, called rapamycin.[118] But again, those results don't appear to translate to humans, and in fact they have translated to far less dramatic results in normal mice. There is currently no evidence that stimulating mTOR has a life-shortening effect on humans. Rather, eating complete protein foods, and especially those rich in leucine such as lean meat, fish, and eggs, should be the cornerstone of your diet.

And not to belabor the point, but once again, we are less likely to overeat when we consume sufficient protein because it leaves us feeling full and satisfied.[119]

COMMON QUESTIONS:

Eating 1 gram of protein per pound of body weight leads me to gain weight and/or I don't feel good. What should I do?

Most people who strive to eat 1 gram of protein per pound of body weight do feel better than they did before adopting that habit. From time to time, though, someone will tell me they just don't feel "right" eating so much protein, and that they feel that they must force themselves to do so, even if their overall caloric intake is in proper range for them. We don't have the exact knowledge to know why that might be. I notice my protein hunger follows the intensity and amount of exercise I do, and while that makes sense based on how protein synthesis works, we don't have any formal studies on training and protein hunger, so take my experience as what it is: anecdotal.

For those of you who struggle to eat 1 gram of quality protein per pound of body weight, there are a few things to consider: Make sure you're eating high-protein foods without excess fat or preservatives. If that does not eliminate the discomfort, then try replacing about a fourth of your protein calories with clean starches, like rice, and with fibrous foods, like salad, broccoli, or apples, while keeping your overall calories approximately the same. Starches are calorie dense, so it won't take much to offset the slightly lower protein intake. Then, make adjustments until you arrive at a way of eating that is sustainable, and makes you feel good.

CICO—calories in, calories out—is a universal law of nutrition. Well, that and we all do need adequate protein and essential fatty acids to survive (which is what this protocol is all about). Other than that, figure out what works for you. And what works best for you may even change over time. I have long made it a point to eat enough protein daily, but I need to eat more vegetables now than I did when I was younger to feel my best.

NUTRITION PROTOCOL

4

Choose Fibrous Vegetables and (Some) Fruit as Your Major Sources of Carbohydrates

WHAT TO DO:

- **Vegetables should form the second major brick in the foundation of your diet and fruit, the third.** If protein is the cornerstone, these foods build on it by helping to ensure enough vitamin, mineral, and other micronutrient intake.
- **These foods are also essential for our fiber intake.** Men should aim for at least 35 grams per day, and women at least 25 grams per day.

HOW IT WORKS:

Many readers know already why vegetables and fruits are so important: They contain vitamins, minerals, and other micronutrients like flavonoids, all of which our bodies need to function optimally.[120] Once you understand how nutrient-rich vegetables and fruits are, you won't think about them the same way again. Eating vegetables isn't a chore; it's a gift.

The fiber in vegetables and fruits is also important.[121] A bit about fiber: It provides support structure for the plants that produce it, be that in the roots, the stems, or the leaves. And it's the part we can't digest when we consume them. Fiber can be insoluble (will not dissolve in water), soluble (will dissolve in water), or prebiotic (feeds bacteria).

We need all three. Insoluble fiber, present in root vegetables and fruits with edible seeds, helps with stool formation. Soluble fiber, present in foods such as avocados, carrots, and Brussels sprouts, collects waste products as it travels through the body, helping to eliminate them. Prebiotic fiber, present in apples, asparagus, onions, and garlic, provides sustenance for the beneficial bacteria in our gut microbiome, which promote intestinal health and also healthy brain functioning via the gut-brain axis.[122] (The foods noted above are just a few examples from each category.)

And they do a lot more. Studies also indicate that dietary fiber reduces the risk of metabolic syndrome, a cluster of symptoms that increase the risk of heart disease and diabetes. The heart-protecting benefits of fiber are widely known. A study that followed 9,776 US men and women for an average of nineteen years found that those who ate the least dietary fiber had a significantly higher risk of coronary heart disease compared to those who ate the most dietary fiber.[123] A review of eleven meta-analyses, which each included several studies, confirmed the link between high fiber consumption and a reduced risk of several cancers, including ovarian, prostate, colon, breast, and pancreatic.[124]

Consuming fiber can also leave us feeling full, simply from the physical bulk of the food in our gut and the slowed gastric emptying that results.[125] It also leaves us less fatigued. That's because consuming adequate fiber helps adjust what's called the postprandial glucose response, the entry of sugar (and fat) into the bloodstream, which can otherwise cause "brain fog" and tiredness. Fiber also blunts post-meal inflammation that often follows eating a dish high in fat and carbs. That inflammation, in which levels of some proteins and hormones rise in the body, can contribute to the risk of heart disease if it occurs with any regularity.

How much fiber should we get? Men should get at least 35 grams per day and women 25 grams per day. Very few people actually do that. In fact, an estimated 95 percent of Americans do not consume recommended amounts of fiber.[126]

Some people fear adding more fiber to their diet because it can cause gas and/or bloating. It's true that a sudden increase in daily fiber intake may temporarily result in both. But once you're eating enough fiber on a regular basis, this usually becomes a non-issue. In one study on the link between bloating, sodium, and a high-fiber diet, the researchers found that while this diet did increase bloating to some extent, an accompanying decrease in sodium lessened that side effect, pointing to the idea that it's often what we add to vegetables that becomes the problem, not the vegetables themselves.[127]

And at risk of sounding like your mother, vegetables require more chewing. You need to slow down and chew them well for them to digest properly, and for you to reap their full benefits.

A few notes on fruit: Some people find that eating fruit at the end of a meal causes some digestive discomfort. Others have no such issue. If you experience this problem, try eating fruit alone, before a meal, or as a snack rather than to cap off a full meal. It may help.

Beyond fiber, these foods contain, as I mentioned, essential vitamins, minerals, and other micronutrients. The words *vitamins and minerals* are thrown around a lot (I did it above). But knowing which ones tend to be lacking in most people's diets, and knowing how to get more of these from food, can make a real difference to our health. Magnesium is largely an under-discussed, beneficial component of many foods. This mineral, the eighth most abundant element on earth,[128] is used by the body for energy production, bone development, making DNA, muscle contraction, nerve impulses, and even for regulating our heartbeat.[129] In fact, it's involved in more than three hundred systems in our body and thousands of crucial biological processes. Yet most people don't get enough of it. It's easy to rectify, and I'm sure you can guess how: by eating enough fruits and especially enough vegetables.

Studies of the so-called Paleo diet, which focuses on fruits, vegetables, lean meat, fish, eggs, and nuts (in other words, foods that likely reflect the diet of a hunter-gatherer living in the Paleolithic era) indicate that we once had a magnesium intake of about 600 milligrams per day, leading researchers to theorize that human metabolism is adjusted to this high level.[130] Health authorities currently recommend 420 milligrams of magnesium daily for adult males and 320 milligrams daily for adult females. Available data indicate that most people consume less than that already low recommended amount. For Americans, the average is about 323 milligrams per day for males and 228 milligrams per day for females. This level is due, in part, to not eating enough foods containing magnesium, but likely also because many foods that would be high in magnesium are grown in soil depleted of this mineral due to modern farming methods.[131] Major or persistent magnesium deficiency can cause heart problems, neurological problems, and also dangerous reductions in calcium and potassium.[132] And we don't know how moderate deficiencies over time may more subtly diminish our health and vitality.

Vegetables and some fish, such as salmon and mackerel, are excellent sources of magnesium. Avocados (technically a fruit) and certain dairy products, such as milk and cheese, also contain magnesium. Among the foods with the highest amount of magnesium are pumpkin seeds, almonds, black beans, and soybeans. And I know it can be hard to feel excited about kale, spinach, and chard, but a few minutes spent enlightening yourself about magnesium will likely change that. Dark, leafy greens are an excellent source of it and very low in calories; one cup of cooked spinach contains more than a third of the recommended daily intake and fewer than 50 calories.

And there are more vitamins and minerals that vegetables offer. Potassium (beets, tomatoes, butternut squash) is integral to muscle contraction and nerve impulses.[133] Calcium (broccoli, kale, edamame, leafy greens) is crucial for our bones and our teeth.[134] Flavonoids, a category that includes a wide number of compounds present in the plant world, can reduce inflammation; the risk of diabetes, heart disease, and breast cancer; antibiotic resistance; the formation of free radicals (atoms that can damage cells and can contribute to cancer formation); oxidative stress, which can contribute to various diseases and conditions including neurodegenerative disorders; and the risk of viral, bacterial, and fungal infections.[135]

We could continue talking about the benefits of high-quality protein, vegetables, and fruits until the cows (and cauliflower) come home. In fact, cruciferous vegetables such as cauliflower and broccoli offer numerous additional benefits such as sulforaphane, which can help scavenge and detoxify endocrine disruptors and generally supports healthy reproductive hormones in women and men,[136] and on and on. I hope that all we've covered in this protocol has inspired you to fill half your lunch or dinner plate with vegetables. Perhaps even add some spinach and tomatoes (though, again, technically a fruit) to your breakfast too.

Though one last note on fruit: Most people, unless they are very lean (less than 10 percent body fat for men and less than 15 percent for women) should probably not be eating more than three servings of fruit per day, especially if they are trying to lose body fat. Too much fruit, despite its fiber and water content, can stimulate hunger. Don't get me wrong, fruit is amazing, and is always a part of a healthy diet. Enjoy it, but don't overdo it.

COMMON QUESTIONS:

Should I take magnesium supplements?

I suggest turning to magnesium supplements such as magnesium bisglycinate or L-threonate before bed only as an if-needed sleep aid, as described in Sleep Protocol 9, and then only if you've tried all the other protocols in chapter 1. For the benefit described here, stick primarily with foods that contain magnesium as a source.

That being said, magnesium supplements can help us get our daily recommended amount of this mineral. Magnesium L-threonate and bisglycinate seem to avoid the issue of gastrointestinal distress that some people experience with this supplement. By contrast, magnesium citrate can cause gastric distress and can sometimes even act as a laxative.

For adults, a 135-milligram magnesium L-threonate or bisglycinate supplement daily before sleep may also help ensure you are obtaining the recommended daily amount. Or you can take it with dinner. Be sure to consult with a physician before adding any supplement into your routine.

NUTRITION PROTOCOL

5

Consume Healthy Fats as Part of Most Meals and Snacks

WHAT TO DO:

- **Most of your fat intake should come from unsaturated fats.** These are present in olives, avocados, olive oil, and avocado oil, among other foods. Cook with olive oil, and use it for your salad dressing. If you need an oil with a higher smoke point for certain recipes, avocado oil is a good choice.
- **Consume omega-3 polyunsaturated fats.** These are present in fatty ocean fish, like salmon with the skin, and in various fish oil and krill supplements. (More on the benefits of omega-3 in Nutrition Protocol 7 of this chapter.)

HOW IT WORKS:

Perhaps no category of food is as feared, misunderstood, and maligned as fat. Part of the problem is terminology: The fact that we call dietary lipids fats brings to mind body fat. The two are not the same but they are easy to conflate.

I want you to create a healthy relationship with fat. The purpose of this protocol is to do that, based on science.

We all need some fat in our diet. The question is not if, but which and how much. Which? It turns out there are quite a few to choose from. And how much? As you learned earlier in this chapter, it depends on the other macronutrients you are eating, or avoiding, according to your overall diet (keto, clean omnivore, vegan, and so on).

And yet we have become wary of this macronutrient. This fear is based less on science than on history. Concerns about a link between fat and heart disease date back to the 1940s and grew in the ensuing decades.[137] In 1990, the USDA Dietary Guidelines recommended that Americans limit fat to 30 percent or less of their total calories and saturated fat to just 10 percent of their total calories, a recommendation that led to a proliferation of low-fat and nonfat products.[138] It soon became clear that these foods, often ultra-processed, were much worse for us than the fat we were now avoiding. These guidelines scared many people away from highly nutritious, high-quality protein foods that also contain some fat, like red meat and eggs. Moreover, we were then living without two crucial benefits that consuming fat provides: the way it slows the rise of glucose in the bloodstream and the way it increases satiety between meals. And Americans, on average, gained weight and suffered from rising rates of heart disease in the following years.

More recently, the pendulum swung the other way with rising interest in ketogenic diets, which involve eating mostly fat, some protein, and extremely few carbohydrates.[139] Interestingly, this diet first originated as a treatment for some forms of epilepsy in the 1920s. It's also been studied as a treatment for schizophrenia[140] and bipolar disorder.[141] As a daily routine, the ketogenic diet is hard to stick with. But this and similar trends helped spread the awareness that many fats, such as monounsaturated and polyunsaturated fats, are good for us.

How can we move forward? Again, by looking at the science. Though a comprehensive review of all types of fat is beyond the scope of this book, a few things are helpful to this discussion. Above we established that fats are made from fatty acids. The body breaks down the fat we eat into these component parts, which are then absorbed into the blood. Once inside the body, fatty acids contribute to the structure and function of cell membranes, help regulate metabolism, and influence hormone production, among other roles.[142] Yes, dietary fat can be more readily converted into body fat, and it's higher in calories per gram than carbs or protein—but at the end of the day, if we are burning as much or more of the calories we eat for energy to meet our metabolic needs, then it doesn't matter if the calories we eat come from fat, carbs, or proteins.

We covered the main types of dietary fat in the introduction to this chapter: monounsaturated, polyunsaturated, saturated. There is also trans fat. A bit more detail on all is warranted. The terms *saturated* and *unsaturated*, and the reason the former are solid at room temp and the latter are not, have to do with their different chemical bonds inside the chains of fatty acids.

The lack of double bonds in saturated fats makes the molecules stack on each other more easily, which makes the fat more stable; this is why products like butter stay solid at room temperature. These fats are hard to digest, which can leave us feeling tired. They can also increase certain forms of cholesterol.

Unsaturated fats are kinked in their structure. When you want to consume fat, these are the ones to prioritize. They contain fatty acids, which trigger circuitries involved with many bodily processes mentioned above.[143] Some fatty acids are directly involved in neuroplasticity, which we can loosely define as the continued ability to learn and form new memories and skills.[144] Fatty acids are also integral to regulating appetite. The presence of fat triggers communication along the gut-brain axis, which prompts the brain to release chemicals that deliver a sense of satiety. In addition, fat in our body releases a hormone called leptin, which activates neural circuitries primarily in the hypothalamus that also result in the feeling of fullness.[145] Leptin is also involved in the signaling pathways related to the menstrual cycle and sperm production.[146] It is one reason why having enough body fat, but not too much, is needed for libido and fertility. It's the signal from the body to the brain that food resources exist in sufficient abundance to potentially bring another member of our species into the world.

The fourth kind of fats, trans fats, are unsaturated, but the type of chemical bond is different from those in the other unsaturated fats. Although trans fats that occur naturally in some foods like meat and some dairy are relatively neutral or even beneficial to our health, when we hear about trans fats it usually refers to industrial-made versions.[147] These types of trans fats negatively impact cardiometabolic health, and were banned from the US food supply in 2018.[148] When you hear about partially hydrogenated vegetable oil, that is an industrial trans fat. Prior to 2018, many commercial products, such as margarine, processed meat, microwave popcorn, and packaged baked goods, made in the US contained trans fat, but no more. Health authorities recommend restricting industrial trans fats to 1 percent of total calories consumed—20 calories of a 2,000-calories-per-day diet, which is less than even one tablespoon. If you travel or live outside the US you'll need to see if industrial trans fats are still used in foods there.

As I note in this protocol, ideally choose monounsaturated fats. Also include some amount of saturated fat.[149] Although some studies have found that switching from saturated fats to polyunsaturated fats reduces the risk of heart disease somewhat,[150] other studies have not confirmed this connection.[151] And a common challenge that can arise when eliminating saturated fat from the diet is that it can lead to an increased consumption of ultra-processed carbohydrates and added sugar (we reach for a processed snack instead of, say, some cheese or full-fat yogurt), which is also detrimental to health.[152] This often happens when someone decides to eliminate meat, and ends up eating more packaged foods to reduce the effort required to prepare high-protein meals. Ultra-processed foods often contain a lot of calories and little to no fiber. I believe it is better to have a little bit of satisfying saturated fat than to replace it with foods that do not trigger a satiety response from the brain, that the body cannot digest effectively, or that lead to overconsumption.

If you're at this part of the protocol still wondering exactly how much fat to incorporate into your diet: Aim for 10 percent or less of your diet to consist of saturated fat. Keeping your overall fat intake to about 30 to 35 percent of your diet will help enable you to receive the benefits of this macronutrient without weight gain. Learn to love the right fats and your hormones, connective tissues, heart, and palate will all thank you.

COMMON QUESTIONS:

Should I consume more fat on certain days or post exercise?

No. Assuming you're eating 30 percent or so of your calories from fat, and that fat is a mix of saturated fats from high CP:C ratio proteins, and otherwise unsaturated fats such as avocados, olive oil or avocado oil, and some nuts and seeds, there is no reason to spike or drop your fat intake. If anything, we need to increase our clean starch intake, not our fat intake, on days we exercise. That's because intense exercise depletes us of glycogen, a sugar that the body makes as a way to store energy, which eating clean starch can replace.

NUTRITION PROTOCOL

6

Consume Low-Sugar Fermented Foods

WHAT TO DO:

- **Consume two to four servings of low-sugar fermented foods per day.** Eating foods like sauerkraut, kimchi, pickles in brine (that require refrigeration), kefir, low-sugar kombucha, miso, and natto supports a healthy gut microbiome, which in turn supports all your bodily functions.

HOW IT WORKS:

The human microbiome—the bacteria that colonize our skin, mouth, digestive system, and the rest of our body—has become a focal point of both health research and health trends in recent years. Data from the Whitehall II study,[153] which has been tracking the health of thousands of British civil servants between the ages of thirty-five and fifty-five since 1985, found that eating fermented dairy foods like yogurt and kefir reduced the risk of death,[154] as long as coronary heart disease and diabetes were not present. In one surprising study of 710 people, consumption of fermented foods was linked to less social anxiety among those who were prone to it.[155] That finding was correlation, not causation, and it's impossible to know whether eating something like sauerkraut made people less anxious. But connections like these start to make mechanistic sense as we learn more about the microbiome.

Recent research suggests that our microbiome starts forming before we are even born.[156] Bacteria we are exposed to during the birth process and in the early months of life continue to build this internal environment, which is then added to by microbes we take in through what we eat, what we drink, the people we come into contact with, the air we breathe, even the pets around us, and the soils we come into contact with. The specific makeup of our microbiome, including how diverse it is, changes according to our diet and our environment.[157] Even exercise affects our microbiome. A review of twenty-eight studies found that moderate-to-high-intensity exercise done for thirty to ninety minutes at least three times per week, for at least two months, "is likely to produce changes in the gut microbiota."[158] The reason for this benefit is not fully understood, but may be connected to the changes our body goes through when we exercise, suggesting that temporarily being pushed out of our comfort zone is good for our gut diversity.[159] Then again, we update our gut microbiome from all sorts of sources around us. The mere act of lacing up our muddy running shoes helps build our microbiome. I know that sounds crazy but that's how the microbiome works: It's an internal reflection of our interactions with the outside world.

Not all bacteria that enter our bodies take up residence in our gut.[160] Some cannot survive the acidic environment, for example. Other bacteria cannot survive in areas with high oxygen concentration. And antibiotics tend to wipe out both the beneficial and detrimental bacteria from our gut.

And it's important to have that beneficial bacteria present there. Studies have found connections between the content of our gut microbiome and many digestive disorders, such as irritable bowel disease and colorectal cancer.

The gut microbiome also appears to influence mood and mental health through the gut-brain axis (introduced in Nutrition Protocol 1).[161] A 2022 review of twenty-four observational studies and nineteen experimental trials, totaling about four thousand participants, identified differences in the beta diversity—which measures how dissimilar the various bacteria types present are to one another—between individuals who had been diagnosed with major depressive disorder and those who had not.[162] Researchers theorize that disruptions to the gut microbiome alter the release of serotonin and dopamine, setting off a cascade that ultimately ends with the release of cytokines, proteins that trigger the immune system into action and heighten inflammation.[163] Specific inflammatory cytokines have been linked to depression.[164]

On the positive side, we know that when our gut bacteria are provided with sufficient L-tryptophan (the amino acid precursor to serotonin) and short-chain fatty acids, they can readily help synthesize serotonin and signal for our brain to do the same, via our vagus nerve.

The Human Microbiome Project, the American Gut Project, the British Gut Project, and other ongoing large collaborative studies are continuing to uncover the function of the gut microbiome—both its role in healthy biological processes and its influence on chronic and acute ailments. Studies also seek to figure out which specific species of microbiota are beneficial and which are not. As a general rule, diversity is the most important feature of a healthy gut microbiome.[165] Diet plays a huge role in ensuring that our gut hosts a wide range of healthy bacteria.[166] Fiber has long been a focus in this endeavor to ensure a healthy microbiome (more about how to prioritize fiber in Nutrition Protocol 4).[167] But fermented foods appear to play an equally if not more significant role as well. Hence this protocol.

Take the study led by Stanford University biologist Justin Sonnenburg comparing how dietary fiber and fermented foods affected the microbiome of thirty-six participants.[168] Half of the individuals consumed a high-fiber diet for ten weeks, increasing their intake of soluble and insoluble fiber by eating more fruits, vegetables, legumes, grains, nuts, and seeds. They also consumed more vegetable protein and decreased the quantity of animal protein and salt. The other half upped their intake of fermented low-sugar foods like yogurt and kefir and also consumed fermented vegetables (sauerkraut, kimchi) and beverages (kombucha and vegetable brine). The researchers collected blood and stool samples before the ten weeks began, at four weeks into the intervention, and at the end of the following six weeks. The participants then began following a diet of their choice—maintaining their study diet or something else—and samples were collected after another four weeks.

Analyses of the blood and stool samples revealed that the group focused on fermented foods experienced a significant decrease in nineteen markers of inflammation, including the cytokines interleukin-6, interleukin-10, and interleukin-12b. The researchers also observed beneficial increases in the diversity of the gut microbiomes, as well as decreases in markers of immune system disruption in the low-sugar fermented food condition. The increase in microbial diversity was notably greater among the fermented foods group compared to the high-fiber group. This diversity lasted through the final four weeks of the study, after participants returned to the diet of their choice, indicating that the change was not due to a temporary passing-through of microbes but rather an "ecosystem remodeling," as the researchers call it in their 2022 report in *Cell.*

COMMON QUESTIONS:

What specific fermented foods should I eat?

Any that require refrigeration and are low in sugar, and have no added sugars are good choices. Sauerkraut and kimchi are both excellent choices. However, take note that any sauerkraut, pickles, and such that are stable on the shelf have not been fermented and are not recommended. Kombucha is also great, though it contains small amounts of alcohol and is often high in sugar, and should therefore be consumed in moderation. Natto and miso, made from fermented soybeans, are also good choices and are widely available.

Many fermented foods can be expensive. Yogurt and apple cider vinegar are lower-cost items and easy to find in your grocery store. Kefir is a yogurt drink that is less common but carried by many markets, and also less expensive than some other fermented products.

It is possible to make fermented foods at home, but the process needs careful attention to avoid contamination with harmful bacteria or anything else that can cause a foodborne illness. Tim Ferriss offered a great protocol for homemade sauerkraut in his book *The 4-Hour Chef*, and that can also be found online. Pickling vegetables in miso is a relatively easy way to make fermented food at home. If you decide to make your own fermented foods, be sure to follow the recipe exactly, including all advised precautions.

I get an unpleasant histamine response from fermented foods—itchy eyes, tingling in my hands, and brain fog. What should I do?

This is not uncommon. I've had this experience too from eating broccoli and onions, and I never knew why. When I hosted Sean Mackey, MD, PhD, and chief of the division of Stanford Pain Medicine, on the *Huberman Lab* podcast, he told me about his experience with gut pain, one that defied all approaches . . . until someone suggested he cut out histamine-containing foods like onions.[169] I can live without onions, but love low-sugar fermented foods and the benefits mentioned above are motivation for me to eat them daily. But they can cause a histamine response. So I have taken the histamine enzyme diamine oxidase (DAO) before these meals. It's inexpensive and it solved the issue for me.

NUTRITION PROTOCOL

7

Consume Fatty Ocean Fish and/or Consider Omega-3 Supplements

WHAT TO DO:

- **Make a point to consume some fatty, cold water fish once or twice a week.** Consider including salmon with the skin, sardines, mackerel, or herring as part of your weekly diet.
- **Take supplements of fish oil or krill oil, or, if you're vegan, algae oil.** Aim to consume 1,000 milligrams of eicosapentaenoic acid (EPA) per day. Some people will benefit from consuming as much as 2 to 3 grams of EPA per day, although for most people getting that 1 gram of EPA per day will suffice. Some may even wish to ask their doctor to prescribe generic or name brand Lovaza, which is high in omega-3 fatty acids (at 465 mg per capsule), and is purified of all metals and other toxins. It is now rather inexpensive to obtain given it is available in generic form. I take it daily.

HOW IT WORKS:

Nutrition Protocol 5 included the somewhat bold suggestion that we build a healthier relationship with fat. The omega-3 fatty acids are among the best forms of fat. These compounds form polyunsaturated fats, which are found in some fish, some leafy greens, beans, many plant-based oils and some other foods.[170]

As discussed earlier, fatty acids, the building blocks of fat, help with metabolism, how our bodies respond to hormones, physical performance, and more.[171] The body can turn calories into stored fat. But we can't make omega-3 fatty acids. We have to get them through our diet.

And we should make sure to do that because the evidence that omega-3 fatty acids are good for us—our brains, in particular—is persuasive. Research has found positive ties between omega-3s and memory, cognition,[172] the maintenance of mental health and heart health,[173] improved outcomes after heart disease treatment,[174] and relief from depression.[175]

Let's get specific. Modern interest in omega-3 fatty acids can be traced largely to two Danish researchers who became curious about the diet followed by the Greenland Inuit.[176] The low incidence of heart disease and diabetes led the researchers to wonder whether something in their diet, which contained large amounts of seal and whale fat, was staving off these illnesses. Their 1971 paper comparing plasma lipid and lipoprotein levels, which are associated with coronary artery disease, among a population of Greenland Inuit and a population of Danish citizens (including a small group of Inuit living in Denmark) led the researchers to speculate about a connection between the high content of unsaturated fat in the Inuit diet and low incidence of coronary artery disease as well as diabetes. The publication launched decades of research about the value of omega-3 fatty acids.

Omega-3 fatty acids have been studied in numerous disease settings, with varying results. Among the more striking findings, aside from the clearly beneficial role in reducing the risk of heart disease, is a link to the reduction of depressive symptoms. In one study, researchers randomized sixty people diagnosed with major depressive disorder to treatment with 1,000 milligrams EPA daily, 20 milligrams of the prescription drug fluoxetine (more commonly known as Prozac), or both for eight weeks.[177] Among the forty-eight patients who completed at least four weeks of study treatment, EPA and fluoxetine were equally effective at treating depression, and the combination yielded better outcomes than either one alone.

I mentioned a few of these foods in Nutrition Protocol 5, but it bears repeating here for the particular benefits of omega-3 fatty acids they contain.

COMMON QUESTIONS:

Fish oil supplements can be expensive. Are they necessary? Which ones are the best?

Indeed they can be expensive and concerns about them turning rancid are real. To get 1 gram or more of EPA per day, make sure the source is fresh and from a reputable, third-party tested supplement company. The liquid fish oil (usually cod, mackerel, anchovies, or some combination) sold in dark bottles to protect from light is most cost-effective. Just be sure to keep the bottle refrigerated after opening or it can go rancid. As I mentioned earlier, these days I take Lovaza, which is a prescription high-dose omega-3 capsule that has been purified of metals and other contaminants. It's available in generic form now so it is inexpensive, but you do need a doctor to prescribe it.

I don't like fish oil or fish. Can algae or krill do the job for omega-3s?

All these are decent sources of omega-3 fatty acids. For those who are allergic to fish oil or don't want to take it for ethical reasons, algae oil supplements are vegan and rich with omega-3.

One warning: I know a fair number of people who tolerate fish oil well but for whom krill-based omega-3 gives them a rash that itches. I am one such person. So proceed with caution.

What about just eating a lot of fish instead of taking supplements?

Again, it is hard to consume enough fish. High-quality fish can be expensive. We also have to be careful about avoiding mercury, which now exists in many species at levels that are too high for frequent human consumption.

King mackerel, swordfish, and bigeye tuna are among the fish with the highest mercury levels. Cold-water fish with the lowest mercury levels and that are excellent sources of omega-3s include inexpensive options, like sardines and herring. These and supplementation are going to be the easiest and most cost-efficient approaches to follow. And maybe some sustainably sourced cod, tilapia, or salmon with the skin on one to two times a week, if you like the taste.

CHAPTER 5

PROTOCOLS

for LIGHT

Of all the science I've studied over the years—as a research neuroscientist, in my role hosting many of the world's most qualified doctors and scientists on my podcast, and in my own real-world experience—light, and the incredible influence it has on every aspect of our health, is the subject that has thrilled and surprised me the most.

As a master's student I worked on the visual pathways that control circadian rhythms, and in graduate school and during my postdoc fellowship, and in my own lab, I researched visual circuits that convert light energy—photons, that is—into conscious visual perception, or what is commonly referred to as eyesight. My lab also spent a few years exploring the connections between our eyes and the cerebellum. Turns out, our eyes and our cerebellum—or "mini brain"—are in an ongoing dialogue that helps us orient in space. We will get back to the cerebellum later when we discuss learning in chapter 6.

But as my lab explored the visual system, papers kept coming out showing how light either supports or damages the health of our cells. In some cases these findings were about how light affects the skin. In other cases, it was about how light impacts our health via our eyes in ways that are separate from eyesight. Given that so much of my training centered around our visual system, that research intrigued me. Not just because it was in my wheelhouse but also because of how actionable it was. It could be applied easily to daily life, and impact health in potent ways. So I voraciously read every one of those studies. I also knew one of the pioneers in this field. Glen Jeffery, PhD, at the University College London, a former colleague of mine from the field of visual system development, began to study how particular types and sources of light either help or hurt human physiology. His lab also studied how light affected longevity.[1] I connected with him periodically to get a sense of what was on the horizon. While his is not the only lab working on the relationship between light and health, Glen is a leader in the formal study of this topic. We have him to thank for taking what were largely anecdotal observations put forth by niche online communities and testing them in controlled studies including clinical trials.

Over those years, I was also spending more and more time indoors, under LED lights—both during the day and at night. Such is life in a lab. My colleagues all did the same. So did my friends in medicine, tech, design, and, once smartphones hit the world full force in 2010, pretty much everyone else. I, and some of my more health-conscious colleagues, started to wonder if all that time indoors under the LED lights was part of the reason a lot of us were feeling so lousy.

Now we know that it almost certainly was. The lack of full-spectrum sunlight, and the use of LED light was no doubt directly damaging our bodies, inside and out, by impairing cellular health. Now of course, I can't be sure it was *all* due to indoor lighting, but at one point my hair started falling out, I was always tired in the afternoon, and my joints ached. And I was exercising and eating well at the time, and my life was no more stressful than it is now.

Eventually I decided to use light as a tool, not just to get my sleep right but to improve other aspects of my health. I was amazed by what happened. My hair grew back—like crazy, in fact. I got far fewer colds and other respiratory infections. My mood even lifted. Mind you, I was in my forties then, and I'm in my fifties now, and still with the addition of a few simple protocols, my general health improved markedly. There are different levers of health but based on the data from Glen's lab and others, I treat my relationship to sunlight and indoor lighting as key levers for health.

My experience is anecdotal, but we now have evidence to support why and precisely how the use of light can improve cellular, organ, and body-wide health. It is an area of health just as crucial as sleep, exercise, or nutrition. Moreover, we now know the best ways to capture the benefits of different types of light. Which is why it deserves its own chapter here.

While light as a tool for health is not discussed as often as it should be, it is not new, and its origins are definitely not fringe; we've long known that there was a connection between sunlight and well-being. And in many regions of the world, hospitals still take patients outside for the age-old practice of sunlight exposure to promote recovery from certain ailments.[2] And photobiomodulation has been studied and used by serious scientists and physicians since the early 1900s.[3] The Danish physician Niels Finsen was actually awarded the Nobel Prize in Physiology or Medicine in 1903 for his discovery that light can be used to treat various diseases including tuberculosis of the skin, or lupus.

Nowadays, photobiomodulation has been shown to be effective for treating acne,[4] accelerating wound healing,[5] and promoting hair growth,[6] as well as reducing pain[7] and even improving blood sugar regulation.[8] Studies have also demonstrated the efficacy of photobiomodulation for offsetting age-related vision loss[9] and for improving hormone health.[10] That's not all; light has also been shown to improve heart[11] and GI tract health[12] and to help combat various autoimmune conditions.[13]

And of course, there are countless positive effects of viewing sunlight on your circadian rhythm. As you recall from chapter 1, viewing low solar angle sunlight in the morning and again in the afternoon sets your sleep-wake cycle correctly, increases your daytime mood, alertness and focus, and immune system function, and promotes better sleep at night. It is not exaggerating to say that light is medicine, especially sunlight.

And like any medicine, the effects of light depend on the type, intensity, duration, and timing of its delivery. For example, whereas sunlight in the morning and daytime is beneficial, viewing bright lights (especially from LED sources) too close to your bedtime spikes your cortisol levels, quashes your melatonin, and disrupts your blood sugar regulation (as discussed in Sleep Protocol 3). That affects your sleep that night and your energy the next morning. And certain wavelengths of light—in particular those emitted by most LED sources—may also accelerate cellular aging and promote disease progression by damaging cells in the retina, cornea, and brain, according to studies in animal models.[14]

While all these effects of light might sound tricky to navigate, it's actually quite simple. You just need to know which types of light are beneficial to view, which are detrimental, and how and when to maximize one and minimize the other. In this chapter, I'll teach you.

What Is Light?

First we need to discuss what light is, exactly.

Obviously, light makes things visible. Any light source, be it the sun, a lamp, a candle flame, or the glow from a phone screen makes things visible because it emits energy. Light sources vary by type and amount of energy; that's what makes them different from one another.

Recall from chapter 1 that light is comprised of a broad range of wavelengths, from very short wavelengths to very long ones. Some of these wavelengths are visible to humans—they make up what we call the visible spectrum of red, green, blue, and so on. Other wavelengths of light, such as ultraviolet and infrared, are invisible to us.

Short wavelengths of light are, as their name suggests, waves of energy where the peaks and the troughs of the wave are very close together. Long wavelengths of light are the opposite; the peaks and troughs of long wavelength light are relatively far apart.

The sun emits an extremely broad range of short, medium, and long wavelengths. The entire visible spectrum is held inside sunlight. That's why sunlight through a prism comes through as a rainbow on the other side. The prism slows down and bends the light, and each wavelength exits at a different angle, spreading the light into the full visible spectrum of red, orange, yellow, green, blue, indigo, and violet.

Green, blue, and purple light are shorter in wavelength compared to yellow, orange, and red light, which are longer. Sunlight (in the absence of a prism) appears white or pale yellow. The sky turns colorful at dawn and dusk because, as you may recall from chapter 1, when the sun is low in the sky, components of the atmosphere reduce the amount of shorter wavelengths reaching our eyes—a process called Rayleigh scattering—leaving us primarily seeing the longer wavelengths of red, orange, and yellow. The sun of course always emits the same wavelengths of energy regardless of where it happens to be in the sky. Which visible wavelengths arrive at our eyes is what determines how the sun appears to us, and the effect it will have on us.

Then there are the invisible wavelengths. Sunlight includes wavelengths shorter than blue or violet that are (unimaginatively) called ultraviolet (UV) light. We can't perceive UV light but it's there, radiating down on us all day. (Though interesting to note that bees can see UV, and squirrels can see it too, possibly to help them detect predators at night. Some species of flying squirrels actually have UV fluorescence that causes their bellies to glow a bubblegum pink.)[15] The sun also emits wavelengths longer than red light, appropriately called infrared (IR) light. We humans can't see IR, but we can feel it as warmth. Though we have engineered technologies to see IR emissions—that's what night vision goggles do.

The sun also emits small amounts of X-ray energy, which is made up of very short wavelength radiation, even shorter than UV. And, like with UV and

IR, we can't see X-rays, but they are there. X-rays pass through our skin but are absorbed by our bones, teeth, and other dense tissues. That's how X-ray machines work: They are designed to send out concentrated X-rays so their patterns of absorption can be captured on film or by a digital sensor, allowing your doctor or dentist to see different structures inside your body that absorb those X-rays to varying degrees.

Whether visible or invisible, these wavelengths travel in a similar pattern—not as a line but, well, as a wave, moving up and down, up and down. Shorter wavelengths of light go through many more up-down-up-down cycles as they travel from one point to another; longer wavelengths go through fewer. Thus, we often refer to short wavelengths of light as high frequency light and long wavelengths of light as low frequency.

Mentions of UV light can trigger concerns, so let me address that now. Whether light exposure is harmful, beneficial, or benign depends on the type, intensity, duration, and timing. All light energy is radiation. Often when people hear the word *radiation* they think *radioactive*. The radiation from visible light is not harmful because it doesn't have enough energy to perturb the atoms in our body. But here's where type, duration, and the other factors matter. Some forms of non-ionizing light radiation can disrupt our cells if we are exposed to too much of it. For example, we need some UV light exposure each day. But excessive exposure can cause genetic mutations in our cells by causing the formation of abnormal bonds in our DNA.[16]

Wavelength and intensity of light are inversely related to one another. Put in practical terms, you can be exposed to a lot of long wavelength light, like red or IR light, without damaging your skin. It takes comparatively less exposure to short wavelength UV light to cause a sunburn. But that doesn't mean short wavelength, high frequency light is inherently bad for us. Again, we come back to this core idea: Dosage matters. We all need some UV light from the sun to reach our skin, where it sets off a cascade of reactions that results in the production of vitamin D, which is critical for calcium absorption, bone health, immune health, and more.[17] But too much UV exposure can lead to a sunburn, as I mentioned above, and cause premature aging of your skin, as well as DNA mutations that lead to certain skin cancers.[18] And because long wavelength IR is so low energy (remember, wavelength and intensity are inversely related), we need relatively long sun exposure times to enjoy its benefits. The challenge is getting enough IR and NIR (infrared and near-infrared) light from the sun without also getting excessive UV exposure, but it can be done. There's a protocol for it.

I'm aware that none of what I've shared with you thus far tells you exactly *how* light can change your cells. As wavelengths travel through space, in that up-and-down cycle, they hit various surfaces, big and small: a mountain range, a tree, this page, your hand. These surfaces absorb or reflect wavelengths. But sometimes they pass right through. Light can pass right through your body, for example, and as it does it can change the molecular properties of the cells it encounters and the components within them, such as in the example of excessive UV-altering DNA structure of, say, skin cells. Here are two more examples, this time with light playing positive roles in cellular function: Studies suggest that red, NIR, and IR light can enhance the functioning of your mitochondria, the energy producing organelles in your cells.[19] Data suggest that NIR and IR may also trigger the release of a gas called nitric oxide that acts on your vascular and lymphatic cells and causes them to dilate, allowing for more lymph fluid and blood to move through them.[20]

There are more examples in the protocols that follow. You'll learn how to use light—in some cases sunlight, and in other cases artificial light of specific wavelengths—to improve your physical and mental health. Also here are recommendations for in-home lighting and light devices that emit or block specific wavelengths of light, which you can use to achieve specific benefits, such as increased morning and daytime energy levels, better glucose regulation, and even better eyesight. In chapter 1, we explored how light helps with sleep; now it's time to see its immediate effects on other important aspects of our health.

As you read these protocols, remember this: While it might seem fantastical that light can do so many positive things for our brain and body, it actually makes perfect sense. Light is energy that the cells in our body can absorb and use. The very first law of thermodynamics is that energy can't be destroyed or created de novo; it can only be converted from one form to another. So let's discuss the ways you can convert light energy into cellular energy, which leads to improvements in physical energy, vision, skin, mood, and heart health . . . and more.

I hope this powerful lever will no longer be overlooked.

Note: *If you are reading this book from beginning to end, you'll realize as you encounter Light Protocols 1, 2, and 3 that these are essentially the same as protocols covered in chapter 1 and chapter 3. You may be thinking, "Does he have a memory issue, or think I have one?" The answer is: no and no.*

The practices I suggest in this chapter are indeed found in earlier ones. But, because many people may read this book out of order, I wanted to be sure that these crucial protocols would not be missed. Moreover, the information that follows is not a carbon copy of the protocols in chapter 1 or chapter 3. I include new information about the mechanisms behind the "critical window" in the first hour after you wake up, whereby your SCN can amplify your morning cortisol levels . . . if and only if you give it the right stimulus. I also cover new information about viewing light at specific times to adjust your cortisol rhythm, so you can avoid what is commonly referred to as "burnout," but is often a mistiming in your daily cortisol peak. I also include more options for indoor lighting—some were mentioned only briefly in previous chapters; others are new. All that said, if you feel you are already versed enough in these first three protocols and most importantly, you are already doing them on a daily basis, feel free to skip to Light Protocol 4.

LIGHT PROTOCOL

1

View Bright Light in the First Hour After Waking to (Further) Increase Your Morning Cortisol Levels

WHAT TO DO:

- **Get morning sunlight in your eyes as soon as possible after waking.** If the sun hasn't risen yet, or is otherwise inaccessible, view a 10,000 lux artificial light. Either one will significantly elevate your post-waking morning cortisol levels, which is highly beneficial *if it occurs in the first hour of your day.*
- **The timing will vary based on when you wake up, and where you live.** Refer to the information below to figure out what's best for you. Ten to thirty minutes is a good general rule, but even if you can only grab five, do it. Some is better than none.

HOW IT WORKS:

It is hard to overstate the positive impact of this protocol on your energy, mood, focus, stress levels, immune system, and, of course, sleep. If you've read chapter 1, you might be thinking: Does this protocol sound familiar? Yes, I'm recommending a similar behavioral tool here, but emphasizing different benefits. Stay with me.

I can hear all the questions running through your head, so for this protocol, let's tackle these first.

You're probably thinking, "Wait—I have to get up and watch the sunrise every day?" No. You don't. If you wake up early enough, and the sky is clear, great! Do that. But most people can't. And you don't need to. The key thing here is to view bright light *in the first hour after waking*. This applies even if your normal wake-up time is noon.

"What if I wake up before the sun is out?" Another question I hear often. Again, not a problem. That is where a 10,000 lux artificial light can really help. It's not a replacement for sunlight, but if you wake up before sunrise, I suggest getting one of these lights and looking at it for ten minutes or so upon waking. Then, if you can, get outside for some early natural light once the sun has risen. If you're off to work at an office before sunrise, these lights are a game changer.

"I can't see the sun where I live, so what should I do?" I have good news for you. You need to get sun*light* in your eyes, but you do not need to see the sun. Some days it's clear, and other days it's overcast. Sunlight still comes through on cloudy days. Maybe you're thinking: "Not where I live!" Really? Consider how bright it is at 8:00 a.m. on a densely clouded winter day in Seattle, which is the northernmost major city in the contiguous US. Then consider what it's like at midnight the night before. Unless you live at one of the earth's poles in winter—which I'm guessing you don't—there is always some sunlight during the daytime. So view it within an hour of waking. Let's keep going with those common questions.

"Can I wear sunglasses?" It's best to view morning sunlight without them. Wearing corrective lenses such as eyeglasses or contact lenses is fine, even if they include UV protection. Don't wear a brimmed hat, however. The neurons in your eyes that you need to stimulate here respond to light coming from above and in front of your eyes, and a brimmed hat will block it.

"Can I blink?" Yes! Never force yourself to stare at sunlight, or any bright light for that matter. It can damage your eyes to do so. People vary in their sensitivity to light, so if this is hard for you, squint and look to the area adjacent to the sun as needed. This shouldn't hurt.

"Can I get my morning sunlight through a window?" While better than nothing, the glass used for most windows filters out too much of the wavelengths of light you need. Thus, go outside. Bring your morning coffee, tea, or a glass of water. Bring your dog, kids, partner, or a friend along with you if you like. Yes, your dog will benefit too. After all, the same circuits and mechanisms that underlie this protocol are present in humans and dogs (and horses, goats, and squirrels, as I've mentioned, and all diurnal mammals). And of course you can walk, jog, skip rope, or do calisthenics as you view bright light too. If you take an hour walk, or schedule a run or a yoga session outside, even better, as sunlight and exercise can synergize to increase your early morning cortisol levels. Whatever you do, just don't spend the whole time looking down at your phone. That will negate the effect you're seeking.

"How long should I view morning sunlight to get the maximum effect?" As I mentioned, the answer depends on sunlight availability but a good general rule of thumb is this: On clear mornings shoot for a minimum of ten minutes, on partially cloudy days, get a minimum of twenty minutes, and on very overcast days, thirty minutes. If you view a 10,000 lux artificial light beforehand, for any of the reasons discussed already, you'll need less time viewing sunlight—about half as much—to get the same effect.

It's hard to be more specific than this because sunlight availability is shaped by the time of day, time of year, weather, and location.

And, once more: "What if I wake up before sunrise, then what?" This is by far the most common question I hear. Unless you have powers that I am not aware of, you will have to wait for the sun to come out to see sunlight. Get your in-the-first-hour-of-waking bright light by viewing a 10,000 lux artificial light. Ten thousand lux artificial light devices are not as good as sunlight, because they don't contain the same array and balance of wavelengths present in sunlight as discussed in the introduction to this chapter. But they will elevate your morning cortisol levels, which is your goal in this protocol.[21] They cost about $100 to $150. Some are portable and suitable for travel. And, again, if you rely on a 10,000 lux light first thing in the morning, you'll still want to get five to twenty minutes or so of natural sunlight exposure to your eyes once the sun comes out. Most people find that having a 10,000 lux light in their bathroom or kitchen works well for their morning routines.

If you do use a 10,000 lux light, you needn't be obsessed with the viewing distance, nor do you have to worry about intermittently stepping or pivoting away from the light while preparing for your day. Just aim to be in front of it at a distance of about one to two feet for at least ten minutes total in the first hour after waking. More is fine, but again people vary in their sensitivity to light and some find that after ten minutes of 10,000 lux light they feel *too* awake! Other people can handle more exposure.

And if you have a question about my schedule: Because I typically wake up before the sun is out, I have a 10,000 lux light in my bathroom and my kitchen. I turn them on within a few minutes of waking and leave them on as I brush my teeth and prepare for my day. Once the sun is up, I go outside and view sunlight. That way, on days when I need to commute to work early or exercise before the sun is up, I know I have already spiked my morning cortisol. And when I travel, I bring a small portable 10,000 lux unit and use it in the same way. It's a fantastic tool but it's not a replacement for sunlight.

"Does viewing my computer screen or phone work to replace morning sunlight or 10,000 lux light?" Alas, no. Your phone screen is far too dim and far too narrow a spectrum to accomplish the effect here. Diabolically, however, your phone or computer screen is plenty bright enough to stimulate cortisol release if it's viewed at night. And that is bad. And your phone or computer is plenty bright enough to suppress your melatonin levels. Also bad!

By now you may be asking (or shouting): "Wait, why in the world would I want to *increase* my cortisol levels? Isn't cortisol a stress hormone? Isn't that a bad thing?" Okay, maybe if you read this book in order, you already know the answer, but I'll repeat it here: Most people think cortisol is a stress hormone to avoid, but you absolutely want to have high cortisol levels in the first hours of your day. The science shows us why.

The Natural Cortisol Cycle

Sleep Protocol 1 explains the science behind how viewing morning sunlight impacts your circadian rhythm. As a brief reminder: When you view sunlight, or a 10,000 lux light, it activates cells in your eyes that convert light into electrical signals. Those signals are relayed to the suprachiasmatic nucleus (SCN), your master circadian clock, located above the roof of your mouth in your hypothalamus. The SCN in turn releases chemical and electrical signals that coordinate the activities of the trillions of twenty-four-hour clocks found in every cell and organ of your body into a coherent set of rhythms. The physiological and psychological benefits that circadian coordination brings about are many.

But the SCN is not a one-trick pony. It serves another crucial role that is seldom discussed but, frankly, just as important. Your SCN can also stimulate a significant increase in your cortisol levels in the first sixty minutes after you wake up. It's time restricted, meaning it can only occur in this short window. If you miss it, it's gone—at least until the next day.

This is not a window you want to miss! Because whereas surges in cortisol are generally not advantageous if they occur in the afternoon, the evening, or at night, as I've mentioned, you actually want your cortisol levels to be very high in the first hours of your day.

Cortisol has gotten a bad rap. It's been labeled the stress hormone and indeed, this hormone made in your adrenal glands is released during times of stress. But cortisol is also released when you wake up each morning. More accurately, you wake up each morning because cortisol is released. You read that right. Cortisol is the hormone that ensures you have the energy to get out of bed and lean into your daily activities. That is because cortisol's fundamental role is to cause the release of stored fuels in your liver and muscles, which shifts the state of your brain and body from sleep to one of physical and mental readiness. The technical term for this process, which you might remember from chapter 3, is called the cortisol awakening response (CAR). Cortisol is not just a stress hormone. It's an energy-releasing hormone. (See Stress Control Protocol 5 if you'd like a reminder.)

When we view cortisol in this way, we start to understand that it's not something to be avoided at all. Rather, it is something to harness and use to our advantage. Our body has designated pathways and mechanisms to do just that. It allows for what's called the healthy twenty-four-hour cortisol curve, which follows the pattern below:

1. Very low in the 1 to 2 hours prior to bedtime
2. At its absolute lowest in the first half of your night's sleep
3. Rising slowly in the second half of your night's sleep
4. Rising sharply in the 30 minutes prior to your desired wake-up time
5. Rising sharply even more in the first 1 to 2 hours after you wake up
6. Peaking about 30 minutes to 3 hours after waking
7. Gradually decreasing across the early and late afternoon
8. Repeat . . .

Countless studies now show that allowing this natural cycle to operate without disruption helps optimize our sleep, cognition, and energy levels as well as mood and immune system function.[22] By contrast, altering this cycle such that evening or nighttime cortisol levels are too high (or morning cortisol levels are too low) can lead to problems in all these areas. Studies of night shift workers have been crucial in uncovering these connections.[23] A chronic disruption to the ideal cycle is referred to as a flattening of the cortisol curve. This flattening causes anxiety, sleep disturbances, low daytime energy, and mood disruptions as well as impaired immune resistance to viral, bacterial, and other infections.[24]

Cortisol and Stress

Keep in mind that just because we are framing cortisol as not purely a stress hormone does not mean it is not related to stress. It is. Stress triggers the release of cortisol.[25] If you experience stress at any point during the day or night, you can and should expect a spike in your cortisol to occur. That's perfectly normal, healthy, and adaptive—because that spike will provide you with the immediate physical and mental energy you need to deal with whatever stressor you might face.[26] Stress-triggered cortisol levels typically return to baseline within about one hour or so. In fact, you can experience a lot of cortisol spikes above baseline per day (or night) before it ever becomes problematic for your health. I'm not suggesting you seek out stress, but as we discussed in chapter 3, humans evolved to deal with it in a variety of forms. Raising kids, traffic, difficult people, the pressures of work, school, or athletics, the state of the world . . . many of these are indeed stressful at times, and cortisol makes sure you have the fuel to deal with each one.

Cortisol spikes that occur shortly before sleep are where problems begin. That increase is often what prevents people from falling asleep, and what causes the classic stress-induced sleep disturbance of waking up at 3:00 a.m. and not falling back asleep. One night of that happening, no biggie. Two nights in a row? Hard, but manageable. However, three or more nights of stress-induced sleep disturbances really start to take a toll on your mental and physical health.

Cortisol and Light

And now we get back to the protocol suggested here. I discussed how to deal with both acute and chronic stress in chapter 3. What we didn't discuss is that when you get your twenty-four-hour cortisol curve correct, it makes both kinds of stress much easier to deal with. And to get your twenty-four-hour cortisol curve correct we need to . . . view morning sunlight (or 10,000 lux light) in the first hour after waking. It not only boosts your morning cortisol levels, but also helps ensure your nighttime cortisol is kept low. This has immediate benefits you can feel within minutes and that last all day, among them improved mood, focus, and energy. Think of it as the optimal start signal for your day. Because from the perspective of your brain and body, that's exactly what it is.

Here are the basics of how it works, plus some additional information pertinent to the twenty-four-hour cortisol cycle. Your cortisol level at any one moment, and your overall twenty-four-hour cortisol cycle, are controlled via the hypothalamic-pituitary-adrenal (HPA) axis, which we discussed in chapter 3. Neurons in an area of your hypothalamus called the PVN (paraventricular nucleus) extend wirelike projections into your pituitary, a gland that resembles two small marbles in a sock hanging out the base of your brain.[27] One of those marbles sits in front of the other, and this is called the anterior pituitary. Your PVN neurons release corticotropin-releasing hormone (CRH) to cause your anterior pituitary cells to release adrenocorticotropic hormone (ACTH) into your bloodstream. Next, the ACTH travels to your adrenal glands and stimulates the release of cortisol into your bloodstream. Voila! Cortisol then causes energy to be released from various organs and cells in your body. Cortisol does many other things, but one more that's relevant here: Unlike adrenaline, which is also released from your adrenal glands and increases your energy level, cortisol can cross the blood-brain barrier. That means it has action on the body, such as mobilizing glucose for fuel, but also can increase the excitability of the neurons in your brain involved in alertness, focus, memory formation, and even motivation.

The PVN also detects when cortisol levels in your blood get high. It then *reduces* its release of CRH, which in turn reduces ACTH release, which results in less cortisol release. This is called a negative feedback loop; when the level of cortisol reaching the brain is very high, less cortisol is triggered to be released. In that way, it is like how many home thermostats work. For example, if the temperature in a room becomes too high from the level you've set, the thermostat shuts the heat off.

This self-regulation process takes a bit of time to take effect, which is why a short-term spike in cortisol is no big deal. An hour or so afterward, you're back to your baseline level, appropriate for that time of day. But with frequent spikes, you start to alter your normal twenty-four-hour cortisol cycle. Cortisol surges at 9:00 p.m. for a few nights in a row and the next thing you know, your next-morning levels are lower than they should be *and* your PVN is then primed to release *more* cortisol later that night.

There is a name for this domino effect. It's called chronic-stress-induced burnout. Alas, for many, this is the norm, especially now that a good number of people lie in bed looking at their phone in the first and last hour of each day, which, for reasons you'll soon understand, sets them up for lower-than-needed cortisol levels in the morning and greater-than-desired cortisol levels at night.

So in a way, a better name for chronic-stress-induced burnout would be "wrongly-timed-cortisol-induced-burnout," because, again, you want your morning cortisol high. I already listed some of the immediate benefits of stimulating cortisol in the hour after waking, but perhaps by now you can also identify another: If you do, you not only get enormous benefits in energy, focus, and mood right away, you also kickstart that crucial negative feedback loop that ensures that your levels of cortisol will be dropping as you head into the afternoon and evening. Your cortisol levels will be very low as you progress into sleep.

That's how all the pieces come together: In that special window in the first hour after you wake up, when your SCN can also stimulate a significant increase in your cortisol levels, you can bypass the negative feedback loop and stimulate the release of more cortisol even though its levels are already high. In fact, your SCN does so both through the HPA pathway and via a separate, parallel pathway involving direct activation of your sympathetic nervous system.[28] We can refer to that second pathway as the MLIC pathway (for morning-light-induced-cortisol pathway). And, as the name indicates, the way to activate the MLIC pathway is by viewing bright light.

As a final note, researchers have studied the use of bright artificial light in the first hour of the day not just for this, but as a therapeutic intervention for seasonal affective disorder (SAD), a diagnosable mood disorder characterized by depression that fluctuates with the seasons, worsening in the colder, darker months.[29] Rates of this condition are particularly high among people who have major depression or bipolar disorder. In one study, people diagnosed with seasonal affective disorder were treated with twenty, forty, or sixty minutes of 10,000 lux light in the morning.[30] Even the shortest exposure was sufficient to relieve depression among the participants, according to a self-reported questionnaire. Other studies have shown similar results.[31] Newer studies have shown that reducing the amount of bright light reaching your eyes in the final one to two hours of your day leads to improvements in mood and sleep, and to various mental and physical performance benefits as well.[32]

In the last ten years, it's become clear that far more people are suffering from SAD or SAD-like symptoms due to device usage in the early and late hours of the day. In chapter 1, we discussed the severe negative effects of shift work on long-term health, and the fact that nowadays most adults and kids—most (!)—qualify as shift workers due to this kind of device usage. How can that be? Well, remember—even the brightest device screens are too dim to trigger meaningful cortisol increases in the first hour of your day, and even the dimmest screens are more than bright enough to trigger cortisol increases at night. That is, unless you filter out the short wavelengths reaching your eyes—which we talk about in the next protocol.

COMMON QUESTIONS:

Does it matter if this light hits my skin or are the eyes all that count here?

This protocol is concerned with viewing light only. Later protocols in this chapter will address the need for sunlight on skin and how to balance that exposure with cautions about sun damage.

LIGHT PROTOCOL

2

View Sunlight in the Late Afternoon and/or Early Evening to Help Buffer Against Negative Effects of Artificial Light at Night

WHAT TO DO:

- **View sunlight in the afternoon and early evening, for five to thirty minutes.** Follow the same general guidelines as for Light Protocol 1. Simply go outside, take off your sunglasses (eyeglasses and contacts are fine), and face in the direction of the setting sun. Don't wear a brimmed hat. And again, don't stare at the sun; blink as needed.
- **Do not replace late afternoon/evening sunlight viewing with a 10,000 lux artificial light.** It's too bright, and the wavelengths these devices emit can mess up your sleep-wake cycle.

HOW IT WORKS:

As discussed in Sleep Protocol 2, melatonin, which facilitates falling and staying asleep, begins to increase in the late afternoon and early evening and sharply rises in the hour before your natural bedtime (which, by the way, tends to arrive about fifteen to sixteen hours after your morning sunlight viewing). It continues to rise into the night, before gradually decreasing as morning approaches. Melatonin levels are lowest in the morning and highest at night. In other words, when cortisol is high, melatonin is low, and when cortisol is low, melatonin is high.[33]

Bright light robustly suppresses melatonin, and it causes the release of cortisol as explained in chapter 3.[34] Blue lights, screen lights, and LEDs, all of which emit lots of short wavelengths, are especially potent at suppressing melatonin. Bright LEDs, commonly used in bathrooms, bedrooms, and hallways, are short-wavelength enriched. It takes less than thirty seconds of bright LED exposure to the eyes to significantly reduce your melatonin levels. So if you pick up your phone at night, or flip on the lights . . . you're exposing yourself to the kind of light that will suppress melatonin. Late afternoon and early evening sunlight viewing helps mitigate these negative effects.

Why do I suggest you not use a 10,000 lux artificial light as a replacement for evening sunlight, when I already suggested it as a replacement for morning sunlight in the previous protocol? The reason has to do with wavelengths, discussed earlier in this chapter. Low solar angle sunlight is lower in UV and the short visible wavelengths, which is why sunrises and sunsets often appear orange, pink, or even deep red. Those longer wavelengths help inform your brain that night is coming, and it should prepare for sleep. Too much short wavelength light—especially if it's bright, and 10,000 lux is bright—will alter your sleep-wake cycle.

You'll notice, just as in the previous protocol, that I'm not suggesting specific times to view late afternoon or early evening sunlight. Again, that is because schedules vary from person to person, and the time of day when the sun sets varies according to your location and the time of year. Luckily, you can get the desired effect without being overly precise about the timing. Just aim to view sunlight at some point after the sun is directly overhead and before it sets.

This doesn't mean that you should avoid sunlight or artificial light during other parts of the day. Researchers from Rush University ran a small study where, for one week, people experienced bright light exposure for up to five hours by combining outdoor exposure to sunlight and indoor exposure to 10,000 lux light during the day.[35] They called it "the bright week." The following week, the light exposure was dimmer; people spent two and a half hours outdoors at most, and wore light-obscuring goggles when they did. That was "the dim week." The researchers found that light-induced melatonin suppression at night was greater during the dim week than during the bright week (though some participants showed greater differences than others). Bright light exposure during the day partially prevented light-induced melatonin suppression at night.

Seems paradoxical, given that light suppresses melatonin, right? Yes, until we look at another mechanism at work here. Another small study from the Netherlands measured melatonin levels, body temperature, and skin blood flow (all markers of circadian rhythmicity) of twelve women and noted how sleepy they reported feeling, according to when they viewed light in the evening and at night.[36] They divided subjects into three groups. One group viewed dim light at night. Another group also viewed dim light at night but also viewed bright lights beforehand, late in the evening. The third group viewed bright light in the early evening, and then dim lights at night. All three groups saw some reduction in melatonin, which is not surprising given that light viewing suppresses melatonin production any time of day or night. But the third group—the group that saw early evening bright light *plus* late-night dim light—had a less dramatic melatonin drop. This again supports the idea that early evening light exposure can partially inoculate us against the negative effects of bright light at night.

These studies may be small, but they point to the importance of viewing sunlight in the late afternoon and early evening, and avoiding bright light exposure at night. It's worth noting that it may be especially important for adolescents to avoid bright light at night, as one study showed that early evening sunlight exposure did not protect them against the melatonin-reducing effects of bright light as it did for adults.[37] This may also mean that adolescents are particularly sensitive to the negative effects of bright artificial lights and screens at night.

The reasons to try to offset the negative effects of bright light at night are not just related to sleep. Animal studies have shown that bright light exposure to the eyes late at night activates pro-depression circuitries.[38] And as we've already covered, human studies have shown strong links between nighttime bright light exposure, cortisol increases, melatonin suppression, and mood disturbances. If you or your child happens to view bright light in the hours before sleep now and again, perhaps from a movie or a night out, that's no cause for concern. If you make a habit of keeping bright artificial lights on late at night, however, and you notice your moods are shifting for the worse, that could be why.

As you're probably realizing, modern life—with all its lighting options and screens everywhere—is not oriented around daylight fluctuations in the way it once was. Humans used to wake up and go to sleep with the sun. We had no choice but to be attuned to the solar cycle. The advent of artificial lighting changed everything, and the shift from incandescent to lower cost LED lighting further exacerbated the issues. In fact, in the last ten years, the amount and type of artificial light exposure humans experience has changed so dramatically that we can honestly say that, as a species, our whole relationship to light has been altered. Yet our biology hasn't changed one bit in thousands of years. Hence this chapter.

COMMON QUESTIONS:

How do I make this work if I'm stuck in the office all day?

There is no need to be obsessive about this—it doesn't have to interfere with your life. Still, by making some concerted effort toward viewing sunlight (or a 10,000 lux lamp) in the mornings, and sunlight in the late afternoons or early evenings, and avoiding bright light at night, you can dramatically improve your mood and energy levels, metabolism, and sleep—which of course bolsters all the rest. So try to get outdoors at these times if you can. Better yet, take a walk in the direction of the sun. Or even just make time to turn toward the sun and pause (and not look at your phone) for a few minutes in the parking lot before leaving work.

LIGHT PROTOCOL

3

Avoid Viewing Bright Light One Hour Before Your Bedtime

WHAT TO DO:

- **In the one hour before your bedtime, use only as much artificial light as necessary to safely carry out your nighttime activities.** That recommendation holds until you wake up the next morning to begin your day.
- **Be especially mindful to avoid viewing bright short wavelength light at this time.** Avoid not just lights that appear blue, but also bright "white" LED lights, fluorescent lights, and screens, because they emit a lot of short wavelengths that stimulate cortisol release and inhibit melatonin.
- **If you can't avoid viewing bright short wavelength light, consider wearing short wavelength light blocking lenses.** Not simply "blue blockers," but these specific lenses. For anyone seeking an easier transition into sleep and better overall sleep, these glasses can be helpful.

HOW IT WORKS:

In the first hour of your day, it takes a lot of bright light to stimulate cortisol release and activate the neural pathways in your brain and body that increase wakefulness. By comparison, in the final hour of your day, it takes very little bright light to wake you up. Moreover, melatonin, the hormone that promotes sleepiness, is potently inhibited by viewing bright light at any time of day or night. That's why viewing bright light at night is a double whammy to your system: It makes you more alert and it makes you less sleepy by at least two different pathways.

The whole light-sensing and cortisol-releasing system is just not the same in the morning and at night.[39] If you have ever felt that you are a vastly different person in the morning and at night, indeed you are. The key to using light as a tool to enhance your health is to understand this dynamic.

It all boils down to knowing when you woke up that morning and how many hours it has been since. Here's a reference you can follow:

A Day in the Light

Phase 1: 0–1 hour after waking: You need to see a lot of bright light (Light Protocol 1).

Phase 2: 6–10 hours after waking: Get some late afternoon or early evening sunlight in your eyes (Light Protocol 2).

Phase 3: 10–14 hours after waking: Start dimming the lights, avoid bright light exposure to your eyes (this protocol).

Phase 4: And finally, sleep . . .

Though by now you may be asking (or shouting), "What is all this '0–1 hour after waking, 6–10 hours after waking, and 1–2 hours before sleep' stuff? No one lives this way! Why can't you just give me a clock time?"

I've said this before, and I'll say it again here: People follow different sleep-wake schedules, with some sleeping from 8:00 p.m. to 4:00 a.m. and others sleeping from 11:00 p.m. to 7:00 a.m. Still others work the night shift. Variation in people's schedules makes it impossible for me to say, "Dim the lights and avoid viewing LED screens between 10:00 p.m. and 5:00 a.m." or even "View bright light within an hour of sunrise."

Also, the length of days varies according to location and time of year, and things like daylight further complicate matters. So I suggest you frame your sleep-wake schedule according to four phases. Once you try this approach to your days, and use light (or avoid it) accordingly, I'm certain it will improve your health and well-being.

It's worth noting again that the clock times corresponding to the four phases will change if you were to, say, sleep in an extra hour or two, or wake up an hour earlier than is typical, or go to sleep an hour earlier or later. Not a problem! When it comes to the effects of light on cortisol and melatonin, we care about your biology, not an alarm. Start phase 1, for example, when you get up to begin your day. The light prescription for each phase does not change. This ought to bring a sense of control over your time—after all, no one wants to have to take care of their health strictly by the clock. Work, school, and other commitments have us doing that already.

In case any of this is confusing, here is how I use this system to structure my days (and nights).

My Phase 1 (as of writing):

I woke up at 7:00 a.m. I usually wake up at 5:45 or 6:00, but I was a bit more tired than usual from a long week of work and travel and I forgot to set my alarm. My sleep tracker told me that I fell asleep last night at about 10:15 p.m. At 7:00 a.m., I went for a walk outside for about twenty minutes, without a hat or sunglasses, and walked east in the direction of the sun. It was light out but overcast, with no hint even of the sun's outline in the sky. But because it was fairly bright, I knew I was getting a decent amount of sunlight in my eyes, and therefore stimulating cortisol release. I was not at all concerned that I had somehow missed the window to use sunlight to boost my cortisol because my usual wake-up time is about 5:45. I know it's about getting light in my eyes in the first hour after waking, not at a specific clock time, that matters.

I returned from my walk and, just to be sure that I spiked my morning cortisol sufficiently, I flipped on a 10,000 lux artificial light that I keep in my kitchen and kept it on while I went about my morning activities. Today was my day off from exercise (yesterday was leg day and generally the day after leg day is a day off from exercise for me; see Exercise Protocol 2).

From 8:00 a.m. until 11:00 a.m., I worked (podcast preparation, emails, and calls) at my desk with the overhead indoor lights on their brightest setting, and I sat near a window. I managed to get a few minutes outside during one of my work calls, and I paced while on the call, which allowed me to get a few extra steps in and a bit more sunlight. Around 11:00 a.m., I paused work to eat lunch, and then went back to work at my desk until about 2:00 p.m. On a less busy day, I might have taken my lunch outside.

My Phase 2:

Given that I woke up at 7:00 a.m., this phase began six hours later at 1:00 p.m., and sure enough I started to feel a little sleepy around that time. I almost always experience a dip in energy about six hours after I wake up, even after a great night's sleep. Some people don't, but I do. I know it correlates, among other things, to the decline in cortisol that is normal, healthy, and expected at this time.

I know better than to push through this dip. I could take a prescription stimulant or slam an energy drink or two at that time, but why? I know there are other tools that won't mess with my sleep. So from 2:00 to 2:30 I did a non-sleep deep rest (NSDR) session, which I described in chapters 1 and 3, and I emerged from it feeling refreshed. I drank some water and had a half cup of strong coffee and then dove back into work until about 5:00 p.m. (I can drink caffeine up until about 2:00 to 2:30 p.m. with no negative effect on my sleep, but for those more caffeine sensitive, take care.)

My Phase 3:

Phase 3 is from ten hours until about fourteen hours after waking, so for today, that meant from 5:00 to 9:00 p.m. I used this time for more work. I also took a brief twenty-minute walk outside, then prepared and ate dinner.

Then I started to wind down for the night. I dim the lights in my home to less than full blast starting in phase 3, and I recently started using the medium and long wavelength only setting in the evenings on lights that switch from full spectrum to medium and long wavelength emitting only. (See Sleep Protocol 3 for more on these bulbs.) They appear yellowish-orange rather than white. Several companies such as Bon Charge and Ra Optics now make LED bulbs that switch from full spectrum to medium and long wavelength emitting only (without having to program them for a specific time). You just flick the standard wall-mounted light switch. I love this simple technology because it's so aligned with what our system needs, and it's easy to use with no Wi-Fi or an app. And because they are LEDs, they last a very long time and are cost-efficient.

My Phase 4:

This phase spans from the period starting fourteen hours after waking until the next morning when the new day starts. Today for me that meant from 9:00 p.m. on. For some time now, I have made it a practice to dim the lights in the final hours before I go to sleep. As I mentioned earlier in this chapter, people vary in their visual sensitivity to light. I am one of those who can be in front of a screen right up until I fall asleep. I have no trouble falling asleep, but it tends to make me wake up three to four hours later. When I started dimming the lights before bedtime, those mid-sleep awakenings all but stopped. I also switched to using long-wavelength-only light bulbs (red light) in the one to two hours before my bedtime. I still might wake up once in the middle of the night to use the bathroom but I have no trouble falling back asleep, and both my device-measured sleep scores and my subjective experience is that I am sleeping much better. If I'm out late or otherwise can't use my typical indoor lighting in the hours before sleep—such as when I stay in a hotel—I wear ROKA Wind Down glasses that filter out short wavelength light. Often I wear them at home too, as I find they simplify this process.

Take note that phase 4 is where most people make seemingly small mistakes that cost them dearly in terms of health and well-being. There are two main reasons. With the advent of smartphones, and an endless stream of news, content, and the many other hooks that technology offers, it's very easy to turn to a device. It's also because most homes and hotels use LED lights nowadays, which emit short wavelengths that disrupt sleep. A bit later in the chapter, I'll explain how to help with this. In the meantime, here are some ways to make phase 4 much easier and more effective:

- **Keep it low and keep it dim.** I suggest that any lighting you use in the final hours before you go to sleep come from desk lamps or floor lamps, that is, low light sources, and that, if possible, you avoid using overhead lights. The neurons in your eyes that signal to your brain that it is daytime are arranged across your neural retina (the light sensing tissue in the back of your eye) and they view the upper visual field, meaning the sky when you are outside and the ceiling when you are indoors.[40] Many people find that using low, dim light sources in the one to two hours before bed makes it much easier to fall and stay asleep.[41] This is pretty easy to do, and can make a big difference.

  You can go further still and use bulbs without short wavelengths, which thus appear yellow-orange, or even go with bulbs that emit purely long wavelengths, and thus appear red. Keep in mind this is not red light therapy. Red light therapy (explained later in this chapter) can be very beneficial for certain aspects of health but is altogether different from what we are discussing here. Medium-wavelength-only bulbs are relatively inexpensive and provide a nice yellow-amber glow. Admittedly, using long-wavelength-only bulbs will make your home look a little space age, but they are a great tool to help you sleep better. Either way, using dim, non-overhead lights without short wavelengths in the last one to two hours before bedtime reduces the activation of the retinal neurons that signal your brain to suppress melatonin and boost cortisol.[42]

As mentioned above, several companies have conveniently engineered bulbs that are full-spectrum-emitting (white) for the daytime, and with a simple flick of the light switch, become medium and long wavelength only emitting (yellow-amber or red). Incandescent versions of these exist too and are best, but they use more energy than LEDs, don't last nearly as long, and are more costly. They are also a bit hard to find.

- **Wear eyeglasses that filter out all short wavelength light.** This approach is very convenient if you don't want to change the lights in your home, or if you don't have control over the lighting conditions in a certain environment, such as on planes, in hotels or airports, out with friends, et cetera. I designed the ROKA Wind Down glasses for use during the final hours before sleep, and I use them at home and when I travel. They differ from traditional blue blockers because they prevent all short wavelength light, not just blue light, from reaching your eyes. (Don't wear them while driving because they make anything that is blue or green much harder to see or even invisible, and that could cause an accident.)
- **Don't worry about moonlight.** You may be wondering if bright moonlight or even a roaring fire will stimulate the wakefulness pathways in your brain. The answer is, perhaps surprisingly, no. Although these are concentrated light sources, a bright full moon is less than 1 lux and while candles, fireplaces, and bonfires mostly emit medium and short wavelength light, it doesn't radiate very far. If you have ever been camping and turned around from a roaring campfire, you've noticed that as soon as you are just a few paces away from it, you need a flashlight in order to see. We discussed the physics of this in chapter 1. So while fire and candles are great nighttime light sources from a cortisol-limiting and melatonin-preserving perspective, they are not very practical. Of course, if you'd like to read by candlelight or gather around a fire with friends, great. Just make sure the flames are extinguished when you're finished. Be careful not to start a fire.

You may be wondering if all this attention to avoiding bright light in the hours before sleep is silly, neurotic biohacking. After all, you can find studies showing that blocking blue light improves people's sleep to varying degrees,[43] and you may be one of those people who can pass out with the TV or computer still at full brightness right in front of you. Indeed, there is considerable variation in the degree to which short wavelength light exposure alters people's sleep.[44] That said, having even just a dim 100 lux overhead light on while you sleep can alter the next-morning glucose levels.[45] And that's while sleeping, with eyes closed. The point is, altered sleep is not the only reason to avoid bright light in phase 4. Nighttime bright light exposure increases blood pressure[46] and heart rate, and has been linked to weight gain and even a risk of obesity.[47] Studies have found nighttime bright light to negatively impact next-day cognitive function[48] and mood[49] independent of bright light's negative effects on sleep.

None of this is surprising to biologists who have studied the so-called non-image-forming visual system or the many opsins other than melanopsin that are present in our skin and other tissues for the last three decades.[50] Myself included. We know, for instance, that the retinal neurons that respond to bright short wavelength light connect not only to your SCN but also to areas of your hypothalamus, such as the supraoptic nucleus, that are directly involved in sleep regulation. (I know, supraoptic sounds like suprachiasmatic but please don't blame me, I didn't name either one.) Your eyes also connect to your thalamus's perihabenular nucleus, which has been nicknamed the anti-reward or disappointment center,[51] given it actively inhibits dopamine release and is thought to increase feelings of depression when activated at night by, you guessed it, bright light.

The broader field of medicine is starting to incorporate these discoveries. Disrupting the light-dark cycle can affect lifespan. An international team of researchers conducted an enormous study in which 88,905 people enrolled in the UK Biobank, a database for collecting long-term health information, were given wearable light sensors for one week.[52] The participants wore these wrist sensors for seven days, during which they went about their normal routine. The sensors recorded light exposure around the clock. At the end of the week, the researchers had data on 13 million hours of light exposure.

They grouped all the data according to daytime and night, categorizing participants according to light exposure during the day (between the hours of 7:30 a.m. and 8:30 p.m.) and light exposure during the night (between the hours of 12:30 a.m. and 6:00 a.m.). They then collected health data over a follow-up period of about eight years. For the 3,750 participants who died during the follow-up period, the researchers categorized mortality data according to cause of death.

They found that the brighter the night and the darker the day, the higher the risk of death; the link was dose dependent! The risk of death by any cause was up to 34 percent higher among those who got the most light exposure at night, compared to those with the least light exposure at night. The reverse was also true. The risk of death (by any cause) was up to 34 percent lower among the participants with the most light exposure during the day compared to those with the least. This connection held despite any other traits including age, sex, physical activity, smoking, drinking, and cardiovascular health.

There's more. The analysis zoomed in on nighttime light exposure, grouping it into half hour increments and matching those increments with mortality data. The brightest lighting between 1:00 a.m. and 6:00 a.m. carried a risk of death by any cause that was 11 to 39 percent higher compared to the darkest lighting during this stretch of time. The risk of death due to cardiometabolic issues (heart attack, stroke, diabetes, nonalcoholic fatty liver disease) was 20 to 67 percent higher for the brightest lighting compared to the darkest lighting during this stretch of the night. The time frame here differs slightly from the one described in this protocol, but the exact times aren't the point; the point is that viewing bright light at night is disruptive to your immediate and long-term health.

It's true that this was a relatively brief study, using just a week's worth of light exposure data. However, about three thousand participants repeated the study up to four times and the light exposure patterns were the same. Several other studies have found similar links.[53] And the sheer volume of light exposure data in this one makes a persuasive case. As the researchers wrote in the 2024 publication of their study in the *Proceedings of the National Academy of Sciences*, "Across the general population, avoiding night light and seeking daylight may lead to reduction in disease burden, especially cardiometabolic diseases, and may increase longevity."

In another large study, published in *Nature Mental Health* in 2023, researchers at the University of Manchester cross-referenced data on mental health with data on light, sleep, and physical activity from 86,722 individuals.[54] Their analysis revealed a link between greater nighttime light exposure and higher risk for several mental health issues, including major depressive disorder, anxiety, post-traumatic stress disorder, and self-harm behavior. Greater daytime light exposure correlated with a reduced risk of these issues. They also found that people who experienced darker nights had fewer mental health symptoms, an effect that occurred independent of daytime light exposure. That is, bright-light-filled mornings and days and dark nights independently and additively promoted better mental health.

These large datasets deliver a clear and important message, one that typically goes unmentioned: Keeping the lights off during the late hours of your night is not just about getting great sleep; it is fundamentally important for your health and well-being.

LIGHT PROTOCOL

4

Expose Your Upper and Lower Body Skin to Sunlight During the Day

WHAT TO DO:

- **Get twenty to thirty minutes of outdoor sunlight exposure to your skin at least three times per week, and ideally every day.** Wear the minimum amount of clothing that allows you to be comfortable and that is appropriate for your environment, without covering your entire body (for example, shirtless with shorts, or shorts and a tank top, or a swimsuit. In some cases, jeans and a short-sleeved T-shirt may be what's called for). It is best that you do not wear a hat during this time. I discuss cold weather options below.

HOW IT WORKS:

There is no substitute for sunlight. You could turn on every light in your home in the morning and daytime, make sure they are full-spectrum incandescent bulbs or wavelength-balanced full spectrum LEDs, view a 10,000 lux artificial light within an hour of waking up, and it still would not replace sunlight.

Each of those technologies can serve as a health-promoting supplement on days when you can't get enough sunlight, and they can help boost the effects of sunlight, but they should not be used as an everyday replacement for sunlight. Think of them the same way you would supplements relative to nutritious food; they can help bridge deficiencies, and in some cases they can afford you a real mental or physical performance advantage. Yet no rational person would ever replace all their food with supplements on a consistent basis. Alas, because most people don't understand how powerful light is as a tool for health, and that sunlight is a uniquely beneficial form of it, they engage with light in a way that is analogous to trying to live solely on supplements.

Actually, in many cases it's even worse than that. People are spending the first hours of their day in sunless, dark, or dim indoor environments, viewing screens, and then continuing their days under artificial lights that seem bright but that are actually dim compared to sunlight. After sundown, they stay under those same lights, which are now far too bright for what is needed at night, and many view mostly short wavelength emitting screens. This is, in no uncertain terms, as bad as living on highly processed junk food. And it's making a lot of people sick, mentally and physically.

Getting sunlight on our skin is as much a cornerstone of health as sleep, exercise, or nutrition. It's hard for most people to fully grasp this, especially given that we all have heard how damaging UV light is for our skin. Yet, we need to embrace what is special and beneficial about sunlight and incorporate it into our daily lives. And no, you do not have to live in California, or run around shirtless or in a bathing suit outside. You simply need to know how the energy present in sunlight impacts *every* cell in your body: your brain, hair, skin, liver, heart, your hormones, neurotransmitters, immune system, and on and on.

And so, on to the science.

Sunlight is the absolute best source of long wavelength light, from the red end of the visible spectrum into non-visible near-infrared and IR wavelengths. It is difficult to overstate how important these longer wavelengths are for our health, in particular for our mitochondria, the energy producing organelles within our cells. (I'll cover the uses of LWL devices that purely emit red, NIR, and IR light in the next protocol.)

Sunlight contains short wavelength UV light, which as we discussed earlier in this chapter, triggers the production of vitamin D in the skin. Although this vitamin (which also acts as a hormone) is available in some foods, supplements can replace sunlight as a stimulus for vitamin D,[55] yet our bodies evolved to use sun-induced vitamin D in multiple ways that supplements may not mimic.

For example, vitamin D is important for hormone health and the reproductive system. A multi-institution study on mice and humans looked at the effects specifically of UVB (the ultraviolet wavelength that penetrates the skin) on reproductive-related hormones and behavior.[56] They found that mice exposed to UVB light for one hour per day showed enhanced mating behavior and physiology—greater attraction for one another, larger ovaries, and more testosterone—in both the male and female mice. Moreover, male mice showed a greater attraction to UVB-treated female mice, likely due to how elevated testosterone and estrogen levels in females impacted their appearance and scent, making them more attractive. More interestingly, the researchers saw similar patterns in people. According to their findings, published in *Cell Reports* in 2021, participants reported increased romantic interest in others following time in the sun. The data also showed heightened testosterone levels linked to this exposure in both men and women. Testosterone and estrogen levels—both of which impact romantic desire and feelings of well-being in men and women—were highest in the longer days of spring and summer relative to shorter winter and fall days.

This effect appears to relate to a molecule called p53 expressed in a type of skin cell called keratinocytes. Mice in which p53 had been removed did not exhibit the same changes following UVB exposure. This detail emphasizes the importance of having sunlight reach not only our eyes, but also our skin.

Here's another: UV light from sunlight also reduces physical pain. In 2017, a group of researchers reported a study in which they exposed mice to UVB (midrange ultraviolet light, abundant in sunlight) radiation and then tested various parameters relating to the HPA axis.[57] This brain pathway is the core mechanism behind our stress response (as discussed in chapters 1 and 3).[58] They found a link between UVB radiation and the stimulation of corticotropin-releasing hormone, which helps us cope with social stress,[59] and endogenous beta endorphins, a type of opioid our body naturally produces in response to psychological distress.[60] Although this work focused on mice, the results point toward a potentially crucial and unappreciated role for sunlight, in particular UV light—which most people generally think of as the aspect of sunlight to be avoided.

Excessive UV light exposure will cause sunburn and increase your risk for certain forms of skin cancer. So, while UV light from the sun has many benefits, it is still important to avoid too much exposure and sunburn.

A Word About Sunscreen

Of course, no one wants a sunburn. One's risk of sunburn and skin cancer varies depending on factors such as skin tone and inherited susceptibility to skin cancer. All dermatologists agree that any amount of sunburn is bad for us, so bear that in mind. And all agree that excessive exposure to sunlight leads to more rapid aging of the skin too. Excessive skin exposure to UV light, in particular, mutates our skin cell DNA and destroys keratinocytes, which give skin its suppleness. So the takeaway message is to avoid sunburn at all costs.

I don't burn easily but if I am going to be outside at a time of day when the UV index is high, I either rely on a physical barrier—hat and long sleeves—or I apply a mineral-based sunscreen that uses zinc oxide (not nano zinc) as the only active ingredient. People debate whether chemical-based sunscreens are bad for hormone health and my read of the literature is yes, they can be; but that debate aside, no one argues whether physical barriers or mineral-based-only sunscreen are useful and safe. It's therefore an obvious choice in my opinion, especially since purely mineral-based sunscreens now come in forms that don't leave a white paste on your skin, are reef- and ocean life–safe, and aren't too expensive. I use Le Rub, which is an all-day mineral-based sunscreen that comes in a metal tube. Why is that relevant? Well, I am among a growing number of people who don't want more microplastics in my body if I can help it. After hosting Shanna Swan, PhD, professor of environmental medicine and public health at Mount Sinai School of Medicine, on my podcast, I did an audit of easy-to-eliminate endocrine disruptors, and I decided to find a non-plastic container, non-endocrine-disrupting sunscreen. Le Rub meets those criteria, smells great, and applies clear, unlike many zinc oxide sunscreens that remain as a white paste on the skin. I liked it so much that I became a partial owner of the company—so I am now very biased, but for the very reason that it's the only sunscreen I'll use.

Definitely check the UV index before spending a lot of time in the sun. A simple web search of "What is the UV index at different times today in [enter city and country]?" will yield you a result in less than ten seconds. It will tell you when to be careful about excess UV exposure.

But don't avoid the sun entirely! Getting sun exposure on your skin not only supports various hormone production pathways as described here, it may also help you live longer. A Swedish study looking at mortality rates among 29,518 women found that greater sun exposure correlated with lower all-cause risk of death.[61] In fact, people who spent the least amount of time in the sun had nearly double the mortality risk during the twenty years of the study compared to those who spent the most time in the sun. Obviously, there are likely to be many factors at play here: More time outside usually means more fresh air, movement, social interaction, et cetera, not just sunlight. Yet the data correlating different amounts of sunlight exposure to health and longevity all seem to point in the same direction: Getting sunlight on your skin is beneficial. Interestingly, that work followed an earlier study of nearly forty thousand women that found a reduction in mortality linked to exposure to ultraviolet light coming directly from the sun, and yet an increase in mortality linked to ultraviolet light from artificial sources.[62]

Why would UV light from sunlight help and yet the (seemingly) same UV light from artificial sources harm us? One idea is that because sunlight has a balance of short, medium, and long wavelengths—each at particular energies and with their own unique health-promoting effects—they synergize. UV without adequate longer wavelengths—such as what comes from most LEDs—is thought to be detrimental to our cells.[63]

I'll dive more into the ways that different wavelengths of light impact our cells in the next protocol, but for now here are some crucial things to know: No single wavelength of light is "bad" or "good." Longer wavelengths of light are absorbed by the water in our mitochondria and help "charge" the mitochondria like batteries, making them more efficient at producing ATP[64] and possibly even helping cells to make more mitochondria. Longer wavelength light also helps offset the negative effects of reactive oxygen species (ROS)—a normal by-product of cellular function that, if in excess, damages our cells.[65] ROS are thought to be a major factor in the reduced energy levels and organ dysfunction we experience with aging.[66] Long wavelength light can pass through our skin, eyelids, our ribs, and even our skull to reach our brain and other internal organs, and so helps to promote their health, largely by improving mitochondrial function as described above.[67] How wild is that?! Sunlight also contains abundant amounts of medium wavelength light—yellows and oranges, or in technical terms about 500 to 620 nanometer light, which has been shown to reduce headache pain, stimulate blood flow, and reduce inflammation.[68]

Artificial lights of course contain some of these wavelengths but not in the same balance as is present in sunlight. Incandescent bulbs are better than LEDs in this respect, but nowadays LEDs and fluorescent lights are almost exclusively used for indoor lighting because they cost less, use less energy, and last longer. Most LEDs are enriched with short wavelengths which, unless balanced out by long wavelength light, have been shown to increase ROS and damage mitochondria.[69] Some LEDs and fluorescent lights even emit small amounts of UV.[70] This all becomes a problem for cellular health when we are under these lights all day and not getting the protective effects of long wavelength light or enough sunlight. It's rather incredible that while so many people are afraid of UV from sunlight, they may be unaware how the many hours of daily (and nightly) exposure to short wavelength light can damage our health. The remedy: balanced wavelength exposure from sunlight, done safely of course. The protocols in this chapter represent the key times and ways to do just that. The other remedy: incandescent rather than LED indoor lighting, and limiting your short wavelength light exposure after nightfall.

Still not convinced that light is medicine? I mentioned above how researchers found that UV light from sunlight reduces physical pain, and there are studies of humans experiencing similar effects. In a study of eighty-nine patients who'd undergone spinal surgery, those who stayed on the bright side of the hospital, and were therefore exposed to 46 percent more intense sunlight than those staying on the dim side of the hospital, reported less pain-related stress and a bit less pain, and required 22 percent less pain medication.[71] Similar results have been reported in the relief of fibromyalgia among women[72] and in a small study of US military veterans, chronic lower back pain.[73] Preliminary research indicates that the underlying mechanism here brings us back to the intrinsically photosensitive retinal ganglion cells, which don't just connect to the SCN but also communicate light information (through a relay station) to the periaqueductal gray area, a region that is crucial to pain modulation.[74]

And, as discussed in other protocols in this chapter, regular, consistent light exposure also enhances mood.[75] Data suggest that individuals exposed to moderate amounts of UVB—which is abundant in sunlight—may have a lower risk for depression.[76] A review of seven different studies evaluating the link between ultraviolet radiation and mood concluded that the evidence supports this beneficial connection.[77]

The simple takeaway here is this: Get some sunlight on your skin for at least thirty minutes per day, as many days per week as possible. How much skin you can directly expose will of course vary by weather, location, and circumstances, but do it. Check the UV index and learn what you need without getting a sunburn. Don't get a sunburn. And while sunlight through a window is not the same as going outside, if you can make your indoor environment brighter from sunlight, do it. Otherwise, think seriously about how much conventional LED light exposure you're getting and, if it's a lot, consider switching to full spectrum LED lights. And given the direct and protective benefits of long wavelength light, consider the next protocol.

COMMON QUESTIONS:

What if I live in a dark, gloomy place or it's a dark, gloomy time of year, as it is in much of the UK, Scandinavia, or the Pacific Northwest, especially during the winter?

I've mentioned this elsewhere in this chapter, but time outside is still essential. Even on a cold, cloud-covered day, you'll get more light exposure outside than from an indoor artificial light source. Cold days make people less inclined to be outside in shorts and short sleeves, and that is okay—but avoid the brimmed hat then so you can get more sun on your face and in your eyes. And if you can't get outside into direct sun, do what you can. Sometimes you can only get time out on a covered balcony. Every little bit counts. It's like getting your daily steps in. You need your daily light exposure too.

As a final note on this: If you live in a region where you just can't get much sunlight exposure to your skin for many days of the year, you would be very wise to get a 10,000 lux artificial light (any brand will do), and a red and IR incandescent light. You might also use bulbs in your lighting fixtures that switch from bright, balanced full spectrum to medium and long wavelengths only simply by using the light switch.

LIGHT PROTOCOL

5

Expose Your Skin and Eyes to Long Wavelength Light (Red, Near-IR, and Infrared)

WHAT TO DO:

- **Use a long-wavelength-light-emitting (LWL) device for ten to thirty minutes, three to seven days per week.** For general health effects (energy, skin appearance, exercise recovery, etc.), the goal is to illuminate the largest area of your skin, face, and head that you can. This will obviously depend on what LWL device you have access to and the amount of time you can devote to this.

HOW IT WORKS:

Red light therapy has become a popular health trend. Red light saunas, red light panels, red light beds, masks, even red-light helmets to promote hair growth . . . the list goes on. Despite their space age look, this is a trend with genuine scientific support behind it. Several leading dermatology journals including *JAMA Dermatology* have published in-depth reviews on the use of red light to treat different skin conditions,[78] and other fields of medicine including ophthalmology are following suit by exploring how red light can be used to offset, or even reverse, age-related decline in organ function. Most of these devices also emit near-infrared (NIR) and/or infrared (IR) light as well. For simplicity and accuracy, I will refer to all such devices collectively as LWL devices. Of course, the exact wavelengths and intensities of light that different LWL devices emit vary. Some also emit short wavelength light. I'll touch on some of the different features to look for when considering use of different photobiomodulation devices at the end of this protocol.

First, let's discuss what photobiomodulation is really about. In the context of light, photobiomodulation involves exposing a portion (or all) of your skin to a specific range of wavelengths, typically long wavelength light, for ten, twenty, or thirty minutes, three to seven days per week. As I mentioned above, for general health effects the goal is to illuminate the largest area of your skin, face, and head that you can. Smaller handheld LWL devices that illuminate a limited area can be helpful for pain reduction and to promote wound healing in specific areas,[79] but the most impressive effects of long wavelength light photobiomodulation are generally achieved with whole-body long-wavelength light exposure using a large LWL panel, or a red light bed or LWL blanket, and by illuminating both sides of your body, either simultaneously or sequentially.

Long wavelength light can penetrate the skin's surface and once inside your body, it can scatter up to 8 centimeters.[80] Longer wavelengths in the infrared range have been shown to even pass through thin clothing such as T-shirts and through your torso.[81] That might sound scary but remember that long wavelength light is low energy non-ionizing radiation, so it is safe, and all evidence points to long wavelength light having a protective and a health-promoting effect on your cells. Put simply, exposing your skin to long wavelength light in this way is a good thing. The main reason? It promotes mitochondrial health.

Mitochondrial health is a term used often these days, so before going any further, let's further define what this means. As discussed several times already in this book, cellular energy is generated in the form of a chemical called adenosine triphosphate, or ATP. Mitochondria are crucial for ATP production, as well as for making our hormones and neurotransmitters. Mitochondria contain an enzyme called cytochrome c oxidase, and it can absorb light.[82] In that way, cytochrome c oxidase is similar to the photopigments in your eye that absorb specific wavelengths of light, and that kick off the cascade of events in your eyes and brain that lead to sight. The difference is that cytochrome c oxidase is inside the cells of your body and brain, and its job is to support the formation of ATP for your cells to use. The way it does that is by moving electrons from one protein to the next inside the mitochondria. (Briefly: Like any compound, proteins are made of molecules; molecules are made of atoms bonded together; atoms are made of subatomic particles including protons, which are positively charged, electrons, which are negatively charged, and neutrons, which carry no charge.) That process releases energy that moves protons, also in the mitochondria, and because protons carry an electrical charge, it sort of works like a battery.

The business of moving protons in mitochondria isn't just about making energy; it takes energy too. The first law of thermodynamics is that energy can't be created or destroyed, it can only be transformed. Long wavelength light energy from the sun that is absorbed by cytochrome c oxidase is transformed by your mitochondria to help create ATP. So, in a loose sense, we are solar powered.

The absorption of long wavelength light by cytochrome c oxidase also causes nitric oxide—a chemical that can impair mitochondrial function—to dislodge from the organelle, which then allows cytochrome c oxidase to use oxygen more efficiently. That enhances something called mitochondrial respiration, a process critical for converting nutrients in our blood into ATP.[83] Bam! Long wavelength light can enhance cellular ATP production through at least two proposed mechanisms.

Long wavelength light also may support mitochondrial energy production through a third mechanism involving the increased action of intracellular melatonin, which can help prevent oxidative damage.[84] Until now we have discussed melatonin only as a hormone produced by the pineal gland that promotes sleepiness. However, many cells throughout our body produce melatonin. Long wavelength light may allow intracellular melatonin to act more effectively as an antioxidant, helping to repair some of the oxidative damage that is a normal consequence of cellular metabolism. One potential benefit of this pathway is that it may reduce some of the harm caused by excessive UV light exposure.[85] As we discuss next, the implications of that are, literally, visible.

How It Affects Your Skin

Long wavelength light can promote the youthful look of skin, reduce acne, and accelerate wound healing.[86] Studies have also investigated long wavelength light as a tool to treat wrinkles, scars, burns, and other causes of discoloration of the skin.

In one study of ninety-three patients, administration of rapid pulses of 590-nanometer light was linked to reduced signs of aging.[87] In another study by the same research group, ninety patients were given pulses of 590-nanometer light in eight treatments over four weeks.[88] The investigators took digital images of the patients at the start of the study and over the following twelve months and found reduced signs of aging in the vast majority of participants. They also evaluated tissue samples from ten of the patients and found increased collagen, a protein that provides structure and elasticity to skin, in all the subjects who received this therapy. The wavelength measuring 590 nanometers is in the orange-red range of the visible spectrum and, as noted above, longer wavelengths (600–850 nm) can pass even deeper into the skin layers. Indeed, investigations found even more impressive reductions in wrinkles following treatment with 633-nanometer (red) light combined with 830-nanometer light, which falls in the near-infrared range.[89]

There also are benefits to combining long wavelength light with short wavelength light, at least for improving skin. Dermatologists at Mount Sinai Medical Center, in New York, treated twenty-two people with mild to moderate acne with eight sessions of light therapy that used alternating exposure to blue (short wavelength) and red (long wavelength) light, for twenty minutes per exposure.[90] Four weeks after the treatment ended, participants showed a 46 percent reduction in acne lesions. At eight weeks post-treatment, the reduction had reached 81 percent. A study from Imperial College of Science, Technology, and Medicine, in London, with 107 patients, reported similar outcomes.[91] That is pretty remarkable if you ask me.

How It Affects Your Metabolism

There's another impressive effect of long wavelength light therapy. Exposing your skin to long wavelength light can reduce your glucose levels, and increase your metabolism. It seems unlikely, but it turns out to be true. All we have to do is look at the data. In a recent study, researchers shined a 670-nanometer light on subjects' backs for fifteen minutes and measured their glucose levels in response to ingestion of a sugary drink—a classic research method to measure blood sugar regulation.[92] They observed a 27.7 percent reduction in glucose in comparison to control subjects that did not receive the light exposure. Measurements of oxygen uptake confirmed that their metabolism had risen significantly, which makes sense given that long wavelength light exposure can increase ATP production by as much as 100 to 200 percent.

I heard some people interpreting this study as meaning that eating under short-wavelength-only light sources like conventional LED lights lowers your metabolism, even going so far as to argue that obesity is on the rise because of short wavelength light overuse. While that *might* be the case, that is not what this study shows. It is reasonable, however, to conclude on the basis of this study that eating outside in the sunlight or even in the shade on a sunny day where long wavelength light is abundant, or eating near a LWL device, may be beneficial for those seeking to improve their blood sugar regulation. Getting exercise and proper nutrition per the recommendations in chapters 2 and 4 are the major factors for healthy blood sugar regulation. Nevertheless, long wavelength light can certainly be used to augment proper exercise and nutrition, and it may be a particularly useful tool for regulating blood sugar and metabolism when exercise is restricted due to injury, weather, travel, and the like.

How It Affects Your Eyesight

The effects go on. Long wavelength light has been helpful in preserving eye health too. First, a little bit about your eyes: The photoreceptor cells in your eyes consume more energy than any other cell in your brain or body.[93] Think about that for a second: more than any other cell, meaning more than all the rest of your brain cells, your liver, even your muscle cells . . . and that is true even if you were to run a marathon and use those muscle cells, every single day! Your photoreceptors are almost always active, even in the dark. The point is your photoreceptors produce and use a ton of energy around the clock. The energy they draw on comes in the form of ATP, and ATP production, as you now know, depends on mitochondria. Not surprisingly, your photoreceptors are packed with mitochondria[94] and they produce a ton of ATP, but with all that ATP production comes a high amount of free radicals, and as I mentioned earlier in this protocol, those impose stress on the cells, which over time damages the mitochondria. Exposure of the eyes to long wavelength light—the red, near-infrared, and infrared end of the spectrum—both reduces the presence of free radicals[95] and helps stimulate the production of ATP by the mechanisms discussed above. So it makes sense that long wavelength light therapy might have a role in preserving or improving our photoreceptors . . . and therefore, our vision.

And indeed, that's what the data show. Work by neuroscientist Glen Jeffery (mentioned at the start of this chapter) investigated whether direct viewing of long wavelength light could improve people's vision. In one study, he and his team enrolled twenty-four people between the ages of twenty-eight and seventy-two to look at a 670-nanometer beam (red light) from a flashlight for three minutes per day for two weeks.[96] Participants under the age of forty showed no change in vision. But those around forty years and older showed a greater ability to discern colors at the end of the experiment. In a second study, the investigators used the same intervention but at a less intense level, meaning the light was not as close to the participants' eyes (though it was still 670 nanometers, or red light) and found that to be sufficient to boost vision for one week, again among those about forty years old and over.[97] The improvement in vision in these studies reached 20 percent among some participants, which is a significant and compelling result. The researchers also observed a reduction in drusen, which are fat deposits that accumulate in the eyes as we age[98] and that are connected to age-related macular degeneration.

Importantly, the second study by Jeffery and colleagues found that the timing of the long wavelength light therapy mattered. The benefit to vision occurred only if the red light was seen in the morning, likely because mitochondrial function changes across the twenty-four-hour cycle, with a particular sensitivity to light then. It is worth noting that the range of benefit was wide; some individuals experienced a greater boost than others. The underlying reasons of who benefits and who doesn't are not yet clear. Studies ongoing in Glen Jeffery's lab are now focused on the use of long wavelength light therapy for advanced macular degeneration, retinitis pigmentosa, and glaucoma.

To be clear: The most common causes of vision loss—cataracts, glaucoma, macular degeneration, and diabetes[99]—are unlikely to be caused by lack of long wavelength light exposure, although that possibility hasn't been ruled out either. All these forms of vision loss are typically associated with aging, and some forms have a clear genetic contribution as well. Everyone should get an annual eye exam and get their eye pressures checked for glaucoma once a year. Do not rely on this protocol as the only way to treat or prevent these conditions. That said, the ability for long wavelength light to slow, halt, or reverse vision loss is gaining more and more support.

Along those lines, you might be wondering how exactly to adopt this protocol. Turns out it's very easy: Expose your face to long wavelength light from a concentrated red light source (not laser!) for five to ten minutes once or twice per week, and do it within three hours of waking. You don't need to put the light source terribly close to your eyes either; it's best you do it at a distance that is comfortable and doesn't force you to close your eyes. However, in this and other long wavelength light protocols, you are welcome to close your eyes. It won't hinder the effect unless you wear dark occluding glasses—the ones that make it look like you're going into a tanning bed (which is UV by the way; I do not recommend those for reasons that ought to be obvious by now). Long wavelength light easily passes through your eyelids to reach your photoreceptors. You can get enough retinal long wavelength light exposure as a consequence of whole body long wavelength light illumination too. There is no evidence that more frequent or longer exposures than five to ten minutes once or twice per week are needed for the visual system benefits, but also no evidence that more would be harmful. Remember, the effects were only observed in people forty and older and only if it was done within one to three hours of waking.

SOURCES TO CONSIDER:

You have a lot of options when it comes to long wavelength light sources for photobiomodulation—for this use, and others. I will discuss these in order from the least to the most costly.

Option 1: The sun.

The sun is rich with long wavelength light and it's zero cost, but you get less long wavelength light exposure on overcast days and for most, it's not practical to expose your whole body to it for ten to thirty minutes, three to seven days per week. And while UV light is less of an issue when the sun is low in the sky around sunrise and sunset, for people who miss those windows of opportunity, you will need to take measures to avoid getting excessive UV exposure. As mentioned above, check the UV index for your location. Of course, never, ever, force yourself to stare at the sun. Blink as needed to protect your eyes. The reflex to do so is the guide to follow. Or close your eyes; remember, long wavelength light radiation will reach your eyes just fine through your eyelids as long as you're not wearing sunglasses. It's fine to wear corrective lens eyeglasses or contacts for the reasons discussed in chapter 1.

Option 2: A LWL device.

There are tons of options out there on the market now, and they vary a lot by cost. It's a bit overwhelming. You'll often see claims from companies that their LWL device is best because it has "more power" than others on the market, but that's a bit misleading. Differences in the intensity of devices are negligible when you consider that just getting closer to a device and/or extending the duration that you use it can compensate for most differences in intensity. Which you decide to use will likely be dictated by your budget and access. Small handheld units the size of a sandwich can cost $500, some full body panels $10,000 to $12,000, and the LWL "red light beds" and capsules can cost from $25,000 to more than $100,000. (Sunshine when the UV is low may be sounding pretty good right now.)

Some people like LWL face masks or helmets for skin or hair, respectively. A review of the research on a phototherapy mask, published in the *Journal of Clinical and Aesthetic Dermatology* in 2018, concluded that this light therapy device was effective for treating acne and psoriasis, healing wounds, and reducing actinic keratosis, rough and scaly skin that can result from years of sun exposure.[100] This study was not funded by the device manufacturer, but it was authored by the head of a private dermatology research institute rather than an academic laboratory research group. That said, there is no reason to think the results with a mask would be any different from the results with a light panel, except that the light is hitting a smaller area of skin. I think the panels are the most versatile as you can expose whatever body areas you want but obviously cost compare and decide for yourself.

After deciding what is affordable for you, the most important factor in selecting a LWL device is that it exclusively emits long wavelength light of about 600 nm or longer. (We don't see infrared light, which is why these are often called red light devices.) Generally speaking, the broader the range of long wavelengths that a device emits, the better the results. In other words, the most effective devices emit red, near-IR, and IR (600–850+ nm) light. The Jeffery lab studies used red light at wavelengths of about 600 to 670 nanometers to produce the visual system benefits, while light at wavelengths of 850 nanometers and above penetrated into and through the body—which again, is a good thing. As another rule, LWL devices that feel warm to the skin at the distance you use them are going to be more effective, because that encourages more blood flow and lymphatic flow, and in doing so helps improve the anti-inflammation effects of long wavelength light. Some LWL devices also include non-UV short wavelength light, which can be helpful for pain relief.

Most LWL devices use LEDs, but a few use incandescent bulbs. Lasers, which deliver a focused ray of light, tend to be higher in intensity—and they are brighter. I don't recommend these for home use. Low-level laser therapy (LLLT) is a medical intervention and anyone using it to address aging or skin issues that are often treated with topical creams or other prescription interventions, such as wounds, acne, or other chronic skin conditions, should consult with a physician to ensure this approach is safe for you.

As mentioned above, I strive to take brief walks outside throughout the day just before or after meals, and pace outside when on work calls, if I can. Obviously I wear clothing during these times, but even with most skin covered, I'm sure to get some long wavelength light exposure, especially on clear days. I also use a JOOVV LWL panel for ten to thirty minutes once a day, generally three to five days per week. The JOOVV panels are medical grade and emit red and IR light; note they are a *Huberman Lab* podcast sponsor. I also really like the LWL incandescent bulbs from SaunaSpace as they generate heat, and emit 600 to 1,000 nanometer light. They make actual red light saunas too using those same bulbs; they look like a small canvas tent with a large-bulb long wavelength light–incandescent panel inside, and they are terrific because they too generate a lot of heat—which is what you want for a sauna session—and have all the features of long wavelength light photobiomodulation.

I confess I am not a fan of most other long wavelength light, or red light, saunas that use LEDs because they generally don't get hot enough to trigger the benefits of dry or wet traditional saunas.[101] Dry heat saunas can have great benefits for cardiovascular health, for growth hormone production, and for enhancing red blood cell production leading to endurance performance enhancement, but those effects are generally seen using temperatures ranging from roughly 180 to 210 degrees Fahrenheit. Most red light saunas just don't get hot enough to create those benefits. Rather than view any one LWL device as "the best," consider what you are able to access and afford, and use that. And remember the best and least expensive long wavelength light emitting source: good ol' sunlight.

CHAPTER 6

PROTOCOLS *for* FOCUS, MOTIVATION, *and* LEARNING

Our ability to get and stay motivated, to focus, and to learn new things is at the heart of what it is to be successful in life. Not just in school and work, but in creative endeavors and athletics. Consider the effort it takes to study for a big test or remember the material needed for a big presentation, or even stick with a new approach to a painting or new musical instrument practice, or try to respond to a social situation in a new way.

The question then becomes, "How?" How can we get motivated when our energy or natural impulses pull us toward apathy, overthinking, or procrastination? How can we tap into heightened focus, on demand? How can we learn faster and more effectively?

It turns out these are states of mind and body that we can learn to deliberately access.

My second year of college is when I first started to discover this. I learned that motivation can happen automatically as the consequence of, say, being excited or intrigued by something but it can also be deliberately fostered.

As I mentioned a bit in the introduction, I went from being a good student in my early life to falling behind my peers in high school. I touched on why that happened, but I make no excuses. Those were ultimately my own choices and actions. And those challenges both in and out of school, and watching my peers face those challenges too—seeing some soar and thrive while others struggled—would all become a blessing in many ways. It forced me to realize that no one was coming to save me and that I had to change things on my own. That realization scared me, but it's what motivated me to turn my life around. I never quite had the exact words for what went through my head at that moment until recently, when a very wise friend and mentor said something and I thought, "THAT! That's what I was hearing in my head! THAT!"

I can't say I came up with it, but it's something that I have heard in my head in fragments, over and over since I was nineteen. I still remind myself of it every day:

Losers take the negative things that happen to them and the feelings that come from things that suck . . . and they wallow and they use it for self- or outward destruction.

Winners however take whatever they feel—even if it sucks—and they transmute those feelings into actions that are good for themselves and for the world.

I chose to do something. And through that choice, I learned that while motivation can result in action, it's possible for action to result in motivation too.

As a sophomore in college, I decided to study as if my life depended on it. I didn't care if I liked the subject. I decided it made no difference, that eventually I would find the right path if I kept moving forward but I was going to move forward no matter what. Sure enough, my motivation to learn grew more and more, and morphed into a desire to get a PhD in a topic I fell in love with, to run a lab, to teach, and to build a career in science. Somewhere early along the way that fear I described dissipated. My love of certain topics and lab skills grew, but it often came *after* I had forced myself to learn them. Sure, sometimes it was there prior—I've always had a love for biology for example—but often it was only after I immersed myself in a subject that

I truly fell in love with it. The hardest courses I took in college turned out to be the ones I loved the most, and years later those subjects would be among the major focuses of my lab. The most useful thing I learned back then was that I realized that I could access the state of urgency that we call motivation whether I loved something or not. Reason and persistence, not excitement, anchored my effort.

And the act of being able to access a state of motivation gave me confidence to tackle what I wanted to go after or what was placed in front of me. I wasn't a grade-chasing automaton; I had a sense of agency over my life and that kept me going.

Just as my motivation grew, so too did my ability to focus and learn. At first, I had to take drastic measures to force myself to do both. While studying biology in university, I would set a timer for several hours and force myself to study without breaks until the timer went off. Having been so checked out in high school, I had a lot of catching up to do. This was extremely difficult at first. Long bouts of studying required a level of focus I did not have back then. But over time, my ability to focus got better—and kept getting better.

I later came to discover that the early stages of focus and learning are supposed to include agitation. That feeling comes from the shift in your brain and body's neurochemical milieu that sets the stage for learning to take place. You are asking your brain to change, and your brain doesn't want to change. Changing is very energetically demanding for brains. This uncomfortable feeling is something I often refer to as "limbic friction." It's not an official scientific term, but it refers to a state of elevated autonomic arousal where you're funneling into focus, and it takes constant or near-constant effort to get there and stay there. It's a mental edge of sorts. Once I understood that this limbic friction was not only normal, but essential, focus and learning became easier. I started seeking it out. And it felt good. I share this backstory simply to help illustrate that motivation, focus, and learning are states of mind and body. They have neural and hormonal underpinnings, much in the same way that

REM sleep has its neural and hormonal underpinnings, as does stress, and so on. And that's good news, because it makes what might otherwise be nebulous, clear. We know what to aim for.

This is a physiology-first approach to focus, motivation, and learning. It's rooted in how we work, which is why the approach works.

In this chapter you'll learn how to enhance your ability to focus by leveraging that. You'll also learn a powerful tool for "getting motivated" that is unlike all others you've likely seen before. And you'll finally get the truth about neuroplasticity—the rewiring of neural circuits that underlies all forms of learning (and forgetting), and that is often referred to simply as *plasticity*. Most everyone has heard of plasticity but honestly, most of the ways I've seen it discussed publicly are flat-out wrong.

Perhaps you've heard that "Every experience you have changes your brain." That is not true. Or "It takes twenty-one days to form a new habit." Wrong again. It can take a few days or a year, based on your level of motivation. Perhaps you've heard that "Your brain makes new neurons for your entire life." (The official term for that is neurogenesis.) Alas, barely any new neurons are added to the brain after puberty except for in your olfactory system, which allows you to smell, and those are mostly to replace neurons you've lost. Starting to get depressed? Well don't, because despite these myths, we all possess a tremendous ability to rewire our brains and to learn at any age.

The key is to understand the *type* of plasticity you're after. What we're talking about here—the rewiring of our brains that occurs as part of learning at any age—is a process that involves *a specific set of steps that must be completed in a specific sequence for learning to occur*.

I call these steps self-directed adaptive plasticity (SDAP). Mastering these steps opens the doors to learning pretty much anything you set your mind to. And that's what this chapter is about.

The Steps and Sequence of SDAP

Let's start with an overview of how SDAP occurs:

Get alert.

SDAP requires you to focus on the material at hand. Alertness sets the stage for focus; it's a precursor. I'll explain all this in the pages ahead.

So get alert and . . .

Get and stay focused.

Focused on what? On implementing a specific strategy during your learning bout.

As you go . . .

Maintain a state of urgency.

Your internal state really matters as you learn. You can't be too relaxed, but you can't be stressed either. I define a state of urgency as simply a state of persistent motivation. It's the state to aim for because it has you stay alert but not too alert and . . .

Embrace errors.

Errors that arise from genuine attempts to do something are key signals for triggering plasticity. Your nervous system is stimulated to rewire largely based on what you fail to do, not what you do correctly.

Rest.

Sleep is when neural rewiring actually occurs, especially during REM sleep the first night after a learning bout. There are other ways you can incorporate rest—like non-sleep deep rest (NSDR) and short breaks—to improve performance.

Repeat.

Consolidate newly learned material or skills through repeat performance, either through physical repetition or taking yourself through the material or skill using your imagination (seriously). Mental self-testing is especially effective for reinforcing newly formed brain connections.

Each of these six steps is valuable in its own right, and can be applied to various areas of life. Thus, although this chapter is framed in the context of plasticity, each of the protocols has other important applications too. I'll explain more as we go.

Types of Neuroplasticity

Before we explore each step of SDAP, let's get clear on what we're talking about when we talk about plasticity.

All sustained behavioral and cognitive change is the result of plasticity. These changes come in two broad types: adaptive and maladaptive. Adaptive changes are desirable—this is the plasticity that accompanies learning a new language or a new artistic or athletic skill. Maladaptive changes are the ones that make life harder. Consider when a brain injury renders someone unable to produce coherent speech, or a traumatic event leaves someone stricken with PTSD. That's still plasticity but obviously not the sort you want.

These two types of plasticity happen in different ways. Maladaptive plasticity, as in the brain injury I described above, tends to occur fast and is hard to undo. Adaptive plasticity, like learning that new language, takes more effort, and reverts somewhat easily, at least at first. I realize that's not convenient but the sooner we accept that reality, the further along we can all be in our efforts to learn new things.

Understanding why and how maladaptive brain changes occur will help illustrate how to get the adaptive brain changes that you want, and make them happen more quickly. Psychologically traumatic events trigger astonishingly fast and stable changes to nervous system wiring.[1] This rewiring happens not just in the brain but in the patterns of brain-to-body and body-to-brain connections, and hormone-control pathways.[2] The duration of a traumatic event can be very brief—no more than a few seconds—yet bring about persistent or recurring anxiety, sleep disturbances, and physical challenges, like chronic pain,[3] rashes,[4] gut issues,[5] and more, that last for years.

This is essentially *one trial learning*. Something happens and we are (seemingly) forever changed. The evolutionary logic is straightforward: One trial learning from traumatic events helps ensure we avoid similar circumstances in the future. It keeps us safe.

How one trial learning happens brings us back to an analogy discussed in chapter 3. Remember the autonomic seesaw? A stress-inducing event or thought causes your autonomic nervous system to increase your sympathetic tone, which makes you alert. That sharpens your focus. If sympathetic tone is too high, however, it feels like anxiety or panic.

When we experience a traumatic event, our brains quickly trigger the release of a lot of adrenaline into our bodies and a lot of norepinephrine in our brains.[6] Together, these two neuromodulators create all the necessary conditions for plasticity to occur. We're not talking about a bit of normal life stress. We're talking about something you perceive as really scary that causes a large and rapid shift in the neurochemical milieu of the body and brain. This shift during a traumatic event may sound like a good thing, because it helps you move away from the person or thing stressing you out, but in the long run many times it's not. If the stress response is too big, it triggers the rapid modification of multiple brain circuitries all at once and can result in an unhealthily low stress threshold going forward.[7] In some cases, one's stress threshold becomes set so low that anxiety and panic arise from innocuous events of everyday life. Undoing the kind of rewiring that results from traumatic events takes dedicated effort. Fortunately, it is possible. I discuss one way to do that in the next chapter.

The conditions experienced during this kind of one-trial learning are also at play in SDAP. "Uh-oh," you may be thinking, "is he going to suggest that I get stressed out to learn?" No. In fact, if you're too stressed, and your sympathetic tone is too elevated, you won't be able to focus, and you absolutely need to focus in order to learn. But you do need to be alert. My point here is that a shift in neurochemical milieu is crucial to achieving that state—alert but calm. Not stressed.

Conditions for Neuroplasticity

SDAP is all about desired forms of learning: a new musical instrument, a new language, a new physical skill, a new healthy habit, et cetera. For SDAP to occur, you must focus intensely on what you are trying to learn. To focus intensely on what you are trying to learn, you have to be alert. And to be alert, your autonomic nervous system has to be in a somewhat sympathetic-dominant state.

That seesaw shift in the nervous system signals to the relevant circuits in your brain and body that what is happening is unique and important, and that they need to change to become better equipped for similar circumstances in the future. Another useful way to think about it is that your brain must get the message that there is a gap between its current configuration and the demands you're facing—a deficit of sorts that it needs to overcome. The deficit is resolved by making new brain connections.

Now of course your neurons don't talk to each other in words. They don't say, "This is important, and we have a deficit between where we're at and where we need to be, so we need to change." Neurons communicate in the language of chemicals and electricity. So this message is communicated electrochemically, as a shift in your brain and body's neurochemical milieu that in turn alters the amount of firing in the brain circuits that need to change for the desired learning to occur. And when it comes to shifting neurochemical milieus—that is largely the job of neuromodulators.

The neuromodulators dopamine, serotonin, adrenaline, norepinephrine, and acetylcholine each serve different purposes, depending on where they are released in your brain or body.[8] It's incorrect to say that dopamine alone drives motivation, for instance, or that serotonin controls mood. It's far more varied and nuanced than that. In terms of plasticity, all these neuromodulators can alter the level of electrochemical activity in the circuits I just described. In other words, these neuromodulators can change the amount and the volume that neurons "talk" to each other.

In fact, in the context of plasticity, you can think of a neuromodulator as a microphone lowered over a specific conversation in a crowded stadium. Like a stadium on game day, brains are noisy. They are busy carrying out all kinds of everyday electrochemical duties. The "microphone" makes a conversation louder against the background noise. This is one common way plasticity occurs. The faster and greater the shift in the activity of a given circuit relative to its previous levels, and relative to the background (more electrochemically active), the more likely that circuit will alter its structure and connections—in other words, the more likely plasticity of the circuit will occur. It's also true that if neural circuits are quieter (less electrochemically active) against the chatter of usual background brain activity, they can weaken.

Different contexts spike the release of different neuromodulators alone or in combination, which amplifies the conversation of the neural circuits active in that context. For example, dopamine is a major neuromodulator released in response to novelty and surprise, which facilitates plasticity for learning and memory.[9] And acetylcholine is released at high levels under conditions of heightened focus, but not all over the brain; rather, it's released specifically at the sites in neural circuits that are active.[10]

Regardless of which neuromodulator or combination of neuromodulators is released, what happens next is largely the same. Since the brain is homeostatic—that is, it seeks balance—rather than maintain high levels of activity, the neurons that are part of a given conversation modify themselves so they become more easily active should that context occur again. They may add more receptors to render themselves capable of capturing more neurotransmitters or they may sprout a tiny neurite, an axonal (output) or dendritic (input) branch that becomes part of a new set of synaptic connections with other nearby neurons.[11] All this changes the threshold for activation of that circuit going forward, and on and on.[12] Voila! That is learning-driven plasticity. Other forms of plasticity involve similar cellular and molecular changes but the conditions that create them are different.

SDAP is about creating this situation of specific neural circuits rewiring in specific ways on purpose. The steps involved in this process are designed to help you do just that.

Where to Begin

Above, I noted that the first step of SDAP is getting alert and the second is getting focused. These two work together in a positive feedback loop.

The cool thing is even the mere act of trying to focus shifts us into a slightly more elevated sympathetic tone, which causes our levels of alertness to increase, which then causes activity in the circuits for focusing to increase, which further causes levels of alertness to, you guessed it, increase. For those who struggle with focus, take solace in the fact that the circuits involved with focus are amenable to plasticity too. As you move through the SDAP process described in this chapter, and practice the various protocols here, you'll learn new things, but you'll also get better at focusing, which will help you to learn more new things, and so on.

There are multiple ways to create the increase in alertness and focus needed for SDAP. I'll cover all your options—behavioral, supplement based, pharmacologic—below.

But remember this: Alertness and focus are necessary but not sufficient for plasticity and learning. To trigger learning, you're also going to have to make errors from genuine attempts, what I refer to as repetitions, or reps. Not deliberate errors, and not half-baked efforts, but rather, errors that emerge from truly exerting yourself to learn new information, new movements, even new modes of thinking. Consider this: If your nervous system can already generate the activity patterns that enable you to do a certain task—perform a dance step, for example, or order coffee in a foreign language—why would it change? It doesn't need to! You're already equipped with the neural circuits to accomplish that task. You need to try, and fail, and try again. This is tough to accept, especially for perfectionists, but all who embrace it thrive. Especially those who come to recognize limbic friction, the slight agitation that accompanies effective learning, as a state to seek, not shy away from.

The importance of making mistakes and trying again doesn't mean you have to toil endlessly. SDAP can be enjoyable. You'll likely experience some limbic friction but guess what? Once you learn to expect it, and you realize that it helps not hinders your ability to learn, you too will be seeking it out.

You may be wondering "Why all these conditions for plasticity? Isn't there a plasticity pill?" No. As I mentioned earlier in this introduction, plasticity is energetically expensive. Strengthening and reshaping neural circuits requires a lot of ATP, the energy our cells need to function.

And this process applies to everyone. It's true that when it comes to neuroplasticity, children have it easier than adults. Their brains are more malleable because almost every experience is novel to them. In fact, many aspects of developmental plasticity emerge with no effort or need to deliberately focus at all. Good examples include the way that a baby's visual and auditory systems are shaped by their early visual and sound experiences. Those things just happen. The automaticity of plasticity in our youth isn't always a blessing however. If a child has a temporary eye injury or if a child's eyes are misaligned due to an imbalance in the muscles that help move the eyes, it can cause longstanding maladaptive changes in brain wiring.

Yet even at an early age, many forms of plasticity still require focus. Cognitive skills like language and motor skills like walking or eating with utensils all take deliberate focus to learn. In that sense, the process for motor and cognitive skill learning is inherently the same for all ages. Your states of mind and body, alongside the agitation you experience from errors while making genuine attempts to learn, are what ensure that your brain gets the message: This thing happening right now is unique and important; we're going to have to rewire.

As You Proceed

An important point for anyone wishing to establish new brain patterns is that following each step of the SDAP process in its proper sequence is more important than any one tool listed here. This will be an important reframing for a lot of people.

I mentioned that there wasn't a pill for plasticity, but people love to think about what they can take to increase neuromodulator levels to heighten focus. Adderall, energy drinks, nicotine, modafinil, microdoses of psilocybin, et cetera, are used by many people working in business, tech, sports performance, finance circles, and beyond to try to focus and learn better. The use of such stimulants is widespread on college campuses and among high school students in the US,[13] and millions of adults use them daily too.

Their widespread use merely speaks to how hard most people find it to focus intensely enough and push through limbic friction. I'm not judging anyone. For example, I, like most adults in the US,[14] use caffeine daily to increase focus. I occasionally rely on other pharmacologic tools for focus too. In this chapter, I'll cover the popular as well as the rarely discussed ones.

That all being said, the main focus here is behavioral tools. They may not seem as sexy, but many rival the pharmacologic tools.

It truly doesn't matter what you use to get alert and focused, as long as it's safe. If you opt to use nicotine or modafinil or meditation or good ol' sleep and hydration, those obviously have different safety profiles. You can use white noise or various sound tones.[15] These all have data to support them in the context of focus and learning. You can cycle different tools in and out, by the day or by the month. The point is: You have choices. Think of them as tools in your SDAP arsenal.

Stick with It

We know a lot more about plasticity now than we did twenty-five or even just five years ago. Prior to the 2000s the widely held belief—even among neuroscience researchers—was that the opportunity for adaptive plasticity mostly closes after age twenty-five.[16]

That idea is now dead. We know people can rewire their brains and learn throughout their lifespans.[17] Also mostly dead is the idea that learning-associated plasticity involves the addition of new neurons. Plasticity in humans is almost exclusively the consequence of changes to existing neural circuits, not adding new neurons to those circuits.[18] And yet, the results you can achieve when you incorporate the best of what we know about SDAP can be extraordinary.

Here is an overview of SDAP, once more:

- Get alert.
- Get and stay focused.
- Maintain a state of urgency.
- Embrace errors that arise from genuine attempts.
- Rest.
- Repeat your performance.

I've listed these again because the steps and the sequence are non-negotiable. Not because I say so, but because that's how our neuroplasticity works. There are things you can do to accelerate the process: all the tools I mentioned above (and more), along with micro-pauses, post-learning-bout NSDR, adjusted sleep protocols, and hypnosis. I cover all these in the pages that follow.

I began this chapter with this basic process because it can be applied to learning anything.

Similar to exercise, SDAP is not easy. But with time, each step becomes familiar. If you think of SDAP this way—as a process that consistently leads to a desired end—it can become a pleasure.

LEARNING PROTOCOL

1

Shift into a State of Alertness and Focus

WHAT TO DO:

- **Getting alert and focused is the first step in SDAP.** You have to be in a state of elevated autonomic (sympathetic) arousal, but not stressed.
- **Use tools to help you achieve this state.** Such tools are many and varied, and fall into three general categories:
    - **Foundational**
    - **Behavioral**
    - **Pharmacological**
- **Put your phone away.** You may think you have an issue with getting focused, but it's likely that you are distracted by something in your surroundings—the smartphone being the major culprit. Studies show that even just having your phone in the same room in a bag behind or under your chair reduces your ability to focus on cognitive tasks and/or increases the energy that it takes.[19]

HOW IT WORKS:

You might be thinking "Why would anyone need a protocol for focus?"

Fair question. Most people can easily get (and stay) focused on texting, scrolling social media, playing a video game, or watching their favorite sports team or TV show for an hour or more, with no protocol required.

But when it comes to SDAP—pushing your brain to understand or do that which it currently cannot understand or do—focusing is hard for most people, young or old.[20] One recent, albeit small, study of fifteen people engaged in a work-related task found that their focus wavered every 3.5 minutes, on average.[21] The latest data say that most people switch tasks every couple of minutes, or even less.[22] And that number drops further when people are trying to focus on challenging material. That is why I refer to a dedicated session of trying to learn something as a learning bout. It is a fight—with the material you're trying to learn, and with yourself as you try to stave off frustration and resist the temptation to quit.

Yet it's in that state of mild agitation that plasticity is sparked. But only if we focus intensely on what it is we are trying to learn.

We can all take solace in the fact that getting and staying focused has always been hard. History shows that we humans have long sought tools to make it easier. In the early 1900s an inventor by the name of Hugo Gernsback designed the Isolator—a metal helmet that covered the entire head and face, with eyeholes and a breathing tube cut into the front.[23] It resembled the helmet of an old-school scuba diving suit. The rationale was simple: Block peripheral vision and outside noise to help people focus. The Isolator did not become popular, but 117 years later it inspired the Helmfon, an oversized motorcycle helmet designed to be worn while seated at a desk, created by industrial design company Hochu rayu.[24] The rationale was the same, all that time later: Block out peripheral vision and outside noise to help people focus. The Helmfon, as you might imagine, also did not gain traction. Even if it had, the advent of social media and other online activities essentially moved the outside noise of the entire world directly into one's central field of view. So much for helmets.

Other long-used tools include non-amphetamine stimulants such as caffeine, which blocks adenosine receptors in the brain that would otherwise trigger sleepiness, and nicotine, which triggers the release of several neuromodulators discussed in the introduction to this chapter. The use of caffeine in the form of tea or coffee dates back more than two thousand years. But coffee and tea didn't become popular in Europe until the seventeenth century, the result of invasions and trade.[25] Today, approximately 90 percent of the world's adults—that's estimated as more than five billion people (!)—drink caffeine every single day. Later I'll explain how to use caffeine specifically to enhance focus, but meanwhile those stats reveal that caffeine is the most popular drug on the planet by a huge margin. (If you're wondering, alcohol and nicotine are in a distant second and third place, respectively.)

Nicotine, mostly in oral forms like pouches, gum, and mints, has made a big comeback as a focus aid in recent years. I recently gave a talk to several thousand undergraduate men and women at an East Coast university and asked the auditorium for a show of hands of "who in here takes nicotine daily?" About 30 percent of them raised their hands. (In a more private setting—a smaller group of about fifty male students—about two-thirds said they use nicotine two or more times per day every day.) This is obviously not a controlled study, nor did I count each hand, but even if these are artificially high estimates, it's still pretty shocking. Or is it? Nicotine is an unusual stimulant because it makes people alert but calm—a highly desirable state for learning. Unless smoked, vaped, dipped, or snuffed, nicotine does not cause cancer, but it is highly addictive and it raises blood pressure.[26] Later, I'll explain how, assuming you're okay with the risks, nicotine can be used to enhance focus. There are a few safer alternatives, some of which work through the same mechanisms.

And there are the amphetamines. First synthesized in Romania in the late 1880s, amphetamines are compounds that increase levels of some of the key neuromodulators discussed in the introduction to this chapter, like norepinephrine and dopamine.[27] These stimulants were initially marketed in the 1930s as a treatment for narcolepsy, but soon hit the college scene when research showed a link with increased scores on intelligence tests.[28] They were also investigated for the treatment of attention deficit hyperactivity disorder (ADHD) and as appetite suppressants starting even back then.[29] A decade later, both German and Allied forces used amphetamines during World War II to stay awake and alert.[30] Recreational use of amphetamines exploded in general popularity starting in the 1950s, partly due to a surplus from World War II. By the 1960s, there was an epidemic of amphetamine dependency and abuse in the United States.[31] They were made illegal for non-prescription use in the early 1970s, classified in the same way as cocaine and morphine, and their use dropped. That is, until the FDA approved amphetamines for the treatment of ADHD in 1996.[32] Drugs marketed for ADHD like Adderall, Vyvanse, et cetera, are amphetamines, and they work quite well to increase alertness and focus. Current exact rates are hard to come by, but it seems that up to 35 percent of college students use stimulants at some point during their undergraduate years.[33] For people without a genuine clinical need for amphetamines, their use can be problematic. They are effective for helping people complete work that relies on skills they already have, but far less effective for learning new skills. They are lousy for contemplative thinking, too, and creative endeavors. And they are very habit forming, and in many cases addictive.

That's the history. And while getting and staying focused has always been hard, it seems it's now harder than ever.

The good news is that accessing a state of focus necessary for SDAP is possible for anyone. It starts with understanding the states of mind and body you're after. You'll recall that negative experiences automatically set off the learning process. No coffee, no tutor, no motivational video or mantra required. The fast, massive increase in sympathetic tone caused by adrenaline and norepinephrine ramps up activity in relevant brain circuits. It's proof that if the right electrochemical systems get triggered, we all have the capacity to focus. Again, I'm not saying seek out stressful situations. But this points to adrenaline and norepinephrine as potent pro-focus and pro-plasticity molecules. That is knowledge we can use.

Work in the 1990s from neuroscientists James McGaugh and Larry Cahill at UC Irvine showed that if adrenaline and norepinephrine are elevated using drugs, exposure to cold water, or emotionally activating visual images, the resulting increase in sympathetic tone opens the door for the learning process.[34] Interestingly, the beta-blocker propranolol, which prevents an increase in sympathetic tone, impairs learning and memory of emotional events.[35] Conversely, if sympathetic tone is artificially increased before, during, or even immediately after a learning bout, memory is enhanced.[36] And not just for emotional events or information.[37]

Importantly, the relationship between autonomic arousal and learning follows an inverted U-shape curve, a finding first documented in 1908 and reconfirmed since.[38] If autonomic arousal is too low, learning doesn't occur. If autonomic arousal is too high, learning also doesn't occur. Only if autonomic arousal is somewhere on the top of the inverted U-shape curve does learning occur.

Keep this in mind anytime you begin SDAP. The key is to enter a learning bout alert but calm, then to move through it in such a way that your level of autonomic arousal continues to increase—but never to the point where you start to feel overly stressed.

The best way I can describe that level of autonomic arousal is if I ask you to imagine the kids' game sometimes called "hot hands." It's where one person places their hands out, palms up, and you put your hands on theirs, palms down. The person with palms up flips their hands over to try and tap the top of your hands before you can pull away. You don't know when they will make their move. You're alert and focused, anticipating something will happen. Learn to recognize that state. That's the ideal level of autonomic arousal for a learning bout. With a bit of practice you'll be able to sense when your autonomic arousal is climbing too high or dropping too low, and keep yourself in that ideal state. In other words, you learn to get better at entering the learning process.

Is Being Focused the Same as Being in a Flow State?

No. Don't confuse this state with a flow state. In flow states we forget the rest of the world (and even ourselves), and we do things as if on autopilot.[39] Flow states are ideal for task performance—executing cognitive and motor skills we have already mastered. We don't learn in flow states, we implement what we already learned.

The person who first described flow states—the Hungarian psychologist Mihaly Csikszentmihalyi—accurately described this feeling as when the challenge of a task is matched with your existing skill level, not too easy, nor too hard . . . just challenging enough to engage you and "an absolute sense of control."[40] That last part—"an absolute sense of control"—means your brain already has the neural circuits in place that it needs to execute the task. And as we discussed above, that means no rewiring . . . no plasticity is triggered, and no learning occurs.

To trigger plasticity and start learning, you must push past your current abilities. You have to get stumped, miss the mark, and most importantly, you have to feel the agitation of making errors. Recognize that as limbic friction, and seek it out.

Ask any elite performer how they got so good at their craft and they will tell you, "Practice, lots of practice." But there are two kinds of practice. There are the hours upon hours spent drilling what we already know how to do and there is the practice of pushing ourselves to learn new skills. The latter is accomplished by making errors through genuine attempts. As the great Twyla Tharp, world-renowned choreographer and dancer, put it, "The more you fail in private, the less you will fail in public."[41] Twyla understands that elite performance requires genuine attempts—failing and failing again (and again), until the gap between one's goal and actual performance is reduced to zero.

The Learning State

The experiments that perhaps best illustrate the vital role of focused attention in learning come from the work of neuroscientist Mike Merzenich, PhD, and his lab at University of California, San Francisco.[42] The studies were done in the 1990s using monkeys and later adapted to studies in humans. The monkeys were trained to place their fingers on a rotating cylinder that had both coarse and fine bumps laid out in rows across its surface.[43]

The monkeys quickly learned that if they detected a difference between the coarse bumps and the fine bumps, they earned a reward. To signal when they noticed that difference, they used their other hand to move a joystick. Over time, the researchers made the task harder by making the difference in the bumps progressively smaller, which required more focus from the monkeys. Not only did the monkeys learn to perform the harder task, but the researchers observed significant changes in the brain areas representing sensations in the fingers that were touching the cylinder. In other words, they observed plasticity associated with that learning. These were adult monkeys, too, showing that plasticity was not just confined to developmental critical periods as had long been believed.

That was interesting but it was just the beginning of the story. In other studies from Merzenich, monkeys had to learn to discriminate between different sound tones. In that case the regions of the brain responsible for hearing changed. Perhaps not surprising, except that the monkeys were experiencing bumps on their fingers at the same time they heard the tones. So why did only the auditory areas of the brain change? Because the monkeys received rewards only for learning sound tones, so that's what they focused on. Together, these two sets of experiments showed that mere experience doesn't cause neuroplasticity. Learning-associated brain plasticity only occurs in the circuits associated with where our attention is placed.

Since those landmark studies, there have been thousands of experiments exploring the conditions required for learning and plasticity. Consider the often-cited studies from neuroscientist Eleanor Maguire, PhD, and colleagues of London taxi drivers, who must learn to navigate the complex streets of their city by memory (this was prior to the advent of GPS and

Google Maps, mind you).[44] They found that, compared to bus drivers, taxi drivers had larger hippocampi, a key brain area for encoding new memories. Then there is the study showing more concentrated patterns of brain activation among professional violinists for finger movements compared to amateurs.[45] And there are studies showing significant brain circuit changes as people learn to juggle,[46] as well as reversion of those newly formed circuits if people don't practice in the first weeks afterward.[47]

All these studies—the taxi drivers, the violinists, the jugglers—suggest that intense focus is a foundational need in order for SDAP to occur. But suggestions aren't proof. There is, however, one study that really hammers home the relationship between focus and plasticity in humans. In 1993, two researchers from Hebrew University in Israel asked people to practice detecting a slight shift in the angle of a line relative to the angles of a bunch of surrounding lines. The people got better at that task.[48] Not surprising. Also not surprising was that when participants were asked to detect a slight shift in the angles of *all* the lines, they got better at that task too. What is surprising is that performance on one task did not improve performance on the other task, despite the fact that what they saw in both tasks was exactly the same. The only difference between the two conditions was what the participants were instructed to pay attention to. The finding leads to a profound insight: that the plasticity they experienced was tied to the act of *looking* for something and not solely to the success of *finding* that something. As the authors concluded, "Learning will occur only in those neurons that are activated by the stimulus and that are at the same time relevant for the task. Which neurons are relevant [for neuroplasticity] is dictated by the mechanism or strategy used for task performance (and not merely a stimulus-response correlation)."

These results, along with the earlier studies mentioned here, point to the crucial role of focus in plasticity and learning.

Which brings us to the common saying "fire together, wire together."[49]

People often use this phrase to capture the idea that habits form from neurons being activated at nearly the exact same time. The thinking goes that neurons firing simultaneously or one after the other causes them to become wired together, which will lead them to readily fire together in the future. But the term "fire together, wire together" is actually unrelated to the kind of learning we are talking about in this chapter—achieving new skills, developing new behavioral patterns, et cetera. This is not a trivial point. This phrase is often attached to the false notion that people can learn when in passive or semi-engaged states. It implies that we can simply expose kids to music to enrich their brain. Not so. It also implies that simply reading or doing something repeatedly is enough to create new brain patterns. Alas, not so. Oh and the "fire together, wire together" phrase is constantly misattributed to psychologist Donald Hebb when in fact it was Carla Shatz, the developmental neurobiologist, who said it first—in the context of developmental brain wiring, not learning.[50] The point is this: Whether young or old, if we want to learn, we need to focus intensely on new information, or in the case of cognitive or motor skills, on our attempt to perform them. The good news is that with the right tools and a little practice, anyone can access focus . . . and learn.

Tools for Focus

As I mentioned in the introduction to this protocol, we humans have long sought tools to make this endeavor easier. Here's where science puts us today.

There are three categories of tools to get alert and focused.

1. Foundational
2. Behavioral
3. Pharmacological

The tools offered here can be used for learning bouts, as described above, or even for what I call work sessions—time when you're not necessarily tackling new information or skills, but grappling with some work or physical challenge that simply requires intense focus.

FOUNDATIONAL TOOLS FOR FOCUS

These tools are the bedrock upon which all the other suggestions in this protocol depend. Without them, the rest of the tools in this protocol will be far less effective. Get the foundational tools right, and you'll greatly amplify the potency of all others you opt to use.

Foundational Tool 1: Sleep

In chapter 1 when I said that sleep is the foundation of mental health, physical health, and performance, that included learning of all kinds. When we do not get enough quality sleep, or if our sleep timing is altered by more than an hour or two from our normal schedule, our levels of alertness get harder to regulate and so focusing becomes an even bigger challenge. Thus, aim to get adequate sleep using the protocols in chapter 1. (See Sleep Protocols 1–6 for a reminder on the basics.)

Foundational Tool 2: NSDR

If you've had less than adequate sleep and you're trying to lock in on a learning bout, consider doing ten, twenty, or, if possible, thirty minutes of non-sleep deep rest (NSDR) at some point prior to starting that learning bout. NSDR, while not a replacement for sleep, is your best bet to restore mental and physical vigor if you didn't get enough sleep. As mentioned in Sleep Protocol 8, NSDR is preferable to naps, because it doesn't create sleep inertia so you won't finish a session feeling groggy, nor does it disrupt your normal sleep schedule. A short nap of thirty minutes or less can also restore mental and physical vigor, but midday napping for more than thirty minutes can really mess up your nighttime sleep. Refer to Sleep Protocol 7 for best practices.

Foundational Tool 3: Stress Control

The other key to an effective learning bout is to make sure you don't show up in a state of excessively high sympathetic tone, or what we commonly call stress. Stressing about something other than what you're trying to learn steals your focus. If you're worrying about your to-do list, it's hard to focus on learning a new song on the guitar. And stressing about what you're trying to learn prevents you from staying in the alert but calm state you're after. Chapter 3 provides tools you can use "offline"—meaning when you aren't actively engaged in a learning bout—as well as tools you can use during a learning bout, such as the physiological sigh. Both types of tools are effective to help maintain your level of arousal near the peak of the inverted U-shape curve that is ideal for learning.

Foundational Tool 4: Nutrition

If you're even mildly dehydrated, your focus won't be at its best.[51] Drink water and, if you need to, add some electrolytes, which aids the rehydration process. The same goes for your blood sugar levels—make sure yours are relatively stable by not reaching for sugary foods when you know you want to be focused.

Chapter 4 described how to eat to fuel your body for all types of activity, and that includes learning bouts and work sessions. Those protocols offered guidelines, but there are options for how you adapt them for your schedule when it comes to learning. For example, in the first two to three hours of my day, I focus best if I'm fasted. I make sure I'm hydrated, and that I'm caffeinated, too, but unless I wake up especially hungry (a rarity for me), I don't eat yet. If I already exercised that morning, however, I eat, and then I start work.

You don't want to be distracted by hunger or thirst during a learning bout, nor do you want to be lethargic from an overly large or starch-and-fat-laden meal. Figure out what is best for you. And don't burn valuable mental energy trying to get conditions perfect. That effort can easily use up the self-control available to us, which tends to be finite. If we're mentally exhausted from trying to be perfect, we'll have nothing left for the actual task, a state that psychologists sometimes refer to as ego depletion.[52] Studies show that if people do a lot of decision-making prior to a mental task, they perform less well on the task compared to those who don't.[53] That means no obsessing over your pre-learning nutrition. You'll short-circuit your ability to learn. (See chapter 4 to make sure you're hydrating and eating right.)

BEHAVIORAL TOOLS FOR FOCUS

The ability to deliberately set and maintain focus is a superpower. It is a skill that carries over to all sorts of professional, educational, physical health, and relational activities, not just to plasticity and learning. That said, one of the best ways to get better at focusing is to engage in learning bouts.

The act of continually adjusting your state of autonomic arousal so it's not too high and not too low, while engaging with new information or new skills is work. It involves a lot of top-down control as neuroscientists say, which as discussed in chapter 3, is a loose reference to how your prefrontal cortex repeatedly directs and redirects your mental attention. And while no magic pill or ninja move will instantly give you that superpower, there are behavioral tools that can significantly improve your ability to focus. Some assist the transition into a state of focus, and others help you stay there.

Behavioral Tool 1: Meditation

Meditation can take many forms. One shown to improve focus is as follows: Set aside about ten to twenty minutes, sit or lie down, close your eyes, and direct your mental attention to the location between your eyes, or concentrate on your breathing, or both. As you strive to maintain those points of focus, thoughts, sensations, and outside noises inevitably distract you. Keep redirecting your attention back to the location between your eyes and/or breathing, over and over again, as many times as needed until the allotted time elapses.

From novice to expert, no one is expected to maintain perfect focus for the whole session. It's the redirecting of your attention that is the key component. It's analogous to the final few repetitions of a weight lifting set. It's what drives the nervous system changes that make it easier to focus the next time you meditate, or in any other activity. It's training; it's what is meant by the phrase "meditation is a practice."

A study by researchers at New York University found that meditating in this way for just thirteen minutes per day improved participants' ability to deliberately focus and to regulate their emotions, two strong indications that this behavioral tool can enhance and speed up learning that requires concentration.[54] Shorter meditations of five minutes per day have also been shown to help.[55] You may be thinking this seems like the micro meditation described in Stress Control Protocol 4, or any other meditation . . . and you would be right. All meditation is perceptual exercise where you intentionally limit what you pay attention to. Remember the Isolator? That was a perceptual filter designed to restrict your visual field—that is, intentionally limit what you pay attention to. Knowing that, it should make sense that what you elect to focus on during a meditation is less important than the act of directing, and redirecting, your attention back to the same place. You can close your eyes and focus on the top of your head, your feet, your lower belly, and your breathing, or you can open your eyes and focus on a point on a wall in front of you (allow yourself to blink as needed, of course).

Studies show improvements in focus stem from all such meditations, because meditation is a perceptual exercise for improving focus.[56] It just so happens that it also helps reduce stress,[57] boost mood,[58] and improve sleep.[59] A recent study even showed that meditation can induce a similar glymphatic washout process—that is, the removal of metabolic waste from the brain—as observed during sleep—albeit to a lesser degree.[60] With a year or more of experience, meditation can allow for profound insights into how our thoughts arise (and pass) and for some people it can be transformative for understanding consciousness, but those are not the immediate benefits. Nor should anyone wanting to improve focus shy away from meditation thinking they have to experience those sorts of major insights for it to "work." Meditation done simply as a perceptual exercise is powerful. And the effects show up fast: less procrastination, less impulsivity, and better learning.

If you are very limited on time, here's a simple ten-breath meditation to try immediately upon waking, while still lying in bed: Keep your eyes closed and focus on your breathing for ten slow breaths. If your mind wanders before you reach ten, restart at one, and do that as many times as needed until you reach ten focused breaths. Then get up.

After a few days, you'll notice improvement. Of course, five minutes, as described in Stress Control Protocol 4, and eventually ten, fifteen, or twenty minutes of meditation would be even more beneficial. I've heard from many people who do this regularly—meaning three to seven times per week—that they can focus better, and redirect their focus if it wanders. You'll experience the other positive effects of meditation explained above, such as stress reduction and improved sleep too. My lab found that just five minutes a day of meditation provided these benefits.[61]

What time of day or night you meditate is far less important than if you do it regularly. In fact, there is no bad time to meditate as long as you're in a safe location. If your back or knees ache from sitting cross-legged on the floor, remember that you don't have to do that. Make yourself comfortable. Sit in a chair or lie down in bed.

In my experience, it is the rare person who adheres to a daily meditation practice consistently over many years. Most become the "I used to meditate every day, I need to get back to it" people, not unlike the "I used to work out every day, I need to get back to it" people. I believe that happens because we shoot for ten to twenty minutes of meditation every day right out the gate. We make progress but then stop when life gets too busy, and the benefits of meditation disappear slowly so we don't notice until the habit is broken that we are struggling to focus.

That is why I suggest you set a *very* low bar, just ten breaths. Do that every morning for two weeks, then shift to doing five minutes of meditation as described in Stress Control Protocol 4. Do that three to seven days per week for a month, then increase the duration to ten minutes, still aiming for three to seven days per week for the next month. Then increase it to fifteen minutes three to seven days per week for the following month, then twenty minutes three to seven days per week . . . indefinitely. Mark the days you do it on your calendar to keep track of your progress.

Or just stick with five minutes if that feels right. Be the person who sticks to things rather than the person talking about all the healthy stuff they used to do.

For the time investment needed, what meditation provides in terms of ability to focus, along with stress reduction, better mood, and improved sleep is extraordinary.

Behavioral Tool 2: Hypnosis

Hypnosis. I know the word alone might cause some readers to hesitate before continuing. But keep reading. Maybe the word hypnosis makes you picture people squawking like a chicken, unaware their friends are laughing until they emerge from a trance. But that is stage hypnosis. Clinical hypnosis is completely different. I wish it was called *directed neuroplasticity* instead of hypnosis.

Clinical hypnosis is supported by solid research as a tool to treat chronic pain, and to help with smoking cessation, sleep challenges, anxiety, even gut health issues.[62] Through decades of research, including brain imaging and randomized controlled trials, Stanford University psychiatrist David Spiegel and his lab discovered that clinical hypnosis stimulates specific types of plasticity that allow for better autonomic self-regulation.[63] For example, hypnosis appears to reduce activity in the part of the brain called the dorsal anterior cingulate cortex, indicating diminished self-monitoring. An accompanying increase in connection between the dorsolateral prefrontal cortex and the insula indicates that the brain is doing a better job of regulating the body. These and other findings point to a state in which people are simultaneously less self-conscious and yet better at self-regulating.

Hypnosis won't allow you to immediately speak a new language or perform the perfect golf swing, but it is very effective for teaching people how to access otherwise inaccessible brain and bodily states, such that they can more easily re-access those states once hypnosis is over. For example, someone with an intense fear of public speaking can experience being alert but calm while onstage in front of a big audience. With just a few sessions and the occasional brush-up session, people can get very good at this kind of autonomic self-regulation. Hypnosis, in other words, is about learning how to set your state of mind.

If you have trouble with focus, or any of the other issues mentioned above, you may consider hiring a licensed clinical hypnotist to work with in person or online. Alternatively, some years back, Dr. Spiegel developed an app called Reveri that provides this tool to all (I'm an advisor for Reveri). It has you listen to a brief recorded hypnosis script (in Dr. Spiegel's voice) on your phone, a few times per week. Reveri has hypnosis scripts for improving focus, and also for improving sleep, reducing chronic pain, and much more. Each takes about eight minutes to complete. If you try Reveri, remember this: It's not magic. It's also not mind control and it's most definitely not stage hypnosis. It is a tool for teaching your brain how to access different states, including focus.

Behavioral Tool 3: 40 Hertz Binaural Beats, 20 Hertz Oscillatory Induction, and White, Brown, and Pink Noise

The use of sound as a tool for focus is all about entrainment, or the matching of our internal rhythms to an external sensory event—in these cases, the frequency of sound waves. You may remember the term entrainment from chapter 1 and chapter 5. There, I talked about entraining your circadian rhythm to light, for example, by viewing bright light in the first hour after waking up. There are also ways to entrain to events in the outside world. For example, when you exercise at roughly the same time of day, you experience an increase in catecholamines and certain hormones at that time. Then after about three days or so, you automatically start to feel an increase in energy just prior to when you usually exercise. Entrainment works based on your nervous system's expectation of certain things happening.

Sound waves can entrain our brain, too, and they do so very quickly. When we hear certain frequencies or rhythms, our brain starts to entrain to the predictable features in the sound by our neurons firing in regular fashion. Scientists have figured out how to leverage that and have created specific sound patterns that increase brain activity in areas that underlie focused states.

One example is binaural beats. Two distinct frequencies of sounds are played in each ear. When that happens, a cluster of neurons in your brainstem called the medial superior olivary nucleus performs a subtraction of the two frequencies. So if a 400 hertz (Hz) sound arrives at one ear and 440 Hz at the other ear, it leads you to perceive a 40 Hz beat. That sound frequency, in particular, has been shown to improve levels of focus, and even certain forms of memory.[64] The precise mechanisms for this are still being parsed but there is evidence that 40 Hz sound can do this in part by causing release of acetylcholine from the medial superior olivary nucleus and the release of dopamine in the striatum, a brain area involved in movement and motivated attention.[65]

Some evidence even shows that 40 Hz sounds can trigger the brain circuits involved in focus and memory to enter what are called gamma oscillation states, a pattern of neural activity that is favorable for learning.[66] (Interestingly, there is parallel evidence that activating these circuits using clinical devices may also help offset some of the early symptoms of age-related cognitive decline in Alzheimer's disease.[67])

Not everyone appears to benefit from this tool however. It seems if people already have elevated levels of these neuromodulators prior to the sound exposure, the benefits of binaural beats are less apparent or even absent.[68] Alas, without doing an fMRI and blood draws, there is no way to know your baseline dopamine and acetylcholine levels. Considering 40 Hz binaural beats are safe and cost nothing (there are dozens of free apps, videos, and audio recordings of these on Apple music, Spotify, and YouTube), why not try them and see? You have nothing to lose and perhaps something significant to gain in your efforts to focus better.

Here's how: Try listening to 40 Hz binaural beats for five minutes prior to a learning bout or work session. Once you determine if that works for you, try listening to the beats continuously throughout. (Of course, if you are trying to learn something that requires you to listen to instructions, you'll only be able to use the 40 Hz tones prior to the learning bout.) Also, note that it's recommended you use headphones for binaural beats as it's the best way to entrain your olivary nucleus and other brain circuits to 40 Hz gamma frequencies.[69]

There are exciting new data suggesting that sounds of about 12 to 20 Hz—which cause the brain to entrain to beta, not gamma, waves—may also improve concentration and reduce mental fatigue.[70] Music with 20 Hz as the dominant frequency may be especially effective here.

I personally have tried 40 Hz binaural beats, using one of the many free binaural beat apps out there (I like BrainWave). I've also used white and pink noise, both of which have been shown to improve focus, albeit in a small number of studies.[71] I've heard anecdotal evidence that brown noise can also be helpful. (In case you're wondering, white noise is noise with all sound frequencies present at equal energy, pink noise sounds less "hissy" than white noise, and brown noise is lower pitched than either white or pink noise.) Brown and pink noise work a bit to increase my focus but I was not terribly impressed by the magnitude of the effect. I have also tried Brain.fm and, for me, it works well (I have no affiliation with Brain.fm, I just like their product). I listen to it while reading, and during learning bouts and even writing sessions lasting anywhere from one to three hours. (I do take a break every fifty to ninety minutes, and avoid looking at my phone in those breaks . . . more on phone use to come.)

Behavioral Tool 4: Music

The data on listening to music to enhance focus is very clear: Silence is best. (That is unless the music is 12–20 Hz binaural beats, per the above.)

If you like to listen to music when reading or learning, music with no lyrics is better.[72] All that said, some people like to work in cafés, in airports, or in busy offices. The backdrop of auditory noise helps them focus. I suspect there is a lot of individual variation when it comes to this. You'll have to experiment and see what works for you, and when.

As I write this I am in a completely silent room and it's early evening—the only audible noise is the air conditioner and the keys of my computer, but this morning I listened to Brain.fm for two full hours while I worked on an earlier part of this chapter. I felt extremely focused during both sessions, so go figure. Be a scientist of yourself, and customize your own protocols for focus. One thing is certain: Sound can be a powerful tool for entraining brain states required for learning.

A note before we continue: Throughout this chapter I've been highlighting the important role that adrenaline and norepinephrine play in focus, and the formation of memories and learning. Soon we will cover ways to boost these and some other closely related neuromodulators, like dopamine, using pharmacology. But first, there are established behavioral tools to significantly and safely increase adrenaline and norepinephrine without taking anything. These won't surprise you because I covered them earlier, in different contexts.

Behavioral Tool 5: Physical Exercise

Physical exercise causes meaningful increases in adrenaline through now-*well*-understood neural circuits, stemming from your motor cortex in your brain all the way down to your adrenal glands near your lower back.[73] Any vigorous physical activity that involves the large musculature of your legs and core (abdominals, lower back, etc.), will trigger the release of adrenaline, in a manner that scales with the intensity of the activity. Think: compound lower body exercises like squats or deadlifts, running, martial arts, tennis, and on and on. Adrenaline does not cross the blood-brain barrier, but it binds to receptors on your vagus nerve—the two-way neural superhighway that bridges your body and brain.[74] That, in turn, stimulates the release of norepinephrine from your locus coeruleus (remember that, from chapter 1?) and other brain areas involved in generating a state of focus.[75] That's one mechanism, but there are others at play, including increased blood flow and brain oxygenation, and lactate-induced elevations in brain-derived neurotrophic factor (BDNF) (which you'll recall from chapter 2 . . . see how all of this comes together?). The effects of all this on your focus and cognition are significant, and can last several hours afterward.

One of the best ways to use exercise as a tool for focus is brief high-intensity interval training (HIIT)—for example, after a five- to ten-minute warm-up, I like to do a thirty-second near-all-out sprint, followed by thirty seconds of rest, and again, for a total of eight sprint-rest cycles.

Other HIIT options work too. You can find dozens of ideas for these online with a simple web search. It's crucial to warm up for a few minutes before the first round and important too that you select a form of exercise that you can perform without getting injured. I like to run outside on a track or use a stationary assault bike, but you may prefer to swim, use a rower, a stair climber, et cetera.

There are also studies showing improved focus and cognition after sustained twenty to forty-five minute cardio training sessions at lower intensity

(60–75 percent of maximum heart rate), although the effects of this on focus appear more transient compared to more intense exercise.[76] That makes sense, given HIIT elevates adrenaline and norepinephrine more than lower intensity steady state cardio.[77]

Fewer studies have explored how focus might be increased after resistance training. But assuming the sessions are not overly long or intense, I would expect them to impart a similar focus-enhancing effect as cardio training sessions (see chapter 2 for more on the ideal duration and intensity for those sessions).

Experiment to find the form of exercise you like best to enhance focus. Make sure to time the duration and adjust the intensity of effort so it doesn't exhaust you.

Behavioral Tool 6: Proper Breathing

Sleep apnea is a condition where people under-breathe during sleep. Nasal obstructions, excessive weight, and certain medications cause it. If you snore, there's a good chance you have sleep apnea.

The result? Your brain is deprived of oxygen at night.

Sleep apnea is a dangerous condition, because the health impacts creep up over time—causing fatigue, cognitive impairments, heart issues, and more.[78] Some of these can be reversed with tools to correct breathing while you sleep, but long-lasting impairments can occur.

Why am I discussing sleep apnea in a protocol on focus? Because many people have daytime apnea that impairs their focus too.[79] Daytime apnea is when you hold your breath while working. Chronic mouth breathers experience the same. When your brain doesn't get enough oxygen, you get tired and you can't focus. To feel alert and focus intensely, you need to fix sleep and any daytime apnea.

Luckily, it's easy to do. First, make sure you're breathing through your nose anytime you don't have to speak, eat, or exercise hard. Second, learn to breathe with your diaphragm, also known as *belly breathing*, in which your belly expands as you inhale. This approach increases the amount of oxygen in the blood and promotes a more relaxed state. You'll be amazed what a difference that will make for your energy levels and focus.

Check right now. If you're mouth breathing, switch to nasal breathing. Does your belly move out as you inhale and move in as you exhale through your nose? If so, great, you're nasal diaphragmatic breathing. If you're having trouble, imagine inhaling through your nose as if trying to direct the air backward—in other words, think about drawing the air "in and back" through your nose at an angle parallel to the roof of your mouth, as opposed to inhaling "up" your nostrils toward the top of your head. I know that sounds weird, but try it. You'll notice that you immediately shift. And no, you don't have to think about your breathing all day. After two to three breaths done consciously that way, it will carry on reflexively. Nasal diaphragmatic breathing in the daytime also helps you default to the right breathing pattern when you sleep, which can help offset sleep apnea, so it's a twofer.

A few other issues with breathing to address here. If you have a badly deviated septum or challenged nasal breathing brought about by cartilage growth in your nasal passages, you need to fix that. The simplest way to open your nasal passages is to, again, practice nasal diaphragmatic breathing. Your sinuses are not fixed, but over time this effort will help open them up. Extreme cases of nasal passage collapse or other blockage may require surgery. People can often achieve some results from wearing a magnetic nose bridge for a few hours a day and/or at night. They gently pull your nasal passages open and lead to instant improvement in airway flow. Yes, they look silly. No, you don't have to wear them in public. And it won't make your nostrils or nose bigger. Intake Breathing makes a product that is easy to use. It certainly helped me breathe better at night and when I wore it for a few hours each day, the improvement in breathing, alertness, and focus was immediate, and significant. (Note: I have no affiliation with Intake Breathing.)

Keep in mind that it's 100 percent normal to be able to breathe more easily through one nostril than the other at any one time, and which nostril switches every ninety minutes or so due to a neural circuit mechanism governed by your autonomic nervous system.[80] That's right: The whole right versus left nostril breathing thing practitioners often talk about in yoga classes is supported by modern science, although the reasons for it remain unclear.

Nasal breathing has been shown to improve learning and memory. The reason is simple. It allows for better blood flow and oxygenation of the brain, and thus elevated activity of neural circuits involved in learning and memory.[81]

So find out if you snore. Again, it's an indicator that you may have sleep apnea. There are lots of free apps that record you while you sleep and track your snoring patterns. If you snore, address it. Try different devices and exercises. You may need to get fitted with a CPAP machine. Talk to your doctor to explore your options. Eliminating sleep apnea is a big deal for your health, and it will powerfully impact your ability to feel alert and focused.

Behavioral Tool 7: Cyclic Hyperventilation

Cyclic hyperventilation might sound familiar, but there's new context for this powerful tool.

It's quite simple. You hyperventilate. Intentionally. Not a bunch of quick shallow breaths—that's panting! Instead do ten to twenty cycles of a big deep inhale through your nose, using diaphragmatic breathing as described in the section above, and exhale, letting the air passively "fall out" from your mouth. You don't have to heave into the inhale to get the effect you're seeking. Work up to it gradually, and focus on long, diaphragmatic inhales through the nose. Increase the vigor after a few repetitions. After ten to twenty breaths this way, you will reliably feel much more alert.

As covered in chapter 3, you can spike your levels of adrenaline and norepinephrine and dopamine—the so-called catecholamines—and thereby increase your alertness and focus, by breathing in this specific way. It works by causing increased discard of carbon dioxide, which is called hypocapnia, and increased alkalinity of your blood pH, which is called alkalosis. That in turn triggers fast and significant increases in adrenaline and norepinephrine release in your body and brain.

If you think breathing to shift catecholamine levels is not very potent, think again. This tool works fast and extremely well to increase alertness, so you can focus on whatever task lies before you. It's a causal relationship. In experiments where people hyperventilated through an air mask with artificially elevated CO_2, their epinephrine and norepinephrine levels did not increase, nor did they achieve alkalosis.[82] This tells us it's not just the mechanics of deep breathing, it's about increased discard of CO_2. By the way, that is why people having a panic attack are told to breathe into a paper bag; it's to encourage them to re-breathe the CO_2 they expelled, and bring their epinephrine and norepinephrine back to baseline.

When you do cyclic hyperventilation, you won't have a panic attack as long as you pay attention to your autonomic state as you do. If you feel alert after ten breaths, stop. If not, do ten more breaths. If you want, complete twenty breaths, then take a long exhale and hold your breath for ten to sixty seconds until you feel the gasp reflex, and then start another round of cyclic hyperventilation. When you're as alert as you want to be, resume normal nasal diaphragmatic breathing.

Sure, cyclic hyperventilation looks a little wacky but so what? It costs nothing, and it works. It may also have benefits for your immune system.[83] Just don't ever do it in or near water, or while driving, because when your CO_2 is low, the impulse to breathe is delayed. People have drowned practicing this breathing pattern as a way to extend how long they can hold their breath underwater.

Behavioral Tool 8: Deliberate Cold Exposure

Deliberate cold exposure works very well to increase alertness and focus for hours afterward. That's not surprising: As you now know, it can more than double or triple your circulating levels of epinephrine and norepinephrine and dopamine—our now-familiar friends, the catecholamines—and it does it within seconds. The data on deliberate cold exposure and learning and memory are mixed because most studies have explored if people can learn during deliberate cold exposure, while they are in the cold.[84] You can already guess what happens there: Deliberate cold exposure generally puts people at the far end of the inverted U-shape curve of autonomic arousal, where focusing ability sharply drops off. That is not the idea here.

This is: Try thirty seconds to three minutes of deliberate cold exposure, then shower and start your learning bout or work session. It's about using deliberate cold exposure to create a long-lasting window of moderate catecholamine increase. Depending on the duration of the cold exposure, the increase in alertness and focus can last for many hours afterward.

The challenge is there is no one-size-fits-all protocol for this one because people's cold tolerance varies.

My suggestion is that if you decide to use deliberate cold exposure as a tool to increase focus, select your method, then choose an uncomfortably cold (for you) but safe temperature. Refer to Stress Control Protocol 2 for more information. If you're using a shower, get all the way under the water. If you're submerging yourself in a plunge or pool, submerge your feet, legs, and torso completely, up to your neck. And yes, put your hands in the water, too, unless you need to grip the sides for safety. The water should be cold, but shouldn't cause pain. Remember that the first ten to thirty seconds are going to feel like mild panic. Your breath will quicken, but then try long, slow, and controlled inhales and exhales. You can opt to distract yourself, or not. It makes no difference. Deliberate cold exposure bypasses most all attempts to reframe the experience as enjoyable. Pretty much the only thing that helps is to remember that it never feels good to be in the cold, but you'll feel great when you get out.

When you do get out, towel off and take a warm or hot shower (or if you're a real masochist, cold), get dressed, and go about your day. Again, to derive the focus-increasing benefits of deliberate cold exposure you don't have to do it immediately before a learning bout or work session because the effects last hours. Enjoy! (Getting out of the cold, that is.)

PHARMACOLOGICAL TOOLS FOR INCREASING FOCUS

"What can I take to focus?" is one of the most common questions I get. So here goes.

Pharmacological Tool 1: Caffeine

With 90 percent of the world's adult population drinking caffeine every day, it's hard to run a study on how caffeine affects alertness and focus . . . because most participants would be caffeine adapted, meaning they drink caffeine just to achieve normal, or what I call baseline, levels of alertness. This is an important concept to understand.

So many people rely on caffeine for basic alertness that pretty much any experiment comparing one group that takes caffeine to another that doesn't ends up telling us more about the effects of caffeine withdrawal in the control group than anything else. Alas, most people just won't quit caffeine for two to three weeks—which is the duration needed to get through the withdrawal—to participate in research. So we are left with very limited studies, all of which point to caffeine as a good way to enhance alertness, but not focus per se.

Let me explain. As we discussed in chapter 1, caffeine staves off fatigue by thwarting the action of adenosine, a molecule that builds up in our brain while we are awake and that causes us to feel sleepy as a result. If you drink caffeine regularly, you're getting some modest focus-enhancing effects, as alertness is a prerequisite for focus.

Caffeine also increases adrenaline and norepinephrine in a dose-dependent manner.[85] A single cup of strong coffee—about 250 milligrams of caffeine—can increase circulating adrenaline by more than 200 percent over baseline levels, and norepinephrine 75 percent over baseline levels.[86] Ingesting caffeine daily also may increase the density of brain dopamine receptors, allowing the same amount of dopamine to impart a greater effect.[87] The largest alertness and focus-enhancing effects of caffeine are likely to be felt if you don't regularly drink caffeine, or if you were to ingest more caffeine than is typical for you.

A note of caution: Remember the inverted U-shape curve that relates arousal and focus? If you are not a regular caffeine user and you suddenly consume 100 to 250 milligrams more caffeine than is typical for you, it will excessively elevate your sympathetic tone, and you may find it challenging to focus.

I drink caffeine every day, usually in the form of cold brewed or hot yerba maté. I have done that for more than three decades, and by now my caffeine tolerance is very high. Like most people, I swear that it helps me focus though it probably just does that by bringing my levels of alertness up to baseline. If I were to stop drinking caffeine, and push through the withdrawal, I could find my non-caffeinated baseline level of alertness . . . but I'm uninterested in doing that experiment. I love yerba maté and I love coffee. I sip caffeine from about an hour after I wake up until about 2:00 p.m. daily, and most days I do at least one, and often two or three, long learning bouts or work sessions in that time frame. You'll need to experiment to see what is best for you. I know people who avoid caffeine entirely, those that only use it as a tool for alertness and focus, and I know many like me who use it every day. (Return to Sleep Protocol 11 for more about how caffeine affects your sleep as you experiment with this tool.)

Pharmacological Tool 2: Theanine

I suggest at some point you try taking 100 milligrams of theanine alongside your caffeine. The caffeine-theanine combination can heighten focus, even for those who consume caffeine regularly.[88] What's more, the combination of theanine and caffeine has been shown to improve task-switching capacity and reduce susceptibility to distractions,[89] in part because it's thought to increase alpha wave brain activity, which allows for selective attention.[90] It also increases levels of the inhibitory transmitter GABA, serotonin, and dopamine, which can help make the alert state created by caffeine feel a little more relaxed. For non-regular caffeine users, it reduces any jitteriness caffeine might cause, as it prevents some of caffeine's vasoconstrictive and blood pressure elevating effects.[91] In fact, even though at doses of 100 to 400 milligrams (depending on someone's body weight and tolerance) caffeine is considered safe for adults without anxiety, taking 100 to 200 milligrams theanine with it may further improve caffeine's safety profile for non-regular and regular users alike.

Theanine may even allow you to get more of a focus-enhancing effect from less caffeine. In one study, people who ingested as little as 40 milligrams of caffeine combined with 100 milligrams theanine experienced improved focus.[92] Keep in mind that most commercially sold 12 ounce coffees deliver about 200 to 300 milligrams of caffeine depending on the roast, and 16 ounce coffees can contain as much as 400 to 500 milligrams.

Together, the caffeine-theanine combination tends to induce the "alert but calm" state of mind favorable for learning bouts. With its focus-enhancing effect, and various health benefits—such as reduced blood pressure and anxiety—I consider theanine a good tool for caffeine users, which means for nearly everyone.

Pharmacological Tool 2: Alpha-GPC

I consider alpha-GPC a valuable tool for increasing focus and energy levels, if it's used correctly and very occasionally.

Even small increases in acetylcholine—a neuromodulator—can improve focus.[93] Alpha-GPC does that by increasing the amount of choline that reaches the brain, which in turn indirectly raises acetylcholine levels.[94] Research has found an enhancement of concentration and cognitive flexibility in subjects who take alpha-GPC about thirty minutes prior to a learning bout,[95] and at least one study showed modest improvement in cognition in people with dementia.[96] Other studies, however, show a minimal effect.[97] The variation in outcomes may reflect people's baseline levels of acetylcholine before they take alpha-GPC, similar to what we discussed earlier with people's baseline levels of dopamine before they listen to 40 Hz binaural beats. If a person's natural levels of a given neuromodulator are already high, adding more may not help. If natural levels of acetylcholine are low to moderate, however, boosting it seems to have a positive effect.[98]

Alpha-GPC is often added to energy drinks, and most nootropic formulas (that is, substances marketed for improving cognition). If you're looking to experiment with ways to increase focus for late afternoon or nighttime work or workouts, and you don't want to disrupt your sleep, you can try 300 to 600 milligrams of alpha-GPC taken thirty minutes or so before you begin. Limit your intake to two to four times per week, because your system will quickly adjust to it.

If you take alpha-GPC, make sure to take 600 milligrams of garlic extract (in capsule form, to avoid the taste and smell of raw garlic) at some point in the same twenty-four hours, to help offset the increase in TMAO that alpha-GPC can cause.[99] TMAO is a metabolite formed by gut bacteria in response to high levels of choline and it can pose a cardiovascular risk if elevated too frequently. Garlic contains an antimicrobial chemical called allicin, which may help offset the buildup of TMAO, and garlic extract is very inexpensive.[100]

Some of you may be wondering if you can combine caffeine and alpha-GPC, or even combine caffeine, theanine, *and* alpha-GPC. Yes, that combination works very well to increase focus and energy levels . . . but it might be too stimulating for some people, raise blood pressure too high, and increase anxiety, too, so don't go from none to all three. I can take 200 to 300 milligrams caffeine, 600 milligrams alpha-GPC, and 100 milligrams theanine together before a particularly demanding exercise session or learning bout. I probably take that combination once or twice a month. And I still practice the foundational tools described in this chapter: getting great sleep, practicing NSDR, exercising, et cetera. Stimulants and things that increase neuromodulators tend to work best on that solid foundation. I can't emphasize that enough: Great sleep is still the most important tool for focus. Pharmacologic stimulants taken when you are very sleep-deprived sets you up for cardiac issues. Supplements should be used to augment a stable foundation. Not just for safety, but because that is how they work best.

Pharmacological Tool 3: L-tyrosine

This amino acid is used in the body to synthesize dopamine, as well as adrenaline, norepinephrine, and certain thyroid hormones.[101] It comes from foods we eat but, as a nonessential amino acid, our body can also make it from other compounds if needed. That said, consuming more L-tyrosine from foods or supplements leads to a net increase in catecholamine levels.

L-tyrosine is abundant in nuts and seeds, meats, and some cheeses. Parmesan Reggiano has so much tyrosine that you can often see the L-tyrosine crystals on the surface of the cheese block. Yes, it's safe to eat those L-tyrosine crystals, and yes, that is one of the reasons some people like certain cheeses so much—the taste combined with the dopamine increase it causes is highly reinforcing.

L-tyrosine gets converted into L-dopa by the rate-limiting enzyme tyrosine hydroxylase, which means flooding your system with L-tyrosine is not sufficient to increase dopamine—the amount of tyrosine hydroxylase is the bottleneck on dopamine production.[102] Nonetheless, there is some evidence that supplementing with L-tyrosine can improve alertness, focus, and learning under certain conditions.[103] The problem is that most studies used ridiculously high dosages of L-tyrosine to observe these effects—as much as 8 grams or more delivered in capsule or pure powder form. I do not suggest taking that much all at once!

Anecdotally, many people find that supplementing L-tyrosine at doses of just 500 to 2,000 milligrams can help improve alertness and focus, but the published studies indicate L-tyrosine supplements really only help when people are stressed or fatigued.[104]

I have tried 500 to 1,000 milligrams L-tyrosine and I've tried *Mucuna pruriens*, an over-the-counter naturally occurring form of L-dopa. Both increased my alertness, focus, and energy levels for a few hours but, at least for me, they both led to a significant dip in energy afterward. Some people love L-tyrosine at 500 to 1,000 milligrams before work or exercise sessions, and swear by the focus-enhancing effects. That is why L-tyrosine is found in a lot of energy drinks and pre-workout formulas. I take it from time to time because it happens to be in one of the energy drinks I sometimes consume. So now to energy drinks.

Pharmacological Tool 4: Energy Drinks

More than a third of the world's adult population consumes at least one energy drink per month, and about 9 percent consumes them every day.[105] Studies of adolescents aged thirteen to nineteen have reported that a quarter of those who regularly consume energy drinks have at least one a day, and another quarter have at least two per day.[106] In 2024, the Centers for Disease Control and Prevention noted that 30 to 50 percent of adolescents report some amount of energy drink consumption.[107] These rates are enormous.

To be clear, if you swallow a capsule of 300 to 600 milligrams of alpha-GPC, another capsule of 100 to 200 milligrams theanine, and down both with 100 to 300 milligrams of caffeine from coffee, tea, or diet soda, you're basically making your own energy drink. But there is an important difference.

Many commercially sold energy drinks contain anywhere from 200 to 400 milligrams caffeine, 400 to 900 milligrams alpha-GPC, and 100 to 200 milligrams theanine *per serving*, and contain one to two servings per can. Many also include L-tyrosine, and more are starting to include huperzine A, an alkaloid that blocks the enzyme that breaks down acetylcholine, leading to overall increases in acetylcholine levels in the brain.[108] Many energy drinks are also now starting to include racetams, a family of synthetic compounds that lead to increased activity of acetylcholine and other neuromodulators in the brain.[109] Now you know why energy drinks are so habit forming: They are carefully engineered neuromodulator-increasing cocktails that taste like candy. They can even cause withdrawal effects if you regularly drink one or more per day, and then try to suddenly stop.

I rarely drink commercially sold energy drinks, preferring instead to get my caffeine from yerba maté or black coffee, and sometimes also taking theanine and/or alpha-GPC in capsule form. If I do have an energy drink, it's usually before a particularly hard workout, as opposed to a learning bout.

I suggest that kids under the age of eighteen avoid energy drinks or preworkout formulas, which are similar. We have no idea how all that neuromodulator augmentation impacts brain wiring. I hear from people young and old saying they "can't focus," only to learn that they drink one to three energy drinks per day, or a 20 ounce coffee every morning. That's likely 600 milligrams of caffeine just to feel baseline levels of alertness.

Homeostasis is a nonnegotiable rule of biology. If you want to boost focus and energy levels from caffeine or other substances, a daily high dose is not recommended. Put differently: Whatever stimulant you take every day will soon be needed to merely reach your baseline levels of alertness. Better in my opinion to use stimulants as an augmentation, not a requirement.

That said, I am not going to give up my daily caffeine. I enjoy the taste and the feeling far too much. I drink just enough of it to bring about a mild increase in my level of alertness. Coffee has also been shown to benefit longevity by a variety of mechanisms, and yerba maté and green tea both have additional health benefits from the antioxidants and polyphenols they contain.[110]

Most days I rely on the foundational tools described here: good sleep, nutrition, and hydration. I practice the brief daily meditation I described, and I add caffeine. These generate the alertness and focus I need for learning bouts, work, and exercise.

I include over-the-counter pharmacologic tools like alpha-GPC and theanine here because they *do work*, and I and many others have derived benefit from them. I also consider them a far safer and less expensive alternative to nicotine and prescription drugs for focus. Which brings me to nicotine.

Pharmacological Tool 5: Nicotine

Ah, nicotine. Humans love the effects of nicotine so much they keep coming up with new delivery methods and every time there is a health hazard associated with one way, they develop another.

This plant alkaloid has been used for centuries to increase focus. It was put into soldiers' kits in the early 1900s because of its known stimulant and stress-reducing effects.[111] By the 1960s, more than half of adults in the United States and Europe smoked tobacco daily, with many starting upon waking and only stopping at bedtime.[112]

Nicotine, the primary psychoactive ingredient in tobacco, increases alertness and focus, and also heart rate and blood pressure,[113] but it has the unique property among stimulants of inducing relaxation.[114] It makes you feel "alert yet calm"—that state where the autonomic seesaw is tilted ever so slightly toward increased sympathetic tone. It's the perfect state for focus. It also didn't hurt tobacco sales that smoking alongside a stranger or asking for a light was an icebreaker, and that nicotine reduces appetite. Pair all that with advertising that romanticized the act of smoking, and the cost, foul odor, stained teeth, and stagnant breath that smoking causes all went largely overlooked.

Of course, until people finally realized that smoking, dipping, chewing, or snuffing tobacco is dangerous. It significantly increases cancer and stroke risk.[115] And yet, that went largely overlooked for a long time too. Public health announcements started to make these risks clear in the mid-1960s, but it was a rather slow and reluctant campaign until the 2000s, when the tobacco industry started to be heavily taxed and regulated.[116] By 2010, the tobacco industry—formerly one of the most powerful in the world—saw its sales plummet. I was born in 1975 and I can still remember people smoking in airports and on planes, and how every dining table had an ashtray on it. Even the squat racks in the first commercial gym I joined back in 1993 had ashtrays molded into them so you could set your cigarette down while you performed your set! How times have changed.

Or have they? From 2005 to 2015, as smoking was progressively banned from most every indoor and even some outdoor public spaces, the use of electronic cigarettes, aka vaping, exploded. Vaping is somewhat safer than smoking, but carries its own risks.[117] Nicotine itself doesn't cause cancer, though the contaminants in vape solutions cause lung damage. Also, since nicotine is highly addictive, people struggle to quit vaping just as much as they struggle to quit cigarettes. Health warnings about vaping have curbed the market significantly in recent years, but because no other substance creates that alert-but-calm state like nicotine does, as they always have, people make sure to find a way to get their fix.

Which is why since 2020 the use of oral nicotine products like pouches, gums, and mints has exploded in popularity.[118] Notice the pattern? I get asked about oral nicotine almost daily. "Is it safe? Is it addictive? Is using four 6 milligram pouches worse than vaping?" Some people even use it when exercising; millions more use it to work. An increasing number of women and teens are using oral nicotine products now too.

So, here is what you need to know about oral nicotine: It absolutely works to sharply increase focus . . . if you take it occasionally. Meaning no more than two to three times a week, at a dose of 1 to 6 milligrams each time. If you take nicotine daily, you'll soon need that same dose just to reach your former baseline levels of alertness, and without it you'll be in a mild state of withdrawal. You'll feel foggy and more tired than usual. And it is very habit forming. That is why so few people can limit their oral nicotine use to 3 to 6 milligrams once per day. I hear from countless people who started with that amount, loved the effect, then increased to 3 milligrams twice per day, and now use 4 to 6 milligrams or even 8 milligram pouches pretty much all day long.

There's more to discuss as you consider this tool. Nicotine may also protect against Parkinson's and Alzheimer's. You read that right. Nicotine may prevent the neuronal degeneration underlying Parkinson's and Alzheimer's disease.[119] Clinical trials show, however, that once these diseases start, nicotine is unlikely to be of benefit.[120] Whether any neuroprotection that nicotine provides is great enough to offset the other health problems nicotine is known to cause is also still unclear. Remember, nicotine itself doesn't cause cancer—it's not mutagenic. But it may accelerate tumor progression.[121] It also raises blood pressure and causes vasoconstriction, which increases heart attack and stroke risk, and because of its vasoconstrictive effects, it has the potential to cause sexual side effects too, especially in men.[122] Experts on oral health are noticing that patients who use nicotine have more gum disease. Experts on skin health observe that it may cause premature aging of skin.[123] Both are likely as a result of its vasoconstriction effect (i.e., reduced blood flow to the gums and skin). That all makes sense, as reducing the blood supply means less oxygen and nutrients get delivered to an organ or tissue, and fewer waste products of cellular metabolism are removed from it.

Curious about the oral nicotine hype, I tried 4 milligrams nicotine gum and it worked to make me feel alert but calm. And it worked quickly, like flipping a switch. The next day, however, I felt a bit less mentally sharp. I also felt I needed to clear my throat a lot. I spoke to an MD friend who works on neural pathways for speech, and he told me that nicotine binds to both nicotinic and muscarinic acetylcholine receptors—the latter of which are abundant in the smooth muscles of the throat, larynx, and pharynx. He explained that after nicotine wears off, those muscles go into a slight spasm. Sure enough, taking 4 milligrams nicotine again fixed all that right away . . . until the next day. That experience was enough for me to end the experiment. Fortunately, the throat issue resolved after about three days.

I share this story because it made me understand the appeal—the focus-enhancing effect of nicotine is remarkable—and yet, people should know all the effects, which I'll recap one more time here to underscore them. There's addiction potential, increase in blood pressure and vasoconstriction, and of course how quickly the cravings begin and many of the positive effects evaporate. I have friends who are otherwise very health conscious, and they need nicotine to do any sort of focused work or exercise. It's become part of the way they just get to baseline. Are they addicted? The classic definition of addiction is continued use despite harm to self or others. One way that I define addiction is something that causes a progressive narrowing of the things that bring you pleasure. According to both definitions, they are not addicted to nicotine (unless you consider the long-term health harms). But I do think they are dependent on it.

As with all things, my motto is this: Do what you want, but know what you're doing. If you want to use nicotine, use the lowest possible dose that is effective for you. Stick to pouches, mints, or gums because the cancer risk appears to be lower than with cigarettes, but be aware that we do not yet have enough data to know this risk conclusively.[124] Limit your use to two to four times per week, and at most 6 milligrams per use (2–4 milligrams would be even better). That is, if you want the potent focus-enhancing effect of nicotine to last.

Pharmacological Tool 6: Prescription Drugs: Adderall, Ritalin, Modafinil and Armodafinil, Sunosi, Wellbutrin

These are the heavy guns for pharmacologically increasing alertness and focus. Collectively, these drugs are referred to as sympathomimetics: They increase levels of sympathetic tone by directly increasing levels of dopamine and norepinephrine in the brain, albeit each through different mechanisms.[125] Some block reuptake of dopamine and norepinephrine at synapses, leading to more availability of these two neuromodulators in the brain; others stimulate more release *and* block reuptake. Some also weakly increase other neuromodulators like serotonin. But they all potently increase alertness and focus.

I hesitated to include these drugs in this book, because they were developed to treat specific clinical conditions like ADHD (Adderall, Vyvanse, and Ritalin), or excessive daytime sleepiness (modafinil and Sunosi), or depression and smoking cessation (Wellbutrin), and they were not developed or marketed for merely increasing alertness and focus. The reality, however, is many millions of people get them prescribed or obtain them illicitly for that purpose. Knowing how they work and their margins of safety therefore feels warranted. Also, I hear often from parents wondering if they should medicate their child for ADHD. Or I hear from someone who thinks they themselves may have mild to severe ADHD, and they want to know what to do about it. They know I am not an MD, but they tell me it is hard to find a US doctor who doesn't almost immediately default to prescribing these medications. They are confused and conflicted about what to do.

Here is what everyone should know: All prescription drugs for focus have side effects. These vary by drug, dosage, and by person in ways that can only be determined empirically, meaning by trial and error. Also—and this is very important—the dosage at which some of these drugs are effective is enormously variable. Adderall works to treat ADHD in some people at 5 milligrams, whereas others need 40 milligrams or even more.[126] It's simply impossible to know how someone will respond, and it requires time to find the minimum effective dose. Of course, all the drugs in this section require a prescription to acquire legally. Illegal and questionably legal sources carry significant risk. Fentanyl—a deadly opioid—has frequently been found in counterfeit Adderall.[127]

The reason I call these "the heavy guns" is they work so well that people quickly become dependent on them, and some, such as the amphetamine-based stimulants like Adderall, carry abuse potential because they can create euphoria.[128] It's also important to note, however, that failure to treat kids or adults who have ADHD puts them at a much higher risk for addiction than not, due to the impulsivity associated with ADHD.[129] That said, amphetamines may stunt growth,[130] cause sleep disturbances,[131] and even lead to psychosis if abused or taken by people with bipolar depression or a predisposition to psychosis.[132] And all these drugs are hard to quit.[133] When someone does try, they often suffer from excessive daytime sleepiness and mood and focus issues, aka withdrawal. It's much worse than caffeine or nicotine withdrawal, which is why most people don't quit—they use these drugs indefinitely. Thus, the decision to medicate a child or adult with Adderall or Vyvanse (both amphetamines) or Ritalin (a non-amphetamine stimulant) needs to be carefully considered.

There are also a lot of nondrug therapies for ADHD that can be effective and/or can help reduce dosage needs. They are the foundational and behavioral tools mentioned above. What about supplements? Can alpha-GPC replace a genuine need for Adderall to treat ADHD? Unlikely, but a lifestyle that follows the foundational behaviors described in the protocols here (sleep, hydration, nutrition that favors stable blood sugar levels and satiety, etc.) along with regular meditation or hypnosis for increased focus, and timed use of caffeine and theanine, may allow people to use a lower dose of a prescription drug for ADHD. There are also many cases where these lifestyle changes have allowed people with ADHD to stop taking their medications and still thrive, or thrive even more. It's all highly individual.

That's ADHD. What about the person who doesn't have ADHD, but wants to use a prescription medication to induce states of intense focus one to three times per week? They may be doing everything else correctly, adhering to the foundational tools I've described in this chapter, but they want an "edge." And what about the many millions of people who, due to smartphones, have what clinicians are now calling *mild ADHD*, which is not a diagnosis but a catch-all for no longer being able to focus? Should they take a sympathomimetic? We can no longer pretend that smartphone-induced mild ADHD doesn't exist. My stance is that we should be aware of all the tools available for focus that are legal, and consider their relative potency and risks.

RITALIN

This non-amphetamine stimulant has largely fallen out of favor for the treatment of ADHD and for focus purposes because it's short acting, and people prefer the stronger, longer lasting effects they get with Adderall and Vyvanse.[134] A recent brain imaging study found that methylphenidate—the active ingredient in Ritalin—did not actually increase activation of attentional networks in the brain.[135] It merely reduced the feeling of fatigue and the effects of sleep deprivation on attention. It also made boring work feel more tolerable, and even rewarding—thus allowing for more sustained effort at tasks. The study didn't look at other stimulants, but this may be a general theme of the drugs covered in this section because few if any stimulants directly increase focus. Raising dopamine levels can reduce background "noise" in the brain, and therefore the tendency to get distracted, and raising norepinephrine increases alertness.[136] Together, that can make trivial things feel more engaging. It's important to know that people with ADHD can focus quite well—they just have a much harder time focusing on things they don't enjoy than do people without ADHD. Alas, much of life requires focusing on things we may prefer not doing. Apparently, stimulants like Ritalin trick the brain into ignoring our preferences.

ADDERALL AND VYVANSE

Make no mistake. These are amphetamines, aka speed, but they are not meth. There is a prescription drug for ADHD called Desoxyn, which is pharmaceutical grade methamphetamine, but it's rarely prescribed due to the addiction and abuse potential.[137] (Only a few hundred prescriptions exist in the US currently.)

Adderall and Vyvanse are similar to each other but the former works faster, within minutes, and lasts four to six hours; whereas Vyvanse's effects come on more slowly and last ten or more hours. An estimated 16.5 million people (adults and kids combined) take these amphetamines every day in the United States.[138] Some for ADHD, and some just to help with focus. They get them with valid prescriptions from board-certified MDs. If that is surprising, consider that despite being 5 percent of the world's population, the US accounts for more than 80 percent of the prescribed Adderall and Vyvanse taken worldwide.[139] You can be sure that it is not all being prescribed for clinical levels of ADHD.

Here is my suggestion: If you are considering using these drugs for focus and don't have diagnosed ADHD (and even if you do), first do an inventory of the foundational and behavioral tools for focus that are listed in this chapter. Are you getting enough sleep and exercise? Are you drinking enough water? Have you tried brief meditation or hypnosis for focus, and perhaps the caffeine, theanine, and/or alpha-GPC combination I described? If not, I suggest you do before resorting to use of prescription-level amphetamines. (Also, see the section "A Note on Phone Management" at the end of this protocol, as the phone is a severe impediment to focusing for many people.)

To be clear, I am not against prescription drugs per se, and if you do take one, don't stop suddenly. Talk to your doctor. Many prescription drugs have their place in treatment, but unless there is a genuine clinical need, using stimulants as powerful as Adderall or Vyvanse on a regular basis will soon cause dependence, and other tools you try will pale in comparison.

MODAFINIL AND ARMODAFINIL

These drugs were designed to treat "excessive daytime sleepiness" caused by narcolepsy or sleep apnea or jet lag. Today, they are commonly prescribed to people simply wishing to improve their focus for work or school. They are not amphetamines, but they can similarly disrupt sleep and appetite, and they still pose some cardiac risk—a feature of all sympathomimetics because they elevate blood pressure and heart rate.[140] These drugs are interesting because while they raise alertness and focus, they also have the rare feature of also improving cognition, in particular executive functions that allow for orchestrated task switching and working memory—the ability to hold relevant information in mind for only as long as is necessary.[141] At the same time, they may impair creative divergent thinking.[142]

In speaking with psychiatrists who prescribe these drugs, I've learned that people's sensitivity to modafinil and armodafinil varies tremendously. Some find 50 milligrams much too stimulating and their sleep is disrupted; others need 200 milligrams to achieve the benefits and sleep just fine. I have tried both armodafinil and modafinil and found they can erase my jet lag but they impair my recall memory. Armodafinil is essentially longer lasting modafinil, but even at the lowest dose of modafinil (I broke a 100 mg tablet in half), I struggled to fall asleep later that night. That said, I have a colleague who takes 100 to 200 milligrams of modafinil four to five times a week, which was prescribed to him for "mild ADHD," and he has no issues sleeping afterward. These drugs used to be expensive—but the release of generic versions made it less than one dollar per 100 milligram pill. That, combined with their mild cognitive-enhancing effects, makes me think that modafinil and armodafinil use will increase in years to come.

SUNOSI

This is a relatively new drug that also acts to increase dopamine and norepinephrine in the brain.[143] It is FDA approved for offsetting excessive daytime sleepiness due to sleep apnea, and recently it performed well in clinical trials for ADHD,[144] making it likely to soon be approved for that purpose as well. I know people have already started using Sunosi by off-label legal prescription either daily for ADHD[145] or occasionally for enhancing focus. Sunosi is not an amphetamine, and thus has less abuse or addictive potential than the other compounds mentioned above. It does not cause euphoria, nor does it seem to cause withdrawal on days it is not taken. Provided the dosing is correct (typically 75–150 mg taken in the morning), it does not seem to disrupt sleep either. Interestingly, Sunosi is a much lower affinity dopamine and epinephrine reuptake inhibitor than Wellbutrin, Adderall, or modafinil and it may have some mild serotonin-increasing effects too. That might explain why people find it less stimulatory and anxiety promoting than other pro-alertness and focus drugs. As with all drugs that increase dopamine, people with conditions that cause mania or psychosis should be cautious about using Sunosi.

WELLBUTRIN

This dopamine and norepinephrine reuptake inhibitor is much more noradrenergic than dopaminergic as compared to the other compounds in this section.[146] This means it raises norepinephrine more than it raises dopamine. It was developed to help with smoking cessation, and to treat depression, while bypassing the sexual side effects caused by many SSRIs. Eventually it was adopted by the ADHD community—a mix of psychiatrists and online patient groups that found it useful for its off-label use to increase focus.[147] At higher dosages—200 milligrams or more—Wellbutrin increases risk of seizures in those who are seizure prone, and it carries the usual anxiety and cardiac health warnings of all sympathomimetics.[148] Because of its low dopamine-promoting activity, it has low abuse risk.

I know many people who take 100 to 150 milligrams of Wellbutrin daily—typically the sustained release versions—purely for its energy and focus increasing effects. I have taken 75 to 150 milligrams specifically for that purpose and it worked well, but I found that Wellbutrin impeded my memory, especially for names. I am not sure why or how, but it was a potent and reproducible effect for me. Fortunately, my memory reverted to normal as soon as the drug wore off. I mention this side effect knowing that everyone responds differently to compounds and simply to illustrate how individual the effects of sympathomimetics can be.

A Note on Phone Management

It's clear we messed up. Smartphones are a great technology for many things: texting, apps, and more. And I do think social media can be used to inform, learn, and teach, and of course for entertainment and social connection (of sorts) too. With most powerful technologies, however, humans tend to go overboard before they course-correct. The time for that course correction is now.

People can't seem to set their phones down and even if they do, their phones still interfere with the ability to think. A study that looked at the effect of having your phone on your desk versus in a bag in the same room versus in an entirely separate room found that having your phone on your desk or even zipped up in a backpack reduces your working memory and fluid intelligence—the ability to figure things out on the fly—compared to when your phone is placed in a different room.[149] The authors of the study were able to disentangle focus—people's ability to direct their attention to a task—from how much mental energy they could devote to what they were focusing on. They found that, even when people could focus on the task at hand, having their phone within physical reach reduced their cognitive ability. Apparently, even if we are not consciously thinking about our phone or seeing notifications, if it's within our physical proximity our brain devotes mental energy to resist the temptation to pick it up. The takeaway thus is simple: To maximize focus, put your smartphone in an entirely different room from where you are.

Another very useful tool is to restrict your social media apps to an old phone that has a completely different phone number. I did this, and now I purposefully limit my time with my "social media phone" to sixty minutes or less per day.

If you do both those things and still find yourself continually looking at your phone, I suggest getting a timed lockbox that has a no-code-out option—meaning there is no way whatsoever to open the box until the timer has elapsed. I use a no-code-out lockbox for my phone, and find it helps for getting work done. I don't have ADHD but I find that once the phone is truly inaccessible, my ability to focus is massively increased.

The best analogy I can come up with for the smartphone as it relates to the topic is this: Just as sleep apnea or daytime apnea reduces the amount of oxygen reaching your brain, smartphones cause attentional and cognitive apnea. They lessen the amount of neural activity in our brain circuits for focus. To focus on a work session or a learning bout of any kind, get your phone far out of reach. Your mild-to-severe ADHD may be more phone-proximity-driven than you realize. Perhaps partially, perhaps entirely. There is only one way to find out!

LEARNING PROTOCOL

2

Use Mental Contrasting to Achieve a "State of Urgency" and Reach Your Goals

WHAT TO DO:

- **Think of being in "a state of urgency," rather than a state of motivation.** Urgency is an experience we are all familiar with. We tend to know what it feels like in our mind and body. Motivation can be vague and ephemeral.
- **The most reliable method to create this state is a psychological tool called mental contrasting.** It asks you to imagine your goals, and the obstacles to achieving them, in a structured way. Even if you're already on your way toward your goals, this strategy can further assist you.

HOW IT WORKS:

"Motivation is everything." We hear this all the time and know it's true, yet people vary in their abilities to get and stay motivated. Especially to do things that require sustained focus and energy.

The tools I mentioned in the previous protocol were based on physiology as the primary lever. The idea is if we increase sympathetic tone and deploy catecholamines, we can create the neurochemical milieu required for plasticity. I made no mention of psychological tools.

Mental contrasting is a psychological tool, and a powerful one.

Imagine being able to instantly switch on a state of urgency whenever you want. Someday we'll have that. I'm certain because my colleague at Stanford, neurologist Joe Parvizi, MD, PhD, conducted incredible experiments showing that if activity in a brain area called the anterior midcingulate cortex (aMCC) is increased, people feel an immediate surge in mental energy and readiness to lean into challenges.[150] Alas, currently the only way to instantly and selectively switch on your aMCC is to drill a hole in your skull, lower an electrode into this region, and pass an electrical current into it. It will be a while—probably five to seven years—before selective aMCC stimulation can be achieved noninvasively. In the meantime, if we want to activate a state of urgency we're going to have to rely on something else. There is a pill to make you feel more alert and focused, but there is no pill that can make you feel motivated to do a specific task.

Fortunately, a solution does exist. It's this psychological tool that can reliably shift your mindset, allowing you to become more mentally and physically able to exert effort. But first we should get clear on what a mindset is.

People use the word mindset all the time nowadays but in the context of motivation psychology, it has a very specific meaning and purpose. Alia Crum, a professor of psychology and researcher who directs her own lab at Stanford, explained it best: "A mindset is a setting for your brain."[151] Meaning, a mindset is a psychological stance that makes certain thoughts and actions easier to access, and other thoughts and actions harder to access. Alia's definition also speaks to the power of mindsets to simultaneously influence different aspects of your physiology—your brain directs many systems, including your nervous system, your hormones, even your immune system, in specific ways.[152] That, in turn, guides our behavior. When we switch to a mindset that embraces a challenge, it activates neural circuitries and chemical reactions that make us feel more capable of running that extra mile, putting in extra study hours, or going for one more hour of piano practice. Physiology is also a lever here, but a secondary one.

You may have heard the term "growth mindset," coined by Stanford psychologist Carol Dweck. The term refers to the belief that ability is not fixed but rather can improve with effort.[153] With a growth mindset, a teenager who is failing calculus understands that studying hard will lead to better comprehension. That state unlocks the possibility for even more: You believe in the effort that learning requires, and take the action that it requires too. Upholding a growth mindset means you actively avoid identity-based and valuation labels of being good or bad at something. You aren't "good" or "bad"; you simply haven't put in the effort and taken the action yet. A growth mindset never says, "I'm not a math person"; it says, "I can get better at math if I work at it." Experiments from Carol and others show that adopting a growth mindset can drive significant improvements in learning, especially when paired with a stress-can-enhance-performance mindset.[154] That last bit—that stress can help with growth—implies that challenge can improve your outcome, rather than limit you.

Maybe you are wondering: If stress is so great for learning, then why aren't we all great learners? We all certainly feel stress. I think it's because for most of us, the feeling we have when we fail at doing something difficult overrides the desire to keep striving. That is one reason I continually share ways for real-time autonomic self-regulation, like the physiological sigh described in chapter 3. These protocols are designed to lower stress not only to help people feel calm, but also to expand people's sense of what's possible to learn. If we have the tools to control stress, we can seek out more challenge.

No matter how well we control our stress, however, we are still left with the challenge of how to activate a growth mindset and stress-can-enhance-performance mindset. In other words: How do we actually get motivated? Should we use self-talk? Watch an inspirational clip on YouTube? Fantasize about achieving our goal? Scare ourselves with the fear of not achieving it? How many milligrams of fear should we take? Just kidding. Sort of.

The answer starts, I believe, with swapping the word *motivation* with *a state of urgency*. Here is why:

- A state of urgency is less prone to parsing than motivation, which immediately raises questions about context. Friedrich Nietzsche offered powerful wisdom when he wrote, "*Hat man sein warum? des Lebens, so verträgt man sich fast mit jedem wie?*"[155] Some readers may be more familiar with the English translation made famous by Austrian neurologist, psychiatrist, and Holocaust survivor Viktor Frankl: "He who has a why to live for can bear with almost any how."[156]

- Sometimes the why is clear. But what about when it isn't? What about the many aspects of learning and life that require persistent effort and for which the why, the deeper meaning and larger purpose, is unclear? Often the why only becomes clear during, or even after, the how. Maybe a person is forced to take a course they hate in order to get a degree. Once they complete the course, however, they may realize the new opportunities have been made accessible to them only because of the material they learned in the course; it wasn't just a means to an end after all. A state of urgency doesn't require you to have all the answers yet.
- A state of urgency stimulates catecholamine release, which further increases sympathetic tone, which therefore increases focus.[157] This helps dim distractions, both internal and external, which improves performance . . . and increases your state of urgency.[158] It's a positive feedback loop.
- It's obvious why a sense of urgency would help you maximize the number of repetitions that you can do in a given time frame. That's huge because genuine attempts are the fundamental unit of all forms of learning.
- It's specific enough that we know what to aim for, experientially, but broad in the sense that it applies to all activities and pursuits. Motivation drives you to try something, a state of urgency keeps you practicing.

So now the question is not, "How do we get motivated?" It's "How do we create a state of urgency?"

The answer is mental contrasting, which is a tool based on the research of Gabriele Oettingen, PhD, a professor at New York University and the University of Hamburg.[159] The term is the result of her deep dive into understanding two psychological tools long thought to be helpful to this topic: positive thinking and visualization. The terms are likely familiar to you. Positive thinking refers to the practice of deliberately holding an optimistic view about an outcome as a way to help that hoped-for result come true. Visualization refers to the practice of imagining a desired future outcome, again as a way to help that result come true. Research had shown that a positive mindset can have beneficial effects on health and well-being.[160]

But as Oettingen and others have discovered, although positive thinking and visualization are great, they often undermine motivation just as easily as they can increase it. And get this: Too much positive thinking about goal outcomes undermines performance.[161] Apparently, visualization causes people's brain reward mechanisms to get sufficiently activated, so they feel less energy to continue to strive for the goal.[162] And positive thinking provides a big but transient boost in motivation.

All that is consistent with what we know about dopamine in the context of goal seeking and rewards. As Anna Lembke, an expert on dopamine, put it, dopamine is about wanting, not about having.[163] That's another downside of positive thinking: It activates the "want" circuitries but not the "have" ones. Anna further pointed out that the neural circuits underlying motivation evolved in times of scarcity, where effort almost always preceded reward—think hunting, gathering, seeking shelter, finding a mate, and so on. Because of the abundance of stimulation in modern life, which was designed to satisfy and even exploit our dopamine circuitry, most of us have recalibrated our motivation and reward circuits to expect more reward from less effort.[164] And while Anna's work has mainly focused on addictive and compulsive behaviors, we've all seen this play out for goals too.[165] Too much reward prior to effort, or too much reward without effort, undermines future effort.

A friend of mine, an MD turned successful startup investor, warned me to be careful about telling too many people about a big goal. Most will respond, he explained, by saying "You would be great at that, go for it!" Unless you have a lot at stake, the reward of all that positive feedback can undermine your drive to actually pursue the goal. I asked him if he thought it would be better if we responded instead by saying, "Don't try, you'll never succeed!" "I don't think that helps either," he replied.

He was right. Oettingen found that if people focus too much on the challenge they'll likely face, that too prevents them from pursuing goals, at least in the long run.

So much for just "Focus on the journey not the destination."

We can thus all be grateful to Oettingen for carrying out experiments that tested various common motivational tools, alone and in combination. She also explored their efficacy for helping people achieve different types of goals: learning cognitive skills, learning physical skills, making better food choices, exercising more, and on and on.[166] She eventually discovered that it is the contrast between visualizing the goal and thinking about the obstacles to achieve it that creates a state of heightened physical and mental energy, and that state is what leads us to be more likely to start—and to persist.[167]

In other words, Oettingen figured out how people can activate a state of urgency. She calls the approach mental contrasting, and she calls the way to implement it WOOP, an acronym that stands for *Wish*, *Outcome*, *Obstacles*, *Plan*.[168] The four steps of WOOP can be done in your head, but it works best if you record your answers. Try writing them down, or hitting the record button on your phone. It works for both short- and long-term goals.

WISH: Name the big, overall goal. What do you want to happen?

For example:

- "I want to learn guitar well enough to play with a band live in front of a thousand people."
- "I want to get a PhD in neuroscience from a top program."
- "I want to learn to speak fluent German."
- "I want to paint well enough to make a living selling my art."

It takes only a few seconds to complete the *W* step in WOOP. You don't need to include a lot of detail, but some helps. For instance, "I want to be happy and successful" is too general. Instead of focusing on what you want to feel, name skills, credentials, and proficiencies that you're hoping to achieve.

OUTCOME: Here is where you think about what you want to feel from having achieved the goal.

For example:

- "I will experience the thrill of performing live with other great musicians and knowing that I'm giving people the live music experience I know and love so much too."
- "I will feel the freedom and excitement of being able to work for any number of different companies exploring for cures to neurodegenerative diseases."
- "I will enjoy going to Germany to visit my spouse's family, be able to relate to them better, and maybe even work and start a life there someday. And I can help our kids become bilingual."
- "I will finally get to indulge my desire to be creative. And I can sleep in late and stay up late painting while listening to music, which is what I always wanted!"

You'll notice this outcome step is aspirational—you're encouraged to daydream about how you want to feel. I gave short examples here but feel free to expand on the many things you look forward to feeling. The reality check is next.

OBSTACLES: Get clear on the obstacles you anticipate en route to your goal.

Be hyperrealistic. Record the roadblocks you might face. Include how you might feel as you do. People's temperaments vary, but you know yourself—so be honest about how you'll react when things don't go to plan.

For example:

- "I tend to be really tired from work at the end of the day. I'm going to feel frustrated when I am too tired to practice guitar or when traffic makes me late to guitar lessons."
- "I will miss the chance to attend weddings and go on fun vacations with my friends because I'll be in the lab doing experiments or studying. I won't have much money because PhD students don't get paid much."
- "It will be a long time before I am truly fluent in German because I learn really slowly. And writing in German is even more difficult than speaking it, so I will get discouraged a lot."
- "The art I make is not likely to appeal to a lot of people because I like melancholy themes and darker tones, and most people seem to buy art that is happy and playful."

Again, feel free to expand as much as you want to for this step.

PLAN: Come up with if-then statements to address the obstacles you anticipated.

These are *action* steps.

For example:

- "On days when I'm too tired to practice guitar after work, I will go to sleep early and get up thirty minutes earlier than usual the next day. That way I can get fifteen to twenty minutes of practice done in the morning. My mind is much sharper then anyway. Playing in the morning also makes me feel good for hours, so maybe work might not feel so exhausting. If I'm late to guitar practice because of traffic, then I will do my best to stay calm and practice in my head on the way there. I will add a few minutes of practice in my car after the lesson to really drill in what I learned."
- "When I can't attend fun events because of time or money restrictions, I will remember that having a PhD in neuroscience puts me at a unique advantage for job choices and long-term financial security because there is so much still to discover about nervous system diseases . . . and we still don't have cures to most all of them. Also, a lot of my friends who make more money than me now are bored with their jobs or have already maximized their earning potential. I will be able to consult and/or invest in biotech companies because I really understand where the field is and where it might grow. Also, I will remember that I love doing experiments."
- "If I feel frustrated at my slow progress learning German, I will remind myself that the frustration is a signal my brain is getting the message to change, and that a lot of learning happens in bursts; it's rarely linear. I will ask my spouse (who is fluent) if we can do an only-in-German dinner once per week as a family, so I and the kids can

practice. I will use AI to generate some free German language quizzes for me that I can listen to when I'm alone in the car."

- "I will remind myself that the best art has always come from people who really care about the work they are doing, and that I really feel and believe in the messages that motivate the art I create. I'll set up a website and social media platform so I can connect with other artists with similar tastes, and learn from them about marketing my work."

You may have noticed what happened there. Mental contrasting quickly moves you from idealizing and making aspirational statements about goals and feelings to concrete action steps . . . and, more importantly, clarity about how you will deal with setbacks. It customizes the process of getting motivated. If you're optimistic and unflappable and start new projects all the time or if you're pessimistic and tend to talk yourself out of things or if it depends on the circumstances or the time of day or the goal, mental contrasting still works. It also serves as a strategy setting session. It's not a pep talk. It's a preparation exercise that has been proven to help people get started and persist in pursuit of their goals. It's also zero cost, and takes around ten minutes at the outset. It's a real gift to us all, and we have Oettingen, along with the students and postdocs that ran the experiments, to thank for it.

In My Experience

I used mental contrasting for a goal that I had been procrastinating on forever. I followed the WOOP process. I typed out the WOOP answers into a word processing document and hit Save. That took about ten minutes.

And it worked spectacularly well for me. It somehow cleared away the laziness and analysis paralysis and all the other stuff that had been holding me back, and I enjoyed two solid work sessions that very day, and then two months of steady effort toward the goal thereafter, even though I was in my busiest season of work and I had many other commitments.

When I started feeling a bit unmotivated again, I reread the document. I made some edits and additions based on new changes in life. That only took about five minutes. I now do mental contrasting for learning goals, for work goals, for fitness goals, and for personal goals too. I reread and update the WOOP documents whenever I am feeling a bit unmotivated. It's become reflexive. I don't share my WOOP answers with anyone, they are for me and for me only, but you can decide if you want to keep yours private or not.

The Mechanisms Behind Mental Contrasting

I was struck that mental contrasting seemed to increase my motivation across the board, not just for my specific goal. I procrastinate far less on everything now. I'm not aware of any data showing that doing mental contrasting rewires specific brain areas, but given what we know about the aMCC, I wonder if it might. Recall how Joe Parvizi conducted incredible experiments showing that if activity in the aMCC is increased, people feel an immediate surge in mental energy and readiness to lean into challenges. Especially since every instance of learning—whether that's a new behavior or a new piece of information—is the consequence of plasticity and our aMCC is the brain structure most closely associated with tenacity.[169] It has been shown to increase in volume in successful dieters, people who push themselves to stick to a new exercise program, and other situations where thinking about and overcoming a challenge is called for. Parvizi discovered the role of the aMCC in 2013, and only recently has it been discussed in the larger field of neuroscience and media, so I doubt that Oettingen was aware of its potential role in WOOP. I look forward to a day soon when someone explores whether the aMCC is activated by going through the steps of the WOOP Protocol. In the meantime, I plan to keep using mental contrasting any time I need to generate a state of urgency for something, and I hope you'll consider it too.

Why Some People Will Avoid Mental Contrasting

This may surprise the dreamers and go-getters, but a lot of people are afraid to strategize around—let alone think about—their big goals. Some of that is cultural[170] but in my observation a lot of people are afraid to change, even if they are unhappy with their current circumstances. It's just not reflexive (and in many cases it feels aversive) for them to do so. Before you conclude that a resistance to change is just the way you're wired, consider the experiment where people preferred to get strong electrical shocks they knew were coming at specific times . . . versus weaker electrical shocks that arrived without warning.[171] The same general conclusion comes from studies of pain. People like what's predictable, even if it isn't good. That defies logic until we remember that our nervous systems are prediction machines that seek to minimize energy expenditure.[172] So, while mental contrasting is merely a mental exploration of a goal, I anticipate some people will shy away from it . . . because change is hard. I hope you don't and instead, go with the data. Put it to work for you. WOOP is a really cool tool to explore new things, and I'm grateful Gabriele Oettingen and colleagues came up with it. And learning to switch on a state of urgency to increase focus and achieve your goals and get things done in life is a valuable superpower, for SDAP and beyond.

LEARNING PROTOCOL

3

Embrace Errors to Improve Your Performance

WHAT TO DO:

- **Embrace the fact that errors are an essential trigger for learning.** Errors that come from genuine attempts to learn something are the signal for plasticity to occur. This is true for all forms of skill development: cognitive, motor, musical, mathematical, et cetera, and why it's an essential step in SDAP.
- **Strive to perform at a level of difficulty just slightly beyond your current ability.** Studies show that the right level is such that it produces an error rate of 15 to 30 percent. The 30 percent level tends to work best for learning motor skills, whereas 15 percent is the approximate level to shoot for with cognitive skills.
- **Don't make errors deliberately.** That won't have the same result. Work on pushing yourself past what you think you can do and using your mistakes as learning tools.

HOW IT WORKS:

If you can do something with proficiency, your nervous system won't change. The gap between your current level of ability (even if it's zero!) and the level you are striving for is what triggers learning and plasticity. No gap, no change.

Before I dive into this protocol, I need to make something clear. There are many forms of learning and plasticity that don't require making errors. Just look at what happens with children. As every parent knows, a toddler learns that ice cream is delicious in a matter of seconds, and never forgets it. They also learn that tablets and phones can display cartoons after seeing them only once. No errors needed. (By contrast, learning to walk, to speak, or to eat with utensils are all examples of learning and plasticity that require errors to eventually master.) Traumatic events, at any age, are also examples of error-independent learning and plasticity. So is the learning that comes from experiencing a welcome surprise. Let's say you drop by a friend's party expecting to say hello and then go home early, but you end up meeting someone you really like there. You can be sure you will remember their name, their job, et cetera. Should a great long-term relationship emerge from it, you'll no doubt maintain fond memories of the party, the friend who hosted it, and the events of the entire weekend when the party occurred.

You can thank dopamine for that. Dopamine helps us learn by linking our memories of prior actions, and the contexts in which they took place, with our sense of whether things went better or worse than we expected—a phenomenon known as *reward prediction error*.[173] It makes perfect sense why this evolved: to help us find and remember the paths we took to life-sustaining resources—food, water, shelter, potential mates, et cetera. Unwelcome surprises, even if they are not traumatic, shape our memories, help us learn, and guide our future actions too. Whereas positive events simultaneously increase dopamine and lower serotonin, negative events do the opposite. Say that instead of meeting a new friend at a party, you unexpectedly run into an old boss you hoped to never see again. That would shape your expectations and motivations around future gatherings at that house. It may even change your feelings about the friend—a phenomenon known to neuroscientists as *context-dependent plasticity*.[174]

Why We Need To Make Mistakes

You'll notice that none of the examples of learning I just described require that we make errors. Stuff happened, for better or worse, and learning occurred. It speaks to the many types of plasticity.

SDAP is different. We *need* to make errors. With errors often comes some amount of agitation, of limbic friction, which by now you know is a good thing because it increases the release of catecholamines that facilitate focus and plasticity. But also, perhaps more importantly, mistakes provide the signal that sets the size and type of neural circuit changes (and thus skill improvement) that follow learning attempts.

I'll use motor skills as an example but the same holds true for all types of skills. Let's say you want to learn tennis. You need to learn to serve the ball. At first, it's likely that you'll hit the ball into the net often. Each time you do, it's an error that you register as objective performance feedback. You adjust your serve accordingly. You may decide "that last serve was too hard, I'll use less force this time" or "perhaps I am gripping the racket too high on the handle, I'll hold it lower" or "I'm throwing the ball too high before I swing," and so on. Even if you have a tennis coach who gives you instructions, you are the only one who has access to the proprioceptive information associated with each serve attempt—by that I mean the awareness of your body's movements. Your nervous system tracks each and every one of those, and compares it to the performance outcome. Some of that is conscious, and some is unconscious, working below your level of awareness.

Remember back in chapter 3, when we discussed what your nervous system does? As you may recall, whether you are asleep or awake, your nervous system is handling the basic stuff of survival, making sure that your heart keeps beating, your lungs keep expanding, your digestion keeps flowing, and so on. It is also letting you perceive the world around you. And, as we also discussed, your nervous system is also a *prediction machine.* It's constantly trying to make causal inferences: "If I do A, then B seems to happen immediately afterward . . . If I don't do X, then Y happens a few hours later . . ." When you are awake, your nervous system is running a ceaseless if-then analysis of you and your actions and feelings, thoughts and memories; of others and their actions and feelings, thoughts and memories; of the world around you, and on and on.

Here is the key thing to remember: Any time your nervous system figures out that one of your actions leads to a successful outcome, it starts to shift the pattern of neural firing that occurred from your conscious awareness into your *implicit motor memory*. It works to make the action automatic. The rationale for that is obvious: Thinking and doing and making associations is metabolically demanding. As is rewiring brain circuitry.[175] The more your brain can make things automatic, the more energy it can devote to other things. This is especially true in the case of skill learning. With maintaining focus, moving into a state of urgency, making errors, and calibrating adjustments, we can all learn to execute new skills. Once we do, we don't need to think about each step. We simply activate performance of the skill. We serve the ball, play the chord, finish the math problem. Voila!

I acknowledge that your reaction to this point might be: "Duh!" But I said there was a key thing to remember. It will forever change the way you approach learning.

First, your brain doesn't work alone here. It needs your second brain. No, not your gut. I'm referring to the mini brain tucked right under your occipital lobe. If you touch the top of your neck where it meets the back of your skull, you're touching the area just above your cerebellum, aka your mini brain. Many people have heard of the cerebellum for its role in balance, but your cerebellum is also crucial for eye movements related to attention, for proprioceptive awareness, for speaking, for estimating time, for your sense of rhythm, and much more. Your cerebellum is also a key site of action for comparing what you are trying to do with what you're currently doing, and sending the rest of your nervous system the signals it needs to close the gap in performance.

I would love to devote a thousand pages to the function of the cerebellum in learning because it is that cool, but I'll keep it (relatively) brief. When you make errors in the context of trying to learn a new skill, you activate neurons in your cerebellum. The bigger the error, the larger the response from your cerebellum. Your cerebellum is kind of like that tennis coach in this regard, except unlike a coach that observes you and makes educated guesses as to what you need to do in order to improve, your cerebellum has full access to both your inner and outer workings: the angles of your limbs and joints, the speed and stretch of your muscles; it knows when you blinked relative to your maximum effort, your level of autonomic arousal, et cetera. Thus, your cerebellum is also uniquely suited to be your coach because of both the *specificity* and the *interconnectedness* of its wiring. Different cerebellar neurons respond to the movement of different parts of the body, even your eyes and lips and tongue. It also encodes how movement of one body area changes the movement of all the others. If you consciously adjust the angle of your elbow and it improves your serve, your cerebellum registers the many other changes that accompanied the elbow adjustment and then makes sure they become part of your serve "motor program" going forward. If your elbow angle adjustment makes things worse, your cerebellum registers that too. With repeated effort, your brain eventually stamps down the exact motor program needed to serve the ball properly.

I wish we all learned about the role of the cerebellum in learning when we were kids. Instead, we watched *Star Wars*, *Harry Potter*, *X-Men*, and Marvel movies, et cetera, which are all wonderful stories, but sadly also embed the false idea in us that skills are things that just need to be activated, as if by magic. Of course, that's fiction. The real-life superpower all of us possess from birth is our ability to focus and learn. We can progress from unskilled to skilled, and from skilled to mastery. Your cerebellum, and the larger neural circuit it participates in, is the coach that guides the entire progression. If that were the message, I believe the frustration that comes from errors would take on a whole new meaning. We would (and should) view errors and the agitation that come from genuine attempts to learn as something to seek out, not to avoid. *Errorful learning*, as some researchers call it, appears to be the most efficient approach to acquiring new skills.[176]

The Goldilocks Zone for Errors

You may be asking, "How many errors are needed? And what kind?" In a study published in 2019, researchers set out to determine the optimal level of difficulty—the Goldilocks zone for learning new skills.[177] They calculated the ideal rate of error using several learning algorithms and found that training progressed much faster when the level of difficulty set was associated with an accuracy rate of about 85 percent (an error rate of 15 percent). A few additional insights emerged from this study. First, when something is too hard such that 50 percent of attempts were unsuccessful, the brain can't seem to capture the right strategy for neural circuit modification. It was much better, the researchers found, to continually adjust the training level to maintain the approximately 15 percent error rate. This was a quantitative modeling study, meaning the findings are based on a simulation, but it was aligned with studies of visual-perception-based decision-making and motor learning.

It works for cognitive tasks too. For example, students who are allowed to figure out how to solve complex math problems on their own—and therefore can make mistakes—tend to do better than students who are told the right way to do it from the start.[178] And we seem to know this intuitively. In one study, researchers at Columbia University asked fifty-two people to play a series of computer games.[179] They were free to choose from a range of games, some of which were easy, some harder, and some impossible to learn. As the task progressed, participants chose increasingly difficult games and preferred to repeat the challenging games rather than repeat the easy ones.

Remember the 15 percent "rule" is an approximate measure. There's no need to become obsessed with maintaining this exact error rate. To put it in simple terms, you want to work at a level at which you're getting things right much of the time, but also wrong some of the time.

This insight can be used in education as well. Given the relationship between errors and plasticity, and the pivotal role of the cerebellum in that process, teachers should consider reserving verbal feedback to students in cases where the students thought they got something right but actually didn't. Otherwise, it's better to give students the opportunity to register their own errors.

The moment immediately following making a mistake is critical for learning. Negative reactions typically occur within 100 milliseconds,[180] but the sympathetic arousal lasts longer and provides the milieu for enhanced focus and plasticity as we have discussed many times now. Which means our systems are primed for learning in those immediate post-error moments. This internal state improves the effectiveness of the whole learning bout. Studies of motor learning show that within-trial errors and across-trial errors both provide valuable signals for plasticity and learning.[181] If you leave a language class or tennis lesson or other learning bout thinking, "Darn, I couldn't seem to get that right on that one part," well, congratulations! The learning process set in motion by within- and across-trial errors was triggered. You'll no doubt come back better next time . . . but only if you do what's in the next protocol.

LEARNING PROTOCOL

4

Prioritize Sleep the Night After a Learning Bout

WHAT TO DO:

- **Get adequate sleep the night after a learning bout.** That's when plasticity actually occurs, and why it's an essential step in the SDAP process.
- **Enhance plasticity by practicing ten to thirty minutes of NSDR at any point after a learning bout.** Done prior, as described in Protocol 1 of this chapter, it will increase your mental and physical vigor.

HOW IT WORKS:

During sleep, our brains rapidly replay what we tried to learn during the day, including what errors to avoid in the future. Brain imaging and electrophysiological recordings show that the very same neural firing sequences that occurred during learning bouts occur again at that time.[182] If the patterns of brain activity in sleep are disrupted, we don't learn as well. Sleep isn't just a time for consolidation, it's also when we build schemas—which are extractions of common themes of movement or ideas that let our brain store information in a more efficient way. They serve as patterns that become part of our foundational understanding of how the world works.

Evidence points to REM sleep in the first night after a learning bout as being the most crucial for the learning consolidation process, a phenomenon known as the *night after learning effect*, but depending on the skill you're trying to master, deep slow wave sleep may matter more.[183] I wouldn't parse things that finely. Rather, do your best to get adequate (for you) sleep every night, but especially in times of striving to master new information and skills. I define adequate sleep in chapter 1, and give you lots of tools to use to achieve it. If you suffer a poor night's sleep, however, don't make things worse by fretting about the learning lost from it. Do NSDR the next morning, and get your sleep schedule back on track that night.

LEARNING PROTOCOL

5

Incorporate Micro Rests into Your Learning Bouts

WHAT TO DO:

- **Pause now and then between repetitions as you practice a new motor or cognitive skill.** These *waking micro rests* have been shown to accelerate learning by increasing repetition density at the level of neural circuit activation.
    - **Short breaks of five to thirty seconds** during a learning bout in which you do nothing at all (meaning, no checking your phone!) can significantly accelerate motor learning.
    - **Short breaks of five to ten minutes** during a learning bout focused on cognitive learning can do the same. These micro rests induce ten to twenty times accelerated replay of the neural circuit firing pattern related to what you are trying to learn.

HOW IT WORKS:

We try to perform a new skill and we fail, and fail again, and get close, but fail again. We get a few nights' adequate sleep, and when we come back for our next attempt, somehow we've improved.

The previous protocol explained how sleep reinforces neural circuit firing patterns that allow our brains to integrate new skills. But recent studies show that a waking micro rest can increase consolidation on fast timescales too—meaning in just seconds to minutes, and even during the learning bout.

The observation that people learn faster if they pause from time to time between repetitions goes back to the late 1800s, when the German psychologist Hermann Ebbinghaus measured his ability to learn new material.[184] He saw that spaced repetitions led to faster and more stable learning than continuous repetition. That was self-experimentation, but many years later, in a study led by National Institutes of Health physiologist Marlene Bönstrup, twenty-seven participants were asked to practice several keyboard-based motor skills, tasks that were well established in the research of memory and learning.[185] Participants had to tap out a sequence of five items using their nondominant hand. They were given thirty-six tries to learn the sequence, with each attempt lasting ten seconds followed by ten seconds of rest. Performance was measured according to both speed and accuracy.

At first, Bönstrup and her colleagues examined the learning curve across all thirty-six attempts of a given sequence. They could see the performance improved rapidly, and then petered out at around the eleventh cycle. That's a familiar pattern. We often get better at a new skill fast and then reach a ceiling when further improvements become harder.

But the researchers noticed something interesting. All along, they had been monitoring the participants' brain waves. During very brief periods of rest between repetitions—lasting about ten seconds—the patterns of brain activity showed a unique signature. They tended to occur in regions connected to our ability to plan our movements. The researchers hypothesized that some form of additional rehearsal was occurring in their brains during the micro-rest periods, and it might be important for plasticity. That mapped well onto Ebbinghaus's observation. A second study, carried out in 2020 by Ethan Buch and others, found that micro rests induce rapid plasticity and learning, most likely because the same neural circuits active during the attempt to perform the motor skill get replayed during the micro rest in between repetitions, but at about twenty-fold the speed and forward and backward.[186] In other words, waking micro rests increase repetition density. This *wakeful consolidation* seems to allow you to integrate the new motor sequence with prior learned sequences. Of course, it's during sleep when our brains really engrave the circuits carrying newly learned information. Nonetheless micro rests of ten to thirty seconds during motor learning bouts, and five to ten minutes during cognitive learning bouts, have been shown to improve many different types of skills.[187]

You may be wondering what to do during the micro rests, and how often to take them. For a learning bout focused on motor learning, the key is to simply pause and not do another rep for five to ten seconds. A bit longer, say fifteen or seventeen or twenty seconds is not a problem, so don't obsess about the exact duration. Just pause for a short time, and then continue. You can draw a bit or just sit there—which sounds boring and might make you feel lazy, but the data say you are learning faster. Yes, you can get up and walk around, use the bathroom, et cetera. Just stay off your phone, web browser, or email . . . !

Introduce micro rests somewhat at random. How often you do them depends on the complexity and the duration of a repetition. Practicing serving a tennis ball is very different, for instance, from practicing an entire song on the piano. I suggest you start the learning bout by doing continuous repetitions one after the other, and when you start to make errors, introduce a pause every third or fifth trial, then go back to continuous repetitions, and then pause after every error or every other or every third error. If you want, you could set a chime to go off at random intervals. A website that offers that feature for free is www.random.org/clock-times and there is another great, no-cost website at www.microbreaks.co/timer.html that lets you set the parameters, including (1) learning bout duration, (2) duration of micro-break, and (3) the tone you want to hear, et cetera. It's terrific for both cognitive and motor skill learning. (Note: I have no affiliation to it but I use it.)

Waking micro rests are a great tool for accelerating learning and plasticity that are based in behavioral and neuroscience-backed data. I suggest trying them.

LEARNING PROTOCOL

6

Increase Retention of New Skills and Information with Mental Rehearsal

WHAT TO DO:

- **Take one to five minutes to reflect on what you read or did during a learning bout at some point after the learning bout concludes.** The key is to test yourself for what you do and do not remember, do or do not comprehend. That's why it's the final step of SDAP.
    - **For cognitive skills and new information**, this can be informal, done simply as a mental exercise, or more formal, such as by having a friend or ChatGPT test you for comprehension on the exact same material.
    - **For motor skills**, think about where you were challenged and made errors.

HOW IT WORKS:

All of learning is anti-forgetting.

On the one hand, that statement is another giant "DUH!" But through the lens of what we know about how humans learn and remember new information and skills, it's a very important concept to integrate.

The human brain can't remember all it senses and perceives. Even though neuromodulators can serve as a sort of highlighter pen for certain experiences, most information is forgotten. Neuroimaging studies have shown that for people who learn to juggle as adults, their brain circuits rewire to reflect the specific skills of juggling but those changes are quickly lost if they don't practice.[188] Both memories and new skills extinguish quickly, in days to weeks, unless they are locked in by rehearsal. The exception to this is, of course, the information related to very emotionally charged events, for reasons partially discussed earlier in this chapter. When adrenaline is very high, a second memory pathway involving our amygdala and other limbic-associated structures opens up and we remember more "snapshots" of whatever took place while in the high arousal state.[189]

Rehearsal in the form of self-testing turns out to be the best way to protect newly acquired skills and information against forgetting. A classic 2006 study from psychologists Henry Roediger and Jeffrey Karpicke compared repeated reading of a passage of text with one-time reading of the text combined with later mental reflection, and found that mental reflection was far superior when it came to both retention and comprehension of the material.[190] That's pretty wild if you think about it. People who spend less time with the actual material but attempt to review what they do and don't remember, and what they do and don't comprehend, can work with it more flexibly. That tells us that what we remember is not simply a matter of how much time we spend with information or in an experience, but that reflection somehow reinforces and enhances the circuits carrying that information or experience.

This research has vast implications for educational settings, particularly for how best to study. We know that underlining and highlighting information only helps us remember it if we also later write down what was highlighted and underlined. It also means that testing—whether by our teacher or ourselves—is not just a form of evaluation to gauge our level of knowledge, it also represents a valuable "anti-forgetting" tool that helps us remember the information for months or years to come.[191]

The takeaway is clear: Tests work. If you're a teacher or coach, yes, this justifies pop and scheduled quizzes. It may help to test on recently learned material in exercises that count toward a grade. And, yes, don't tell the students that until after the quiz.

For those without a teacher or coach navigating SDAP, reflect on what you learned, and most of all: self test! You can do so informally or formally. AI is a great tool for this. Ask ChatGPT to quiz you on a given set of material as a teacher would. Or simply take a few minutes and test your level of recall or physical skill on your own. Try to find where your ability drops off. It takes only a few minutes and is immensely valuable. You'll learn faster and retain more of what you learn.

CHAPTER 7

PROTOCOLS

for PERSONAL GROWTH

Thus far I've focused on protocols, and the science they're based on, for bolstering key pillars of your health and performance: sleep, exercise, nutrition, stress management, light exposure, as well as focus, motivation, and learning. You'll notice I did so mostly through the lens of biology, not psychology. Even when talking about mindsets or ways to generate a sense of urgency, the emphasis unabashedly has been on the biological underpinnings of what makes these protocols work. That reflects my training and interests, but as I mentioned in the introduction it's also an essential part of how these protocols work. They are customizable to your needs. When you know how a machine works—how the parts fit together—you come away knowing which aspects you can modify.

We, however, are *not* machines. We think and feel, and hope and fear, and more. That needs attention too. The quality of our lives is strongly driven by our emotional lives, our relationships to others and to ourselves. After all, what good is it feeling vital and rested, focused and resilient, fit and capable, if we don't also enjoy our time with others, and with ourselves? We just can't overlook these aspects of life.

Scores of data now tell us the obvious: that social connection is vital to our health and longevity.[1] Like all the other Old World primates, we have an immense need to care for and be cared for by others.[2] Our nervous system evolved to crave and require these types of interactions we consciously or unconsciously register as safety.[3] Not just safety from harm, but also the sort of safety that makes us feel capable of seeking out challenges: healthy risk-taking in our work, new goals in our hobbies, going on adventures; all things that give us a sense that life, our life, matters.

Equally important but far less discussed is our relationship to ourselves. That's an admittedly squishy term. What I mean is how we talk to ourselves, and how we think about ourselves—the decisions we make, the paths we choose. In fact, this chapter could have been called "Protocols for Thinking." My goal here is not to get you to second-guess yourself. Quite the opposite. It's about clearing the clutter from your mind so you can think better. It's about moving forward on the right path and not mindlessly slaving away on the wrong one.

What are thoughts anyway?

Marcus Aurelius famously said, "Our life is what our thoughts make it"[4] and nearly identical statements were made by René Descartes,[5] the Buddha,[6] Ralph Waldo Emerson,[7] William Shakespeare,[8] and in the Bible.[9] Most people would agree their thoughts are a crucial feature of their experience of life but few ever stop to ask, "What are thoughts?" Most neuroscience textbooks don't even attempt to answer that question. They include chapters on sensation, perception, emotions, behaviors, even memories and dreams, but not a single textbook that I am aware of provides a good explanation of what thoughts are. Fortunately, researchers are starting to figure it out.

Jennifer Groh, PhD, neuroscientist at Duke University, researches how our brain maps, or *represents*, to use the neuroscience term, the world around us.[10] That makes her particularly well suited to answer the question "What are thoughts?" because thoughts are representations too. They are estimates, approximations, best guesses. She explained to me, "When we are thinking, we are running simulations with the sensory and motor infrastructure of our brain." She gave me the following example, posed as a brief series of questions. If you want, you can answer them now as well.

Think of a cat.

What comes to mind first?

Chances are the partial or complete mental image of a cat, or maybe the sound of a cat. Something cattish.

Now ask yourself: What color is the cat?

What next comes to mind?

For me, it was a gray cat and very soon afterward, the smell of kitty litter, which I intensely dislike. Then a memory of the laundry room in the house where I grew up, which is where my sister's cat Samantha often slept.

The point is that anything that we focus on—an image seen or imagined, a song, a memory, and so on—causes the sensory areas of our brain to become active. That means our visual areas, auditory areas, the areas involved in processing touch, et cetera, all ramp up their levels of electrical activity. And while each of these areas has a different name and a different job in representing the world around us, they are all extensively interconnected too. They don't work in isolation. They work as parts of what are called distributed networks. Which sensory area is activated first and which ones follow depends on what "seeds" the thought. In the above example it was the word *cat* but think about the extremely soft fur of a chinchilla. That may set off a thought that activates the touch area of your brain, and you might experience a simulation of touch, what neuroscientists call somatosensation. From there, the patterns of brain activity expand.

Regardless of where it starts, focusing on something—anything—causes your brain to call up memories, as well as any potential motor actions you might take in relation to it. In some, it also conjures up emotions related to that thing. This "simulation" aspect of human brain function is vitally important. Not just as a way to navigate our lives, but for how we eventually come to make sense of our different life experiences. It is among our most valuable mental resources and a key feature of what sets us apart from the other species on earth.

As Groh explained, "Humans don't hear or see any better than a macaque monkey. What we do have is more brain areas devoted to each of the same senses, which makes our brain capable of building up very elaborate simulations of what we perceive." In other words, the more we focus on something the richer the simulation of that thing becomes. That valuable mental resource is adaptive. It's what allows us to make predictions of "If A then B, and if B then maybe C" and so on. It's what allows us to imagine solutions to certain problems, and to build tools and technologies to overcome them. It's what gave us electricity, planes, the internet, smartphones, and so much more.

Our brains can only run a certain number of simulations at once. Groh described an experiment she does that illustrates this, and why. She stops one of her class lectures midway through and asks her students to try to think of a word totally unrelated to what they have been discussing. Sounds easy, right? Wrong. Eventually the students come up with a word, but it takes significantly more time and effort than if she asked them to think of a word related to what they have been discussing. It's as if thoughts are roads: The more time you spend thinking about something, the farther you travel down that road. Sounds obvious, but is it true? Yes. Neuroimaging and direct recordings of brain electrical activity confirm that as thought-triggered simulations get more elaborate, they outcompete other simulations.[11] Neuroscientists call these *attractor states*, which is when brain activity increases in a certain set of circuits and as it does, activity in other circuits diminishes.[12]

Incidentally, this phenomenon may be what led to the idea that humans only use a small percentage of our brain at any one time—which unfortunately made it seem like we were dumber than we could be if only we used more of our brains. Now that you understand a bit about how thoughts work, it should be obvious why that's a silly idea. Who would want too many thoughts happening at once?!

Thought competition and attractor states are vital, in fact. Groh used a great example to explain why. Think about when you're driving and you say to someone, "Hold that thought for a second, I need to change lanes." You are reflexively limiting the amount of information coming in so you can switch simulations—from talking and listening, to driving and navigating. You are allocating resources to different brain circuits.

So maybe you're now asking, "What in the world does that mean for improving our relationship to ourselves?" Turns out: everything. Improving our relationship to ourselves is about being intentional with what thoughts we sow.

Gone unchecked, our thoughts grow, and grow, and grow. This can be a good or a bad thing for our mental and physical health and how we show up in the world.

It's important you know that your thoughts occur downstream of your perceptions. It's hard to overstate how strong this link really is. The way we see our lives, the way we narrate our lives and the events of the world at large to ourselves, shapes the thoughts we have. If you tell yourself that every time you try to do something new, you fail—well, your thoughts will reflect that perception. This realization is the first step in having control over them. So yes, I'm saying you *can* control your thoughts. Below I explain how. I promise none of what follows is about the power of positive thinking. I will not be guiding you through a series of manifestations. The first protocol in this section is, of course, a science-supported tool.

The other protocols that follow are about resolving a tension that exists for many people, regardless of age or stage of life, which is the push-pull between "needing to perform outward roles in life" and "being true to oneself." That is one of the most common challenges I hear from people and it can produce varying degrees of confusion, conflict, and in some cases, crippling paralysis. I've often been asked by people forty and younger who are not already wholeheartedly committed to a career path, "What should I study, do, or be?" By contrast, people older than forty usually ask me about making meaning of their life.

With all the books and news articles and podcasts out there about finding a sense of purpose, I started to wonder: How can science help us answer these questions? It turns out there is a way. In my opinion, it's been best addressed by James Hollis, an eighty-six-year-old Jungian psychologist with more than five decades of clinical experience treating patients of all ages and backgrounds. He has helped them build their best life by taking specific steps daily. He's not a life coach, mind you. He's a credentialed therapist who has also authored twenty-two books on this subject. He was a guest on the *Huberman Lab* podcast in 2024, and I personally have used the tools he described then every day since our conversation to great benefit.[13] They resolve the tension between "needing to perform outward roles in life" and "being true to oneself." Hollis's "Daily Protocols for Creating Your Best Life," as I refer to them in this chapter, are something I wish I had heard long before that conversation. They help us make decisions aligned with our interests, and reduce a lot of second-guessing that can arise when we consider such actions. No matter your age or level of contentment with your life, I am certain these protocols will be of great benefit for you too.

Finally, I include a protocol related to resolving inner conflicts that stem from unresolved pain. Formal trauma therapies are beyond the scope of this book and usually require working with a licensed practitioner, whether that's done in talk therapy, eye movement desensitization and reprocessing (often just called EMDR), hypnosis, psychedelics, or other modality. But there is a heavily researched approach to self-healing that has been shown time and time again to work in these cases, to lighten or even remove the chainmail these experiences cast upon us. It takes very little time, it's confidential, and requires no signing up for anything. It also costs nothing. It only requires that you are willing to confront the thing that is weighing on you. I provide the specific and most effective protocol for that here.

In short, what follows will set you up for more success in all the protocols listed up until now—and for whatever else you decide to focus on and achieve in your life. It will improve your self-understanding in ways that unburden your mind.

PERSONAL GROWTH PROTOCOL

1

Replace Mind Wandering with Present-Tethered Awareness

WHAT TO DO:

- **Throughout your day, periodically ask yourself if your thoughts are focused on the present.** For example: "Are my thoughts focused on what I am doing and where I am, or are they related to the past or future?" Be honest in your response.
- **If your thoughts are elsewhere, re-tether them to the present.** Ask questions anchored in your current surroundings, such as these: "How cold or warm is it in this room? What does it smell like? How many people in line in front of me are on their phone?" That seemingly trivial line of inquiry returns your perceptions to the present because they can only be answered right here, and now.

HOW IT WORKS:

Most people would like to be happier. Among the many benefits, a better mood allows us to access more focus and creativity, enhances our rational assessment of information, and improves countless objective health metrics.[14] On the flip side, psychologist Jamil Zaki's lab at Stanford has shown that a cynical mindset significantly limits people's problem-solving abilities, creativity, and physical health.[15] Similar reductions in problem-solving abilities and creativity have been shown among people with low mood.[16] Fortunately, there is now good, actionable science on how to be happier *and* how to avoid unhappiness. Both involve—you guessed it—controlling your thoughts. But not by suppressing bad thoughts, or replacing them with positive ones. Quite the opposite in fact. Let me explain.

The 2010s marked an interesting shift in the Western perspective on happiness, and life goals generally. The change was catalyzed in part by a prominent study by Nobel Prize–winning psychologist Daniel Kahneman showing that beyond a certain threshold income level, having more money does not increase happiness.[17] (If you want to know, in 2010 that threshold amount was $75,000 annually—equal to about $110,000 today.) I confess, those results always gave me pause because let's face it: Money may not buy happiness, but it sure can help buffer against many common forms of stress, some obvious ones being housing, food, and healthcare. Turns out, there is a rarely mentioned aspect of the Kahneman study that found that more income did not increase daily happiness but it did improve people's overall sense of life satisfaction. Nevertheless, the notion that money can't buy happiness stuck around. I would argue one of the reasons for that is because it came at the same time as a rising interest in "mindfulness." That interest was accompanied by the idea that being "present" to our daily experiences, a mindset long embraced in Eastern traditions, is vital to our well-being. Just as important as material wealth, if not more so.[18]

The 2010s also brought a growing interest in the neural and psychological changes associated with mindfulness and also meditation, both of which are intended to help with being present. These practices are by no means new; they had existed in Eastern cultures for thousands of years, experienced fleeting popularity in the US in the 1970s, and then became trendy again. Now some fifteen to twenty years later, mindfulness is a familiar term, and meditation is a common practice. We also have a lot of data from lab studies and clinical trials showing that our level of "presence" is not just the outcome but a *cause* of happiness, both in the short and long term.[19] Okay, so we should "be present." Got it. But the whole "be present" thing is another pretty squishy term. Even for scientists wishing to study our level of presence, defining it is no easy task.

To shift away from catchy phrases like "Be Here Now" (I love that phrase by the way) and run actual experiments, capture data, and suggest actionable tools on the basis of those data, scientists needed to create an operational definition of presence. They also needed to study it in the real world, which is not easy. Such studies were done by a few pioneering scientists to whom we owe a debt of gratitude, such as Richard Davidson, PhD, from the University of Wisconsin–Madison, and Matthew Killingsworth, PhD, and Dan Gilbert, PhD, from Harvard.

In 2010, Killingsworth and Gilbert published what is now considered a landmark study in *Science*.[20] First, they created an app to collect real-time information on participants' thoughts and feelings as they went about their day. The app sent question prompts to people at random moments during waking hours, such as, "How are you feeling right now?" and "What are you doing right now?" Every prompt also included the question "Are you thinking about something other than what you're currently doing?" The researchers amassed a database of nearly 250,000 responses from around 5,000 people ages eighteen to eighty-eight from eighty-three different countries.

Then they dove in. Killingsworth and Gilbert analyzed the responses from 2,250 adults, most from the US, to look for any connections between the specific activity they were doing, their level of presence with that activity, and their mood. Their results showed that for nearly 50 percent of our waking lives, our minds are elsewhere, thinking about times and places and things that have nothing to do with the present. But the researchers also showed the firm connection between presence and happiness. When study participants were focused on specific activities and on their immediate physical surroundings, they were happier. Even when those specific activities were boring or unpleasant, that focus was still a buffer against unhappiness. "A wandering mind is an unhappy mind," the researchers wrote in a summary of their study.[21]

But perhaps the most interesting finding from the study was the causative link between mind wandering and unhappiness. When it came to feeling happy, mind wandering was a much bigger deterrent than whatever they were doing. It didn't even matter what they were thinking about. Being present during a less enjoyable activity seemed to make people happier than daydreaming about pleasant things unrelated to the present activity. When we are focused on the present moment, we are happier. This is the power of present-tethered awareness.

While that study has some obvious limitations—for a start, it's based on subjective self-reports—it is notable for a few reasons. First, it has a real-world context. It drew from large sample sizes. And it has readily implementable findings. It tells us that one of the most powerful determinants of our current and future levels of "happiness" is giving what we are doing as much of our undivided attention as we can. Notice I didn't say all our attention. Fully focusing 100 percent of our mental attention can happen, and that can be great—we discussed ways to do just that in the previous chapter. But it appears that the mere act of periodically devoting a bit more of your attention to the present can be of meaningful benefit to your level of happiness. The data tell us that striving to anchor your thoughts to the present forms the scaffolding of your well-being. So if you'd like to be happy, and you want your children to be happy, find ways to practice present-tethered awareness alone or together. The questions included in the protocol above are a good way to start.

Of course, feeling sad, disappointed, angry, et cetera, is sometimes warranted. It's also healthy.[22] Suppressing negative feelings has consistently been shown to lead to poorer mental and physical health outcomes.[23] The problem is when we get stuck in those low-mood states too long.

Studies that followed supported general findings from this landmark study but brought some important revisions too. There are benefits to letting your mind wander too. Daydreaming during familiar activities that don't require much attention generally supports our well-being and creativity. As someone who daydreams during cleaning tasks, long drives, and hikes, I find that reassuring. It also helps explain why people report getting some of their best insights while in the shower, while doing routine tasks such as washing dishes or mowing the lawn, while on walks or commuting, and so on. A 2017 analysis by Shaghayegh Konjedi and Reza Maleeh confirmed, however, that mind wandering during emotionally or physically challenging negative experiences was detrimental to people's immediate and future mood, just as the earlier study had concluded.[24]

The takeaway is clear: Whenever you can, bring your thoughts back to what you are doing. Don't chastise yourself for letting your mind wander but understand its negative impact on your mood. Use the simple recommendation above to re-tether your mind to the present.

If you tend to daydream, try to do so during activities that don't require much focus. In today's world, where the first seconds of waiting in line at the store, airport, or a doctor's office has us immediately reaching for our smartphone to text or scroll, a bit of good old-fashioned daydreaming is probably a better idea.

Getting Off Your Phone

Is browsing social media and the internet violating present-tethered awareness?

As that 2010 study discussed above indicates, people's minds were already wandering about 50 percent of their waking hours before social media became such a prominent—arguably even *dominant*—feature of modern life that it is now. Tech companies just figured out how to get people to devote a significant percentage of that time to scrolling on their social media platforms.

My view is that, in moderation, meaning about an hour or so per day, engaging on social media platforms can be great for learning, social interaction, and entertainment. The key is to not use social media to blunt your present-tethered awareness. We are starting to see the damage to mental and physical health that this can cause.[25] Put simply, scrolling can become just another form of mood-lowering mind wandering. The algorithms are strong. Their superpower is to get you to use them for as long as possible. Your superpower is your ability to consciously redirect your thoughts to specific activities and your immediate physical surroundings. That's a skill worth developing. If the benefits of doing so for your mood and well-being are not incentive enough, perhaps the longevity benefits I'll describe next will be.

One of the causes of aging is the shortening of our telomeres, small molecular structures that form protective caps on the ends of our chromosomes in each of our cells. In cell types that duplicate, such as our immune cells, as telomeres get shorter, they stop dividing. At that point they become what are called *zombie cells*, and they secrete inflammatory molecules that damage nearby cells. Preclinical studies suggest that this zombie cell–induced damage may be a factor in aging and age-related illnesses such as cancer, dementia, and heart disease.[26] Conversely, having cells with longer telomeres is a biomarker of youthful, healthy, and (for cell types that replicate) division-competent cells.[27]

With that knowledge in hand, UCSF psychologist Elissa Epel and colleagues conducted a study where they measured the average telomere length of immune cells from women who scored either high, moderate, or low on measures of mind wandering.[28] She discovered that the women engaged in the greatest amount of task-irrelevant thought throughout the day had telomeres that were on average two hundred base pairs (a base pair is a functional unit of DNA) shorter than the telomeres of women with low amounts of mind wandering. We all lose about 50 telomere base pairs for each year of life, so the difference between being someone who is present and someone whose mind wanders was equivalent to about four years of additional aging. This was an especially remarkable finding because the benefits appeared independent of variables known to impact longevity, such as body mass index and stress level. The takeaway: Make the effort to be present in your daily activities, tasks, and relationships. Doing so provides an actionable way to improve your mental and physical health and, potentially, your lifespan.

This doesn't mean you have to be a Luddite. Texting a friend, sending a work email, or updating a family schedule on your phone can definitely be about the "here and now." So is scrolling for education or entertainment. *The thing to be wary of is texting and scrolling or doing anything out of boredom or avoidance.* Ask yourself: "Am I numbing out or getting drawn in by things that I can't actually have an impact on?" If you answer yes, that's a good indicator that you are engaged in deleterious mind wandering. Retired Navy SEAL and two-time world-record-holding athlete Andy Stumpf talks about this in his book *Drownproof.*[29] And he shared a tool that I have found immensely useful, even life-changing. Here it is: Take a sheet of paper and draw a line down the middle from top to bottom. On the left side, list all the things that concern you at that moment. On the right side, list all the things you can actually control, and what you can do to directly impact your life that day, right then and there. Try it. You'll be amazed at what you learn about your mental preoccupations and reflexes, and what it opens up in terms of your ability to better direct your mind and actions. Doing this exercise makes you keenly aware of what really matters to you. And it gives you a heightened sense of agency around those things. It places you in a great mental stance to lean into the important stuff in your life. It also makes time spent relaxing on the couch or doing nothing feel restorative again. It's a simple tool, but a super valuable one. Yes, it's a good idea to do it every few weeks or once a month, but it's quick: five minutes at most. Do it.

Getting Out of Your Head

I am a fan of certain forms of structured introspection. I'm referring to journaling, therapy with a well-trained expert who offers useful points of action, or other deliberate, timed self-reflection done within a specific framework.

There are very good data to support those practices as tools for mental health.[30] What none of us want, however, is to be stuck in our own heads and feeling anxious. Turns out, we don't have to. We just need to understand a bit more neuroscience. And then apply that knowledge.

Your brain has cells that are grouped into circuits, which in turn are grouped into networks. Think of a network sort of like a setting for your brain: You have sleep networks, feeding networks, language networks, math networks, and on and on. And you have a network that turns on when you do nothing, aptly named the default mode network, or DMN. It was discovered to be active when people were getting their brains scanned, in between moments where they were asked to focus on certain tasks.[31] That alone wasn't terribly surprising. What was surprising was that the DMN is hyperactive in ruminators, people with cognitive impairments like Alzheimer's disease, and in depressed patients.[32] More than a decade of studies now show that many antidepressants work in part by dampening activity in the DMN.[33] Guess what? So does dancing, exercising, socializing with friends, drawing . . . essentially anything that requires your attention.[34] That's the key takeaway about the DMN. You can't just "turn it off" or even reduce its activity unless you do something to activate a competing brain network, such as the salience network—a different collection of circuits that, you guessed it, become active when you focus your attention on something external to you.[35]

So while your DMN has important healthy functions, like simulating what other people are thinking or feeling, which is useful for some kinds of social interactions, to stop ruminating and to alleviate depressive states, you want to actively inhibit your DMN. Practicing present-tethered awareness is the way to do that too. If you are too much in your own head, feeling anxious or depressed, you would do well to focus outside yourself, literally on your surroundings. Better yet, engage in an activity that forces you to do that, such as exercising, reading a book, or listening to a podcast or music. If you feel your mind is still looping even while doing those things and that you can't seem to turn off that dominant inner narrative, try the exercise Andy Stumpf wrote about. Of course, clinical major depression deserves professional support. But for anyone seeking to be happier, more fulfilled, and more on track in life, learning to recognize what thoughts are, understanding how we can direct them, and then directing them to the present, especially toward the things in the present we can have a positive impact on . . . that's the ticket to a great life.

PERSONAL GROWTH PROTOCOL

2

Apply James Hollis's Guide to Creating Your Best Life

WHAT TO DO: Practice these two things every single day.

1. **Apply the Shut Up. Suit Up. Show Up motto to your everyday life.** These are science-based tools to help bring your outward and inner lives into alignment.
   - **Shut Up:** Don't whine, instead incorporate a daily gratitude practice into your routine.
   - **Suit Up:** Use a task-switching protocol to move between tasks associated with your outward roles.
   - **Show Up:** Fulfilling our outward roles moves our life forward. That is what gives you real confidence.
2. **Allow your internal maps to update.** The best way to do this is to exit what neuroscientists and psychologists call stimulus-response mode. Here are two ways to do so:
   - **Engage in an activity unrelated to any ambitions or outward roles.** Draw, read, think, stare at the sky, go biking . . . whatever it is, this is just for you.
   - **Simply close your eyes and let your thoughts emerge.** Practice not doing anything about them. At least not in those moments. While this sounds passive, it allows your mind to reconnect to what's most important to you.

HOW IT WORKS:

A great outward life requires that we show up and perform well in roles at school and work, and in our relationships. That requires we handle our responsibilities, even when we don't feel like it. A great inner life requires that we pursue the roles at school and work and in our relationships that are right for us, not just out of duty. When our outward and inner lives are aligned, life is good. When they conflict, things take more energy. We second-guess ourselves. We ruminate. We feel more tired from less effort. Psychologist James Hollis has developed a simple way for us to understand, and integrate, our outward and inner lives. It's a daily practice. It's for everyone, regardless of individual differences. It's applicable in both good and hard times. It's good, actionable science on how to be happier and how to avoid wasting valuable years of your life.

The key, as Hollis says, is to never expect your best self to emerge by default. Hollis has a simple motto he recites to himself every morning, and throughout the day. He recommends his patients write it down and carry it with them, and recite it to themselves every morning, and throughout the day too.

This protocol is named after his motto: "Shut Up. Suit Up. Show Up." While that might sound harsh, it's not what it seems. The motto is the inspiration for a collection of science-based tools that can help you build your best life. Let me explain.

Shut Up

This means don't whine; there is always someone suffering more than you. Instead, adopt a daily gratitude practice—and do it the way the science has shown to be effective (more on that below). It's especially important to avoid whining and practice gratitude when you are feeling overwhelmed or down. I know many people are probably thinking, "So I'm supposed to suppress my feelings?" Hollis is a psychologist not a coach. He's all about acknowledging feelings. But he also is aware of what it takes to build a life that brings a person lasting joy. So stay with me.

Suit Up

This means be prepared. Take the steps you can each day to arrive at your outward roles as best you are able. This sometimes looks like self-care: Get adequate sleep and don't overbook yourself. It can also look like work: Finish your assignments, be on time, keep your belongings in order, schedule your kids' activities, and so on. Homework doesn't end when we finish school.

Show Up

This means hold yourself accountable for your work, for how you act in relationships, and indeed for all the outward roles you take on in life. You are in the driver's seat, so to speak.

Now before you tell me all that just sounds like Boomer diligence, consider this: Our inner narratives about our self-worth, and our self-esteem, are strongly impacted from fulfilling these outward roles.[36] Now is that the whole picture? Of course not. There are many factors at play when it comes to how we talk and think and feel about ourselves. But this is a significant fraction of it. Alas, just telling yourself, "You are enough just as you are," won't lead you to believe it . . . unless you are fulfilling these outward roles. This is what Hollis points out. If you're a member of a sports team, you show up to practice and work hard, with the subsequent feeling of pride in yourself. If you're a parent, you work hard at doing right by your child, with the subsequent satisfaction of having given that your all.

Holding ourselves accountable to our chosen roles also leads us into a state of thankfulness for the opportunity to perform well in them. Hollis explained to me that this state is the most important aspect of the practice. We choose a role, we commit to it, we do well, and then we are lifted into gratitude. Giving our roles our best each day becomes an act of gratitude—the act of living our life becomes a devotional practice of being thankful. Sound corny? Perfect! Because it's not about saying it. It's about the actions associated with each of the sentences. Let's get to it.

Shut Up, Redefined

At first glance, you might think that "shut up" means stop complaining. But what Hollis is after here is replacing complaining with something more beneficial. And the suggestion is more nuanced than simply "feel grateful." Rather, try spending a short amount of time each day thinking about something that causes you to feel grateful that you would not be aware of without some effort. This is not a simple gratitude list. It's about searching for something we would otherwise be unaware of or take for granted. Take a minute, or five. The data tell us this dedicated effort is positively transformative for your health, and more.[37]

In many ways, gratitude is a lot like hydration, but for your emotional well-being. Its importance for basic daily functioning is overlooked. People think of it as an extra, but it's foundational to high performance. Of all the things I've covered on my podcast, this is the tool that surprised me the most in terms of its potency. Thinking back to what we now know about thoughts—what they are and how they grow and compete with one another—it makes sense. When we are seeding thoughts of gratitude, we suppress negative thoughts. We also run simulations from a place of security and stability, rather than a place of lack. Much more feels possible from that place. So forget the idea that if you do a gratitude practice daily you'll become complacent. Actually, the opposite happens. Even a short gratitude practice of a few minutes has been shown to elevate motivation and mood, and can even improve memory recall and cognitive ability.[38]

Gratitude tends to increase other positive feelings and states, like happiness and optimism too.[39] And there is evidence that this link is causative. In a 2003 study by psychologists Robert Emmons and Michael McCullough,

192 undergraduates were randomly assigned to one of three groups, each of which was asked to reflect on the past week by writing about (1) up to five things they were grateful for; (2) up to five things that were a hassle (a dirty kitchen, doing poorly on a test, etc.); or (3) five events that affected them in some way in the past week (attending a concert, cleaning a closet, and so on).[40] All three groups also rated their mood, any physical symptoms they were experiencing, such as headaches, congestion, sore muscles, nausea, skin irritation, poor appetite, or other minor issues, and how they reacted to any offers of help over the past week. A second study followed the same design but with daily writing instead of weekly. And a third study randomly assigned people with neuromuscular disease to either the first writing group or a control group that did only the self-rating part of the study.

All three studies—weekly reflecting, daily reflecting, and reflecting among people coping with a serious illness—showed that deliberately exercising gratitude was associated with more optimism, fewer minor health issues, more exercising, a greater tendency to lend emotional support to others, and other benefits. Among the participants with neuromuscular disease, those in the gratitude writing group slept better and felt more connected to others. Importantly, the data analysis showed that these outcomes were the specific result of inducing gratitude in oneself and not a side effect of the study as a whole.

Gratitude is also good for the heart. One study of eighty-six adults looked at changes in blood pressure and heart rate in response to a stimulus and alongside participants' responses to questions intended to gauge their level of gratitude.[41] The researchers found no connection between trait gratitude and cardiovascular reactivity. However, participants with higher levels of state gratitude tended to not experience the same spikes in blood pressure that the other participants did. A review of nineteen studies, including a total of 2,951 participants, found links between gratitude and a lower risk of cardiovascular disease and a greater likelihood of healthy behaviors, such as maintaining a good diet and adhering to prescription medication.[42]

It's important to note this refers to what psychologists call state gratitude, as opposed to trait gratitude. The latter is a personality trait. Some people have a disposition that is just naturally more grateful.[43] And yes, they do better in life.[44] State gratitude, meanwhile, is about appreciation for what we are given. For most people, state gratitude needs to be cultivated intentionally. It does not emerge by default.

Some data even suggest a link between gratitude and mortality. A study published in *JAMA Psychiatry* in 2024 looked at data on 49,275 female registered nurses from across the US, obtained through the Nurses' Health Study, which has been ongoing since 1976.[45] Specifically, the researchers, from Harvard and the University of British Columbia, focused on responses to a six-item questionnaire about gratitude that enrollees first completed in 2016 and the 4,608 deaths that occurred between 2016 and 2019. The analysis showed a link between gratitude and mortality: The greater the gratitude, the less likely a person was to die during the time frame of the study. "This study provides the first empirical evidence suggesting that experiencing grateful affect is associated with increased longevity in older adults," the authors wrote.

The benefits of this practice are astounding, but if you're curious as to how to actually feel gratitude, psychologist Robert Emmons, professor emeritus at University of California, Davis, and a pioneer in the research of gratitude and positive psychology, tells us how. He found that gratitude comes from a two-step cognitive process:

> (a) recognizing that one has obtained a positive outcome [in some area of life], and
> (b) recognizing that there is an external source for this positive outcome.

Cultivating gratitude requires commitment. So Hollis's recommendation of pausing each day to acknowledge what we are grateful for is a logical starting point. But weaving together some compelling research suggests ways to make this protocol even more effective.

First, pioneering neuroscientist Antonio Damasio and colleagues investigated brain regions associated with gratitude by asking participants to listen to stories from genocide survivors who received lifesaving assistance from strangers and to imagine how they would feel about that care, rating their level of gratitude for each incident of assistance.[46] The researchers found that participants documented feelings of gratitude correlated with brain activity in the anterior cingulate cortex and the medial prefrontal cortex, regions associated with values, morals, and theory of mind (which refers to the ability to understand what another person might be thinking). The approach taken in this study is important. Note that the participants here were not thinking about their own lives. They were putting themselves in other people's shoes.

The final clue here comes from a study in which participants wrote letters of gratitude to their coworkers, unbeknownst to that coworker.[47] When the coworkers received these letters, researchers were on call. They took brain images while the coworkers listened to what had been written about them. Like in the prior study, hearing these feelings of gratitude correlated with prefrontal cortex activation, suggesting that the recipients were experiencing their *own* gratitude.

All of these findings point toward the importance of practicing gratitude. Make it nonnegotiable for a few minutes each day. Try Hollis's method. Or put yourself in the mindset of others experiencing feelings of gratitude through story or solicit examples of when your friends, family, and colleagues felt grateful for you.

You can also seek out stories that are powerful for you—such as in documentaries or in books or movies—where you observe someone sharing gratitude for actions performed by others. This approach is likely to be as effective as listing what you personally are grateful for, as is often recommended in journaling practices. It is aligned with how our brains link observing gratitude to our internal sense of reward.[48] We are clearly wired to feel better from observing and receiving genuine gratitude.

Suit Up, Redefined

"Suit up" may sound somewhat, well, obvious: We all know to shower, get dressed for school or work, pack our lunch and perhaps the kids' too, and get on with the day. But this isn't about any of that. It's about what neuroscientists call task switching.

Task switching is an essential aspect of role fulfillment but is rarely discussed. Moving our attention from one chore or job or activity to another is fundamental to being effective in whatever outward roles we perform. Good task switchers are more focused and they are calmer when things get busy.[49] They are often the kind of people about which others say, "I don't know how they do it all, much less so gracefully . . ."

Neuroscience has a lot to say about task switching, and it has everything to do with our earlier discussion about thoughts. As we spend more time doing a task, and the internal simulations around that task get more and more elaborate, a greater and greater *switch cost* accumulates.[50] That means that it gets harder to move on from that task, and those internal simulations, to a new task, and new internal simulations. Switch costs are real and significant, reducing our mental and physical performance by anywhere from 15 to 40 percent. Sometimes it's a slowing of response times, other times it's a reduction in accuracy, or both.[51] Think of it this way: Doing something for a long time gets you deep into a neural trench, so to speak, and getting out of that trench requires more time and more energy. Some people seem to intuitively know about this aspect of brain function, and always add a few minutes between tasks to get out of a neural trench. Others of us make the false assumption that we can hop between tasks and be at our best. You know who doesn't? Athletes, cognitive athletes (like professional chess players), and creative artists.

They are famed for their stereotyped rituals around both practice and competitions. They know how to "get into frame," "reset between points," and on and on.[52] Six-time Mr. Olympia winner Dorian Yates—known for his brief but extremely intense training (which, by the way, was based in large part on Mike Mentzer's principles I described in chapter 2)—told me he ironed his clothes prior to every workout . . . not just for the appearance but as a mental preparation ritual for what was to come. He was actively steering his mind.[53] Loads of books on high performance have delved into such practices and found that, when it comes to routines to harness our mental and physical resources so we can apply them with the utmost focus and effectiveness, what works best is what can be ritualized, not necessarily the specific thoughts or actions.[54] It's not that you take three slow breaths emphasizing the exhale to slow your heart rate or intentionally blink fast five times before you sit down to work, it's that you do something that you can do most anywhere, anytime and that you have decided is *your* ritual. Pick one, and design your own task-switching ritual.

Studies across a range of sports and cognitive tasks, like public speaking or test taking, show that stereotyped physical actions are the most effective task-switching rituals, as opposed to just mental mantras or self-talk. Think of the way a baseball player taps the bat on home plate before the first pitch. These may "shake off" the neural residue of the thoughts and actions related to your prior activity by shutting down the specific circuits involved in it. This is a distributed phenomenon, which means it does not happen in a single region of the brain, but it does critically involve your basal ganglia, which control "go" circuits that generate action commands for your brain and body, as well as "no go" circuits responsible for suppressing specific actions.[55]

Your own short task-switching ritual will make you more effective at moving from one task to the next, which has outsized positive benefits in all your outward roles.

So when Hollis talks about "suiting up," and getting prepared for your outward roles, or when former Navy SEAL Jocko Willink talks about putting out your workout clothes the night before an early morning session,[56] or when the great choreographer Twyla Tharp talks about ritualizing the transition into and out of her legendarily long and repetitive dance practices, they are all talking about the same thing: the importance of having a ritualized task-switching protocol.[57]

To be an effective task switcher, you also need to *not* do certain things. Nowadays we fill every second between activities—sets in the gym, the wait for food to arrive at a restaurant, the drive to pick up the kids from school, and so on—with smartphone use. Then we wonder why we are struggling to manage it all. We are overscheduled, overstimulated, and overtired. On days when we do sleep well, our task-switching abilities are vastly improved, but most of us need, and can benefit from, "anytime" actions to help us task switch to be ready and at our best for when we "show up."

Show Up, Redefined

This task-switching protocol can add benefit to our cognitive, emotional, and physical capabilities.[58] And yes, many of the things that you may already do—taking a few long exhale breaths as you return home at the end of the day, or before getting into work mode when you arrive at the office or into workout mode when you step inside the gym—are about this whole notion.

So make it work for you. And remember that the ritual between tasks associated with different outward roles can be exactly the same. Same for every switch. It's yours; do whatever works. This tool, as I said above, places the locus of control inside us. It moves us away from the need for conditions outside us to always be optimal to tackle our outward roles. It puts us in charge of how we start our tasks, and gives us confidence to continue.

I'm guessing that when you first read Shut Up. Suit Up. Show Up., you probably weren't thinking about gratitude practices, or about your basal ganglia, but what makes Hollis's approach uniquely powerful is that it balances introspection with action. It's neither coddling nor harsh. And it's realistic to the demands of life we all have to meet, as well as the internal challenges most all of us feel at some point or another. I take comfort in the fact that there are science-backed tools to help foster Shut Up. Suit Up. Show Up.

We're an oddly fortunate species. On the one hand we are born with unmatched cognitive capacity, as well as the ability, through neuroplasticity, to continually learn. No other creature alive has that and yet, because of those very gifts, we can get stuck in our own heads on big decisions before we make them or sometimes wake up one day to realize we took the wrong path after we did. Building your best life requires making Shut Up. Suit Up. Show Up. a daily practice, just as Hollis suggests. But we have to look inward, too, to assess if we are acting in alignment with our values and our desires. And to know, with confidence, what those values and desires are, and that they are worthy of our time and attention. There's a clear way to do that. Here's how that is done:

Take time every day to update your internal maps.

The other piece of the puzzle is to make sure you know yourself well. Your fears, hopes, aspirations. This kind of self-knowledge is hard to come by. The combination of life's demands and the ever-present noise of modern life can make it hard to simply know ourselves.

That's where the second part of this protocol comes in. Is this necessary? Yes. People who excessively focus on excelling in outward roles often feel unfulfilled or they end up neglecting other important areas of life. Yet those who are excessively focused on self-knowledge and self-care—another admittedly squishy term—often put off taking action that would allow their careers and relationships to thrive. There needs to be a balance.

The solution, Hollis explains, is to incorporate a second daily practice of exiting the stimulus-response mode that our outward roles—employee, parent, spouse, et cetera—require of us, giving us a chance to direct our attention inward instead. This protocol is like leaving the highway to take a local road: You benefit from the scenery, absence of high-speed traffic, and the insights that inevitably come from this change of pace. This pause allows us to separate what we think other people think about us from what we actually know to be true. That separation improves our awareness of what we want and clarifies what might make our lives genuinely more meaningful and more aligned with who we are.

There are two surefire ways to go about exiting the stimulus-response mode. First, engage in an activity unrelated to any ambitions or outward roles. Draw, read, think, stare at the sky . . . whatever it is, take time each day for this activity. The key is that the activity doesn't involve any other people, or their expectations or projections of you, or even your dog or cat. That means social media is out; so is posting photos from this activity. This is about you and you alone. Even just ten minutes can make a meaningful difference.

Second, simply close your eyes and ask how you're feeling, and watch for what brings you joy or makes you uncomfortable.

Try one, or both. Each is a way to better know who you are as an individual, and better understand what distinguishes you from others.

Swiss psychiatrist Carl Jung believed that this process is a core aspect of human existence.[59] Hollis's writings and lectures, too, often focus on the importance of this process as a foundation for any other relationship we may have.

These insights might sound wishy-washy or even self-indulgent, but they are neither. Pausing from the constant need to respond to this or that stimulus gives us the chance to hear, then question, what we have internalized from others, and to hear, then acknowledge, what we know to be true for us, irrespective of what others say. To not explore and continually seek to know our true selves in this way, Hollis explains, is to not live life fully. In his clinical experience, not periodically exiting the stimulus-response mode is what causes people to make choices that can seriously harm themselves or others in the long run.

A different perspective on the benefit of this protocol comes from psychologist Alfred Adler, who believed the need to spend time alone is crucial for us to avoid an *inferiority complex*, a term he coined.[60] As Adler saw it, the feeling that we aren't as good as other people is something that gets internalized as we grow up. Maybe someone made fun of us for a particular piece of clothing we wore, maybe a parent compared us to an older brother or sister . . . we all encounter things like this. They are part of life. The problem is that we tend to take them on board. When someone teases us for how we look, we may end up thinking we look bad. When someone expresses disappointment in a grade, we may end up thinking we're not smart. You get the idea. The result is a whole lot of negative opinions about ourselves that we did not create but that we treat as our own thoughts. Adler saw self-encouragement as a powerful way out of this dynamic.[61]

But how? What would impactful self-encouragement even look like if—as we discussed several times already in chapters 3 and 6—positive self-talk isn't effective?

The answer is: Get yourself out of stimulus-response mode. Not forever. We have to fulfill our roles after all. Just for brief periods of time, but daily. Take a few minutes alone without inputs from others or even your phone.

Spending time alone can help quiet negative voices we've internalized so that we can better hear our own inner voice. It's a skill to learn to hear your own inner voice, and understand it. But it is one well worth cultivating.

This isn't to suggest that we already have the answers to every challenge. Sometimes we need to ask for help, and encouragement, from others. Psychotherapy, for instance, can be extremely beneficial. Data show that it can improve symptoms of psychological difficulties, that these improvements remain stable for years, and that these patients use less healthcare than the population at large after completing therapy.[62]

Still, for all these reasons, alone time tends to cause peaceful feelings, even for extroverts. Researchers from the Netherlands and the UK asked

178 people to keep a daily diary for twenty-one days in which they noted how much time they spent in solitude each day, regardless of the activity they were doing, among other reflections.[63] On average, days with more hours in solitude were lonelier for the participants. However, the researchers found that choice made the difference. People were happier being alone when that was what *they chose*. And across the entire study group, days with more alone time were less stressful. People tended to feel more themselves and more free from external pressure on days when they had comparably more solitude.

Combining alone time with activities that aren't part of the daily demands of life (work, errands, and such) adds to the benefit, because these "extra" activities also tend to be good for our mental health. In September 2023, *Nature Medicine* published a remarkable study by an international group of researchers in which they looked at data from five long-term studies conducted in sixteen countries enrolling more than 93,000 people.[64] This analysis found that having a hobby was tied to fewer depressive symptoms, greater happiness, and a greater sense of life satisfaction. The more time spent with these pursuits, the greater these benefits. This study focused on older adults, so one might wonder whether the benefits of a hobby are because they give people who've left the workforce something to do. But the percentage of retirees ranged from 56 percent to 99 percent among the studies included in the analysis, which means that some of the participants still held a job; the benefits cannot be explained by the notion that the hobby is simply replacing a career. Carving out time to pursue our personal interests is good for our health, whether we are still in the workforce or not.

We need time to get to know ourselves. Constantly reacting to external demands leaves no space for thoughts and feelings to surface into our full awareness. It can be tempting to think that who we are is what we do, who we know, where we live—that these are the ingredients of our identity. But when we exit the stimulus-response mode, we can tune in to questions, or even answers, that have been quietly brewing but not fully acknowledged.

Hollis speaks about these pauses as moments to "recollect," as in re-collect ourselves. I would encourage you to try it.

If you find it hard to just . . . sit there in silence, then try a different entry point. I often turn to drawing. There is no outside demand about what I draw or how I draw it. For you, it may be playing an instrument or gardening. "But those activities have to be done correctly, and I can't introspect while doing them," you might say. I get it. There is a format to many such activities, and there are often metrics by which to gauge your success at them. But that doesn't matter. The key thing is that what you're doing is not about occupying an outward role that others place on you; it's about just being you.

It is easy to fall into the trap of thinking we don't have time for these things. We do. There is always time, if not every day then at least a few times each week. I have an immensely demanding schedule and have for the last thirty or so years. I try to step away from my devices and stand or sit quietly for at least five minutes per day. Time with hobbies can be admittedly more sporadic, based on my work schedule, but I aim to spend at least an hour a week doing something completely unrelated to work or the routine demands of life.

By stepping away, you'll develop a closer relationship with your own inner voice. Insights and ideas inevitably surface. Not always right away, but everyone I know who does this protocol has described a moment when something related to a thought they had during solo time days prior suddenly shot to the surface of their awareness. The idea was a clear "go," a call to action. Or a clear "no go," a call to halt certain patterns in their life going forward—either small or large. Somehow what was previously suppressed or hidden from their awareness became clear. And it changed their life for the better.

Stories like that are not uncommon, and become the norm when we take the time to regularly exit the stimulus-response mode. They speak to the incredible power of our unconscious mind, but also to our brain as a whole. Most of us have barely tapped into our capacity to link our outward roles and inner narratives, to balance comfort and striving, and to build a life that is uniquely ours. Hollis has said, "Ask large questions, you'll live a large and interesting journey."[65] To be clear, I don't think we are all meant to be artists, just as I don't think we are all meant to be engineers. I know for certain, however, that we all have an inner and an outward life, and that learning to understand and bridge the two is key to our sense of fulfillment. That, as I understand it, is what Hollis means when he talks about creating our best possible life.

COMMON QUESTIONS:

When should I pause for gratitude? In the morning, before I go to work? At night, before I go to bed?

There is no time of day that is best for a gratitude practice. But it may work best if you decide on a specific time and place to do so, as a way to boost that conscious awareness and to help yourself stay committed.

Would going for a walk work as a way to exit the stimulus response?

Absolutely, as long as you are not turning the walk into a physically demanding exercise (see Exercise Protocol 1 for more about walking, and Exercise Protocol 3 for more about how to know when movement tips over into cardio work). And leave the phone at home. The point here is to give yourself some aimless time where the only variable worth measuring is your connection to yourself.

PERSONAL GROWTH PROTOCOL

3

Resolve Inner Pain Points Through Expressive Writing

WHAT TO DO:

- **Write for fifteen to twenty minutes about a challenging experience that affected your life.** Do this exercise four times, once per day for four consecutive days. Keep in mind:
  - Do not write for longer than twenty minutes. Set a timer and stop even if you feel you could keep going.
  - Do not worry about the quality of your writing. No one will read this but you.
  - Write about what happened, what you felt at the time, what you feel now, and any lasting repercussions, however large or small, from this experience. Be honest about everything you felt, and everything you still feel.

HOW IT WORKS:

Not everyone has experienced trauma, but if you have, I encourage you to seek out the resources to address it. Whether it happened in childhood or adulthood, trauma and the shadow it leaves can be utterly destructive to our relationship to ourselves, and ultimately to those around us. It can lead to self- or outwardly destructive patterns.[66]

How do we know if we have trauma? Trauma has a specific definition. As Paul Conti, MD, an expert on trauma, explains, it's a negative event, or set of events, that happens to you or that you observe that causes changes in your brain that significantly reduce your functionality in other areas of life.[67] Symptoms of this can show up in our behavior as hypervigilance, dissociation, or both. It can manifest as sleep disruptions, irritability, or even OCD-like or ADHD-like symptoms.[68] It can also lead to substance abuse. The challenge is that all the symptoms of trauma can arise from other causes as well. There is no blood test or even brain image to rule in or rule out psychological trauma. Not yet anyway.

For now, the only way to know if you have trauma is to seek out a formal assessment from a qualified psychologist or psychiatrist, and as Dr. Conti pointed out, "Always engage the best possible self-care, in or out of treatment." I pressed him a bit more on this.

"As people seek out help, is there anything they can do on their own?" I asked.

Turns out there is. And at first Dr. Conti's answer surprised me. Until I looked at the peer-reviewed data on it. The protocol? Expressive writing. But not a journal entry, or a poem, or a novel. Rather, a very specific form of repetitive recall of a troubling event or events. This is the protocol I mentioned in chapter 6, as a way to undo the kind of rewiring that happens in their wake.

Social psychologist James Pennebaker developed the research for this protocol, beginning with a study in the 1980s.[69] He and a colleague asked forty-six participants, all university students, to write about traumatic life events once a day for four days consecutively. For comparison, another group followed the same writing schedule but focused only on trivial occurrences. The researchers collected health records and recorded moods and physical symptoms self-reported by the participants. People writing about traumatic events experienced a decline in mood and an increase in blood pressure immediately following the exercise. But over the following six months, they had fewer visits to the university health center.

Two years later, Pennebaker followed up with another study in which fifty students did the same exercise: Write about a traumatic experience or trivial topic four days in a row.[70] This time, though, the researchers did not use self-reported data. Instead, alongside measuring blood pressure and heart rates before and after the writing exercise, the researchers also collected blood samples and tested blood for two markers of immune system function. Here, again, the exercise proved beneficial to health and mood. Writing about trauma, the researchers concluded, boosted immune function, led to less physical illness, and reduced stress.

A deluge of work on journaling about difficult experiences followed. More than 1,400 papers on expressive writing are now part of the scientific literature, with interest increasing in the forty years since Pennebaker's first studies.[71] A 2004 meta-analysis of nine papers confirmed the improvements in health tied to this type of expressive writing.[72] Among the groups for which this approach has shown a benefit are adolescents, people undergoing cancer treatment, caregivers, people suffering from post-traumatic stress disorder, people experiencing depression, along with many others. Expressive writing isn't a cure. But decades of data provide undeniable evidence that it helps with mental health—and physical health.

Why? What is going on under the surface that makes this simple act work? The mechanisms behind this are multiple, but studies suggest that the most powerful lies in how this type of writing affects the prefrontal cortex. Creating cohesive narratives that are honest—that is, truthful, even when the experience is painful to recount—appears to stimulate this region of the brain in a way that benefits us both psychologically and physically.

Let's zero in on the "honest" part of the equation. A study from 2017 shows the hardwiring of this trait to the prefrontal cortex. Researchers from the University of Zurich, the University of Chicago, and Harvard University gave the 145 study participants a cash reward every time they won a die-rolling game.[73] Only the person who threw the die knew their own results. The test was rigged in a way that put the chances of winning any round at 50 percent.

Here's where the experiment gets interesting: During the challenge, the researchers applied transcranial stimulation (a noninvasive application of a weak electric current to the scalp) to the prefrontal cortex of half the participants. Specifically, this electric current reached the dorsolateral region of the prefrontal cortex, an area activated when we are choosing whether or not to be honest. The group with this stimulation reported winning 58 percent of their rolls, which meant they had lied approximately 15 percent of the time. The group without this stimulation reported winning 68 percent of the time, which meant they had lied about their rolls about 37 percent of the time. The full study included more tests to gain insight into what exactly was going on here. The researchers concluded that this brain region regulates honesty specifically when lying would benefit us.

The amygdala, by contrast, is connected to stress, fear, and anxiety. People under duress tend to have heightened activity in this part of the brain.[74] Activation of the amygdala triggers the release of adrenaline and cortisol,[75] which are crucial for responding to challenges and processing the memory of them. That helps when we're faced with similar challenges in the future. But the overabundance of these chemicals appears to affect the immune system, decreasing our ability to mount an immune response over time.[76]

The specific journaling exercise pioneered by Pennebaker likely works because it avoids activating the amygdala and instead connects to the prefrontal cortex. An added benefit is that any time spent with tasks that deliberately engage the prefrontal cortex may improve brain plasticity, which has a long-term benefit on cognitive function (for more on this link, turn back to chapter 6).[77]

This type of journaling is not necessarily comfortable. It asks us to revisit the most difficult experiences in our lives—four times. But the point of this exercise is not to feel good in the short term. The point is to create a better relationship with our past, with our emotions about the past, and with ourselves. And remember, this isn't about moving through current conflicts or other difficulties but rather about moving past old wounds that hold us back.

As for doing the writing exercise four times, for four days in a row, the reason is simple. That time frame allows us greater depth of reflection. It takes time to process old wounds, partly because they are just that—wounds. Sticking with this exercise for four days gives you the chance to see how you felt about it then and how you feel about it now, but without that internal dialogue becoming an open-ended rumination, which ends up occupying even more mental real estate. The idea here is to deal with those past pains in a way that lets you make peace with them, and then move forward. Four days is a low commitment. And Pennebaker himself has given this advice: If it doesn't work for you, then stop doing it.[78]

COMMON QUESTIONS:

Does it matter what time of day this exercise is done?

No. There is nothing about the mechanisms behind expressive writing that draws on physiological changes associated with day and night. Do this protocol at whatever time of day you're able to set aside the time, about fifteen to twenty minutes, plus perhaps a few minutes to recover before moving to the next part of your day.

I did this as described here and I don't feel any better about the past.

This exercise is not designed to resolve emotional pain entirely. It has physical and psychological health benefits, but it is not a cure. Therapy or other interventions are often needed in order to work through emotional pain so that it no longer affects us negatively. Meditation, EMDR, hypnosis, exercise, and other techniques are all widely available. I cannot say what approach will work for you but if you are suffering from emotional pain, then do not hesitate to seek professional help.

PERSONAL GROWTH PROTOCOL

4

Reframe Loss to Effectively Move Through Grief

WHAT TO DO:

- **Understand grief as a lack of reward.** Over time, your brain has learned to predict certain events, like our expectation of someone's voice or smell. It is a process that draws on our expectation of a "reward" that is no longer there.
- **Spend ten to thirty minutes a day to deeply feel your attachment to the person, animal, or thing you are grieving.** Do not try to reduce the intensity of your reaction to this attachment. Experience it fully.
- **Avoid what-if thoughts.** Try not to dwell on how else a situation might have gone.

HOW IT WORKS:

Losing people, animals, and things is part of life. It's healthy and normal to experience grief in the wake of those events, provided it eventually wanes. What's "eventually"? That depends. The loss of a parent or sibling is devastating. The loss of a keepsake can be, too, but in a very different way. These are obviously not the same. But no matter who or what we lose, grief has some hallmark features because in every case it is a fracture in our reward-prediction brain circuitry. What's more, it requires our brain to remap; these circuits, which once had us expecting someone we love to walk in the room, are still there, even if that someone is no longer there. We must reorganize our awareness of what's now in our proximity and come to learn what actions related to the person or thing lost are no longer, well, actionable.

The purpose of this protocol is not to intellectualize, avoid, nor exacerbate grief. It's to ensure you don't get stuck in what is called maladaptive grief, also called complicated or prolonged grief disorder, in which grief interferes with life long after the loss initially occurred, which can be extremely detrimental to your physical and mental health.[79]

I want to note too that this protocol should not replace tools and insights derived from extensive studies of bereavement, like cognitive behavioral therapy for prolonged grief,[80] which call for being wary about heavy drinking in the year or two immediately following a death,[81] and for doing things that keep you in the flow of life like still holding dinner plans and getting exercise.[82] Rather, it offers an understanding about grief, based in neuroscience, that may help you cope with these strong and difficult feelings that come in after loss.

The first component of this framework requires a shift in thinking: Consider grief not as a state of sadness but rather as a state of longing. Brain-imaging studies have found that grief activates regions and circuitries that are involved with motivation and craving. A study led by neuroscientist and grief researcher Mary-Frances O'Connor, at UCLA, proved just that. O'Connor and her team imaged the brains of twenty-three women who were actively experiencing grief, eleven of whom were experiencing a state referred to as prolonged or complicated grief,[83] generally defined as intense, debilitating, and unrelieved grief lasting more than a year. The women viewed photographs of the deceased and words related to their death as brain images were taken using functional magnetic resonance imaging.

Brain images of the women with complicated grief showed activity in pathways connected to motivation and reward during moments when the women reported feelings of yearning. These neural circuitries lead to the release of chemicals that make us feel good, like dopamine, serotonin, and oxytocin, keeping us motivated to obtain things that are good for us, like food and social connections. Specifically, the images showed activation of the nucleus accumbens, which releases dopamine during social interactions.[84] This (at the time) surprising observation led the researchers to hypothesize that grief is akin to searching for a reward that never arrives. We stay motivated to keep finding it, but we don't—and can't. That makes sense to anyone who has experienced grief but until O'Connor's work, neuroscientists were unaware that grief was tied to reward anticipation circuits in the brain.

We all experience loss. This is a lesser example than the one described above, but simply for example: Anyone who's lost a large bill knows what it's like to look in their wallet and not find it. You can tell yourself it's just money, and you will get over it, but the loss of it brings the sudden understanding that whatever it made possible is now gone. Translate that to more emotional losses, such as a loved one or a friend or a pet. Suddenly our neural circuitry around that attachment is no longer actionable. The pathways that used to fire are still there, but they aren't useful anymore. What is possible has changed. The circuit of anticipation and action resolution remains open. And that's painful.

But motivation circuitries aren't the only ones at play in this state of longing. Our brains contain cells dedicated to mapping the world we move through—think of it like a sort of mental map of where things are.[85] Likewise, we also map our relationships, keeping track of the ties that connect us, albeit with different brain cells.

Studies have found some overlap among neurons we use to orient ourselves in space and time and those we use to understand our relationships to other people.[86] Researchers at Dartmouth College found that physical distance, proximity in time, and social closeness activate the same region of the brain, namely the inferior parietal lobe.[87] The circuitries that store information about the distance from your bed to the bathroom, from your house to the supermarket, and from your town to Paris overlap with circuitries that store information about how close another person is to you socially.

Rewiring the neural circuitries that orient us with regard to the people in our lives takes time. We experience this physically often: If you've ever rearranged the furniture in your living room, for example, you know that it can take time to remember that the couch isn't where it used to be. Grieving includes a similar reorientation but, of course, with heightened emotionality. We have to get used to our loved one not being where we always found them—arriving home from work at 6:00 p.m., at the other end of the phone, across from us at the dinner table. We no longer experience the rush of chemicals we once did when that happened, what our brain registered as a reward. Grief exists where these circuitries contradict with reality, what O'Connor refers to as the "Gone-But-Also-Everlasting" theory of grief.[88] It takes time for our brains to update. Thus grief is not only a disruption to our circuitries connected to motivation and reward, but also a difficult learning process.

Avoidance makes this learning process even harder because it prevents us from incorporating new information into the map.[89] If we are refusing to face reality, then our brains can't integrate it. As O'Connor has written, "Learning requires experience, and avoidance of things that remind the bereaved of the loved one's death or absence will prevent accommodation of the information."[90]

Instead, allowing ourselves to really feel our attachment to a person we've lost, a pet who's died, or even a missing object that held sentimental value, without denying what happened, gives our brains a chance to decouple the object of our love from our current environment and our brain's expectation of being able to interact with the person (or pet) that was lost. This decoupling—accepting a death while also savoring the memories and the essence (meaning our internal representation of the person themselves)—allows us to hold on to these important feelings without triggering a prediction that, say, the person will be waiting for us in the kitchen when we arrive home from work. Taking time to feel this attachment allows our brains to consolidate new memories and create maps, or expectations, about our lives.

Some researchers suggest what they call grief rituals as a way to "be" with a deceased loved one.[91] A person might light a candle, spend time with a photograph, or write a letter to the person, for example. Visiting a grave can be understood as a grief ritual. These ceremonial acts allow us to experience feelings of loss in a way that helps us begin to separate the person (or other object of our grief) from our new reality.

Finally, a word about counterfactual thinking that sometimes arises during the grief process, those "what-if" thoughts that have us imagining a different outcome if only we'd come home earlier, taken a different route, said a kind word, or spent more time with them. A psychologist friend of mine once told me "if only" are the two most destructive words we can think, say, or write. Had I known that long ago, I would have saved myself a lot of pain, and had I known the modern neuroscience of grief, I would have understood that pain I felt (and sometimes still feel) is one of yearning, a natural reflex to act—call, write, see that person—that is impossible to carry out.

It's a mistake to wonder why we still aren't over that pain, to suppress it. But the biggest mistake is to ruminate in "if only." That type of thinking inhibits the grief process. It's a lie about an alternate reality that truly blocks recovery. In one study, researchers examined links between counterfactual thoughts and symptoms stemming from prolonged grief and depression among fifty-nine people suffering a recent loss.[92] They found a strong correlation. People who engaged in what-if thinking experienced a longer period of grieving and symptoms of depression.

Besides, grief is hard enough without the guilt. Psychology, philosophy, religion—all these disciplines have considered grief, tried to help us understand why we experience it and how to live with it. The protocol above is one of neuroscience's offerings. Understand that grief is like a craving for a reward that is no longer coming. Make space to feel the deep attachment, whether through small rituals or just finding moments in your day to pause and fully experience your feelings. This time will allow your brain circuitries to rewire, creating memories along with new mental maps. Finally, resist engaging in counterfactual thinking, which can prolong suffering, trigger feelings of guilt, and exacerbate any depressive symptoms arising during this period.

COMMON QUESTIONS

What is a healthy amount of time for grief?

Psychologists tend to consider prolonged grief to be grief that is debilitating and lasts more than a year. With prolonged grief, people feel depressed and hopeless, often stop engaging socially, and may have little appetite.

Not all grief is like this, but it's hard to put a time frame on when any grief should end, since the process is so personal. It's more important to understand what healthy grieving is, rather than putting a time frame on the process. Allow yourself the time and space to be with your deep feelings of attachment and closeness and let the process unfold

What I can say, though, is that one day, you might be walking along and remember someone you lost, and you might experience that person—not just the memory of them, but *them*—as a completely positive presence that somehow (and I don't have any science to explain this) is fully integrated into who and where you are now, right at that moment. Meaning: You know they are gone, and yet they are still very present. The remapping has occurred. That's happened in my life many times over. To me, that is the end stage of the grief process, one that fortunately never subsides. It just takes some time to get there.

Before You Turn the Last Page

Although this is the end of the book, I hope you see it as a beginning—the start of a new direction for your health that is rooted in a deeper understanding of the incredible thing that is the human brain and body, and how each and every one of us can improve our mental and physical health and learn new things that rewire our nervous system. As I mentioned in the introduction, each of our lives is its own kind of laboratory. There is no question that there are hardwired aspects of the human brain and body, common to us all, and thank goodness for those aspects. They are much of what the protocols in this book are based on, and why they work.

But we should all also acknowledge our individuality. So whether you are working on improving your sleep or stress control, changing your exercise regimen or nutrition to get leaner, stronger, more mobile, or all the above, it's important that you honor the universal aspects of human biology but also feel free to make adjustments to suit your needs. The right way to do that—the scientific approach that is—is to become a systematic observer of you. Record your results. Then raise hypotheses, ask questions, and make changes one at a time to customize the protocols to, again, suit your needs. For reasons stated at the outset, I included a lot of science in this book. Even if you don't remember each and every mechanism, what you do recall, even vaguely, will afford you a greater sense of control over your health. My not-so-hidden wish is that you have also come to appreciate, perhaps even marvel in (as I do), the beauty and utility of biology. Together your body and brain are a miracle of astonishing precision and possibilities. They are to be honored and explored for your well-being and so you can better serve others with more vigor, joy, and meaning along the way.

Thank you for embarking on this learning journey with me and for taking your health and well-being seriously.

And, as always, thank you for your interest in science.

Acknowledgments

The idea to write a book of some sort first came up during a trip to London in 2012 when my then-girlfriend Keegan said, "You should write a book about science and about health because people don't know about the sunlight stuff, and they are confused about what to do or take for their health." (I just might have been talking about sunlight viewing and a few other things during that trip . . .)

Thank you, Keegan, for the encouragement to write what eventually became *Protocols*, and for all your love and support. Huge love and my deepest gratitude for you, Costello, and Zoë (and Zissa!), now and forever.

Also, THANK YOU:

Rob Mohr, producer of the *Huberman Lab* podcast, cofounder of Scicomm, my brother-in-arms, and the ever-steady rudder in smooth or choppy waters. It's impossible to overstate the positive impact of your friendship and support. And to Marla and Viv for being so gracious with Rob's time spent on the HLP and *Protocols*.

Celeste Fine, for being far more than a book agent. You're a true fighter on behalf of authors. I appreciate your razor-sharp mind, your balance of scrappiness and poise, and the ways you are evolving the publishing landscape. You're also my top pick to survive the apocalypse and emerge saying, "Okay, so this is what we are going to do next . . ."

Jessica Wapner, for working with me to shape the structure, content, and delivery of this book. Could. Not. Have. Done. It. Without. You!

Emily Graff, for your editing virtuosity, immense patience, ideas for this book, and encouragement to "keep going!" . . . and for allowing time for my dog stories and many tangents on Zoom calls.

Richard Rhorer, for your immense patience and optimism and for being such a champion of this project. My meetings with you and with Emily remain some of my fondest memories of working on *Protocols*.

Thank you also to Ben Kaslow-Zieve at Park, Fine & Brower, for all your efforts. Thank you, too, to Katie McClimon, Jessica Preeg, Carah Gideon, Suzanne Donnahue, Elizabeth Breeden, Jenny Carrow, Shayna Holmes, Laura Jarrett, and everyone at Simon Element and Simon & Schuster, for your efforts too.

Mike Blabac, for your fastidious eye on all things brand and photos and aesthetic, for your dry humor, and for your friendship. I have such respect for you and the way you show up in life. There is a reason Ken Block and so many others loved and love working with you and trust you to showcase them and their craft—it's the heart and soul you put into everything.

Ian Mackey, for juggling the endless mechanics and anchor points of the HLP, for stoically taking my hazing, and for laughing at anyone who acts entitled. Ever grateful you took the leap of faith to join Scicomm and, above all, for your friendship.

Chris Ray, for your insane work ethic. I've never seen anything like it (perhaps matched only by Martin!). For your insistence on perfection and style and for doing it all with such grace and fortitude. And for your friendship.

Martin Fobes, for your insistence on quality, your work ethic (you and Chris truly raise the bar!), and for doing it all with a smile, and for your friendship. The HLP would not be what it is without you, nor would this book have ever been finished.

Greg Annunziata, for your friendship, for working around the clock (literally) on my behalf, and for the endless planning, travels, and adventures. You and Coby are family, and I wouldn't have it any other way.

Special thank you to: Nick Norwitz, Andy Galpin, Alan Aragon, and Samer Hattar for lending your expertise and providing invaluable input and suggestions to make earlier versions of this book better. The readers of this book have directly benefited as a result of your hard work.

Wendy Kranz, for helping me glimpse into my possible futures way back when and for teaching me how to step into the unknown, in full stride.

Martha Beck: Wild! . . . How our paths converged. There are simply no words for how much I appreciate your love and guidance.

Greg Carroll and Jim Thiebaud, for stepping in as the wiser older brother figures that I (and so many other guys) needed way back when . . . and, as life would have it, again in my thirties, and in my forties. Greg, I hope in the next life you get the childhood you had to forego to take care of the rest of us. You more than deserve it. Jim, thanks for giving me my first black coffee, journal, pen, and the Crimpshrine tape. I've never been the same.

Tim Armstrong, for bringing such sheer honesty, bravery, and passion to your art and to every aspect of life, for shining a light on human nature, for teaching me how to navigate this gig, and for soundtracking reality. Your music, advice, and friendship have been (and remain) a lifeline.

Elvis Cortez, for your friendship, for finding Costello, and for Strummer, and for quietly demonstrating what dedication and HARD WORK really looks like.

Toby Morse, for your friendship and the incredible energy and positivity you bring to all you do. You're one of a kind. And to Moon and Max and Stella. Love your punk rawk family!

Rick Rubin, for teaching me how to remove energy blocks and distractions, for your friendship, and for the Joe Strummer stories. Huge love for you, Muriel, and Ra.

Lex Fridman, for encouraging me to start a podcast, for being a loyal brother and friend, and for continually taking calculated risks to grow. And for pushing me to be braver.

Joe Rogan, for your friendship and guidance, and for being such an unstoppable and fearless renegade creative. You have forever changed the game of public discourse. It's been an honor to witness, and it's opened the doors for so many others, including me. Thank you.

Frank and Krista Speno, for your friendship and support, and for the utterly beautiful example of family and all its workings.

Ryan Soave, for teaching me yoga nidra, for healing so many people, for your irreverent humor, and of course for your friendship.

Coleman Ruiz, for teaching me that it all starts with remaining expressionless in the freezing cold and for modeling true vulnerability and resilience. And for your friendship.

Eddie Penny, for encouraging me to start reading the Bible and pray, for reminding me not to look to humans for what only God can do and provide, and for being a constant watchdog against evil and darkness. A lot of people talk about faith, but you exemplify what it is to go ALL IN. Thank you.

Harper Carroll, for your love and support. The brilliance, love, and passion you bring to all you do is unmatched. Evvie too. Grateful for you both.

Eddie Chang, for your friendship and for that extraordinarily brilliant mind of yours. For the countless hours we've spent talking about neuroscience and life path selection. I feel blessed to understand the significance of your scientific and clinical work and to also know the depth and rigor (and soul) you bring to it . . . and to your family and friends. You're truly N of 1.

Jocko Willink, for modeling what discipline of mind and action doesn't just sound like but looks like, EVERY. SINGLE. DAY. For your friendship, humor, and for keeping the hardcore energy flowing. Oi!

Cameron Hanes, for your friendship and for always raising the bar. I don't think people understand what it takes to make it through one of your typical days. Correction: They *don't* understand. But I've seen it and it's super inspiring. I'll never forget at the 2024 Olympic Trials, the runners seeing you in the stands during their victory laps, stopping and coming up to thank you. That's not an accident; that's you making the most of all God's gifts and lessons. I strive harder every day because of your example.

Ken Rideout, for your friendship and for the way you care for your family and friends. You're a super athlete but it's your love for Shelby, Tensae, and the boys that makes me honored to know you, much less to be able to call you a friend.

Kelly Boys, for your friendship, love, support, and irreverent sarcasm, and for leading the nidra/NSDR mission with such grace and purpose. I admire and appreciate the way you approach all you do.

Jeff Cavaliere, for your friendship and for being such a great colleague and source of encouragement. For the work you do—it's kept me out of the hurt locker, mobile and strong.

David and Sophie and Vivian and Lucas, for taking me and Costello in and for always giving me a seat at the dinner table even if I never let anyone know if I'm showing up.

Steve Fish and Layla, for the middle of the night calls and incredible support and friendship.

Gary Holl, for your friendship all these (thirty-six!) years, the encouragement to go big, and for modeling what diligence and consistency (in everything!) looks like. Much love to you and Victoria.

Jacob Rosenberg, for your friendship, for having the foresight to record everything way back when (!), and for reminding me of how themes link up over time to ultimately create each of our life stories. Much love to your whole family.

Joel Rosenberg, you're an inspiration to people at every age to never stop learning and moving!

Michael Muller, for your friendship, for taking me out of the cage in Lupe, and for keeping the fire going at all hours, and for always being on call for an emergency or adventure.

Nolan Williams, for your friendship and for amazing contributions to science and treatments for PTSD and addiction. You are missed.

Andre Valente, for your friendship, encouragement to teach publicly, and for being such an incredible (yet quiet and humble) ambassador for science and scientists.

Khalil Rafati, no, your name does not get to be in all capital letters—ha! But thank you for the way you genuinely lift up all those around you, for being the one to always say the forbidden thing simply so people can feel *more* relaxed. And to Taylor, for also being a dear friend and the one who keeps things from going off the rails.

Brian Mackenzie, for your friendship and for always peering out over that next edge to build and discover new tools. For keeping an eye out for danger and for staying true to your mission and encouraging me to do the same.

Tyler Ramsey (and Jackie and River and Violet!) for all the love, friendship, support, and constant flood of good vibes.

Gabrielle Lyon, for your friendship and for always checking in on me.

Diana, for your love and friendship, and the constant reminder that some people not only can but must eat ice cream and doughnuts once per week.

Ari and Sharon, for the decades now of friendship, love, and support at every turn.

James Sexton, for your advice, friendship, and humor, and sharing more punk and movie references and quotes per unit time than anyone else I know.

Eleni, for helping me get off to college and steer myself right, and for teaching me about love and dedication.

Hilary and Mark, for your support and friendship.

Marc Andreessen and Laura Arrillaga-Andreessen, for your friendship and support and the endless ways you support science and medicine and more.

Tess, for your friendship and insights that only the children of scientists could possibly understand!

Michael Englander, for your friendship and support and for asking the truly big questions at the heart of it all.

Neggy Rismanchi, for all your love and support all these years.

Julian Retana, for helping to build the flagship studio in Topanga and for friendship.

Julia (Gulia), for your love and friendship and endless humor. And for your loyalty and advocacy. My immense respect and love.

Whitney Cummings, for your friendship and for teaching me how to navigate this crazy life and town. For the real conversations and laughter. So much love for you, Henry, Mona, and Frank.

Justin Mager, for your friendship and guidance.

Chris Williamson, for your friendship and for breathing so much life into the podcast (everyone)sphere!

MJL: I wouldn't have made it very far without your support, much less here. THANK YOU.

Paul Conti, for the many incredible conversations and support, insights into the human mind, and for helping me better understand mine.

And to the many other friends that gave and continue to give love and support along the way: THANK YOU: EJ Chichilnisky, Dave Morin, David Berson, Bill Guido, Rachel Wong, Jeff Goldberg, Chris and Denise Niell, Matt Walker, Hoby Darling, Chris Voss, Rhonda Patrick, Shawn Ryan, Tom and Lisa Bilyeu, Craig and Keli Koniver, Adam Haidary, Steven Bartlett, Jay Shetty, Mark Hyman, Lewis Howes, Ben Bruno, Josh Trachtenberg, Rich Roll, Tim Ferriss, Laird Hamilton and Gabby Reece, Pat Dossett, Brooke Jaye, Mark Bell, Nsima Inyang, Derek, Rory Cordial, Peter Attia, Julia Allison, Tom Segura, Bert Kreischer, Luca Padua, DJ Shipley, Marcus and Amber Capone, Noelle Fischer, Rich and Kristen Diviney, John Joseph, Darin Olien, Orin Snyder, Jimmy Asci, Mark Kalan, Benjamin Reese, Mark Whiteley, Dusty Brown, Erik Gambatese, Larissa Martinez, Bob Peters, Ari Emmanuel and

Ben Davis at WME, Justin Edbrooke and Ethan Kurtzman at CAA, Michael Kives . . . and on and on and on.

Immense thanks to my scientific mentors. There are really no words to express my gratitude to Harry Carlisle, Barbara Chapman, and Ben Barres for teaching me how to do science right and for being more than just mentors—for being guides for me in science and life. I miss you each and all so much.

My Portland family: Jocelyn, Henry, Nina, Sunny, Daniel: for all the encouragement, laughs, and love.

Deanna F., for all your care and guidance. Incalculable.

Emmy, Baya, Lennon, for your love and support. Huge love for you now and forever.

Stanford and Stanford Medicine, for being so supportive of the HLP and for being such pillars of excellence. It's an extraordinary thing to be surrounded by so many brilliant and mission-driven people.

The members of the "original" Huberman Lab—the staff, students, postdocs, and all those who came through and contributed to the experiments and culture of hard work and playful discovery. I am immensely grateful for your (often heroic) efforts and for you each as people as well.

Aunt Sue, for your love and all the animal photos and advice on life. I am blessed to have you in my corner and I love you.

Rick, Dan, Gena, Maddie, for your love and support and always being there to encourage.

And all the Argentine relatives for the love and messages, laughter and reminders to come visit in Buenos Aires.

Mom, for instilling in me a desire and drive to help the world, not just because one can and should but because we feel we absolutely must.

Dad, for instilling in me a love of science and discovery.

Mike, for your encouragement and support. Mette, for your encouragement and support.

Isabel, for helping me research HLP episodes, the eye rolls, for making family gatherings so joyful, and for your dry sense of humor.

Lara, for the laughs and love, loyalty, and friendship. Love you, Leff.

Emily, for your love, your seemingly endless patience and support, your optics on people and life that only someone as grounded, calm, and yet observant could possibly have. For being so genuinely kind and expressing your wish to make life easier for me. I am so blessed to have you and Nino and Strummer in my life.

All the HLP guests: Thank you for sharing so much valuable knowledge with the public, for trusting me to showcase your voices, and for allowing me to be in the role of student. I am truly blessed to be able to sit and learn from you much less to be able to share that with so many people.

HLP listeners and readers of this book: Thank you for embracing the material—including my occasional stumbling and perpetual lack of succinctness. I appreciate your openness to science, to protocols, to learning, and to your commitment to improving yourself and, in doing so, the world.

God. Acknowledging out loud that I am a scientist who also has faith was once scary.

No more. Thank you.

Notes

A note to the reader about the references below:

Specific statements or mention of specific studies in the main text are numerically referenced below. For each chapter, general references such as textbooks, comprehensive reviews, and book chapters are also cited early on. Where a set of findings or general conclusion is discussed in the text, multiple references (and often textbooks and chapters also) are listed together. Anyone interested in the substantiation of a specific statement or general theme within a chapter should see the specific references cited at the end of that sentence and within the preceding paragraphs, as well as the general book chapter and review materials for that chapter, and relevant references therein.

Introduction

[1] Konstantinos I. Avgerinos et al., "Effects of Creatine Supplementation on Cognitive Function of Healthy Individuals: A Systematic Review of Randomized Controlled Trials," *Experimental Gerontology* 108 (2018): 166–73, https://doi.org/10.1016/j.exger.2018.04.013.

Chapter 1: Protocols for Sleep

[1] Meir H. Kryger et al., *Kryger's Principles and Practice of Sleep Medicine*, 7th ed. (Elsevier UK, 2022); Alexander J. Scott et al., "Improving Sleep Quality Leads to Better Mental Health: A Meta-Analysis of Randomised Controlled Trials," *Sleep Medicine Reviews* 60 (December 2021): 101556, https://doi.org/10.1016/j.smrv.2021.101556; Esther Yuet Ying Lau et al., "A Longitudinal Investigation of the Bidirectional Relationship of Sleep Quality with Emotional Stability and Social Cynicism in a Large Community Sample," *Sleep Health* 7, no. 3 (2021): 384–89, https://doi.org/10.1016/j.sleh.2021.03.007. Luciana Besedovsky et al., "Sleep and Immune Function," *Pflügers Archiv: European Journal of Physiology* 463 (2012): 121–37, https://doi.org/10.1007/s00424-011-1044-0; Ken A. Paller et al., "Memory and Sleep: How Sleep Cognition Can Change the Waking Mind for the Better," *Annual Review of Psychology* 72 (January 2021): 123–50, https://doi.org/10.1146/annurev-psych-010419-050815; Bryce A. Mander et al., "Wake Deterioration and Sleep Restoration of Human Learning," *Current Biology* 21, no. 5 (2011): R183–84, https://doi.org/https://doi.org/10.1016/j.cub.2011.01.019.

[2] Healthy People 2030, "Increase the Proportion of Adults Who Get Enough Sleep—SH-03," data from the National Health Interview Survey, accessed September 30, 2024, https://health.gov/healthypeople/objectives-and-data/browse-objectives/sleep/increase-proportion-adults-who-get-enough-sleep-sh-03/data?tab=data-table#data-table.

[3] Endurance O. Evbayekha et al., "Sleep Deprivation Is Associated with Increased Risk for Hypertensive Heart Disease: A Nationwide Population-Based Cohort Study," *Cureus* 14, no. 12 (2022): e33005, https://doi.org/10.7759/cureus.33005; Chun Seng Phua et al., "Relationship Between Sleep Duration and Risk Factors for Stroke," *Frontiers in Neurology* 8 (August 2017): 392, https://doi.org/10.3389/fneur.2017.00392; Eve Van Cauter et al., "The Impact of Sleep Deprivation on Hormones and Metabolism," *Medscape Neurology*, April 28, 2005, https://www.medscape.org/viewarticle/502825; Ali Darraj, "The Link Between Sleeping and Type 2 Diabetes: A Systematic Review," *Cureus* 15, no. 11 (2023): e48228, https://doi.org/10.7759/cureus.48228; Yuan Pan et al., "The Association Between Sleep Deprivation and the Risk of Cardiovascular Diseases: A Systematic Meta-Analysis," *Biomedical*

Reports 19, no. 5 (September 2023): 78, https://doi.org10.3892/br.2023.1660; Francesco P. Cappuccio and Michelle A. Miller, "Sleep and Cardio-Metabolic Disease," *Current Cardiology Reports* 19, no. 11 (September 2017): 110, https://doi.org/0.1007/s11886-017-0916-0; Peter Y. Liu and Radha T. Reddy, "Sleep, Testosterone and Cortisol Balance, and Ageing Men," *Reviews in Endocrine and Metabolic Disorders* 23 (September 2022): 1323–39, https://doi.org/10.1007/s11154-022-09755-4; Peter Y. Liu et al., "Clamping Cortisol and Testosterone Mitigates the Development of Insulin Resistance During Sleep Restriction in Men," *Journal of Clinical Endocrinology and Metabolism* 106, no. 9 (May 2021): e3436-48, https://doi.org/10.1210/clinem/dgab375; Suling Zhang et al., "Effects of Sleep Deprivation on Heart Rate Variability: A Systematic Review and Meta-Analysis," *Frontiers in Neurology—Sleep Disorders* 16 (2025): 1556784, https://doi.org/10.1177/25424823251391704; Jaruwan Vierra et al., "Effects of Sleep Deprivation and 4-7-8 Breathing Control on Heart Rate Variability, Blood Pressure, Blood Glucose, and Endothelial Function in Healthy Young Adults," *Physiological Reports* 10, no. 13 (July 2022): e15389, https://doi.org/10.14814/phy2.15389.

[4] Vijay Kumar Chattu et al., "The Global Problem of Insufficient Sleep and Its Serious Public Health Implications," *Healthcare* 7, no. 1 (2019): 1, https://doi.org/10.3390/healthcare7010001; Healthy People 2030, "Sleep," accessed September 30, 2024, https://health.gov/healthypeople/objectives-and-data/browse-objectives/sleep; Alberto R. Ramos et al., "Sleep Deprivation, Sleep Disorders, and Chronic Disease," *Preventing Chronic Disease* 20 (August 2023): 230197, https://dx.doi.org/10.5888/pcd20.230197.

[5] Matthew Walker, *Why We Sleep: Unlocking the Power of Sleep and Dreams* (Scribner, 2017).

[6] "2025 Sleep in America Poll," National Sleep Foundation, March 6, 2025, https://www.thensf.org/wp-content/uploads/2025/03/NSF_SIA_2025-Report_final.pdf.

[7] Nathaniel F. Watson et al., "Joint Consensus Statement of the American Academy of Sleep Medicine and Sleep Research Society on the Recommended Amount of Sleep for a Healthy Adult: Methodology and Discussion," *Journal of Clinical Sleep Medicine* 11, no. 8 (2015): 931–52, https://doi.org/10.5664/jcsm.4950.

[8] Healthy People 2030, "Increase the Proportion."

[9] Tanner J. Bommersbach et al., "Insufficient Sleep Among US Adolescents Across Behavioral Risk Groups," *JAMA* 335, no. 13 (March 2026): 1173–76, https://doi.org/10.1001/jama.2026.1417.

[10] J. Miguel Cisneros-Franco et al., "Critical Periods of Brain Development," *Handbook of Clinical Neurology* 173 (2020): 75–88, https://doi.org/10.1016/B978-0-444-64150-2.00009-5.

[11] Valerie J. Sydnor et al., "Investigating Hierarchical Critical Periods in Human Neurodevelopment," *Neuropsychopharmacology* 51, no. 1 (January 2026): 67–85, https://doi.org/10.1038/s41386-025-02246-5; Takao K. Hensch, "Critical Period Regulation," *Annual Review of Neuroscience* 27 (July 2004): 549–79, https://doi.org/10.1146/annurev.neuro.27.070203.144327; Eric I. Knudsen, "Sensitive Periods in the Development of the Brain and Behavior," *Journal of Cognitive Neuroscience* 16, no. 8 (October 2004): 1412–25, https://doi.org/0.1162/0898929042304796; Bart Larsen et al., "A Critical Period Plasticity Framework for the Sensorimotor-Association Axis of Cortical Neurodevelopment," *Trends in Neurosciences* 46, no. 10 (October 2023): 847–62, https://doi.org10.1016/j.tins.2023.07.007.

[12] Bommersbach, "Insufficient Sleep"; Maria Fiore et al., "Digital Devices and Sleep Use in Adolescents: An Umbrella Review," *International Journal of Environmental Research and Public Health* 22, no. 10 (October 2025): 1517, https://doi.org/10.3390/ijerph22101517.

[13] Isabel Silva and Daniela Costa, "Consequences of Shift Work and Night Work: A Literature Review," *Healthcare* 11, no. 10 (2023): 1410, https://doi.org/10.3390/healthcare11101410.

[14] Cheng Wang et al., "The Association Between Blue Light Exposure and Incidence of Type 2 Diabetes: A Prospective Study of UK Biobank," *Environmental Research* 246 (April 2024): 118070, https://doi.org/10.1016/j.envres.2023.118070; Izere Salomon et al., "Artificial Light Exposure at Night: A Hidden Risk Factor for Type 2 Diabetes," *Sleep Medicine: X* 10 (June 14, 2025): 100146, https://doi.org/10.1016

/j.sleepx.2025.100146; Cappuccio, "Sleep and Cardio-Metabolic Disease," 110; Zhang, "Effects of Sleep Deprivation on Heart Rate Variability: A Systematic Review and Meta-Analysis," 1556784.

15 Andrew Huberman, "Dr. Satchin Panda: Intermittent Fasting to Improve Health, Cognition and Longevity," *Huberman Lab* (podcast audio), March 13, 2023, https://www.hubermanlab.com/episode/dr-satchin-panda-intermittent-fasting-to-improve-health-cognition-and-longevity.

16 Diego Robles Mazzotti et al., "Human Longevity Is Associated with Regular Sleep Patterns, Maintenance of Slow Wave Sleep, and Favorable Lipid Profile," *Frontiers in Aging Neuroscience* 6 (June 2014): 134, https://doi.org/10.3389/fnagi.2014.00134.

17 Melinda A. Ma and Elizabeth H. Morrison, "Neuroanatomy, Nucleus Suprachiasmatic," StatPearls, last updated July 24, 2023, https://www.ncbi.nlm.nih.gov/books/NBK546664/.

18 Rong-Chi Huang, "The Discoveries of Molecular Mechanisms for the Circadian Rhythm: The 2017 Nobel Prize in Physiology or Medicine," *Biomedical Journal* 41, no. 1 (2018): 5–8, https://doi.org/10.1016/j.bj.2018.02.003.

19 Martha Hotz Vitaterna et al., "Overview of Circadian Rhythms," *Alcohol Research & Health* 25, no. 2 (2001): 85–93, https://pmc.ncbi.nlm.nih.gov/articles/PMC6707128/.

20 Roberto Refinetti, "Circadian Rhythmicity of Body Temperature and Metabolism," *Temperature* 7, no. 4 (2020): 321–62, https://doi.org/10.1080/23328940.2020.1743605; Davide Gnocchi and Giovannella Bruscalupi, "Circadian Rhythms and Hormonal Homeostasis: Pathophysiological Implications," *Biology* 6, no. 1 (2017): 10, https://doi.org/10.3390/biology6010010; Sujana Reddy et al., "Physiology, Circadian Rhythm," StatPearls, last updated May 1, 2023, https://www.ncbi.nlm.nih.gov/books/NBK519507/.

21 Hitoshi Okamura, "Clock Genes in Cell Clocks: Roles, Actions, and Mysteries," *Journal of Biological Rhythms* 19, no. 5 (2004): 339–458, https://doi.org/10.1177/0748730404269169.

22 "Mammoth Cave," Collections & Exhibits, University of Chicago Library, 2016, https://www.lib.uchicago.edu/collex/exhibits/discovering-beauty/mammoth-cave/.

23 Kristin D. Hussey, "Timeless Spaces: Field Experiences in the Physiological Study of Circadian Rhythms, 1938–1963," *History and Philosophy of the Life Sciences* 45, article no. 17 (2023), https://doi.org/10.1007/s40656-023-00571-w.

24 Maria-Angeles Bonmati-Carrion et al., "Living Without Temporal Cues: A Case Study," *Frontiers in Physiology* 11 (February 2020): 11, https://doi.org/10.3389/fphys.2020.00011; Jürgen Aschoff, "Circadian Rhythms in Man," *Science* 148, no. 3676 (1965): 1427–32, https://doi.org/10.1126/science.148.3676.1427.

25 Ma and Morrison, "Neuroanatomy."

26 F. K. Stephan and I. Zucker, "Circadian Rhythms in Drinking Behavior and Locomotor Activity of Rats Are Eliminated by Hypothalamic Lesions," *Proceedings of the National Academy of Sciences U. S. A.* 69, no. 6 (1972): 1583–86, https://doi.org/10.1073/pnas.69.6.1583; Robert Y. Moore and Victor B. Eichler, "Loss of a Circadian Adrenal Corticosterone Rhythm Following Suprachiasmatic Lesions in the Rat," *Brain Research* 42, no. 1 (July 1972): 201–06, https://doi.org/10.1016/0006-8993(72)90054-6.

27 Robert M. Haugh and William Markesbery, "Hypothalamic Astrocytoma: Syndrome of Hyperphagia, Obesity, and Disturbances of Behavior and Endocrine and Autonomic Function," *JAMA Neurology* 40, no. 9 (September 1983): 560–63, https://doi.org/10.1001/archneur.1983.04050080060011.

28 Ehab Tousson and Hilmar Meissl, "Suprachiasmatic Nuclei Grafts Restore the Circadian Rhythm in the Paraventricular Nucleus of the Hypothalamus," *Journal of Neuroscience* 24, no. 12 (2004): 2983–88, https://doi.org/10.1523/JNEUROSCI.5044-03.2004.

29 Charles A. Czeisler et al., "Stability, Precision and Near-24-Hour Period of the Human Circadian Pacemaker," *Science* 284, no. 5423 (1999): 2177–81, https://doi.org/10.1126/science.284.5423.2177. Kryger et al., *Kryger's Principles.*

[30] Kryger et al., *Kryger's Principles*; Anita Jagota et al., "Morning and Evening Circadian Oscillations in the Suprachiasmatic Nucleus in Vitro," *Nature Neuroscience* 3 (2000): 372–76, https://doi.org/10.1038/73943; Horacio O. De La Iglesia et al., "Antiphase Oscillation of the Left and Right Suprachiasmatic Nuclei," Science 290, no. 5492 (2000): 799–801, https://doi.org/10.1126/science.290.5492.799.

[31] Stephanie J. Crowley and Charmane I. Eastman, "Phase Advancing Human Circadian Rhythms with Morning Bright Light, Afternoon Melatonin, and Gradually Shifted Sleep: Can We Reduce Morning Bright Light Duration?," *Sleep Medicine* 16, no. 2 (February 2015): 288–97, https://doi.org/10.1016/j.sleep.2014.12.004.

[32] Renske Lok et al., "Perils of the Nighttime: Impact of Behavioral Timing and Preference on Mental Health in 73,888 Community-Dwelling Adults," *Psychiatry Research* 337 (July 2024): 115956, https://doi.org/10.1016/j.psychres.2024.115956; Kristen L. Knutson and Malcolm von Schantz, "Associations Between Chronotype, Morbidity and Mortality in the UK Biobank Cohort," *Chronobiology International* 35, no. 8 (2018): 1045–53, https://doi.org/10.1080/07420528.2018.1454458; Raha West et al., "Sleep Duration, Chronotype, Health and Lifestyle Factors Affect Cognition: A UK Biobank Cross-Sectional Study," *BMJ Public Health* 2, no. 1 (July 2024): e001000, https://doi.org/10.1136/bmjph-2024-001000.

[33] Mohit Gupta et al., "Neuroanatomy, Visual Pathway," StatPearls, last updated March 23, 2026, https://www.ncbi.nlm.nih.gov/books/NBK553189/; Onkar S. Dhande and Andrew D. Huberman, "Retinal Ganglion Cell Maps in the Brain: Implications for Visual Processing," *Current Opinion in Neurobiology* 24, no. 1 (February 2014): 113–42, http://doi.org/10.1016/j.conb.2013.08.006; Alyssa M. Rivera and Andrew D. Huberman, "Neuroscience: A Chromatic Retinal Circuit Encodes Sunrise and Sunset for the Brain," *Current Biology* 30, no. 7 (April 2020): R316–18, http://doi.org/10.1016/j.cub.2020.02.090.

[34] Ignacio Provencio et al., "Melanopsin: An Opsin in Melanophores, Brain, and Eye," *Proceedings of the National Academy of Sciences* 95, no. 1 (1998): 340–45, https://doi.org/10.1073/pnas.95.1.340; Rivera and Huberman, "Neuroscience"; Sara S. Patterson et al., "S-Cone Circuits in the Primate Retina for Non-Image-Forming Vision," *Seminars in Cell & Developmental Biology* 126 (June 2022): 66–70, https://doi.org/10.1016/j.semcdb.2021.05.004.

[35] Ignacio Provencio et al., "A Novel Human Opsin in the Inner Retina," *Journal of Neuroscience* 20, no. 2 (January 2000): 600–605, https://doi.org/10.1523/JNEUROSCI.20-02-00600.2000; Ignacio Provencio et al., "Photoreceptive Net in the Mammalian Retina," *Nature* 415, no. 493 (January 2002): 493, https://doi.org/10.1038/415493a; Rivera and Huberman, "Neuroscience."

[36] Provencio et al., "Melanopsin"; Provencio et al., "A Novel Human Opsin."

[37] Akihisa Terakita and Takashi Nagata, "Functional Properties of Opsins and Their Contribution to Light-Sensing Physiology," *Zoological Science* 31, no. 10 (2014): 653–59, https://doi.org/10.2108/zs140094.

[38] Provencio et al., "A Novel Human Opsin"; Ignacio Provencio et al., "Photoreceptive Net in the Mammalian Retina. This Mesh of Cells May Explain How Some Blind Mice Can Still Tell Day from Night," *Nature* 415, no. 6871 (January 2002): 493, https://doi.org /10.1038 /415493a.

[39] David M. Berson et al., "Phototransduction by Retinal Ganglion Cells That Set the Circadian Clock," *Science* 295, no. 5557 (February 2002): 1070–73, https://doi.org/10.1126/science.1067262; S. Hattar et al., "Melanopsin-Containing Retinal Ganglion Cells: Architecture, Projections, and Intrinsic Photosensitivity," *Science* 295, no. 5557 (February 2002): 1065–70, https://doi.org/10.1126/science.1069609.

[40] Sara S. Patterson et al., "S-Cone Circuits in the Primate Retina for Non-Image-Forming Vision," *Seminars in Cell & Developmental Biology* 126 (June 2022): 66–70, https://doi.org/10.1016/j.semcdb.2021.05.004; Rivera and Huberman, "Neuroscience."

[41] Mohamed Boubekri et al., "Impact of Windows and Daylight Exposure on Overall Health and Sleep Quality of Office Workers: A Case-Control Pilot Study," *Journal of Clinical Sleep Medicine* 10, no. 6 (2014): 603–11, https://doi.org/10.5664/jcsm.3780.

[42] Till Roenneberg et al., "Life Between Clocks: Daily Temporal Patterns of Human Chronotypes," *Journal of Biological Rhythms* 18, no. 1 (2003): 80–90, https://doi.org/10.1177/0748730402239679.

[43] Christine Blume et al., "Effects of Light on Human Circadian Rhythms, Sleep and Mood," Somnologie 23, no. 3 (2019): 147–56, https://doi.org /10.1007 /s11818-019-00215-x.

[44] Blume et al., "Effects of Light"; Manuel Spitschan and Johannes Zauner, "Light Exposure as a Modifiable Determinant of Mental Health," Current Psychiatry Reports 28, no. 1 (April 2026): 24, https://doi.org/10.1007/s11920-026-01671-7.

[45] Majd A. Alnawwar et al., "The Effect of Physical Activity on Sleep Quality and Sleep Disorder: A Systematic Review," *Cureus* 15, no. 8 (2023): e43595, https://doi.org/10.7759/cureus.43595; Masahiro Banno et al., "Exercise Can Improve Sleep Quality: A Systematic Review and Meta-Analysis," *PeerJ* 6 (July 2018): e5172, https://doi.org/10.7717/peerj.5172.

[46] Christian Cajochen, "Alerting Effects of Light," *Sleep Medicine Reviews* 11, no. 6 (2007): 453–64, https://doi.org/10.1016/j.smrv.2007.07.009.

[47] Vitaterna et al., "Overview of Circadian Rhythms"; Joshua J. Gooley et al., "Exposure to Room Light Before Bedtime Suppresses Melatonin Onset and Shortens Melatonin Duration in Humans," *Journal of Clinical Endocrinology & Metabolism* 96, no. 3 (2011): E463–72, https://doi.org/10.1210/jc.2010-2098.

[48] Shan Jiang et al., "Role of the Paraventricular Nucleus of the Hypothalamus in Sleep–Wake Regulation," *Brain Science Advances* 8, no. 3 (2022): 197–209, https://doi.org/10.26599/BSA.2022.9050017.

[49] Christophe Ribelayga and Stuart C. Mangel, "A Circadian Clock and Light/Dark Adaptation Differentially Regulate Adenosine in the Mammalian Retina," *Journal of Neuroscience* 25, no. 1 (2005): 215–22, https://doi.org/10.1523/jneurosci.3138-04.2005; Tarja Porkka-Heiskanen et al., "Adenosine: A Mediator of the Sleep-Inducing Effects of Prolonged Wakefulness," *Science* 276, no. 5316 (May 1997): 1265–68, https://doi.org/10.1126/science.276.5316.1265; Radhika Basheer et al., "Adenosine and Sleep-Wake Regulation," *Progress in Neurobiology* 73, no. 6 (August 2004): 379–96, https://doi.org/10.1016/j.pneurobio.2004.06.004.

[50] Aarti Jagannath et al., "Adenosine Integrates Light and Sleep Signalling for the Regulation of Circadian Timing in Mice," *Nature Communications* 12, article no. 2113 (2021), https://doi.org/10.1038/s41467-021-22179-z; Carolin Franziska Reichert et al., "Adenosine, Caffeine, and Sleep–Wake Regulation: State of the Science and Perspectives," *Journal of Sleep Research* 31, no. 4 (2022): e13579, https://doi.org/10.1111/jsr.13597.

[51] Kenneth P. Wright Jr. et al., "Entrainment of the Human Circadian Clock to the Natural Light-Dark Cycle," *Current Biology* 23, no. 16 (2013): 1554–58, https://doi.org/10.1016/j.cub.2013.06.039.

[52] Jasleen Kaur et al., "Physiology, Cortisol," StatPearls, last updated December 1, 2025, https://www.ncbi.nlm.nih.gov/books/NBK538239/.

[53] Catherine J. Dunlavey, "Introduction to the Hypothalamic-Pituitary-Adrenal Axis: Healthy and Dysregulated Stress Responses, Developmental Stress and Neurodegeneration," *Journal of Undergraduate Neuroscience Education* 16, no. 2 (2018): R59–60, https://www.ncbi.nlm.nih.gov/pmc/articles/PMC6057754/.

[54] Kaur et al., "Physiology, Cortisol"; Dunlavey, "Introduction to the Hypothalamic-Pituitary-Adrenal Axis"; Sarah Leach and Kazuhiro Suzuki, "Adrenergic Signaling in Circadian Control of Immunity," *Frontiers in Immunology* 11 (June 2020): 1235, https://doi.org/10.3389/fimmu.2020.01235.

[55] Christoph Szeska et al., "A Vagal Route to Memory: Evidence from Invasive and Non-Invasive Electrical Vagus Nerve Stimulation Studies and Areas for Future Clinical Application," *Frontiers in Human Neuroscience* 19 (2025): 1595737, https://doi.org/10.3389/fnhum.2025.1595737; T. Miyashita and C. L. Williams, "Epinephrine Administration Increases Neural Impulses Propagates along the Vagus Nerve: Role of Peripheral Beta-adrenergic Receptors," *Neurobiology of Learning and Memory* 85, no. 2 (March 2006): 116–124, https://doi.org/10.1016/j.nlm.2005.08.013.

[56] Jennifer A. Ross and Elisabeth J. Van Bockstaele, "The Locus Coeruleus-Norepinephrine System in Stress and Arousal: Unraveling Historical, Current, and Future Perspectives," *Frontiers in Psychiatry* 11 (January 2021): 601519, https://doi.org/10.3389/fpsyt.2020.601519.

[57] Kaur et al., "Physiology, Cortisol."

[58] Sharon Chan and Miguel Debono, "Replication of Cortisol Circadian Rhythm: New Advances in Hydrocortisone Replacement Therapy," *Therapeutic Advances in Endocrinology and Metabolism* 1, no. 3 (2010): 129–38, https://doi.org/10.1177/2042018810380214; Elliot D. Weitzman et al., "Twenty-Four Hour Pattern of the Episodic Secretion of Cortisol in Normal Subjects," *Journal of Clinical Endocrinology and Metabolism* 33, no. 1 (July 1971): 14–22, https://doi.org/10.1210/jcem-33-1-14.

[59] Weitzman et al., "Twenty-Four Hour Pattern"; Katja Petrowski et al., "The Effects of Post-Awakening Light Exposure on the Cortisol Awakening Response in Healthy Male Individuals," *Psychoneuroendocrinology* 108 (2019): 28–34, https://doi.org/10.1016/j.psyneuen.2019.05.016; E. Van Cauter et al., "Effects of Gender and Age on the Levels of Circadian Rhythmicity of Plasma Cortisol," *Journal of Clinical Endocrinology and Metabolism* 81, no. 7 (July 1996): 2468–73, https://doi.org/10.1210/jcem.81.7.8675562; Ines Wilhelm et al., "Is the Cortisol Awakening Rise a Response to Awakening?," *Psychoneuroendocrinology* 32, no. 4 (May 2007): 358–66, https://doi.org/10.1016/j.psyneuen.2007.01.008; Timothy M. Brown et al., "Recommendations for Daytime, Evening, and Nighttime Indoor Light Exposure to Best Support Physiology, Sleep, and Wakefulness in Healthy Adults," *PLOS Biology* 20, no. 3 (2022): e3001571, https://doi.org/10.1371/journal.pbio.3001571.

[60] Rachel Leproult et al., "Transition from Dim to Bright Light in the Morning Induces an Immediate Elevation of Cortisol Levels," *Journal of Clinical Endocrinology & Metabolism* 86, no. 1 (2001): 151–57, https://doi.org/10.1210/jcem.86.1.7102; Weitzman, "Twenty-Four Hour Pattern"; Katja Petrowski et al., "The Effects of Post-Awakening Light Exposure on the Cortisol Awakening Response in Healthy Male Individuals," *Psychoneuroendocrinology* 108 (October 2019): 28–34, https://doi.org/10.1016/j.psyneuen.2019.05.016.

[61] Nora A. O'Byrne et al., "Sleep and Circadian Regulation of Cortisol: A Short Review," *Current Opinion in Endocrine and Metabolic Research* 18 (June 2021): 178–86, https://doi.org/10.1016/j.coemr.2021.03.011; Petrowski et al., "Effects of Post-Awakening Light"; Van Cauter et al., "Effects of Gender and Age"; Wilhelm, "Is the Cortisol Awakening"; Brown, "Recommendations for Daytime;" Kaur, "Physiology, Cortisol."

[62] Berson, "Phototransduction"; Xiwu Zhao et al., "Prolonged Inner Retinal Photoreception Depends on the Visual Retinoid Cycle," *Journal of Neuroscience* 36, no. 15 (April 2016): 4209–17, https://doi.org/10.1523/JNEUROSCI.2629-14.2016.

[63] Vincent M. Cassone, "Avian Circadian Organization: A Chorus of Clocks," *Frontiers in Neuroendocrinology* 35, no. 1 (January 2014): 76–88, https://doi.org/10.1016/j.yfrne.2013.10.002; Deng Pan et al., "Melanopsin-Mediated Optical Entrainment Regulates Circadian Rhythms in Vertebrates," *Communications Biology* 6, no. 1054 (October 2023), https://doi.org/10.1038/s42003-023-05432-7.

[64] Lily Yan et al., "Two Antiphase Oscillations Occur in Each Suprachiasmatic Nucleus of Behaviorally Split Hamsters," *Journal of Neuroscience* 25, no. 39 (2005): 9017–26, https://doi.org/10.1523/JNEUROSCI.2538-05.2005; Jagota et al., "Morning and Evening"; De La Iglesia et al., "Antiphase Oscillation"; Colin S. Pittendrigh and Serge Daan, "A Functional Analysis of Circadian Pacemakers in Nocturnal Rodents. V. Pacemaker Structure: A Clock for All Seasons," *Journal of Comparative Physiology A* 103, no. 3 (1976): 333–55, https://doi.org/10.1007/BF01417856.

[65] Ashna Ramkisoensing et al., "Enhanced Phase Resetting in the Synchronized Suprachiasmatic Nucleus Network," *Journal of Biological Rhythms* 29, no. 1 (2014): 4–15, https://doi.org/10.1177/0748730413516750; Andries Kalsbeek et al., "Circadian Disruption and SCN Control of Energy Metabolism," *FEBS Letters* 585, no. 10 (2011): 1412–26, https://doi.org/10.1016/j.febslet.2011.03.021; Pittendrigh and Daan, "Functional Analysis."

[66] Jamie M. Zeitzer et al., "Effectiveness of Evening Phototherapy for Insomnia Is Reduced by Bright Daytime Light Exposure," *Sleep Medicine* 12, no. 8 (2011): 805–7, https://doi.org/10.1016/j.sleep.2011.02.005; Marije te Kulve et al., "Early Evening Light Mitigates Sleep Compromising Physiological and Alerting Responses to Subsequent Late Evening Light," *Scientific Reports* 9, no. 16064 (2019), https://doi.org/10.1038/s41598-019-52352-w.

[67] Shadab A. Rahman et al., "Circadian Phase Resetting by a Single Short-Duration Light Exposure," *JCI Insight* 2, no. 7 (2017): e89494, https://doi.org/10.1172/jci.insight.89494.

[68] Rahman et al., "Circadian Phase Resetting"; Sat Bir S. Khalsa et al., "A Phase Response Curve to Single Bright Light Pulses in Human Subjects," *Journal of Physiology* 549, no. 3 (June 2003): 945–52, https://doi.org/10.1113/jphysiol.2003.040477; Andrew J. K. Phillips et al., "High Sensitivity and Interindividual Variability in the Response of the Human Circadian System to Evening Light," *Proceedings of the National Academy of Sciences U. S. A.* 116, no. 24 (2019): 12019–24, https://doi.org/10.1073/pnas.1901824116; Jamie M. Zeitzer et al., "Sensitivity of the Human Circadian Pacemaker to Nocturnal Light: Melatonin Phase Resetting and Suppression," *Journal of Physiology* 526, no. 3 (August 2000): 695–702, https://doi.org/10.1111/j.1469-7793.2000.00695.

[69] te Kulve et al., "Early Evening Light"; Tomoaki Kozaki et al., "Effects of Day-Time Exposure to Different Light Intensities on Light-Induced Melatonin Suppression at Night," *Journal of Physiological Anthropology* 34, no. 27 (2015), https://doi.org/10.1186/s40101-015-0067-1.

[70] Mariana G. Figueiro and Mark S. Rea, "The Effects of Red and Blue Lights on Circadian Variations in Cortisol, Alpha Amylase, and Melatonin," *International Journal of Endocrinology* 2010 (June 2010): 829351, https://doi.org/10.1155/2010/829351; Sebastian Babilon et al., "Study Protocol for Measuring the Impact of (Quasi-)Monochromatic Light on Post-Awakening Cortisol Secretion Under Controlled Laboratory Conditions," *PLOS One* 17, no. 5 (2022): e0267659, https://doi.org/10.1371/journal.pone.0267659; Sonia Ancoli-Israel et al., "Effect of Light Treatment on Sleep and Circadian Rhythms in Demented Nursing Home Patients," *Journal of the American Geriatrics Society* 50, no. 2 (2002): 282–89, https://doi.org/10.1046/j.1532-5415.2002.50060.x.

[71] Jiexiu Zhao et al., "Red Light and the Sleep Quality and Endurance of Chinese Female Basketball Players," *Journal of Athletic Training* 47, no. 6 (November–December 2012): 673–78, http://doi.org/10.4085/1062-6050-47.6.08; Emiliano Terán et al., "Home lighting, Blue-Light Filtering, and Their Effects on Melatonin Suppression," *Scientific Reports* 16 (2026): 2850, https://doi.org/10.1038/s41598-025-29882-7.

[72] Ana Sanchez-Cano et al., "Comparative Effects of Red and Blue LED Light on Melatonin Levels During Three-Hour Exposure in Healthy Adults," *Life* 15, no. 5 (April 2025): 715, https://doi.org/10.3390/life15050715.

[73] Lynne Peeples, "The Surprising Science Behind Red-Light Therapy—and How It Really Works," *Nature* 651 (March 2026): 871–74, https://doi.org/10.1038/d41586-026-00878-1; Emiliano Terán et al., "Home Lighting, Blue-Light Filtering, and Their Effects on Melatonin Suppression," *Scientific Reports* 16, no. 2850 (January 2026), https://doi.org/10.1038/s41598-025-29882-7; Edward M. Barrett and Glen Jeffery, "LED Lighting (350–650nm) Undermines Human Visual Performance Unless Supplemented by Wider Spectra (400–1500nm+) like Daylight," *Scientific Reports* 16, no. 1 (January 2026): 3061, https://doi.org/10.1038/s41598-026-35389-6.

[74] Diego Carlos Fernandez et al., "Light Affects Mood and Learning Through Distinct Retina-Brain Pathways," *Cell* 175, no. 1 (2018): 71–84.e18, https://doi.org/10.1016/j.cell.2018.08.004.

[75] Laura-Joy Boulos et al., "Translating the Habenula—from Rodents to Humans," *Biological Psychiatry* 81, no. 4 (2016): 296–305, https://doi.org/10.1016/j.biopsych.2016.06.003.

[76] Jessica L. Ables et al., "Understanding the Habenula: A Major Node in Circuits Regulating Emotion and Motivation," *Pharmacological Research* 190 (April 2023): 106734, https://doi.org/10.1016/j.phrs.2023.106734; Sarah Cameron et al., "The Disappointment Centre of the Brain Gets Exciting: A Systematic Review of Habenula Dysfunction in Depression," *Translational Psychiatry* 14, no. 1 (2024): 499, https://doi.org/10.1038/s41398-024-03199-x; Liang Yang et al., "Stress Dynamically Modulates Neuronal Autophagy to Gate Depression Onset," *Nature* 641 (2025): 427–37, https://doi.org/10.1038/s41586-025-08807-4.

[77] Christophe D. Proulx et al., "Reward Processing by the Lateral Habenula in Normal and Depressive Behaviors," *Nature Neuroscience* 17, no. 9 (2014): 1146–52, https://doi.org/10.1038/nn.3779.

[78] Tara A. LeGates et al., "Aberrant Light Directly Impairs Mood and Learning Through Melanopsin-Expressing Neurons," *Nature* 491 (November 2012): 594–98; Fernandez et al., "Light Affects Mood"; Tenley Weil et al., "Daily Changes in Light Influence Mood via Inhibitory Networks Within the Thalamic Perihabenular Nucleus," *Science Advances* 8, no. 23 (June 2022), https://doi.org/10.1126/sciadv.abn3567; Christian Kaiser et al., "The Human Habenula Is Responsive to Changes in Luminance and Circadian Rhythm," *NeuroImage* 189 (2019): 581–88, https://doi.org/10.1016/j.neuroimage.2019.01.064.

[79] Grace E. Guindon et al., "Turn Off That Night Light! Light-at-Night as a Stressor for Adolescents," *Frontiers in Neuroscience* 18, no. 1 (July 2024): 1451219, https://doi.org/10.3389/fnins.2024.1451219; Christopher J. Young et al., "Circadian Influences on the Habenula and Their Potential Contribution to Neuropsychiatric Disorders," *Frontiers in Behavioral Neuroscience* 15, no. 1 (January 2022): 815700, https://doi.org/10.3389/fnbeh.2021.815700.

[80] Kryger et al., *Kryger's Principles and Practices of Sleep Medicine*; Mats Gillberg and Torbjörn Åkerstedt, "Body Temperature and Sleep at Different Times of Day," *Sleep* 5, no. 4 (1982): 378–88, https://doi.org/10.1093/sleep/5.4.378; Victor E. Del Bene, "Temperature," in *Clinical Methods: The History, Physical, and Laboratory Examinations*, 3rd ed., ed. H. Kenneth Walker et al. (Butterworths, 1990), https://www.ncbi.nlm.nih.gov/books/NBK331/.

[81] Leon Lack et al., "Chronotype Differences in Circadian Rhythms of Temperature, Melatonin, and Sleepiness as Measured in a Modified Constant Routine Protocol," *Nature and Science of Sleep* 1 (November 2009): 1–8, https://doi.org/10.2147/nss.s6234.

[82] Michael Bauer et al., "The Potential Influence of LED Lighting on Mental Illness," *World Journal of Biological Psychiatry* 19, no. 1 (2018): 59–73, https://doi.org/10.1080/15622975.2017.1417639.

[83] Yu-Sheng Shen, "Multiple Pathways and Mediation Effects of Built Environment on Kidney Disease Rate Via Mitigation of Atmospheric Threats," *Science of the Total Environment* 833 (August 2022): 155177, https://doi.org/10.1016/j.scitotenv.2022.155177; Manman Chen et al., "Artificial Light at Night and Risk of Depression: A Systematic Review and Meta-Analysis," *Environmental Health and Preventive Medicine* 29 (December 2024): 73, https://doi.org/10.1265/ehpm.24-00257; Xiaomeng Li et al., "Light at Night Exposure and Risk of Depression: A Meta-Analysis of Observational Studies," *Journal of Global Health* 15 (2025): 04304, https://doi.org/10.7189/jogh.15.04304.

[84] Sean W. Cain et al., "Evening Home Lighting Adversely Impacts the Circadian System and Sleep," *Scientific Reports* 10, no. 1 (2020): 19110, https://doi.org /10.1038 /s41598-020-75622-4.

[85] Blume et al., "Effects of Light."

[86] S. Paruthi et al., "Consensus Statement of the American Academy of Sleep Medicine on the Recommended Amount of Sleep for Healthy Children: Methodology and Discussion," *Journal of Clinical Sleep Medicine* 12 (November 2016): 1549–61, https://doi.org/10.5664/jcsm.6288.

[87] Melissa A. Woortman et al., "Day/Night Fluctuations of Breast Milk Bioactive Factors and Microbiome," *Frontiers in Nutrition* 12 (2025), https://doi.org/10.3389/fnut.2025.1618784.

[88] Ellen R. Stothard et al., "Circadian Entrainment to the Natural Light-Dark Cycle Across Seasons and the Weekend," *Current Biology* 27, no. 4 (2017): 508–13, https://doi.org/10.1016/j.cub.2016.12.041.

[89] Samuel E. Jones et al., "Genome-Wide Association Analyses of Chronotype in 697,828 Individuals Provides Insights into Circadian Rhythms," *Nature Communications* 10, article no. 343 (2019), https://doi.org/10.1038/s41467-018-08259-7.

[90] Freda Patterson et al., "Interactive Effects of Sleep Duration and Morning/Evening Preference on Cardiovascular Risk Factors," *European Journal of Public Health* 28, no. 1 (2018): 155–61, https://doi.org/10.1093/eurpub/ckx029.

[91] Ilona Merikanto et al., "Associations of Chronotype and Sleep with Cardiovascular Diseases and Type 2 Diabetes," *Chronobiology International* 30, no. 4 (2013): 470–77, https://doi.org/10.3109/07420528.2012.741171.

[92] Rosa Levandovski et al., "Depression Scores Associate with Chronotype and Social Jetlag in a Rural Population," *Chronobiology International* 28, no. 9 (2011): 771–78, https://doi.org/10.3109/07420528.2011.602445.

[93] Elise R. Facer-Childs et al., "Resetting the Late Timing of 'Night Owls' Has a Positive Impact on Mental Health and Performance," *Sleep Medicine* 60 (August 2019): 236–47, https://doi.org/10.1016/j.sleep.2019.05.001.

[94] Y. Takahashi et al., "Growth Hormone Secretion During Sleep," *Journal of Clinical Investigation* 47, no. 9 (1968): 2079–90, https://doi.org/10.1172/JCI105893.

[95] Weihao Wang et al., "The GH-IGF-1 Axis in Circadian Rhythm," *Frontiers in Molecular Neuroscience* 14 (September 2021): 742294, https://doi.org/10.3389/fnmol.2021.742294.

[96] Joshua E. Brinkman et al., "Physiology, Growth Hormone (Archived)," StatPearls, last updated May 1, 2023, https://www.ncbi.nlm.nih.gov/books/NBK482141/.

[97] Nikola Chung et al., "Does the Proximity of Meals to Bedtime Influence the Sleep of Young Adults? A Cross-Sectional Survey of University Students," *International Journal of Environmental Research and Public Health* 17, no. 8 (April 2020): 2677, https://doi.org/10.3390/ijerph17082677.

[98] Li-Ming Yan et al., "Chronobiological Perspectives: Association Between Meal Timing and Sleep Quality," *PLOS One* 19, no. 8 (August 2024): e0308172, https://doi.org/10.1371/journal.pone.0308172.

[99] Arcady A. Putilov et al., "Single-Item Chronotyping (SIC), a Method to Self-Assess Diurnal Types by Using 6 Simple Charts," *Personality and Individual Differences* 168 (2021): 110353, https://doi.org/10.1016/j.paid.2020.110353.

[100] Christer Hublin and Jaakko Kaprio, "Chronotype and Mortality—a 37-Year Follow-Up Study in Finnish Adults," *Chronobiology International* 40, no. 7 (2023): 841–49, https://doi.org/10.1080/07420528.2023.2215342.

[101] Rikie M. Scholtens et al., "Physiological Melatonin Levels in Healthy Older People: A Systematic Review," *Journal of Psychosomatic Research* 86 (July 2016): 20–27, https://doi.org/10.1016/j.jpsychores.2016.05.005; L. Thiélbot, "Physiology of the Pineal Body," *Progress in Brain Research* 10 (1965): 479–88, https://doi.org/10.1016/S0079-6123(08)63466-4; K. P. Minneman and R. J. Wurtman, "The Pharmacology of the Pineal Gland," *Annual Reviews of Pharmacology and Toxicology* 16 (April 1976): 33–51, https://doi.org/10.1146/annurev.pa.16.040176.000341; Josephine Arendt et al., "Physiology of the Pineal Gland and Melatonin," in *Endotext* [internet], ed. K. R. Feingold et al. (MDText.com, 2022).

[102] Jennifer A. Shekleton et al., "Improved Neurobehavioral Performance During the Wake Maintenance Zone," *Journal of Clinical Sleep Medicine* 9, no. 4 (April 2013): 353–62, https://doi.org/10.5664/jcsm.2588; Jan de Zeeuw et al., "The Alerting Effect of the Wake Maintenance Zone During 40 Hours of Sleep Deprivation," *Scientific Reports* 8, no. 1 (July 2018): 11012, https://doi.org/10.1038/s41598-018-29380-z.

[103] Gina Poe, in discussion with the author; Dante Picchioni et al., "Increased Rates of Brain Protein Synthesis During [N1,N2] Sleep: L-[1-^{11}C]leucine PET Studies in Human Subjects," *Journal of Cerebral Blood Flow & Metabolism* 43, no. 1 (2023): 59–71, https://doi.org/10.1177/0271678X221121873.

[104] Matthew P. Walker et al., "Sleep-Dependent Learning and Memory Consolidation," *Neuron* 44, no. 1 (2004): 121–33, https://doi.org/10.1016/j.neuron.2004.08.031.

[105] Matthew P. Walker and Robert Stickgold, "Sleep, Memory, and Plasticity," *Annual Review of Psychology* 57 (January 2006): 139–66, https://doi.org/10.1146/annurev.psych.56.091103.070307.

[106] Mia Michaela Pal, "Glutamate: The Master Neurotransmitter and Its Implications in Chronic Stress and Mood Disorders," *Frontiers in Human Neuroscience* 15 (October 28, 2021): 722323, https://doi.org/10.3389/fnhum.2021.722323; Roberto Malinow and Robert C. Malenka, "AMPA Receptor Trafficking and Synaptic Plasticity," *Annual Review of Neuroscience* 25 (2002): 103–26, https://doi.org/10.1146/annurev.neuro.25.112701.142758.

[107] Eve Van Cauter and Laurence Plat, "Physiology of Growth Hormone Secretion During Sleep," *Journal of Pediatrics* 128, no. 5 (1996): S32–37, https://doi.org/10.1016/s0022-3476(96)70008-2; Lauren M. Hablitz and Maiken Nedergaard, "The Glymphatic System: A Novel Component of Fundamental Neurobiology," *Journal of Neuroscience* 41, no. 37 (2021): 7698–711, https://doi.org/10.1523/JNEUROSCI.0619-21.2021.

[108] Andy R. Eugene and Jolanta Masiak, "The Neuroprotective Aspects of Sleep," *MEDtube Science* 3, no. 1 (2015): 35–40, https://pmc.ncbi.nlm.nih.gov/articles/PMC4651462/; Brinkman et al., "Physiology, Growth Hormone (Archived)"; Joshua E. Brinkman et al., "Physiology of Sleep," StatPearls, last updated April 3, 2023, https://www.ncbi.nlm.nih.gov/books/NBK482512/.

[109] Aakash K. Patel et al., "Physiology, Sleep Stages," StatPearls, last updated January 26, 2024, https://www.ncbi.nlm.nih.gov/books/NBK526132/.

[110] Oliver Cameron Reddy and Ysbrand D. van der Werf, "The Sleeping Brain: Harnessing the Power of the Glymphatic System Through Lifestyle Choices," *Brain Sciences* 10, no. 11 (2020): 868, https://doi.org/10.3390/brainsci10110868.

[111] Helene Benveniste et al., "The Glymphatic System and Waste Clearance with Brain Aging," *Gerontology* 65, no. 2 (2018): 106–19, https://doi.org/10.1159/000490349; Hablitz and Nedergaard, "The Glymphatic System."

[112] John Peever and Patrick M. Fuller, "The Biology of REM Sleep," *Current Biology* 27, no. 22 (2017): R1237–48, https://doi.org/10.1016/j.cub.2017.10.026.

[113] Patricia L. Brooks and John H. Peever, "Unraveling the Mechanisms of REM Sleep Atonia," *Sleep* 31, no. 11 (2008): 1492–97, https://doi.org/10.1093/sleep/31.11.1492.

[114] Mark S. Blumberg and Alan M. Plumeau, "A New View of 'Dream Enactment' in REM Sleep Behavior Disorder," *Sleep Medicine Reviews* 30 (December 2016): 34–42, https://doi.org/10.1016/j.smrv.2015.12.002; Patricia L. Brooks and John H. Peever, "Unraveling the Mechanisms of REM Sleep Atonia," *Sleep* 31, no. 11 (2008): 1492–97, https://doi.org/10.1093/sleep/31.11.1492.

[115] Jerome C. J. Fryer, "Is a Purpose of REM Sleep Atonia to Help Regenerate Intervertebral Disc Volumetric Loss?," *Journal of Circadian Rhythms* 7, article no. 1 (January 2009), https://doi.org/10.1186/1740-3391-7-1.

[116] Hai-Lin Chen et al., "Rapid Eye Movement Sleep During Early Life: A Comprehensive Narrative Review," *International Journal of Environmental Research and Public Health* 19, no. 20 (2022): 13101, https://doi.org/10.3390/ijerph192013101.

[117] Carissa Gardiner et al., "The Effect of Alcohol on Subsequent Sleep in Healthy Adults: A Systematic Review and Meta-Analysis," *Sleep Medicine Reviews* 80 (April 2025): 102030, https://doi.org/10.1016/j.smrv.2024.102030; Leela McKinnon et al., "Sound Reasons for Unsound Sleep: Comparative Support for the Sentinel Hypothesis in Industrial and Nonindustrial Groups," *Evolution, Medicine, and Public Health* 11, no. 1 (November 2022): 53–66, https://doi.org/10.1093/emph/eoac039; Rob Velzeboer et al., "Cannabis and Sleep Architecture: A Systematic Review and Meta-Analysis," *Sleep Medicine Reviews* 84 (December 2025): 102164, https://doi.org/10.1016/j.smrv.2025.102164; Irwin Feinberg et al., "Effects of Marijuana Extract and Tetrahydrocannabinol on Electroencephalographic

Sleep Patterns," *Clinical Pharmacology and Therapeutics* 19, no. 6 (June 1976): 782–94, https://doi.org/10.1002/cpt1976196782.

118 Elahhe Afkhamnejad and Sandhya Kumar, "The Role of Prescription Drugs in REM Sleep (P1.109)," *Neurology* 90, no. S15 (April 2018), https://doi.org/10.1212/WNL.90.15_supplement.P1.109; Gardiner et al., "Effect of Alcohol."

119 Dimitris Repantis et al., "REM Sleep in Acutely Traumatized Individuals and Interventions for the Secondary Prevention of Post-Traumatic Stress Disorder," *European Journal of Psychotraumatology* 6, no. 1 (2020): 1740492, https://doi.org/10.1080/20008198.2020.1740492.

120 William D. S. Killgore, "Effects of Sleep Deprivation on Cognition," *Progress in Brain Research* 185 (2010): 105–29, https://doi.org/10.1016/B978-0-444-53702-7.00007-5.

121 Matthew P. Pase et al., "Sleep Architecture and the Risk of Incident Dementia in the Community," *Neurology* 89, no. 12 (2017): 1244–50, https://doi.org/10.1212/WNL.0000000000004373.

122 Eileen B. Leary et al., "Association of Rapid Eye Movement Sleep with Mortality in Middle-Aged and Older Adults," *JAMA Neurology* 77, no. 10 (2020): 1241–51, https://doi.org/10.1001/jamaneurol.2020.2108.

123 Kelly Baron et al., "Circadian Phase Alignment and Sleep Duration in Overweight Adults: Associations with Cardiometabolic Risk Factors," *Sleep* 47, no. S1 (2024): A7–8, https://doi.org/10.1093/sleep/zsae067.0017; Andrew J. K. Phillips et al., "Irregular Sleep/Wake Patterns Are Associated with Poorer Academic Performance and Delayed Circadian and Sleep/Wake Timing," *Scientific Reports* 7, no. 1 (2017): 3216, https://doi.org/10.1038/s41598-017-03171-4.

124 Yinyan Gao et al., "Association Between Shift Work and Risk of Type 2 Diabetes Mellitus: A Systematic Review and Dose-Response Meta-Analysis of Observational Studies," *Chronobiology International* 37, no. 1 (2020): 29–46, https://doi.org/10.1080/07420528.2019.1683570; Johanna Samulin Erdem et al., "Night Shift Work and Indicators of Cardiovascular Risk: A Systematic Review and Meta-Analysis," *Environmental Research* 276 (July 2025): 121503, https://doi.org/10.1016/j.envres.2025.121503; Qi-Jun Wu et al., "Shift Work and Health Outcomes: An Umbrella Review of Systematic Reviews and Meta-Analyses of Epidemiological Studies," *Journal of Clinical Sleep Medicine* 18 (2022): 653–62, https://doi.org/10.5664/jcsm.9642; Minzhi Xu et al., "Lifestyle Factors in the Association of Shift Work and Depression and Anxiety," *JAMA Network Open* 6, no. 8 (2023): e2328798, https://doi.org/10.1001/jamanetworkopen.2023.28798.

125 Thomas Vlasak et al., "Neurocognitive Impairment in Night and Shift Workers: A Meta-Analysis of Observational Studies," *Occupational & Environmental Medicine* 79, no. 6 (2022): 365–72, https://doi.org/10.1136/oemed-2021-107847; Kneginja Richter et al., "Shiftwork and Alcohol Consumption: A Systematic Review of the Literature," *European Addiction Research* 27, no. 1 (2021): 9–15, https://doi.org/10.1159/000507573.

126 Rea Alonzo et al., "Does Shiftwork Impact Cognitive Performance? Findings from the Canadian Longitudinal Study on Aging (CLSA)," *International Journal of Environmental Research and Public Health* 19, no. 16 (2022): 10124, https://doi.org/10.3390/ijerph191610124.

127 Drew Dawson and Kathryn Reid, "Fatigue, Alcohol and Performance Impairment," *Nature* 388 (1997): 235, https://doi.org/10.1038/40775.

128 Jijo Varughese and Richard P. Allen, "Fatal Accidents Following Changes in Daylight Savings Time: The American Experience," *Sleep Medicine* 2, no. 1 (January 2001): 31–36, https://doi.org/10.1016/S1389-9457(00)00032-0.

129 Amneet Sandhu et al., "Daylight Savings Time and Myocardial Infarction," *Open Heart* 1, no. 1 (2014): e000019, https://doi.org/10.1136/openhrt-2013-000019.

130 Birgitte T. Hansen et al., "Daylight Savings Time Transitions and the Incidence Rate of Unipolar Depressive Episodes," *Epidemiology* 28, no. 3 (May 2017): 346–53, https://doi.org/10.1097/EDE.0000000000000580.

[131] Porkka-Heiskanen et al., "Adenosine"; Basheer et al., "Adenosine and Sleep-Wake Regulation."

[132] M. H. Hagenauer et al., "Adolescent Changes in the Homeostatic and Circadian Regulation of Sleep," *Developmental Neuroscience* 31, no. 4 (2009): 276–84, https://doi.org/10.1159/000216538.

[133] Stephanie J. Crowley et al., "Sleep, Circadian Rhythms, and Delayed Phase in Adolescence," *Sleep Medicine* 8, no. 6 (September 2007): 602–12, https://doi.org/10.1016/j.sleep.2006.12.002; Mary A. Carskadon et al., "Association Between Puberty and Delayed Phase Preference," *Sleep* 16, no. 3 (May 1993): 258–62, https://doi.org/10.1093/sleep/16.3.258; M. H. Hagenauer et al., "Adolescent Changes in the Homeostatic and Circadian Regulation of Sleep," *Developmental Neuroscience* 31, no. 4 (2009): 276–84, https://doi.org/10.1159/000216538.

[134] Adolescent Sleep Working Group, Committee on Adolescence, Council on School Health, "School Start Times for Adolescents," *Pediatrics* 134, no. 3 (2014): 642–49, https://doi.org/10.1542/peds.2014-1697.

[135] Robert D. Foss et al., "School Start Times and Teenage Driver Motor Vehicle Crashes," *Accident Analysis & Prevention* 126 (May 2019): 54–63, https://doi.org/10.1016/j.aap.2018.03.031.

[136] Anne G. Wheaton et al., "Short Sleep Duration Among Middle School and High School Students—United States, 2015," *Morbidity and Mortality Weekly Report* 67, no. 3 (2018): 85–90, https://doi.org/10.15585/mmwr.mm6703a1.

[137] Sara Uccella et al., "Sleep Deprivation and Insomnia in Adolescence: Implications for Mental Health," *Brain Sciences* 13, no. 4 (2023): 569, https://doi.org/10.3390/brainsci13040569; Wheaton et al., "Short Sleep Duration."

[138] Junxin Li et al., "Sleep in Normal Aging," *Sleep Medicine Clinics* 13, no. 1 (2018): 1–11, https://doi.org/10.1016/j.jsmc.2017.09.001.

[139] Judith A. Floyd et al., "Changes in REM-Sleep Percentage over the Adult Lifespan," *Sleep* 30, no. 7 (2007): 829–36, https://doi.org/10.1093/sleep/30.7.829.

[140] Allison G. Harvey and Suzanna Payne, "The Management of Unwanted Pre-Sleep Thoughts in Insomnia: Distraction with Imagery Versus General Distraction," *Behaviour Research and Therapy* 40, no. 3 (2002): 267–77, https://doi.org/10.1016/s0005-7967(01)00012-2.

[141] Allison G. Harvey, "The Attempted Suppression of Presleep Cognitive Activity in Insomnia," *Cognitive Therapy and Research* 27 (2003): 593–602, https://doi.org/10.1023/A:1026322310019.

[142] Nami Ohmura et al., "A Method to Soothe and Promote Sleep in Crying Infants Utilizing the Transport Response," *Current Biology* 32, no. 20 (October 2022): 4521–29.e4, https://doi.org/10.1016/j.cub.2022.08.041; Aurore A. Perrault et al., "Whole-Night Continuous Rocking Entrains Spontaneous Neural Oscillations with Benefits for Sleep and Memory," *Current Biology* 29, no. 3 (February 2019): 402–11.e3, https://doi.org/10.1016/j.cub.2018.12.028.

[143] Patricia J. Murphy and Scott S. Campbell, "Nighttime Drop in Body Temperature: A Physiological Trigger for Sleep Onset?," *Sleep* 20, no. 7 (1997): 505–11, https://doi.org/10.1093/sleep/20.7.505.

[144] Scott S. Campbell and Roger J. Broughton, "Rapid Decline in Body Temperature Before Sleep: Fluffing the Physiological Pillow?," *Chronobiology International* 11, no. 2 (1994): 126–31, https://doi.org/10.3109/07420529409055899.

[145] Yaqian Fan et al., "How Temperature Influences Sleep," *International Journal of Molecular Sciences* 23, no. 20 (2022): 12191, https://doi.org/10.3390/ijms232012191; Shreyas S. Joshi et al., "The Importance of Temperature and Thermoregulation for Optimal Human Sleep," *Energy and Buildings* 131 (November 1, 2016): 153–57, https://doi.org/10.1016/j.enbuild.2016.09.020; Kryger et al., *Kryger's Principles and Practices of Sleep Medicine.*

[146] Edward C. Harding et al., "The Temperature Dependence of Sleep," *Frontiers in Neuroscience* 13 (April 23, 2019): 336, https://doi.org/10.3389/fnins.2019.00336.

[147] Harding et al., "Temperature Dependence of Sleep."

[148] A. Cagnacci et al., "Melatonin: A Major Regulator of the Circadian Rhythm of Core Temperature in Humans," *Journal of Clinical Endocrinology & Metabolism* 75, no. 2 (1992): 447–52, https://doi.org/10.1210/jcem.75.2.1639946.

[149] James K. Wyatt et al., "Circadian Temperature and Melatonin Rhythms, Sleep, and Neurobehavioral Function in Humans Living on a 20-h Day," *American Journal of Physiology* 277, no. 4 (1999): R1152–63, https://doi.org/10.1152/ajpregu.1999.277.4.r1152; Kurt Kräuchi et al., "Thermoregulatory Effects of Melatonin in Relation to Sleepiness," *Chronobiology International* 23, no. 1–2 (2006): 475–84, https://doi.org/10.1080/07420520500545854; Stephen Deacon and Josephine Arendt, "Melatonin-Induced Temperature Suppression and Its Acute Phase-Shifting Effects Correlate in a Dose-Dependent Manner in Humans," *Brain Research* 688, no. 1–2 (1995): 77–85, https://doi.org/10.1016/0006-8993(95)96872-i.

[150] Ronald Szymusiak, "Body Temperature and Sleep," *Handbook of Clinical Neurology* 156 (2018): 341–51, https://doi.org/10.1016/B978-0-444-63912-7.00020-5.

[151] Takafumi Maeda et al., "Effects of Bathing-Induced Changes in Body Temperature on Sleep," *Journal of Physiological Anthropology* 42, article no. 20 (2023), https://doi.org/10.1186/s40101-023-00337-0.

[152] Harding, "Temperature Dependence of Sleep."

[153] Jeong-Whun Kim et al., "Polysomnographic Evidence of Enhanced Sleep Quality with Adaptive Thermal Regulation," *Healthcare* (Basel) 13, no. 19 (October 2025): 2521, https://doi.org/10.3390/healthcare13192521.

[154] Stephen R. Morairty et al., "Selective Increases in Non-Rapid Eye Movement Sleep Following Whole Body Heating in Rats," *Brain Research* 617, no. 1 (1993): 10–16, https://doi.org/10.1016/0006-8993(93)90606-n.

[155] Fang Wang et al., "The Effect of Meditative Movement on Sleep Quality: A Systematic Review," *Sleep Medicine Reviews* 30 (December 2016): 43–52, https://doi.org/10.1016/j.smrv.2015.12.001.

[156] Kazue Okamoto-Mizuno and Koh Mizuno, "Effects of Thermal Environment on Sleep and Circadian Rhythm," *Journal of Physiological Anthropology* 31, article no. 14 (2012), https://doi.org/10.1186/1880-6805-31-14.

[157] J. P. Libert et al., "Effect of Continuous Heat Exposure on Sleep Stages in Humans," *Sleep* 11, no. 2 (1988): 195–209, https://doi.org/10.1093/sleep/11.2.195.

[158] Pier Luigi Parmeggiani, "Interaction Between Sleep and Thermoregulation: An Aspect of the Control of Behavioral States," *Sleep* 10, no. 5 (1987): 426–35, https://doi.org/10.1093/sleep/10.5.426.

[159] Okamoto-Mizuno and Mizuno, "Effects of Thermal Environment."

[160] Mats Gillberg and Torbjörn Åkerstedt, "Body Temperature and Sleep at Different Times of Day," *Sleep* 5, no. 4 (1982): 378–88, https://doi.org/10.1093/sleep/5.4.378; Institute of Medicine Committee on Military Nutrition Research, "Physiological Responses to Exercise in the Heat," in *Nutritional Needs in Hot Environments: Applications for Military Personnel in Field Operations* (Washington, DC: National Academies Press, 1993), https://www.ncbi.nlm.nih.gov/books/NBK236240/.

[161] Janna Mantua and Rebecca M. C. Spencer, "Exploring the Nap Paradox: Are Mid-Day Sleep Bouts a Friend or Foe?," *Sleep Medicine* 37, no. 1 (September 2017): 88–97, https://doi.org/10.1016/j.sleep.2017.01.019; Pengqiang Du et al., "Multiple Health Outcomes of Daytime Napping: A Comprehensive Umbrella Review," *Public Health Reviews* 47, no. 1 (February 2026): 1609013, https://doi.org/10.3389/phrs.2026.1609013; Yves Dauvilliers and Alain Buguet, "Hypersomnia," *Dialogues in Clinical Neuroscience* 7, no. 4 (December 2005): 347–56, https://doi.org/10.31887/DCNS.2005.7.4/ydauvilliers.

[162] Matthew P. Walker, "Sleep, Memory and Emotion," *Progress in Brain Research* 185 (2010): 49–68, https://doi.org/10.1016/B978-0-444-53702-7.00004-X.

[163] Patel et al., "Physiology, Sleep Stages."

[164] Ninad Gujar et al., "A Role for REM Sleep in Recalibrating the Sensitivity of the Human Brain to Specific Emotions," *Cerebral Cortex* 21, no. 1 (2011): 115–23, https://doi.org/10.1093/cercor/bhq064.

[165] Thomas V. Dunwiddie and Susan A. Masino, "The Role and Regulation of Adenosine in the Central Nervous System," *Annual Review of Neuroscience* 24 (March 2001): 31–55, https://doi.org/10.1146/annurev.neuro.24.1.31.

[166] Theresa E. Bjorness and Robert W. Greene, "Adenosine and Sleep," *Current Neuropharmacology* 7, no. 3 (2009): 238–45, https://doi.org/10.2174/157015909789152182.

[167] Dunwiddie and Masino, "Role and Regulation of Adenosine"; Porkka-Heiskanen et al., "Adenosine."

[168] Mark R. Rosekind et al., "Alertness Management: Strategic Naps in Operational Settings," *Journal of Sleep Research* 4, no. S2 (1995): 62–66, https://doi.org/10.1111/j.1365-2869.1995.tb00229.x.

[169] Erin J. Wamsley, "Memory Consolidation During Waking Rest," *Trends in Cognitive Sciences* 23, no. 3 (March 2019):171–73, https://doi.org/10.1016/j.tics.2018.12.007; Olivia King and Jessica Nicosia, "The Effects of Wakeful Rest on Memory Consolidation in an Online Study," *Frontiers in Psychology* 13 (October 2022): 932592, https://doi.org/10.3389/fpsyg.2022.932592; Anika T. Löwe et al., "N2 Sleep Promotes the Occurrence of 'Aha' Moments in a Perceptual Insight Task," *PLOS Biology* 23, no. 6 (2025): e3003185, https://doi.org/10.1371/journal.pbio.3003185.

[170] Kryger et al., *Kryger's Principles.*

[171] Maher Souabni et al., "Benefits and Risks of Napping in Older Adults: A Systematic Review," *Frontiers in Aging Neuroscience* 14 (October 2022): 1000707, https://doi.org/10.3389/fnagi.2022.1000707.

[172] Omar Boukhris et al., "The Acute Effects of Nonsleep Deep Rest on Perceptual Responses, Physical, and Cognitive Performance in Physically Active Participants," *Applied Psychology: Health and Well-Being* 16, no. 4 (November 2024): 1967–87, https://doi.org/10.1111/aphw.12571; Shashank Ghai et al., "Effects of Yoga Nidra on Stress, Anxiety, and Depression: A Systematic Review and Meta-Analysis," *Annals of the New York Academy of Sciences* 1556, no. 1 (February 2026): e70149, https://doi.org/10.1111/nyas.70149; V. Kachera et al., "The Effects of Yoga Nidra Practice on EEG: A Systematic Review," *medRxiv* (June 2025), https://doi.org/10.1101/2025.06.16.25329676; Karuna Datta et al., "Improved Sleep, Cognitive Processing and Enhanced Learning and Memory Task Accuracy with Yoga Nidra Practice in Novices," *PLOS One* 18, no. 12 (December 2023): e0294678, https://doi.org/10.1371/journal.pone.0294678.

[173] Julia C. Basso et al., "Brief, Daily Meditation Enhances Attention, Memory, Mood, and Emotional Regulation in Non-Experienced Meditators," *Behavioural Brain Research* 356 (January 2019): 208–20, https://doi.org/10.1016/j.bbr.2018.08.023; Daniel Goleman and Richard J. Davidson, *Altered Traits: Science Reveals How Meditation Changes Your Mind, Brain, and Body* (Avery, 2017); Simon B. Goldberg et al., "Sitting and Active Meditation Practice: Utilization and Associations with Outcomes in Naturalistic and Clinical Trial Data," *Mindfulness* 17 (2026): 1120–37, https://doi.org/10.1007/s12671-026-02787-w; Simon B. Goldberg et al., "Mindfulness-Based Interventions for Psychiatric Disorders: A Systematic Review and Meta-Analysis," *Clinical Psychology Review* 59 (February 2018): 52–60, https://doi.org/10.1016/j.cpr.2017.10.011.

[174] Camila Ferreira-Vorkapic et al., "The Impact of Yoga Nidra and Seated Meditation on the Mental Health of College Professors," *International Journal of Yoga* 11, no. 3 (2018): 215–23, https://doi.org/10.4103/ijoy.IJOY_57_17; Seithikurippu R. Pandi-Perumal et al., "The Origin and Clinical Relevance of Yoga Nidra," *Sleep and Vigilance* 6, no. 1 (2022): 61–84, https://doi.org/10.1007/s41782-022-00202-7.

[175] Pandi-Perumal et al., "Origin and Clinical Relevance."

[176] Troels W. Kjaer et al., "Increased Dopamine Tone During Meditation-Induced Change of Consciousness," *Cognitive Brain Research* 13, no. 2 (2002): 255–59, https://doi.org/10.1016/s0926-6410(01)00106-9.

[177] Ferreira-Vorkapic et al., "Impact of Yoga Nidra"; Heather Eastman-Mueller et al., "iRest Yoga-Nidra on the College Campus: Changes in Stress, Depression, Worry, and Mindfulness," *International*

Journal of Yoga Therapy 23, no. 2 (2013): 15–24, https://doi.org/10.17761/ijyt.23.2.r8735770101m8277; Roberta Anderson et al., "Using Yoga Nidra to Improve Stress in Psychiatric Nurses in a Pilot Study," *Journal of Integrative and Complementary Medicine* 23, no. 6 (2017): 494–95, https://doi.org/10.1089/acm.2017.0046; Khushboo Nayak and Kedarmal Verma, "Yoga-Nidra as a Mental Health Booster: A Narrative Review," *Journal of Ayurveda and Integrative Medicine* 14, no. 6 (2023): 100842, https://doi.org/10.1016/j.jaim.2023.100842; Datta et al., "Improved Sleep, Cognitive Processing."

178 Melis Yilmaz Balban et al., "Brief Structured Respiration Practices Enhance Mood and Reduce Physiological Arousal," *Cell Reports Medicine* 4, no. 1 (2023): 100895, https://doi.org/10.1016/j.xcrm.2022.100895; Andrea Zaccaro et al., "How Breath-Control Can Change Your Life: A Systematic Review on Psycho-Physiological Correlates of Slow Breathing," *Frontiers in Human Neuroscience* 12 (September 2018): 353, https://doi.org/10.3389/fnhum.2018.00353; Melis Yilmaz Balban et al., "Human Responses to Visually Evoked Threat," *Current Biology* 31, no. 3 (February 2021): 601–12, https://doi.org/ 10.1016/j.cub.2020.11.035.

179 "#NSDR (Non-Sleep Deep Rest) with Dr. Andrew Huberman," Virtusan, YouTube, September 11, 2022, https://www.youtube.com/watch?v=AKGrmY8OSHM; "20 Minute Non-Sleep Deep Rest (NSDR) to Restore Mental & Physical Energy | Dr. Andrew Huberman," Huberman Lab Clips, YouTube, April 26, 2024, https://www.youtube.com/watch?v=hEypv90GzDE.

180 Karuna Datta et al., "*Yoga Nidra* Practice Shows Improvement in Sleep in Patients with Chronic Insomnia: A Randomized Controlled Trial," *National Medical Journal of India* 34, no. 3 (2021): 143–50, https://doi.org/10.25259/NMJI_63_19.

181 Prashant Kaul et al., "Meditation Acutely Improves Psychomotor Vigilance, and May Decrease Sleep Need," *Behavioral and Brain Functions* 6, article no. 47 (July 2010), https://doi.org/10.1186/1744-9081-6-47.

182 Boukhris et al., "Acute Effects of Nonsleep Deep Rest."

183 Ji Won Yeom and Chul-Hyun Cho, "Herbal and Natural Supplements for Improving Sleep: A Literature Review," *Psychiatry Investigation* 21, no. 8 (2024): 810–21, https://doi.org/10.30773/pi.2024.0121; Monica Kazlausky Esquivel and Brittany Ghosn, "Current Evidence on Common Dietary Supplements for Sleep Quality," *American Journal of Lifestyle Medicine* 18, no. 3 (2024): 323–27, https://doi.org/10.1177/15598276241227915; Vicky Chan and Kenneth Lo, "Efficacy of Dietary Supplements on Improving Sleep Quality: A Systematic Review and Meta-Analysis," *Postgraduate Medical Journal* 98, no. 1158 (2022): 285–93, https://doi.org/10.1136/postgradmedj-2020-139319.

184 Victor Navarro et al., "The Contents of Herbal and Dietary Supplements Implicated in Liver Injury in the United States Are Frequently Mislabeled," *Hepatology Communications* 3, no. 6 (June 2019): 792–94, https://doi.org/10.1002/hep4.1346; Pieter A. Cohen et al., "Quantity of Melatonin and CBD in Melatonin Gummies Sold in the US," *JAMA* 329, no. 16 (April 2023): 1401–2, https://doi.org/10.1001/jama.2023.2296.

185 Inna Slutsky et al., "Enhancement of Learning and Memory by Elevating Brain Magnesium," *Neuron* 65, no. 2 (2010): 165–77, https://doi.org/10.1016/j.neuron.2009.12.026.

186 Heather A. Hausenblas et al., "Magnesium-L-Threonate Improves Sleep Quality and Daytime Functioning in Adults with Self-Reported Sleep Problems: A Randomized Controlled Trial," *Sleep Medicine: X* 8 (December 15, 2024): 100121, https://doi.org/10.1016/j.sleepx.2024.100121.

187 A. N. Panche et al., "Flavonoids: An Overview," *Journal of Nutritional Science* 5 (December 29, 2016): e47, https://doi.org/10.1017/jns.2016.41; A. N. Panche et al., "Flavonoids: An Overview—CORRIGENDUM in Figure 1," *Journal of Nutritional Science* 14 (January 29, 2025): e11, https://doi.org/10.1017/jns.2024.73; Bahare Salehi et al., "The Therapeutic Potential of Apigenin," *International Journal of Molecular Sciences* 20, no. 6 (2019): 1305, https://doi.org/10.3390/ijms20061305.

188 Daniel J. Kramer and Adiv A. Johnson, "Apigenin: A Natural Molecule at the Intersection of Sleep and Aging," *Frontiers in Nutrition* 11 (February 26, 2024): 1359176, https://doi.org/10.3389/fnut.2024.1359176.

[189] P. Zanoli et al., "Behavioral Characterisation of the Flavonoids Apigenin and Chrysin," *Fitoterapia* 71, suppl. 1 (2000): S117–23, https://doi.org/10.1016/s0367-326x(00)00186-6; Nicholas K. Chow et al., "Telemetry as a Tool to Measure Sedative Effects of a Valerian Root Extract and Its Single Constituents in Mice," *Planta Medica* 77, no. 8 (2011): 795–803, https://doi.org/10.1055/s-0030-1250589.

[190] Suzanna M. Zick et al., "Preliminary Examination of the Efficacy and Safety of a Standardized Chamomile Extract for Chronic Primary Insomnia: A Randomized Placebo-Controlled Pilot Study," *BMC Complementary and Alternative Medicine* 11, article no. 78 (2011), https://doi.org/10.1186/1472-6882-11-78; Pandi-Perumal et al., "Origin and Clinical Relevance."

[191] Rebeka Olga Mátyus et al., "Promising, but Not Completely Conclusive—The Effect of L-Theanine on Cognitive Performance Based on the Systematic Review and Meta-Analysis of Randomized Placebo-Controlled Clinical Trials," *Journal of Clinical Medicine* 14, no. 21 (October 2025): 7710, https://doi.org/10.3390/jcm14217710.

[192] Chiara M. Portas et al., "Serotonin and the Sleep/Wake Cycle: Special Emphasis on Microdialysis Studies," Progress in Neurobiology 60, no. 1 (2000): 13–35, https://doi.org /10.1016 /s0301-0082(98)00097-5; Nobuhiro Kawai et al., "The Sleep-Promoting and Hypothermic Effects of Glycine Are Mediated by NMDA Receptors in the Suprachiasmatic Nucleus," *Neuropsychopharmacology* 40, no. 6 (2015): 1405–16, https://doi.org/10.1038/npp.2014.326.

[193] Claude Gottesmann, "GABA Mechanisms and Sleep," *Neuroscience* 111, no. 2 (2002): 231–39, https://doi.org/10.1016/s0306-4522(02)00034-9.

[194] Rebecca B. Costello et al., "The Effectiveness of Melatonin for Promoting Healthy Sleep: A Rapid Evidence Assessment of the Literature," *Nutrition Journal* 13, article no. 106 (November 7, 2014), https://doi.org/10.1186/1475-2891-13-106; Eduardo Ferracioli-Oda et al., "Meta-Analysis: Melatonin for the Treatment of Primary Sleep Disorders," *PLOS One* 8, no. 5 (2013): e63773, https://doi.org/10.1371/journal.pone.0063773; Lucreția Anghel et al., "Benefits and Adverse Events of Melatonin Use in the Elderly (Review)," *Experimental and Therapeutic Medicine* 23, no. 3 (2022): 219, https://doi.org/10.3892/etm.2022.11142; Daniel P. Cardinali et al., "Melatonin's Benefits and Risks as a Therapy for Sleep Disturbances in the Elderly: Current Insights," *Nature and Science of Sleep* 14 (October 2022): 1843–55, https://doi.org/10.2147/NSS.S380465.

[195] Glenna A. Dowling et al., "Melatonin and Bright-Light Treatment for Rest-Activity Disruption in Institutionalized Patients with Alzheimer's Disease," *Journal of the American Geriatrics Society* 56, no. 2 (2008): 239–46, https://doi.org/10.1111/j.1532-5415.2007.01543.x.

[196] Glyn Howatson et al., "Effect of Tart Cherry Juice (*Prunus cerasus*) on Melatonin Levels and Enhanced Sleep Quality," *European Journal of Nutrition* 51, no. 8 (2012): 909–16, https://doi.org/10.1007/s00394-011-0263-7.

[197] Hsiao-Han Lin et al., "Effect of Kiwifruit Consumption on Sleep Quality in Adults with Sleep Problems," *Asia Pacific Journal of Clinical Nutrition* 20, no. 2 (2011): 169–74, https://pubmed.ncbi.nlm.nih.gov/21669584/.

[198] "Supplement and Vitamin Certification," NSF, n.d., https://www.nsf.org/consumer-resources/articles/supplement-vitamin-certification; "Dietary Supplement Verification Program," United States Pharmacopeia (USP), n.d., https://www.usp.org/verification-services/dietary-supplements-verification-program.

[199] Natalie L. Hauglund et al., "Norepinephrine-Mediated Slow Vasomotion Drives Glymphatic Clearance During Sleep," *Cell* 188, no. 3 (February 2025): 606–22, https://doi.org/10.1016/j.cell.2024.11.027.

[200] Alan N. Bateson, "The Benzodiazepine Site of the GABAA Receptor: An Old Target with New Potential?," *Sleep Medicine* 5, suppl. 1 (2004): S9–15, https://doi.org/10.1016/s1389-9457(04)90002-0.

[201] Kalyanakrishnan Ramakrishnan and Dewey C. Scheid, "Treatment Options for Insomnia," *American Family Physician* 76, no. 4 (2007): 517–26, https://pubmed.ncbi.nlm.nih.gov/17853625/; Connor G.

Bounds and Preeti Patel, "Benzodiazepines," StatPearls, last updated January 30, 2024, https://www.ncbi.nlm.nih.gov/books/NBK470159/.

[202] Judy Wagner and Mary L. Wagner, "Non-Benzodiazepines for the Treatment of Insomnia," *Sleep Medicine Reviews* 4, no. 6 (2000): 551–81, https://doi.org/10.1053/smrv.2000.0126.

[203] "FDA Requires Stronger Warnings About Rare but Serious Incidents Related to Certain Prescription Insomnia Medicines," US Food & Drug Administration, April 30, 2019, https://www.prnewswire.com/news-releases/fda-requires-stronger-warnings-about-rare-but-serious-incidents-related-to-certain-prescription-insomnia-medicines-300840960.html.

[204] Hauglund et al., "Norepinephrine-Mediated Slow Vasomotion."

[205] Molly S. Clark et al., "FPIN's Clinical Inquiries: Antidepressants for the Treatment of Insomnia in Patients with Depression," *American Family Physician* 84, no. 9 (2011): 1–2, https://pubmed.ncbi.nlm.nih.gov/22164891/.

[206] Andrea Fagiolini et al., "Rediscovering Trazodone for the Treatment of Major Depressive Disorder," *CNS Drugs* 26, no. 12 (December 2012): 1033–49, https://doi.org/10.1007/s40263-012-0010-5.

[207] Adam Wichniak et al., "Effects of Antidepressants on Sleep," *Current Psychiatry Reports* 19, no. 9 (August 2017): 63, https://doi.org/10.1007/s11920-017-0816-4; Takashi Maruki et al., "Efficacy and Safety of Each Class of Sleep Medication for Major Depressive Disorder with Insomnia Symptoms: A Systematic Review and Meta-Analysis of Double-Blind Randomized Controlled Trials," *Psychiatry and Clinical Neurosciences* 79, no. 6 (June 2025): 306–18, https://doi.org/10.1111/pcn.13811; Stephen Wilson and Svetoslav Argyropoulos, "Antidepressants and Sleep: A Qualitative Review of the Literature," *Drugs* 65, no. 7 (2005): 927–47, https://doi.org/10.2165/00003495-200565070-00003.

[208] Costello et al., "Effectiveness of Melatonin"; Akira Kuriyama et al., "Ramelteon for the Treatment of Insomnia in Adults: A Systematic Review and Meta-Analysis," *Sleep Medicine* 15, no. 4 (2014): 385–92, https://doi.org/10.1016/j.sleep.2013.11.788.

[209] Guan Jian Liu et al., "Efficacy and Tolerability of Gabapentin in Adults with Sleep Disturbance in Medical Illness: A Systematic Review and Meta-Analysis," *Frontiers in Neurology* 8 (July 2017): 316, https://doi.org/10.3389/fneur.2017.00316; Russell P. Rosenberg et al., "A Randomized, Double-Blind, Single-Dose, Placebo-Controlled, Multicenter, Polysomnographic Study of Gabapentin in Transient Insomnia Induced by Sleep Phase Advance," *Journal of Clinical Sleep Medicine* 10, no. 10 (October 2014): 1093–100, https://doi.org/10.5664/jcsm.4108; Heike Benes et al., "Long-Term Safety and Efficacy of Cabergoline for the Treatment of Idiopathic Restless Legs Syndrome: Results from an Open-Label 6-Month Clinical Trial," *Sleep* 27, no. 4 (June 2004): 674–82, https://doi.org/10.1093/sleep/27.4.674; Birgit Högl et al., "The Effect of Cabergoline on Sleep, Periodic Leg Movements in Sleep, and Early Morning Motor Function in Patients with Parkinson's Disease," *Neuropsychopharmacology* 28 (May 2003): 1866–70, https://doi.org/10.1038/sj.npp.1300250.

[210] S. Nishino et al., "Hypocretin/Orexin and Narcolepsy: New Basic and Clinical Insights," Acta Physiologica 198, no. 3 (March 2010): 209–222.

[211] Rebeka Bustamante Rocha et al., "Dual Orexin Receptor Antagonists for the Treatment of Insomnia: Systematic Review and Network Meta-Analysis," *Arquivos de Neuro-Psiquiatria* 81, no. 5 (2023): 475–83, https://doi.org/10.1055/s-0043-1768667.

[212] Clemens Muehlan et al., "The Orexin Story and Orexin Receptor Antagonists for the Treatment of Insomnia," *Journal of Sleep Research* 32, no. 6 (2023): e13902, https://doi.org/10.1111/jsr.13902; Cecilio Álamo et al., "Orexinergic Receptor Antagonists as a New Therapeutic Target to Overcome Limitations of Current Pharmacological Treatment of Insomnia Disorder," *Actas Españolas de Psiquiatría* 52, no. 2 (2024): 172–82, https://doi.org/10.62641/aep.v52i2.1659.

[213] Bustamante Rocha et al., "Dual Orexin Receptor Antagonists."

[214] Morgan Adams Rhodes, "Lemborexant (Dayvigo) for the Treatment of Insomnia," *American Family Physician* 103, no. 4 (2021): 241–42, https://pubmed.ncbi.nlm.nih.gov/33587572/.

[215] Dunwiddie and Masino, "Role and Regulation of Adenosine."

[216] Reichert et al., "Adenosine, Caffeine, and Sleep–Wake Regulation."

[217] Deborah Blum, "How a Lawsuit Against Coca-Cola Convinced Americans to Love Caffeine," *Time*, September 25, 2018, https://time.com/5405132/coca-cola-trial-caffeine-history/.

[218] Ludy T. Benjamin Jr. et al., "Coca-Cola, Caffeine, and Mental Deficiency: Harry Hollingworth and the Chattanooga Trial of 1911," *Journal of the History of the Behavioral Sciences* 27, no. 1 (1991): 42–55, https://doi.org/10.1002/1520-6696.

[219] Benjamin Jr. et al., "Coca-Cola, Caffeine, and Mental Deficiency."

[220] Ian Clark and Hans Peter Landolt, "Coffee, Caffeine, and Sleep: A Systematic Review of Epidemiological Studies and Randomized Controlled Trials," *Sleep Medicine Reviews* 31 (February 2017): 70–78, https://doi.org/10.1016/j.smrv.2016.01.006.

[221] Carissa Gardiner et al., "The Effect of Caffeine on Subsequent Sleep: A Systematic Review and Meta-Analysis," *Sleep Medicine Reviews* 69 (June 2023): 101764, https://doi.org/10.1016/j.smrv.2023.101764; Clark and Landolt, "Coffee, Caffeine, and Sleep."

[222] N. D. Volkow et al., "Caffeine Increases Striatal Dopamine D_2/D_3 Receptor Availability in the Human Brain," *Translational Psychiatry* 5, no. 4 (2015): e549, https://doi.org/10.1038/tp.2015.46.

[223] Astrid Nehlig and Sylvette Boyet, "Dose-Response Study of Caffeine Effects on Cerebral Functional Activity with a Specific Focus on Dependence," *Brain Research* 858, no. 1 (2000): 71–77, https://doi.org/10.1016/s0006-8993(99)02480-4.

[224] Joaquim A. Ribeiro and Ana M. Sebastião, "Caffeine and Adenosine," *Journal of Alzheimer's Disease* 20, no. S1 (2010): S3–15, https://doi.org/10.3233/JAD-2010-1379.

[225] "Coffee & Sleep: How Does Caffeine Work & Its Effects on Sleep | Matt Walker & Andrew Huberman," Huberman Lab Clips, YouTube, October 1, 2021, https://www.youtube.com/watch?v=bFdBJ2v6sps&t=291s.

[226] Porkka-Heiskanen et al., "Adenosine"; Basheer et al., "Adenosine and Sleep-Wake Regulation."

[227] Yu Zhang et al., "Coffee and Tea Intake, Dementia Risk, and Cognitive Function," *JAMA* 335, no. 11 (2025): 961–74, https://doi.org/10.1001/jama.2025.27259; Miaomiao Yang et al., "Association of Unsweetened and Sweetened Coffee Consumption with Risk of Cardiovascular Disease: A Prospective Cohort Study," *Nutrition, Metabolism and Cardiovascular Diseases* 36, No. 6 (June 2026): 104539, https://doi.org/10.1016/j.numecd.2026.104539; Robin Poole et al., "Coffee Consumption and Health: Umbrella Review of Meta-Analyses of Multiple Health Outcomes," *BMJ* 359, no. 1 (November 2017): j5024, https://doi.org/10.1136/bmj.j5024.

[228] Diane C. Mitchell et al., "Beverage Caffeine Intakes in the U.S.," *Food and Chemical Toxicology* 63 (January 2014): 136–42, https://doi.org/10.1016/j.fct.2013.10.042; Jack E. James, "Caffeine and Cognitive Performance: Persistent Methodological Challenges in Caffeine Research," *Pharmacology Biochemistry and Behavior* 124 (September 2014): 117–22, https://doi.org/10.1016/j.pbb.2014.05.019.

[229] J. V. Rétey et al., "A Genetic Variation in the Adenosine A_{2A} Receptor Gene (*ADORA2A*) Contributes to Individual Sensitivity to Caffeine Effects on Sleep," *Clinical Pharmacology & Therapeutics* 81, no. 5 (2007): 692–98, https://doi.org/10.1038/sj.clpt.6100102.

[230] Janine Weibel et al., "The Impact of Daily Caffeine Intake on Nighttime Sleep in Young Adult Men," *Scientific Reports* 11, article no. 4668 (2021), https://doi.org/10.1038/s41598-021-84088-x.

[231] Yang Zhang et al., "Caffeine and Diuresis During Rest and Exercise: A Meta-Analysis," *Journal of Science and Medicine in Sport* 18, no. 5 (September 2015): 569–74, https://doi.org/10.1016/j.jsams.2014.07.017.

[232] Mayo Clinic Staff, "Caffeine Content for Coffee, Tea, Soda and More," Mayo Clinic, February 6, 2025, https://www.mayoclinic.org/healthy-lifestyle/nutrition-and-healthy-eating/in-depth/caffeine/art-

20049372; "Caffeine Chart," Center for Science in the Public Interest, last updated March–April 2025, https://www.cspinet.org/caffeine-chart.

233 Luigi Barrea et al., "Coffee Consumption, Health Benefits and Side Effects: A Narrative Review and Update for Dietitians and Nutritionists," *Critical Reviews in Food Science and Nutrition* 63, no. 9 (2023): 1238–61, https://doi.org/10.1080/10408398.2021.1963207; Xuan Wang et al., "Coffee Drinking Timing and Mortality in US Adults," *European Heart Journal* 46, no. 8 (February 2025): 749–59, https://doi.org/10.1093/eurheartj/ehae871.

234 Kitty Pham et al., "High Coffee Consumption, Brain Volume and Risk of Dementia and Stroke," *Nutritional Neuroscience* 25, no. 10 (2022): 2111–22, https://doi.org/10.1080/1028415X.2021.1945858.

235 Poole et al., "Coffee Consumption and Health"; Erratum, Poole et al., "Coffee Consumption and Health," *BMJ* 360 (January 12, 2018): k194, https://doi.org/10.1136/bmj.k194.

236 Sun-Young Kim et al., "Anti-Obesity Effects of Yerba Mate (*Ilex paraguariensis*): A Randomized, Double-Blind, Placebo-Controlled Clinical Trial," *BMC Complementary and Alternative Medicine* 15 (September 25, 2015): 338, https://doi.org/10.1186/s12906-015-0859-1; Paolo Manghi et al., "Coffee Consumption Is Associated with Intestinal *Lawsonibacter asaccharolyticus* Abundance and Prevalence across Multiple Cohorts," *Nature Microbiology* 9, no. 12 (December 2024): 3120–34, https://doi.org/10.1038/s41564-024-01858-9.

237 Office of the U.S. Surgeon General, *Alcohol and Cancer Risk: The U.S. Surgeon General's Advisory*, 2025, https://www.hhs.gov/sites/default/files/oash-alcohol-cancer-risk.pdf.

238 D. L. Williams et al., "Dose-Response Effects of Ethanol on the Sleep of Young Women," *Journal of Studies on Alcohol and Drugs* 44, no. 3 (1983): 515–23, https://doi.org/10.15288/jsa.1983.44.515; Ian M. Colrain et al., "Alcohol and the Sleeping Brain," *Handbook of Clinical Neurology* 125 (2014): 415–31, https://doi.org/10.1016/B978-0-444-62619-6.00024-0.

239 Eliza Van Reen et al., "Effects of Alcohol on Sleep and the Sleep Electroencephalogram in Healthy Young Women," *Alcohol: Clinical & Experimental Research* 30, no. 6 (2006): 974–81, https://doi.org/10.1111/j.1530-0277.2006.00111.x; Julie K. M. Chan et al., "The Acute Effects of Alcohol on Sleep Architecture in Late Adolescence," *Alcohol: Clinical & Experimental Research* 37, no. 10 (2013): 1720–28, https://doi.org/10.1111/acer.12141.

240 Patricia N. Prinz et al., "Effect of Alcohol on Sleep and Nighttime Plasma Growth Hormone and Cortisol Concentrations," *Journal of Clinical Endocrinology & Metabolism* 51, no. 4 (1980): 759–64, https://doi.org/10.1210/jcem-51-4-759; A. C. Ekman et al., "Ethanol Decreases Nocturnal Plasma Levels of Thyrotropin and Growth Hormone but Not Those of Thyroid Hormones or Prolactin in Man," *Journal of Clinical Endocrinology & Metabolism* 81, no. 7 (1996): 2627–32, https://doi.org/10.1210/jcem.81.7.8675588.

241 Marco Zaffanello et al., "Complex Relationship Between Growth Hormone and Sleep in Children: Insights, Discrepancies, and Implications," *Frontiers in Endocrinology* 14 (January 24, 2024): 1332114, https://doi.org/10.3389/fendo.2023.1332114; Rafael Luboshitzky et al., "Disruption of the Nocturnal Testosterone Rhythm by Sleep Fragmentation in Normal Men," *Journal of Clinical Endocrinology & Metabolism* 86, no. 3 (2001): 1134–39, https://doi.org/10.1210/jcem.86.3.7296.

242 Subhajit Chakravorty et al., "Alcohol Dependence and Its Relationship with Insomnia and Other Sleep Disorders," *Alcohol: Clinical & Experimental Research* 40, no. 11 (2016): 2271–82, https://doi.org/10.1111/acer.13217.

243 Ian M. Colrain et al., "Impact of Alcoholism on Sleep Architecture and EEG Power Spectra in Men and Women," *Sleep* 32, no. 10 (2009): 1341–52, https://doi.org/10.1093/sleep/32.10.1341.

244 Colrain et al., "Alcohol and the Sleeping Brain."

245 Robert E. Roberts et al., "Chronic Insomnia and Its Negative Consequences for Health and Functioning of Adolescents: A 12-Month Prospective Study," *Journal of Adolescent Health* 42, no. 3 (2008): 294–302, https://doi.org/10.1016/j.jadohealth.2007.09.016.

[246] Eric O. Johnson et al., "Epidemiology of DSM-IV Insomnia in Adolescence: Lifetime Prevalence, Chronicity, and an Emergent Gender Difference," *Pediatrics* 117, no. 2 (2006): e247–56, https://doi.org/10.1542/peds.2004-2629; Sofia de Sá et al., "The Influence of Smartphones on Adolescent Sleep: A Systematic Literature Review," *Nursing Reports* 13, no. 2 (2023): 612–21, https://doi.org/10.3390/nursrep13020054.

[247] Liese Exelmans and Jan Van den Bulck, "Bedtime Mobile Phone Use and Sleep in Adults," *Social Science & Medicine* 148 (January 2016): 93–101, https://doi.org/10.1016/j.socscimed.2015.11.037.

[248] Lindsay M. Squeglia, "Alcohol and the Developing Adolescent Brain," *World Psychiatry* 19, no. 3 (2020): 393–94, https://doi.org/10.1002/wps.20786.

[249] Jeffrey S. Wojtowicz, "Long-Term Health Outcomes of Regular, Moderate Red Wine Consumption," *Cureus* 15, no. 10 (2023): e46786, https://doi.org/10.7759/cureus.46786.

[250] Scott Shannon et al., "Cannabidiol in Anxiety and Sleep: A Large Case Series," *Permanente Journal* 23, no. 1 (2019), https://doi.org/10.7812/TPP/18-041.

[251] Lucy H. Silmore et al., "Food Effects on the Formulation, Dosing, and Administration of Cannabidiol (CBD) in Humans: A Systematic Review of Clinical Studies," *Pharmacotherapy* 41, no. 4 (April 2021): 405–20, https://doi.org/10.1002/phar.2512; Ehsan Moazen-Zadeh et al., "Pharmacokinetics of Cannabidiol: A Systematic Review and Meta-Regression Analysis," *Cannabis and Cannabinoid Research* 9, no. 4 (August 2024): 939–66, https://doi.org/10.1089/can.2023.0025.

[252] Priyamvada Sharma et al., "Chemistry, Metabolism, and Toxicology of Cannabis: Clinical Implications," *Iranian Journal of Psychiatry* 7, no. 4 (2012): 149–56, https://pubmed.ncbi.nlm.nih.gov/23408483/.

[253] Andréia Pucinelli de Sousa Queiroz et al., "Cognitive Effects of Cannabis Use: A Comprehensive Review Across Domains," *Neurology International* 17, no. 7 (2025): 107, https://doi.org/10.3390/neurolint17070107; Ana Julia de Lima Bomfim et al., "Effects of the Acute and Chronic Administration of Cannabidiol on Cognition in Humans and Animals: A Systematic Review," *Cannabis & Cannabinoid Research* 8, no. 6 (2023): 955–73, https://doi.org/10.1089/can.2023.0086.

[254] C. Austin Zamarripa et al., "Assessment of Orally Administered Δ9-Tetrahydrocannabinol When Coadministered with Cannabidiol on Δ9-Tetrahydrocannabinol Pharmacokinetics and Pharmacodynamics in Healthy Adults: A Randomized Clinical Trial," *JAMA Network Open* 6, no. 2 (2023): e2254752, https://doi.org/10.1001/jamanetworkopen.2022.54752.

[255] Thomas Schierenbeck et al., "Effect of Illicit Recreational Drugs upon Sleep: Cocaine, Ecstasy and Marijuana," *Sleep Medicine Reviews* 12, no. 5 (2008): 381–89, https://doi.org/10.1016/j.smrv.2007.12.004.

[256] Anu-Katriina Pesonen et al., "REM Sleep Fragmentation Associated with Depressive Symptoms and Genetic Risk for Depression in a Community-Based Sample of Adolescents," *Journal of Affective Disorders* 245 (February 15, 2019): 757–63, https://doi.org/10.1016/j.jad.2018.11.077; Leary et al., "Association of Rapid Eye Movement Sleep."

[257] Joshua Feriante and Shantanu Singh, "REM Rebound Effect," StatPearls, last updated September 12, 2024, https://www.ncbi.nlm.nih.gov/books/NBK560713/.

[258] N. Kuhathasan et al., "The Use of Cannabinoids for Sleep: A Critical Review on Clinical Trials," *Experimental and Clinical Psychopharmacology* 27, no. 4 (2019): 383–401, https://doi.org/10.1037/pha0000285.

[259] Evan Winiger et al., "Novel Methods of Cannabis Use and Lower Sleep Duration Among High School Students," *Cannabis* 5, no. 2 (2022): 66–73, https://doi.org/10.26828/cannabis/2022.02.006.

[260] Anthony N. Nicholson et al., "Effect of Delta-9-Tetrahydrocannabinol and Cannabidiol on Nocturnal Sleep and Early-Morning Behavior in Young Adults," *Journal of Clinical Psychopharmacology* 24, no. 3 (2004): 305–13, https://doi.org/10.1097/01.jcp.0000125688.05091.8f.

[261] Evan A. Winiger and John K. Hewitt, "Prenatal Cannabis Exposure and Sleep Outcomes in Children 9–10 Years of Age in the Adolescent Brain Cognitive Development SM Study," *Sleep Health* 6, no. 6 (2020): 787–89, https://doi.org/10.1016/j.sleh.2020.05.006.

[262] Kelly C. Young-Wolff et al., "Prenatal Cannabis Use and Maternal Pregnancy Outcomes," *JAMA Internal Medicine* 184, no. 9 (2024): 1083–93, https://doi.org/10.1001/jamainternmed.2024.3270.

[263] Kelly C. Young-Wolff et al., "Rates of Prenatal Cannabis Use Among Pregnant Women Before and During the COVID-19 Pandemic," JAMA 326, no. 17 (2021): 1745–47, https://doi.org/10.1001/jama.2021.16328.

[264] Mohammad R. Hayatbakhsh et al., "Birth Outcomes Associated with Cannabis Use Before and During Pregnancy," *Pediatric Research* 71, no. 2 (2012): 215–19, https://doi.org/10.1038/pr.2011.25.

[265] B. Adam Crosland et al., "Risk of Adverse Neonatal Outcomes After Combined Prenatal Cannabis and Nicotine Exposure," *JAMA Network Open* 7, no. 5 (2024): e2410151, https://doi.org/10.1001/jamanetworkopen.2024.10151.

[266] Shannon et al., "Cannabidiol in Anxiety and Sleep."

[267] Juan G. Perez et al., "Cannabinoids for Anxiety and Sleep Disturbances: A Scoping Review," Medical Cannabis and Cannabinoids 8, no. 1 (October 2025): 219–237, https://doi.org/10.1159/000548890.

[268] Andrea J. Narayan et al., "Cannabidiol for Moderate–Severe Insomnia: A Randomized Controlled Pilot Trial of 150 mg of Nightly Dosing," *Journal of Clinical Sleep Medicine* 20, no. 5 (2024): 753–63, https://doi.org/10.5664/jcsm.10998.

[269] Tabea Schoeler et al., "Rates and Correlates of Cannabis-Associated Psychotic Symptoms in Over 230,000 People Who Use Cannabis," *Translational Psychiatry* 12, no. 1 (2022): 369, https://doi.org/10.1038/s41398-022-02112-8; Alessio Fiorentini et al., "Substance-Induced Psychoses: An Updated Literature Review," *Frontiers in Psychiatry* 12 (December 22, 2021): 694863, https://doi.org/10.3389/fpsyt.2021.694863; Nadia Solowij and Robert Battisti, "The Chronic Effects of Cannabis on Memory in Humans: A Review," *Current Drug Abuse Reviews* 1, no. 1 (2008): 81–98, https://doi.org/10.2174/1874473710801010081.

[270] Michael Gradisar et al., "The Sleep and Technology Use of Americans: Findings from the National Sleep Foundation's 2011 Sleep in America Poll," *Journal of Clinical Sleep Medicine* 9, no. 12 (2013): 1291–99, https://doi.org/10.5664/jcsm.3272.

[271] Anne-Marie Chang et al., "Evening Use of Light-Emitting eReaders Negatively Affects Sleep, Circadian Timing, and Next-Morning Alertness," *Proceedings of the National Academy of Sciences* 112, no. 4 (2015): 1232–37, https://doi.org/10.1073/pnas.1418490112.

[272] Michael Bauer et al., "The Potential Influence of LED Lighting on Mental Illness."

[273] T. A. Bedrosian and R. J. Nelson, "Influence of the Modern Light Environment on Mood," *Molecular Psychiatry* 18, no. 7 (2013): 751–57, https://doi.org/10.1038/mp.2013.70.

[274] Richard R. Bootzin, "Stimulus Control Treatment for Insomnia," *Proceedings, 80th Annual Convention, APA, 1972.*

Chapter 2: Protocols for Exercise

[1] Hans Selye, "Stress and the General Adaptation Syndrome," *British Medical Journal* 1, no. 4667 (June 1950): 1383–92, https://doi.org/10.1136/bmj.1.4667.1383.

[2] *Nautilus Bulletin* 1, ArthurJonesExercise.com, http://www.arthurjonesexercise.com/Bulletin1/37.PDF; *Nautilus Bulletin* 2, ArthurJonesExercise.com, http://www.arthurjonesexercise.com/Bulletin2/Bulletin2.html.

[3] Kate Neudecker, "This Golden Era Bodybuilder Trained Just Twice a Week—and New Science Proves It Works," *Men's Health*, September 22, 2025, https://www.menshealth.com/uk/building-muscle/train-smarter/a67959687/mike-mentzer-heavy-duty-workout/.

[4] Robert W. Morton et al., "Training for Strength and Hypertrophy: An Evidence-Based Approach," *Current Opinion in Physiology* 10 (2019): 90–95; Andrew Huberman, "Guest Series | Dr. Lauren Colenso-Semple: The Most Effective Weight Training, Cardio & Nutrition for Women," *Huberman Lab* (podcast audio), February 16, 2026, https://www.hubermanlab.com/episode/the-most-effective-weight-training-cardio-and-nutrition-for-women-lauren-colenso-semple.

[5] Andrew Huberman, "Guest Series | Dr. Andy Galpin: How to Assess & Improve All Aspects of Your Fitness," *Huberman Lab* (podcast audio), January 18, 2023, https://www.hubermanlab.com/episode/dr-andy-galpin-how-to-assess-improve-all-aspects-of-your-fitness.

[6] Charles M. Tipton, "The History of 'Exercise Is Medicine' in Ancient Civilizations," *Advances in Physiology Education* 38, no. 2 (2014): 109–17, https://doi.org/10.1152/advan.00136.2013.

[7] Michael Noetel et al., "Effect of Exercise for Depression: Systematic Review and Network Meta-Analysis of Randomised Controlled Trials," *BMJ* 384, no. 1 (February 2024): e075847, https://doi.org/10.1136/bmj-2023-075847; James A. Blumenthal et al., "Exercise and Pharmacotherapy in the Treatment of Major Depressive Disorder," *Psychosomatic Medicine* 69 (September 2007): 587–96, https://doi.org/10.1097/PSY.0b013e318148c19a; J. A. Blumenthal et al., "Effects of Exercise Training on Older Patients with Major Depression," *Archives of Internal Medicine* 159, no. 19 (October 1999): 2349–56, https://doi.org/10.1001/archinte.159.19.2349; Gary Cooney, "Exercise for Depression," *Journal of Evidence-Based Medicine* 6, no. 4 (November 2013): 307–8, https://doi.org/10.1111/jebm.12076; Siri Kvam et al., "Exercise as a Treatment for Depression: A Meta-Analysis," *Journal of Affective Disorders* 202 (September 2016): 67–86, https://doi.org/10.1016/j.jad.2016.03.063; Ben Singh et al., "Effectiveness of Physical Activity Interventions for Improving Depression, Anxiety and Distress: An Overview of Systematic Reviews," *British Journal of Sports Medicine* 57, no. 18 (2023): 1203–9, https://doi.org/10.1136/bjsports-2022-106195.

[8] Bente Klarlund Pedersen and Anders Dyhr Toft, "Effects of Exercise on Lymphocytes and Cytokines," *British Journal of Sports Medicine* 34 (2000): 246–51, https://doi.org/10.1136/bjsm.34.4.246.

[9] Jerzy A. Zoladz, *Muscle and Exercise Physiology* (Academic Press, 2018); Scott Powers and Edward Howley, *Exercise Physiology: Theory and Application to Fitness and Performance*, 10th ed. (McGraw Hill, 2017); MoTrPAC Study Group et al., "Temporal Dynamics of the Multi-Omic Response to Endurance Exercise Training," *Nature* 629 (May 2024): 174–83, https://doi.org/10.1038/s41586-023-06877-w; Anna Maria Koman et al., "The Beneficial Effects of Aerobic Exercise on Human Systems and Organs: A Literature Review," *Journal of Education, Health and Sport* 73 (June 2024): 51710, https://doi.org/10.12775/JEHS.2024.73.51710; MoTrPAC Study Group et al., "Multi-Omic, Multi-Tissue Responses to Acute Exercise in Sedentary Adults: Findings from the Molecular Transducers of Physical Activity Consortium," bioRxiv, March 20, 2026, https://www.biorxiv.org/content/10.64898/2026.02.27.702183v2.full; Kévin Contrepois et al., "Molecular Choreography of Acute Exercise," *Cell* 181, no. 5 (May 2020): 1112–30.e16, https://doi.org/10.1016/j.cell.2020.04.043.

[10] Silvia Grimanesa Revelo Herrera and Jose E. Leon-Rojas, "The Effect of Aerobic Exercise in Neuroplasticity, Learning, and Cognition: A Systematic Review," *Cureus* 16, no. 2 (2024): e54021, https://doi.org/10.7759/cureus.54021; Xueyang Li et al., "Physical Exercise for Brain Plasticity Promotion: An Overview of the Underlying Oscillatory Mechanism," *Frontiers in Neuroscience* 18 (August 2024): 1440975, https://doi.org/10.3389/fnins.2024.1440975; Lamia Ben Ezzdine et al., "Physical Activity and Neuroplasticity in Neurodegenerative Disorders: A Comprehensive Review of Exercise Interventions, Cognitive Training, and AI Applications," *Frontiers in Neuroscience* 19 (February 2025), https://doi.org/10.3389/fnins.2025.1502417.

[11] Kirk I. Erickson et al., "Exercise Training Increases Size of Hippocampus and Improves Memory," *Proceedings of the National Academy of Sciences* 108, no. 7 (2011): 3017–22, https://doi.org/10.1073/pnas.1015950108.

[12] K. I. Erickson et al., "Physical Activity Predicts Gray Matter Volume in Late Adulthood: The Cardiovascular Health Study," *Neurology* 75, no. 16 (2010): 1415–22, https://doi.org/10.1212/WNL.0b013e3181f88359; Tibor Hortobágyi et al., "Functional Relevance of Resistance Training-

Induced Neuroplasticity in Health and Disease," *Neuroscience and Biobehavioral Reviews* 122 (March 2021): 79–91, https://doi.org/10.1016/j.neubiorev.2020.12.019; Fabian Herold et al., "Functional and/or Structural Brain Changes in Response to Resistance Exercises and Resistance Training Lead to Cognitive Improvements - A Systematic Review," *European Review of Aging and Physical Activity* 16, no. 10 (2019), https://doi.org/10.1186/s11556-019-0217-2; Orgesa Qipo et al., "Dose-Response Relationship of Resistance Training and the Effects on Circulating Biomarkers of Inflammation or Neuroplasticity In Older Adults: A Systematic Review and Meta-Analysis," *Ageing Research Reviews* 113 (January 2026): 102917, https://doi.org/10.1016/j.arr.2025.102917.

13 Rodolfo R. Llinás, *I of the Vortex: From Neurons to Self* (MIT Press, 2002), https://mitpress.mit.edu/9780262621632/i-of-the-vortex/.

14 Emily Zhao et al., "The Role of Mobility as a Protective Factor of Cognitive Functioning in Aging Adults: A Review," *Sports Health* 6, no. 1 (2014): 63–69, https://doi.org/10.1177/1941738113477832.

15 Adria Quigley et al., "Effects of Exercise on Cognitive Performance in Older Adults: A Narrative Review of the Evidence, Possible Biological Mechanisms, and Recommendations for Exercise Prescription," *Journal of Aging Research* 2020 (May 14, 2020): 1407896, https://doi.org/10.1155/2020/1407896; Ahmed Disouky et al., "Human Hippocampal Neurogenesis in Adulthood, Ageing and Alzheimer's Disease," *Nature* 652 (2026): 1264–73, https://doi.org/10.1038/s41586-026-10169-4.

16 Ziyue Aiden Wang et al., "Brain-Wide Analysis Reveals Movement Encoding Structured Across and Within Brain Areas," *Nature Neuroscience* 29 (2026): 147–58, https://doi.org/10.1038/s41593-025-02114-x.

17 Li et al., "Physical Exercise for Brain Plasticity"; Ezzdine et al., "Physical Activity and Neuroplasticity."

18 Magdalena Miranda et al., "Brain-Derived Neurotrophic Factor: A Key Molecule for Memory in the Healthy and the Pathological Brain," *Frontiers in Cellular Neuroscience* 13 (August 2019): 363, https://doi.org/10.3389/fncel.2019.00363; Carla Cunha et al., "A Simple Role for BDNF in Learning and Memory?," *Frontiers in Molecular Neuroscience* 3 (February 2010): 1, https://doi.org/10.3389/neuro.02.001.2010.

19 Kristin L. Szuhany et al., "A Meta-Analytic Review of the Effects of Exercise on Brain-Derived Neurotrophic Factor," *Journal of Psychiatric Research* 60 (January 2015): 56–64, https://doi.org/10.1016/j.jpsychires.2014.10.003.

20 Siresha Bathina and Undurti N. Das, "Brain-Derived Neurotrophic Factor and Its Clinical Implications," *Archives of Medical Science* 11, no. 6 (2015): 1164–78, https://doi.org/10.5114/aoms.2015.56342.

21 Hassane Zouhal et al., "Catecholamines and the Effects of Exercise, Training and Gender," *Sports Medicine* 38, no. 5 (2008): 401–23, https://doi.org/10.2165/00007256-200838050-00004; Joanna Kruk et al., "Physical Exercise and Catecholamines Response: Benefits and Health Risk: Possible Mechanisms," *Free Radical Research* 54, no. 2–3 (2020): 105–25, https://doi.org/10.1080/10715762.2020.1726343; William J. Kraemer and Nicholas A. Ratamess, "Hormonal Responses and Adaptations to Resistance Exercise and Training," *Sports Medicine* 35 (April 2005): 339–61, https://doi.org/10.2165/00007256-200535040-00004; Nikolaos Athanasiou et al., "Endocrine Responses of the Stress System to Different Types of Exercise," *Reviews in Endocrine and Metabolic Disorders* 24 (2023): 251–66, https://doi.org/10.1007/s11154-022-09758-1; David Walzik et al., "Molecular Insights of Exercise Therapy in Disease Prevention and Treatment," *Signal Transduction and Targeted Therapy* 9, no. 138 (May 2024), https://doi.org/10.1038/s41392-024-01841-0; R. S. Staron et al., "Skeletal Muscle Adaptations During Early Phase of Heavy-Resistance Training in Men and Women," *Journal of Applied Physiology* 76, no. 3 (1994): 1247–55, https://doi.org/10.1152/jappl.1994.76.3.1247; Vedat Çinar et al., "Impact of Different Exercise Modalities on Neuroendocrine Well-Being Markers Among University Students: A Study of Renalase and Catecholamine Responses," *Frontiers in Physiology* 16 (April 2025): 1591132, https://doi.org/10.3389/fphys.2025.1591132.

22 Bernward Winter et al., "High Impact Running Improves Learning," *Neurobiology of Learning and Memory* 87, no. 4 (2007): 597–609, https://doi.org/10.1016/j.nlm.2006.11.003.

[23] Hortobágyi et al., "Functional Relevance"; Herold et al., "Functional and/or Structural Brain Changes."

[24] Jessica R. Alley et al., "Effects of Resistance Exercise Timing on Sleep Architecture and Nocturnal Blood Pressure," *Journal of Strength and Conditioning Research* 29, no. 5 (2015): 1378–85, https://doi.org/10.1519/JSC.0000000000000750; Giselle S. Passos et al., "Effect of Acute Physical Exercise on Patients with Chronic Primary Insomnia," *Journal of Clinical Sleep Medicine* 6, no. 3 (2010): 270–75, https://doi.org/10.5664/jcsm.27825; Majd A. Alnawwar et al., "The Effect of Physical Activity on Sleep Quality and Sleep Disorder: A Systematic Review," *Cureus* 15, no. 8 (2023): e43595, https://doi.org/10.7759/cureus.43595.

[25] Passos et al., "Effect of Acute Physical Exercise."

[26] Lynette L. Craft and Frank M. Perna, "The Benefits of Exercise for the Clinically Depressed," *Primary Care Companion to the Journal of Clinical Psychiatry* 6, no. 3 (2004): 104–11, https://doi.org/10.4088/pcc.v06n0301; Chaoxin Ji et al., "Physical Exercise Ameliorates Anxiety, Depression and Sleep Quality in College Students: Experimental Evidence from Exercise Intensity and Frequency," *Behavioral Sciences* 12, no. 3 (2022): 61, https://doi.org/10.3390/bs12030061.

[27] Insung Park et al., "Exercise Improves the Quality of Slow-Wave Sleep by Increasing Slow-Wave Stability," *Scientific Reports* 11, article no. 4410 (2021), https://doi.org/10.1038/s41598-021-83817-6.

[28] Justy Reed and Deniz S. Ones, "The Effect of Acute Aerobic Exercise on Positive Activated Affect: A Meta-Analysis," *Psychology of Sport and Exercise* 7, no. 5 (2006): 477–514, https://doi.org/10.1016/j.psychsport.2005.11.003.

[29] Emma Childs and Harriet de Wit, "Regular Exercise Is Associated with Emotional Resilience to Acute Stress in Healthy Adults," *Frontiers in Physiology* 5 (May 2014): 161, https://doi.org/10.3389/fphys.2014.00161.

[30] R. E. Thayer et al., "Self-Regulation of Mood: Strategies for Changing a Bad Mood, Raising Energy, and Reducing Tension," *Journal of Personality and Social Psychology* 67, no. 5 (1994): 910–25, https://doi.org/10.1037/0022-3514.67.5.910.

[31] D. Scully et al., "Physical Exercise and Psychological Well Being: A Critical Review," *British Journal of Sports Medicine* 32, no. 2 (1998): 111–20, https://doi.org/10.1136/bjsm.32.2.111.

[32] Childs and de Wit, "Emotional Resilience to Acute Stress."

[33] Bonnie G. Berger and Robert W. Motl, "Exercise and Mood: A Selective Review and Synthesis of Research Employing the Profile of Mood States," *Journal of Applied Sport Psychology* 12, no. 1 (2000): 69–92, https://doi.org/10.1080/10413200008404214.

[34] Adilson Marques et al., "Bidirectional Association between Physical Activity and Dopamine Across Adulthood—a Systematic Review," *Brain Sciences* 11, no. 7 (2021): 829, https://doi.org/10.3390/brainsci11070829; Hamed Alizadeh Pahlavani, "Possible Role of Exercise Therapy on Depression: Effector Neurotransmitters as Key Players," *Behavioural Brain Research* 459 (February 29, 2024): 114791, https://doi.org/10.1016/j.bbr.2023.114791; Çinar, "Impact of Different Exercise Modalities."

[35] Lan Yan et al., "Physical Exercise Mediates Cortical Synaptic Protein Lactylation to Improve Stress Resilience," *Cell Metabolism* 36, no. 9 (September 2024): 2104–17.e4, https://doi.org/10.1016/j.cmet.2024.07.018.

[36] Kathleen K. A. Cho et al., "Long-Range Inhibition Synchronizes and Updates Prefrontal Task Activity," *Nature* 617, no. 7961 (April 2023): 548–54, https://doi.org/10.1038/s41586-023-06012-9.

[37] Richard P. Dum et al., "The Mind-Body Problem: Circuits That Link the Cerebral Cortex to the Adrenal Medulla," *Proceedings of the National Academy of Sciences* 116, no. 51 (2019): 26321–28, https://doi.org/10.1073/pnas.1902297116.

[38] Teiko Miyashita and Cedric L. Williams, "Epinephrine Administration Increases Neural Impulses Propagated Along the Vagus Nerve: Role of Peripheral β-Adrenergic Receptors," *Neurobiology of Learning and Memory* 85, no. 2 (March 2006): 116–24, https://doi.org/10.1016/j.nlm.2005.08.013;

D. L. Hassert et al., "The Effects of Peripheral Vagal Nerve Stimulation at a Memory-Modulating Intensity on Norepinephrine Output in the Basolateral Amygdala," *Behavioral Neuroscience* 118, no. 1 (February 2004): 79–88, https://doi.org/10.1037/0735-7044.118.1.79; R. N. Holdefer and R. A. Jensen, "The Effects of Peripheral D-Amphetamine, 4-OH Amphetamine, and Epinephrine on Maintained Discharge in the Locus Coeruleus with Reference to the Modulation of Learning and Memory by These Substances," *Brain Research* 417, no. 1 (August 1987): 108–17, https://doi.org/10.1016/0006-8993(87)90184-3; Gina R. Poe et al., "Locus Coeruleus: A New Look at the Blue Spot," *Nature Reviews Neuroscience* 21 (September 2020): 644–59, https://doi.org/10.1038/s41583-020-0360-9; Mei Hao et al., "Neural Circuit Connections and Functions of Locus Coeruleus–Norepinephrine System," *International Journal of Molecular Sciences* 26, no. 22 (November 2025): 11163, https://doi.org/10.3390/ijms262211163; Avi K. Matarasso et al., "Stimulus-Dependent Dopamine Dynamics from Locus Coeruleus Axons," preprint available on bioRxiv (2025), https://doi.org/10.1101/2025.09.15.676390.

39 Morgan Kindel et al., "Exercise-Induced Activation of Ventromedial Hypothalamic Steroidogenic Factor-1 Neurons Mediates Improvements in Endurance," *Neuron* 114, no. 9 (February 2026): 606–22.e17, https://doi.org/10.1016/j.neuron.2025.12.033; Teppei Fujikawa et al., "SF-1 Expression in the Hypothalamus Is Required for Beneficial Metabolic Effects of Exercise," *eLife* (November 2016): e18206, https://doi.org/10.7554/eLife.18206.

40 Ralph S. Paffenbarger et al., "Physical Activity, All-Cause Mortality, and Longevity of College Alumni," *New England Journal of Medicine* 314, no. 10 (1986): 605–13, https://doi.org/10.1056/NEJM198603063141003.

41 Trine Moholdt et al., "Sustained Physical Activity, Not Weight Loss, Associated with Improved Survival in Coronary Heart Disease," *Journal of the American College of Cardiology* 71, no. 10 (2018): 1094–101, https://doi.org/10.1016/j.jacc.2018.01.011; Erratum, Moholdt et al., "Sustained Physical Activity," *Journal of the American College of Cardiology* 71, no. 13 (2018): 1499, https://doi.org/10.1016/j.jacc.2018.03.013.

42 Steven N. Blair et al., "Influences of Cardiorespiratory Fitness and Other Precursors on Cardiovascular Disease and All-Cause Mortality in Men and Women," *JAMA* 276, no. 3 (1996): 205–10, https://doi.org/10.1001/jama.1996.03540030039029.

43 Stephen R. Bird and John A. Hawley, "Update on the Effects of Physical Activity on Insulin Sensitivity in Humans," *BMJ Open Sport & Exercise Medicine* 2 (March 1, 2017): e000143, https://doi.org/10.1136/bmjsem-2016-000143; Kedi Gao and Youliang Lin, "Insulin Resistance Mediates the Association Between Physical Activity and Mortality in US Adults with Metabolic Syndrome," *Scientific Reports* 15, article no. 18872 (2025), https://doi.org/10.1038/s41598-025-02921-z; Contrepois et al., "Molecular Choreography of Acute Exercise"; Lykke Sylow et al., "The Many Actions of Insulin in Skeletal Muscle, the Paramount Tissue Determining Glycemia," *Cell Metabolism* 33, no. 4 (April 2021): 758–80, https://doi.org/10.1016/j.cmet.2021.03.020.

44 L. B. Borghouts and H. A. Keizer, "Exercise and Insulin Sensitivity: A Review," *International Journal of Sports Medicine* 21, no. 1 (2000): 1–12, https://doi.org/10.1055/s-2000-8847; Contrepois et al., "Molecular Choreography of Acute Exercise"; Sylow et al., "Many Actions of Insulin."

45 Vighnesh Vetrivel Venkatasamy et al., "Effect of Physical Activity on Insulin Resistance, Inflammation and Oxidative Stress in Diabetes Mellitus," *Journal of Clinical and Diagnostic Research* 7, no. 8 (2013): 1764–66, https://doi.org/10.7860/JCDR/2013/6518.3306.

46 Sylow et al., "Many Actions of Insulin"; Erik A. Richter and Mark Hargreaves, "Exercise, GLUT4, and Skeletal Muscle Glucose Uptake," Physiological Reviews 93, no. 3 (July 2013): 993–1017, https://doi.org/10.1152/physrev.00038.2012; Stephen M. Cornish and Matthew J. Barnes, "Editorial: Nutrition and Muscle Recovery After Exercise," *Frontiers in Sports and Active Living* 6 (April 2024): 1413822, https://doi.org/10.3389/fspor.2024.1413822; Lifeng Wang et al., "From Food Supplements to Functional Foods: Emerging Perspectives on Post-Exercise Recovery Nutrition," *Nutrients* 16, no. 23 (November 2024): 4081, https://doi.org/10.3390/nu16234081.

[47] Carl-Detlef Reimers et al., "Does Physical Activity Increase Life Expectancy? A Review of the Literature," *Journal of Aging Research* 2012, no. 1 (2012): 243958, https://doi.org/10.1155/2012/243958.

[48] Liisa Byberg et al., "Total Mortality After Changes in Leisure Time Physical Activity in 50 Year Old Men: 35 Year Follow-Up of Population Based Cohort," *BMJ* 338 (March 5, 2009): b688, https://doi.org/10.1136/bmj.b688.

[49] Gabriel Nasri Marzuca-Nassr et al., "Muscle Mass and Strength Gains Following Resistance Exercise Training in Older Adults 65–75 Years and Older Adults Above 85 Years," *International Journal of Sport Nutrition and Exercise Metabolism* 34, no. 1 (October 2023): 11–19, https://doi.org/10.1123/ijsnem.2023-0087.

[50] Amanda E. Paluch et al., "Steps per Day and All-Cause Mortality in Middle-Aged Adults in the Coronary Artery Risk Development in Young Adults Study," *JAMA Network Open* 4, no. 9 (2021): e2124516, https://doi.org/10.1001/jamanetworkopen.2021.24516.

[51] Kosuke Inoue et al., "Association of Daily Step Patterns with Mortality in US Adults," *JAMA Network Open* 6, no. 3 (2023): e235174, https://doi.org/10.1001/jamanetworkopen.2023.5174.

[52] Borja del Pozo Cruz et al., "Association of Daily Step Count and Intensity with Incident Dementia in 78,430 Adults Living in the UK," *JAMA Neurology* 79, no. 10 (2022): 1059–63, https://doi.org/10.1001/jamaneurol.2022.2672.

[53] P. Bernard et al., "Effects of a Six-Month Walking Intervention on Depression in Inactive Post-Menopausal Women: A Randomized Controlled Trial," *Aging & Mental Health* 19, no. 6 (2015): 485–92, https://doi.org/10.1080/13607863.2014.948806.

[54] Marcel Ballin et al., "Daily Step Count and Incident Diabetes in Community-Dwelling 70-Year-Olds: A Prospective Cohort Study," *BMC Public Health* 20, article no. 1830 (2020), https://doi.org/10.1186/s12889-020-09929-2.

[55] Elaine M. Murtagh et al., "The Effect of Walking on Risk Factors for Cardiovascular Disease: An Updated Systematic Review and Meta-Analysis of Randomised Control Trials," *Preventive Medicine* 72 (March 2015): 34–43, https://doi.org/10.1016/j.ypmed.2014.12.041.

[56] Anne McTiernan et al., "Physical Activity in Cancer Prevention and Survival: A Systematic Review," *Medicine & Science in Sports & Exercise* 51, no. 6 (2019): 1252–61, https://doi.org/10.1249/MSS.0000000000001937.

[57] Hiral Master et al., "Association of Step Counts over Time with the Risk of Chronic Disease in the *All of Us* Research Program," *Nature Medicine* 28 (2022): 2301–8, https://doi.org/10.1038/s41591-022-02012-w.

[58] Sébastien Herzig and Reuben J. Shaw, "AMPK: Guardian of Metabolism and Mitochondrial Homeostasis," *Nature Reviews Molecular Cell Biology* 19, no. 2 (2018): 121–35, https://doi.org/10.1038/nrm.2017.95.

[59] Sibylle Jäger et al., "AMP-Activated Protein Kinase (AMPK) Action in Skeletal Muscle via Direct Phosphorylation of PGC-1α," *Proceedings of the National Academy of Sciences of the United States of America* 104, no. 29 (July 2007): 12017–22, https://doi.org/10.1073/pnas.0705070104; Sandra Galic et al., "Hematopoietic AMPK β1 Reduces Mouse Adipose Tissue Macrophage Inflammation and Insulin Resistance in Obesity," *Journal of Clinical Investigation* 121, no. 12 (December 2011): 4903–15, https://doi.org/10.1172/JCI58577; Jianhui Li et al., "AMPK Alters Proteasome Phosphorylation Status and Prevents Persistent Proteasome Condensates," *bioRxiv* (July 2025), https://www.biorxiv.org/content/10.1101/2025.07.01.662652v1.

[60] Aidan J. Buffey et al., "The Acute Effects of Interrupting Prolonged Sitting Time in Adults with Standing and Light-Intensity Walking on Biomarkers of Cardiometabolic Health in Adults: A Systematic Review and Meta-Analysis," *Sports Medicine* 52 (2022): 1765–87, https://doi.org/10.1007/s40279-022-01649-4.

[61] Tobias Engeroff et al., "After Dinner Rest a While, After Supper Walk a Mile? A Systematic Review with Meta-Analysis on the Acute Postprandial Glycemic Response to Exercise Before and After Meal Ingestion in Healthy Subjects and Patients with Impaired Glucose Tolerance," *Sports Medicine* 53 (2023): 849–69, https://doi.org/10.1007/s40279-022-01808-7; Yasuyo Hijikata and Seika Yamada, "Walking Just After a Meal Seems to Be More Effective for Weight Loss Than Waiting for One Hour to Walk After a Meal," *International Journal of General Medicine* 4 (June 2011): 447–50, https://doi.org/10.2147/IJGM.S18837.

[62] Engeroff et al., "After Dinner Rest a While."

[63] Marc T. Hamilton et al., "A Potent Physiological Method to Magnify and Sustain Soleus Oxidative Metabolism Improves Glucose and Lipid Regulation," *iScience* 25, no. 9 (2022): 104869, https://doi.org/10.1016/j.isci.2022.104869.

[64] James A. Levine and Jennifer M. Miller, "The Energy Expenditure of Using a 'Walk-and-Work' Desk for Office Workers with Obesity," *British Journal of Sports Medicine* 41 (2007): 558–61, https://doi.org/10.1136/bjsm.2006.032755.

[65] Zoltan Ungvari et al., "The Multifaceted Benefits of Walking for Healthy Aging: From Blue Zones to Molecular Mechanisms," *GeroScience* 45, no. 6 (2023): 3211–39, https://doi.org/10.1007/s11357-023-00873-8.

[66] Diederick C. Niehorster, "Optic Flow: A History," *i-Perception* 12, no. 6 (2021): 20416695211055766, https://doi.org/10.1177/20416695211055766.

[67] Heekyung Jung and Andrew D. Huberman, "An Unbiased View of Neural Networks: More Than Meets the Eye," *Neuron* 100, no. 5 (2018): 1019–21, https://doi.org/10.1016/j.neuron.2018.11.038.

[68] Francine Shapiro, "The Role of Eye Movement Desensitization and Reprocessing (EMDR) Therapy in Medicine: Addressing the Psychological and Physical Symptoms Stemming from Adverse Life Experiences," *Permanente Journal* 18, no. 1 (Winter 2014): 71–77, https://doi.org/10.7812/TPP/13-098.

[69] Francine Shapiro, "Efficacy of the Eye Movement Desensitization Procedure in Treatment of Traumatic Memories," *Journal of Traumatic Stress* 2, no. 2 (1989): 199–223, https://doi.org/10.1002/jts.2490020207.

[70] Marco Pagani et al., "Eye Movement Desensitization and Reprocessing and Slow Wave Sleep: A Putative Mechanism of Action," *Frontiers in Psychology* 8 (November 2017), https://doi.org/10.3389/fpsyg.2017.01935; Leonard S. Milling et al., "A Meta-Analysis of Hypnotic Interventions for Depression Symptoms: High Hopes for Hypnosis?," *American Journal of Clinical Hypnosis* 61, no. 3 (December 2018): 227–43, https://doi.org/10.1080/00029157.2018.1489777; Siobhan K. O'Toole et al., "A Meta-Analysis of Hypnotherapeutic Techniques in the Treatment of PTSD Symptoms," *Journal of Traumatic Stress* 29, no. 1 (February 2016): 97–100, https://doi.org/10.1002/jts.22077.

[71] Ji-Woo Seok and Joong Il Kim, "The Efficacy of Eye Movement Desensitization and Reprocessing Treatment for Depression: A Meta-Analysis and Meta-Regression of Randomized Controlled Trials," *Journal of Clinical Medicine* 13, no. 18 (September 23, 2024): 5633, https://doi.org/10.3390/jcm13185633; Bessel A. van der Kolk et al., "A Randomized Clinical Trial of Eye Movement Desensitization and Reprocessing (EMDR), Fluoxetine, and Pill Placebo in the Treatment of Posttraumatic Stress Disorder: Treatment Effects and Long-Term Maintenance," *Journal of Clinical Psychiatry* 68, no. 1 (January 2007): 37–46, https://doi.org/10.4088/jcp.v68n0105.

[72] Sonja Sudimac et al., "How Nature Nurtures: Amygdala Activity Decreases as the Result of a One-Hour Walk in Nature," *Molecular Psychiatry* 27, no. 11 (2022): 4446–52, https://doi.org/10.1038/s41380-022-01720-6.

[73] Mathew P. White et al., "Spending at Least 120 Minutes a Week in Nature Is Associated with Good Health and Wellbeing," *Scientific Reports* 9, article no. 7730 (June 2019), https://doi.org/10.1038/s41598-019-44097-3.

[74] Xiaorong Bai et al., "Effect of Brisk Walking on Health-Related Physical Fitness Balance and Life Satisfaction Among the Elderly: A Systematic Review," *Frontiers in Public Health* 9 (January 31, 2022): 829367, https://doi.org/10.3389/fpubh.2021.829367.

[75] Ungvari et al., "Walking for Healthy Aging."

[76] Ying Gao et al., "Enhanced Muscle Activity During Interrupted Sitting Improves Glycemic Control in Overweight and Obese Men," *Scandinavian Journal of Medicine and Science in Sports* 34, no. 4 (April 2024): e14628, https://doi.org/10.1111/sms.14628.

[77] Patricia Huston and Bruce McFarlane, "Health Benefits of Tai Chi: What Is the Evidence?," *Canadian Family Physician* 62, no. 11 (2016): 881–90, https://pubmed.ncbi.nlm.nih.gov/28661865/; Guo-Yan Yang et al., "Determining the Safety and Effectiveness of Tai Chi: A Critical Overview of 210 Systematic Reviews of Controlled Clinical Trials," *Systematic Reviews* 11, article no. 260 (December 3, 2022), https://doi.org/10.1186/s13643-022-02100-5.

[78] William J. Kraemer and Nicholas A. Ratamess, "Fundamentals of Resistance Training: Progression and Exercise Prescription," *Medicine & Science in Sports & Exercise* 36, no. 4 (2004): 674–88, https://doi.org/10.1249/01.mss.0000121945.36635.61; Brad J. Schoenfeld et al., "Effects of Resistance Training Frequency on Measures of Muscle Hypertrophy: A Systematic Review and Meta-Analysis," *Sports Medicine* 46, no. 11 (April 2016): 1689–97, https://doi.org/10.1007/s40279-016-0543-8; Eneko Baz-Valle et al., "A Systematic Review of the Effects of Different Resistance Training Volumes on Muscle Hypertrophy," *Journal of Human Kinetics* 81 (February 2022): 199–210, https://doi.org/10.2478/hukin-2022-0017.

[79] Andrew Huberman, "Pavel Tsatsouline: The Correct Way to Build Strength, Endurance & Flexibility at Any Age," *Huberman Lab* (podcast audio), February 10, 2025, https://www.hubermanlab.com/episode/pavel-tsatsouline-build-strength-endurance-flexibility-at-any-age.

[80] Andrew Huberman, "Dr. Kelly Starrett: How to Improve Your Mobility, Posture & Flexibility," *Huberman Lab* (podcast audio), December 2024, https://www.hubermanlab.com/episode/dr-kelly-starrett-how-to-improve-your-mobility-posture-flexibility.

[81] Zouhal et al., "Catecholamines and the Effects."

[82] Richard P. Dum et al., "Motor, Cognitive, and Affective Areas of the Cerebral Cortex Influence the Adrenal Medulla," *Proceedings of the National Academy of Sciences* 113, no. 35 (August 2016): 9922–27, https://doi.org/10.1073/pnas.1605044113.

[83] James W. Krieger, "Single vs. Multiple Sets of Resistance Exercise for Muscle Hypertrophy: A Meta-Analysis," *Journal of Strength and Conditioning Research* 24, no. 4 (April 2010): 1150–59, https://doi.org/10.1519/JSC.0b013e3181d4d436.

[84] Mark D. Peterson et al., "Maximizing Strength Development in Athletes: A Meta-Analysis to Determine the Dose-Response Relationship," *Journal of Strength and Conditioning Research* 18, no. 2 (2004): 377–82, https://doi.org/10.1519/00124278-200405000-00031; Brad J. Schoenfeld et al., "Dose-Response Relationship Between Weekly Resistance Training Volume and Increases in Muscle Mass," *Journal of Sports Sciences* 35, no. 11 (June 2017): 1073–82, https://doi.org/10.1080/02640414.2016.1210197; Baz-Valle et al., "Systematic Review of the Effects"; Roberto Bernzárdez-Vázquez et al., "Resistance Training Variables for Optimization of Muscle Hypertrophy: An Umbrella Review," *Frontiers in Sports and Active Living* 4 (July 2022): 949021, https://doi.org/10.3389/fspor.2022.949021; Brad Jon Schoenfeld et al., "How Many Times per Week Should a Muscle Be Trained to Maximize Muscle Hypertrophy? A Systematic Review and Meta-Analysis," *Journal of Sports Sciences* 37, no. 11 (2019): 1286–95, https://doi.org/10.1080/02640414.2018.1555906.

[85] Helene Pedersen et al., "High-Frequency Resistance Training Improves Maximal Lower-Limb Strength More Than Low Frequency," *European Journal of Sport Science* 24, no. 5 (2024): 557–65, https://doi.org/10.1002/ejsc.12055.

[86] Kraemer and Ratamess, "Hormonal Responses and Adaptations"; William J. Kraemer et al., "Effects of Heavy-Resistance Training on Hormonal Response Patterns in Younger vs. Older Men,"

Journal of Applied Physiology 87, no. 3 (1999), https://journals.physiology.org/doi/full/10.1152/jappl.1999.87.3.982; William J. Kraemer et al., "Recovery Responses of Testosterone, Growth Hormone, and IGF-1 After Resistance Exercise," *Journal of Applied Physiology* 122, no. 3 (2017): 549–58, https://journals.physiology.org/doi/full/10.1152/japplphysiol.00599.2016; Simon Haunhorst et al., "Acute Effects of Heavy Resistance Exercise on Biomarkers of Neuroendocrine-Immune Regulation in Healthy Adults: A Systematic Review," *Exercise Immunology Review* 28 (2022): 36–52, PMID: 35452397.

[87] Mary I. Jumbelic, "Traumatic Asphyxia in Weightlifters," *Journal of Forensic Sciences* 52, no. 3 (April 2007): 702–5, https://doi.org/10.1111/j.1556-4029.2007.00429.x.

[88] Simeon P. Cairns, "Lactic Acid and Exercise Performance," *Sports Medicine* 36, no. 4 (2006): 279–91.

[89] Brad J. Schoenfeld et al., "Strength and Hypertrophy Adaptations between Low- vs. High-Load Resistance Training," *Journal of Strength and Conditioning Research* 31, no. 12 (December 2017): 3508–23, https://doi.org/10.1519/jsc.0000000000002200.

[90] Brad J. Schoenfeld et al., "Differential Effects of Heavy Versus Moderate Loads on Measures of Strength and Hypertrophy In Resistance-Trained Men," *Journal of Sports Science and Medicine* 15, no. 4 (December 2016): 715–22.

[91] Brad S. Currier et al., "American College of Sports Medicine Position Stand. Resistance Training Prescription for Muscle Function, Hypertrophy, and Physical Performance in Healthy Adults: An Overview of Reviews," *Medicine and Science in Sports and Exercise* 58, no. 4 (March 2026): 851, https://doi.org/10.1249/MSS.0000000000003897.

[92] Brad J. Schoenfeld, "The Mechanisms of Muscle Hypertrophy and Their Application to Resistance Training," *Journal of Strength and Conditioning Research* 24, no. 10 (October 2010): 2857–72, https://doi.org/10.1519/JSC.0b013e3181e840f3; Henning Wackerhage et al., "Stimuli and Sensors That Initiate Skeletal Muscle Hypertrophy Following Resistance Exercise," *Journal of Applied Physiology* 126, no. 1 (2019): 30–43, https://doi.org/10.1152/japplphysiol.00685.20; Carl Juneau, "Training for Hypertrophy: The Case Against Muscle Damage," Stronger by Science, accessed May 20, 2026, https://www.strongerbyscience.com/muscle-damage.

[93] A. Chesley et al., "Changes in Human Muscle Protein Synthesis After Resistance Exercise," *Journal of Applied Physiology* 73, no. 4 (1992): 1383–88, https://doi.org/10.1152/jappl.1992.73.4.1383; J. Duncan MacDougall et al., "The Time Course for Elevated Muscle Protein Synthesis Following Heavy Resistance Exercise," *Canadian Journal of Applied Physiology* 20, no. 4 (1995): 480–86, https://doi.org/10.1139/h95-038.

[94] Eric R. Helms et al., "Effect of Small and Large Energy Surpluses on Strength, Muscle, and Skinfold Thickness in Resistance-Trained Individuals: A Parallel Groups Design," *Sports Medicine—Open* 9, no. 1 (November 2023), https://doi.org/10.1186/s40798-023-00651-y.

[95] Gary John Slater et al., "Is an Energy Surplus Required to Maximize Skeletal Muscle Hypertrophy Associated with Resistance Training," *Frontiers in Nutrition* 6 (2019), https://doi.org/10.3389/fnut.2019.00131.

[96] F. I. Katch and W. D. McArdle, "Validity of Body Composition Prediction Equations for College Men and Women," *American Journal of Clinical Nutrition* 28, no. 2 (1975): 105–9, https://doi.org/10.1093/ajcn/28.2.105.

[97] C. Roth et al., "Lean Mass Sparing in Resistance-Trained Athletes During Caloric Restriction: The Role of Resistance Training Volume," *European Journal of Applied Physiology*, February 11, 2022, https://doi.org/10.1007/s00421-022-04896-5.

[98] R. Pratley et al., "Strength Training Increases Resting Metabolic Rate and Norepinephrine Levels in Healthy 50- to 65-Yr-Old Men," *Journal of Applied Physiology* 76, no. 1 (January 1994): 133–37, https://doi.org/10.1152/jappl.1994.76.1.133.

[99] Yasuko Manabe et al., "Exercise Training-Induced Adaptations Associated with Increases in Skeletal Muscle Glycogen Content," *FEBS Journal* 280, no. 3 (February 2013): 916–26, https://doi.org/10.1111/febs.12085.

[100] Colin D. Wilborn and Darryn S. Willoughby, "The Role of Dietary Protein Intake and Resistance Training on Myosin Heavy Chain Expression," *Journal of the International Society of Sports Nutrition* 1, no. 2 (December 2004), https://doi.org/10.1186/1550-2783-1-2-27.

[101] Erik A. Richter and Mark Hargreaves, "Exercise, GLUT4, and Skeletal Muscle Glucose Uptake," *Physiological Reviews* 93, no. 3 (2013): 993–1017, https://doi.org/10.1152/physrev.00038.2012; Erik A. Richter, "Is GLUT4 Translocation the Answer to Exercise-Stimulated Muscle Glucose Uptake?," *American Journal of Physiology* 320, no. 3 (February 2021): E240–43, https://doi.org/10.1152/ajpendo.00503.2020; Kendra D. Sticka et al., "Exercise Increases Glucose Transporter-4 Levels on Peripheral Blood Mononuclear Cells," *Medicine & Science in Sports & Exercise* 50, no. 5 (May 2019): 938–44, https://doi.org/10.1249/MSS.0000000000001528; John L. Ivy, "Muscle Glycogen Synthesis Before and After Exercise," *Sports Medicine* 11, no. 1 (1991): 6–19, https://doi.org/10.2165/00007256-199111010-00002; Jorn Trommelen et al., "The Anabolic Response to Protein Ingestion During Recovery from Exercise Has No Upper Limit in Magnitude and Duration In Vivo in Humans," *Cell Reports Medicine* 4, no. 12 (December 2023): 101324, https://doi.org/10.1016/j.xcrm.2023.101324; Andrew M. Holwerda, "Dose-Dependent Increases in Whole-Body Net Protein Balance and Dietary Protein-Derived Amino Acid Incorporation into Myofibrillar Protein During Recovery from Resistance Exercise in Older Men," *Journal of Nutrition* 149, no. 2 (February 2019): 221–30, https://doi.org/10.1093/jn/nxy263.

[102] Chen Xu et al., "The Effects of Creatine Supplementation on Cognitive Function in Adults: A Systematic Review and Meta-Analysis," *Frontiers in Nutrition* 11 (July 12, 2024): 1424972, https://doi.org/10.3389/fnut.2024.1424972; Chen Xu et al., "Corrigendum: The Effects of Creatine Supplementation," *Frontiers in Nutrition* 12 (February 17, 2025): 1570800, https://doi.org/10.3389/fnut.2025.1570800.

[103] Ali Gordji-Nejad et al., "Single Dose Creatine Improves Cognitive Performance and Induces Changes in Cerebral High Energy Phosphates During Sleep Deprivation," *Scientific Reports* 14, article no. 4937 (2024), https://doi.org/10.1038/s41598-024-54249-9.

[104] Elham Kabiri Naeini et al., "Effect of Creatine Supplementation on Kidney Function: A Systematic Review and Meta-Analysis," *BMC Nephrology* 26, article no. 622 (2025), https://doi.org/10.1186/s12882-025-04558-6.

[105] Mohammadyasin Lak et al., "Does Creatine Cause Hair Loss? A 12-Week Randomized Controlled Trial," *Journal of the International Society of Sports Nutrition* 22, no. S1 (2025): 2495229, https://doi.org/10.1080/15502783.2025.2495229.

[106] Nanci S. Guest et al., "International Society of Sports Nutrition Position Stand: Caffeine and Exercise Performance," *Journal of the International Society of Sports Nutrition* 18, no. 1 (2021), https://doi.org/10.1186/s12970-020-00383-4.

[107] Zhaolong Wang et al., "Effects of the Combined Supplementation of Caffeine and *Rhodiola rosea* with Resistance Training on Lower Limb Explosive Power in Male Volleyball Players," *Nutrients* 17, no. 4 (2025): 681, https://doi.org/10.3390/nu17040681; Xiaolin Wang et al., "The Effect of *Rhodiola rosea* Supplementation on Endurance Performance and Related Biomarkers: A Systematic Review and Meta-Analysis," *Frontiers in Nutrition* 12 (September 25, 2025): 1645346, https://doi.org/10.3389/fnut.2025.1645346; Grant M. Tinsley et al., "*Rhodiola rosea* as an Adaptogen to Enhance Exercise Performance: A Review of the Literature," *British Journal of Nutrition* 131, no. 3 (August 2023): 461–73, https://doi.org/10.1017/s0007114523001988.

[108] Ilkka Heinonen, "Cardiac Output Limits Maximal Oxygen Consumption, but What Limits Maximal Cardiac Output?," *Experimental Physiology* 110, no. 5 (2025): 666–74, https://doi.org/10.1113/EP091594.

[109] Kyle Fulghum and Bradford G. Hill, "Metabolic Mechanisms of Exercise-Induced Cardiac Remodeling," *Frontiers in Cardiovascular Medicine* 5 (September 10, 2018): 127, https://doi.org/10.3389/fcvm.2018.00127; Huihua Chen et al., "Exercise Training Maintains Cardiovascular Health: Signaling Pathways Involved and Potential Therapeutics," *Signal Transduction and Targeted Therapy* 7, article no. 306 (2022), https://doi.org/10.1038/s41392-022-01153-1; Kansan Roh et al., "Exercise-

Induced Cardiac Lymphatic Remodeling Mitigates Inflammation in the Aging Heart," *Aging Cell* 24, no. 6 (June 2025): e70043, https://doi.org/10.1111/acel.70043.

[110] Majd A. Alnawwar et al., "The Effect of Physical Activity on Sleep Quality and Sleep Disorder: A Systematic Review," *Cureus* 15, no. 8 (2023): e43595, https://doi.org/10.7759/cureus.43595; Weicheng Li et al., "Influence of Aerobic Exercise on Depression in Young People: A Meta-Analysis," *BMC Psychiatry* 24, article no. 571 (August 2024), https://doi.org/10.1186/s12888-024-06013-6; James A. Blumenthal et al., "Exercise and Pharmacotherapy in the Treatment of Major Depressive Disorder," *Psychosomatic Medicine* 69, no. 7 (2007): 587–96, https://doi.org/10.1097/PSY.0b013e318148c19a.

[111] Hirofumi Tanaka et al., "Age-Predicted Maximal Heart Rate Revisited," *Journal of the American College of Cardiology* 37, no. 1 (2001): 153–56, https://doi.org/10.1016/s0735-1097(00)01054-8; Martha Gulati et al., "Heart Rate Response to Exercise Stress Testing in Asymptomatic Women: The St. James Women Take Heart Project," *Circulation* 122, no. 2 (2010): 130–37, https://doi.org/10.1161/CIRCULATIONAHA.110.939249.

[112] Øystein Sylta et al., "From Heart-Rate Data to Training Quantification: A Comparison of 3 Methods of Training-Intensity Analysis," *International Journal of Sports Physiology and Performance* 9, no. 1 (2014): 100–107, https://doi.org/10.1123/IJSPP.2013-0298.

[113] Andrea D'Amuri et al., "Effectiveness of High-Intensity Interval Training for Weight Loss in Adults with Obesity: A Randomised Controlled Non-Inferiority Trial," *BMJ Open Sport & Exercise Medicine* 7, no. 3 (2021): e001021, https://doi.org/10.1136/bmjsem-2020-001021.

[114] Stephen H. Boutcher, "High-Intensity Intermittent Exercise and Fat Loss," *Journal of Obesity* 2011 (November 2010): 868305, https://doi.org/10.1155/2011/868305.

[115] Kenneth H. Cooper, "A Means of Assessing Maximal Oxygen Intake: Correlation Between Field and Treadmill Testing," *JAMA* 203, no. 3 (1968): 201–4, https://doi.org/10.1001/jama.1968.03140030033008.

[116] Steve Magness, "Longevity and Vo2max? Does It Actually Matter?," Steve Magness Substack, November 10, 2025, https://stevemagness.substack.com/p/longevity-and-vo2max-does-it-actually.

[117] Dorthe Stensvold et al., "Effect of Exercise Training for Five Years on All Cause Mortality in Older Adults—the Generation 100 Study: Randomised Controlled Trial," *BMJ* 371 (2020): m3485, https://doi.org/10.1136/bmj.m3485.

[118] Ole Johan Kemi and Ulrik Wisløff, "High-Intensity Aerobic Exercise Training Improves the Heart in Health and Disease," *Journal of Cardiopulmonary Rehabilitation and Prevention* 30, no. 1 (January 2010): 2–11, https://doi.org/10.1097/hcr.0b013e3181c56b89.

[119] Knut Sindre Mølmen et al., "Effects of Exercise Training on Mitochondrial and Capillary Growth in Human Skeletal Muscle: A Systematic Review and Meta-Regression," *Sports Medicine* 55, no. 1 (October 2024), https://doi.org/10.1007/s40279-024-02120-2.

[120] Neil L. Coplan et al., "Exercise-Related Changes in Serum Catecholamines and Potassium: Effect of Sustained Exercise Above and Below Lactate Threshold," *American Heart Journal* 117, no. 5 (May 1989): 1070–75, https://doi.org/10.1016/0002-8703(89)90864-8.

[121] Zoladz, *Muscle and Exercise Physiology*; Powers and Howley, *Exercise Physiology*; Koman et al., "Beneficial Effects of Aerobic Exercise"; MoTrPAC Study Group et al., "Multi-Omic, Multi-Tissue Responses"; Contrepois et al., "Molecular Choreography of Acute Exercise"; Kraemer and Ratamess, "Hormonal Responses and Adaptations"; Zouhal et al., "Catecholamines and the Effects"; Athanasiou et al., "Endocrine Responses of the Stress System"; Hellsten, "Cardiovascular Adaptations to Exercise Training"; Mark Ross et al., "Exercise-Induced Skeletal Muscle Angiogenesis," *European Journal of Applied Physiology* 123, no. 7 (July 2023): 1415–32, https://doi.org/10.1007/s00421-022-05128-6; David A. Hood et al., "Exercise and the Regulation of Mitochondrial Turnover," *Progress in Molecular Biology and Translational Science* 135 (2015): 99–127, https://doi.org/10.1016/bs.pmbts.2015.07.007; Tao Cai et al., "The Role of Exercise-Mediated Mitochondrial Quality Control Remodeling in Aging,"

Frontiers in Cell and Developmental Biology 14 (March 2026): 1792645, https://doi.org/10.3389/fcell.2026.1792645; Julia C. Basso and Wendy A. Suzuki, "The Effects of Acute Exercise on Mood, Cognition, Neurophysiology, and Neurochemical Pathways," *Brain Plasticity* 2, no. 2 (March 2017): 127–52, https://doi.org/10.3233/BPL-160040; Bret H. Goodpaster and Lauren M. Sparks, "Metabolic Flexibility in Health and Disease," *Cell Metabolism* 25, no. 5 (May 2017): 1027–36; Mølmen et al., "Effects of Exercise Training on Mitochondrial"; Joanna Kruk et al., "Physical Exercise and Catecholamines Response: Benefits and Health Risk: Possible Mechanisms," *Free Radical Research* 54, no. 2–3 (February 2020): 105–25, https://doi.org/10.1080/10715762.2020.1726343.

[122] David P. Swain and Barry A. Franklin, "Comparison of Cardioprotective Benefits of Vigorous Versus Moderate Intensity Aerobic Exercise," *American Journal of Cardiology* 97, no. 1 (January 2006): 141–47, https://doi.org/10.1016/j.amjcard.2005.07.130.

[123] Laura Weiglein et al., "The 1-Mile Walk Test Is a Valid Predictor of VO_2max and Is a Reliable Alternative Fitness Test to the 1.5-Mile Run in U.S. Air Force Males," *Military Medicine* 176, no. 6 (June 2011): 669–73, https://doi.org/10.7205/milmed-d-10-00444.

[124] Sverre Valstad et al., "Comparison of Long and Short High-Intensity Interval Exercise Bouts on Running Performance, Physiological and Perceptual Responses," *Sports Medicine International Open* 2, no. 01 (December 2017): E20–27, https://doi.org/10.1055/s-0043-124429.

[125] Kyle Mandsager et al., "Association of Cardiorespiratory Fitness with Long-Term Mortality Among Adults Undergoing Exercise Treadmill Testing," *JAMA Network Open* 1, no. 6 (October 2018): e183605, https://doi.org/10.1001/jamanetworkopen.2018.3605; Prathiyankara Shailendra et al., "Resistance Training and Mortality Risk: A Systematic Review and Meta-Analysis," *American Journal of Preventive Medicine* 63, no. 2 (May 2022): 277–85, https://doi.org/10.1016/j.amepre.2022.03.020.

[126] G. A. Dudley and R. Djamil, "Incompatibility of Endurance- and Strength-Training Modes of Exercise," *Journal of Applied Physiology* 59, no. 5 (November 1985): 1446–51, https://doi.org/10.1152/jappl.1985.59.5.1446.

[127] Tao Wang and Shumin Bo, "Optimizing Concurrent Training Programs: A Review on Factors That Enhance Muscle Strength," *Medicine* 103, no. 52 (December 2024): e41055, https://doi.org/10.1097/md.0000000000041055.

[128] Abdulmenaf Korkutata et al., "The Impact of Exercise on Sleep and Sleep Disorders," *npj Biological Timing and Sleep* 2, article no. 5 (2025), https://doi.org/10.1038/s44323-024-00018-w; Ali Gordji-Nejad et al., "Single Dose Creatine Improves Cognitive Performance and Induces Changes in Cerebral High Energy Phosphates During Sleep Deprivation," *Scientific Reports* 14, no. 1 (February 28, 2024): 4937, https://doi.org/10.1038/s41598-024-54249-9.

[129] Jonathan Charest and Michael A. Grandner, "Sleep and Athletic Performance: Impacts on Physical Performance, Mental Performance, Injury Risk and Recovery, and Mental Health," *Sleep Medicine Clinics* 15, no. 1 (2020): 41–57, https://doi.org/10.1016/j.jsmc.2019.11.005.

[130] Shahab Alizadeh et al., "Resistance Training Induces Improvements in Range of Motion: A Systematic Review and Meta-Analysis," *Sports Medicine* 53, no. 3 (January 2023): 707–22, https://doi.org/10.1007/s40279-022-01804-x; Morton Rosenfeldt et al., "Comparison of Resistance Training vs Static Stretching on Flexibility and Maximal Strength in Healthy Physically Active Adults," *BMC Sports Science, Medicine and Rehabilitation* 16 (June 2024): 142, https://doi.org/10.1186/s13102-024-00934-1; Sebastian Vetter et al., "The Effects of Eccentric Strength Training on Flexibility and Strength in Healthy Samples and Laboratory Settings: A Systematic Review," *Frontiers in Physiology* 13 (April 2022): 873370, https://doi.org/10.3389/fphys.2022.873370; Francesco Favre et al., "Influence of Resistance Training on Joint Flexibility in Healthy Adults: A Systematic Review, Meta-Analysis, and Meta-Regression," *Journal of Strength & Conditioning Research* 39, no. 3 (December 2024): 386–97, https://doi.org/10.1519/JSC.0000000000005000.

[131] Milo Wolf et al., "Lengthened Partial Repetitions Elicit Similar Muscular Adaptations as Full Range of Motion Repetitions During Resistance Training in Trained Individuals," *PeerJ* 13 (February

2025): e18904, https://doi.org/10.7717/peerj.18904; Alizadeh et al., "Resistance Training Induces Improvements."

Chapter 3: Protocols for Stress Control

[1] Modupe Akinola et al., "Adaptive Appraisals of Anxiety Moderate the Association Between Cortisol Reactivity and Performance in Salary Negotiations," *PLOS One* 11, no. 12 (December 2016): e0167977, https://doi.org/10.1371/journal.pone.0167977; Alia J. Crum et al., "Rethinking Stress: The Role of Mindsets in Determining the Stress Response," *Journal of Personality and Social Psychology* 104, no. 4 (April 2013): 716–33, https://doi.org/10.1037/a0031201; Alia Crum et al., "The Role of Stress Mindset in Shaping Cognitive, Emotional, and Physiological Responses to Challenging and Threatening Stress," *Anxiety, Stress, & Coping* 30, no. 4 (January 2017): 379–95, https://doi.org/10.1080/10615806.2016.1275585; Alia J. Crum et al., "Optimizing Stress: An Integrated Intervention for Regulating Stress Responses," *Emotion* 20, no. 1 (February 2020): 120–25, https://doi.org/10.1037/emo0000670; Alia J. Crum et al., "Evaluation of the 'Rethink Stress' Mindset Intervention: A Metacognitive Approach to Changing Mindsets," *Journal of Experimental Psychology* 153, no. 9 (2023): 2603–22, http://doi.org/10.1037/xge0001396; Roman Dunce et al., "Acute Exposure to Stress Improves Performance in Trace Eyeblink Conditioning and Spatial Learning Tasks in Healthy Men," *Learning & Memory* 14, no. 5 (May 2007): 329–35, https://doi.org/10.1101/lm.483807; Jeremy P. Jamieson et al., "Mind over Matter: Reappraising Arousal Improves Cardiovascular and Cognitive Responses to Stress," *Journal of Experimental Psychology: General* 141, no. 3 (September 2011): 417–22, https://doi.org/10.1037/a0025719; Eric N. Smith et al., "Stress, Mindsets, and Success in Navy SEALs Special Warfare Training," *Frontiers in Psychology* 10 (January 2020): 2962, https://doi.org/10.3389/fpsyg.2019.02962; Allison Wood Brooks, "Get Excited: Reappraising Pre-Performance Anxiety as Excitement," *Journal of Experimental Psychology: General* 143, no. 3 (2014): 1144–58, https://doi.org/10.1037/a0035325.

[2] J. A. Easterbrook, "The Effect of Emotion on Cue Utilization and the Organization of Behavior," *Psychological Review* 66, no. 3 (May 1959): 183–201, https://doi.org/10.1037/h0047707; Robert J. Hockey, "Stress and the Cognitive Components of Skilled Performance," in *Human Stress and Cognition: An Information Processing Approach*, ed. Vernon Hamilton (John Wiley & Sons, 1979); Lorraine Hope et al., "Witnesses in Action: The Effect of Physical Exertion on Recall and Recognition," *Psychological Science* 23, no. 4 (2012): 386–90, https://doi.org/10.1177/0956797611431463; Jessica Wapner, "Secrets to Surviving Stressful Times," *Scientific American Mind* 32, no. 1 (January 2021): 14, https://www.scientificamerican.com/article/vision-and-breathing-may-be-the-secrets-to-surviving-2020/; R. J. Miller and Masatoshi Takahama, "Effects of Relaxation and Aversive Visual Stimulation on Dark Focus Accommodation," *Ophthalmic and Physiological Optics* 7 (July 1987): 219–23, https://doi.org/10.1111/j.1475-1313.1987.tb00736.x; Edward C. Godnig, "Tunnel Vision: Its Causes and Treatment Strategies," *Journal of Behavioral Optometry* 14, no. 4 (2003): 95–99, https://www.oepf.org/wp-content/uploads/2021/08/14-420Godnig1.pdf.

[3] Lindsay D. Salay et al., "A Midline Thalamic Circuit Determines Reactions to Visual Threat," *Nature* 557, no. 7704 (May 2018): 183–89, https://doi.org/10.1038/s41586-018-0078-2; Joseph E. LeDoux and Daniel S. Pine, "Using Neuroscience to Help Understand Fear and Anxiety: A Two-System Framework," *American Journal of Psychiatry* 173, no. 11 (November 2016): 1083–93, https://doi.org/10.1176/appi.ajp.2016.16030353.

[4] Huda Akil et al., "Stress Fitness: A Neuroscientific Approach to Building Emotional Resilience," *Neuron* (2026), https://doi.org/10.1016/j.neuron.2026.03.032; Bruce S. McEwen, "Stress, Adaptation, and Disease: Allostasis and Allostatic Load," *Annals of the New York Academy of Sciences* 840 (1998): 33–34, https://doi.org/10.1111/j.1749-6632.1998.tb09546.x; Rachel Gilgoff et al., "The Stress Phenotyping Framework: A Multidisciplinary Biobehavioral Approach for Assessing and Therapeutically Targeting Maladapted Stress Physiology," *Stress* 27, no. 1 (January 2024): 2327333, https://doi.org/10.1080/10253890.2024.2327333.

[5] Regula Zueger et al., "Testosterone and Cortisol Responses to Acute and Prolonged Stress During Officer Training School," *Stress* 26, no. 1 (2023), https://doi.org/10.1080/10253890.2023.2199886; Yaxin Fan et al., "Salivary Testosterone and Cortisol Response in Acute Stress Modulated by Seven Sessions of Mindfulness Meditation in Young Males," *Stress* 27, no. 1 (2024), https://doi.org/10.1080/10253890.2024.2316041.

[6] Amna Alotiby, "Immunology of Stress: A Review Article," *Journal of Clinical Medicine* 13, no. 21 (2024): 6394, https://doi.org/10.3390/jcm13216394.

[7] Brynn E. Sherman et al., "Hippocampal Mechanisms Support Cortisol-Induced Memory Enhancements," *Journal of Neuroscience* 43, no. 43 (October 2023): JN-23, https://doi.org/10.1523/jneurosci.0916-23.2023; William J. Kraemer and Nicholas A. Ratamess, "Hormonal Responses and Adaptations to Resistance Exercise and Training," *Sports Medicine* 35, no. 4 (2005): 339–61, https://doi.org/10.2165/00007256-200535040-00004; Truls Raastad et al., "Hormonal Responses to High- and Moderate-Intensity Strength Exercise," *European Journal of Applied Physiology* 82 (May 2000): 121–28, https://doi.org/10.1007/s004210050661; David C. Cumming et al., "Reproductive Hormone Responses to Resistance Exercise," *Medicine & Science in Sports & Exercise* 19, no. 3 (June 1987): 234–38; Stuart F. White et al., "Putting the Flight in 'Fight-or-Flight': Testosterone Reactivity to Skydiving Is Modulated by Autonomic Activation," *Biological Psychology* 143 (April 2019): 93–102, https://doi.org/10.1016/j.biopsycho.2019.02.012; S. D. Richter et al., "Time Kinetics of the Endocrine Response to Acute Psychological Stress," *Journal of Clinical Endocrinology and Metabolism* 81, no. 5 (May 1996): 1956–60, https://doi.org/10.1210/jcem.81.5.8626864; F. S. Dhabhar and B. S. McEwen, "Acute Stress Enhances While Chronic Stress Suppresses Cell-Mediated Immunity In Vivo: A Potential Role for Leukocyte Trafficking," *Brain, Behavior, and Immunity* 11, no. 4 (December 1997): 286–306, https://doi.org/10.1006/brbi.1997.0508; Firdaus S. Dhabhar, "Enhancing Versus Suppressive Effects of Stress on Immune Function: Implications for Immunoprotection and Immunopathology," *Neuroimmunomodulation* 16, no. 5 (2009): 300–317, https://doi.org/10.1159/000216188; Firdaus S. Dhabhar, "Effects of Stress on Immune Function: The Good, the Bad, and the Beautiful," *Immunologic Research* 58 (2014): 193–210, https://doi.org/10.1007/s12026-014-8517-0; Suzanne C. Segerstrom and Gregory E. Miller, "Psychological Stress and the Human Immune System: A Meta-Analytic Study of 30 Years of Inquiry," *Psychological Bulletin* 130, no. 4 (2004): 601–30, https://doi.org/10.1037/0033-2909.130.4.601; Larry Cahill et al., "β-Adrenergic Activation and Memory for Emotional Events," *Nature* 371 (1994): 702–4, https://doi.org/10.1038/371702a0; Marian Joëls et al., "Learning Under Stress: How Does It Work?," *Trends in Cognitive Sciences* 10, no. 4 (April 2006): 152–58, https://doi.org/10.1016/j.tics.2006.02.002; Carmen Sandi and M. Teresa Pinelo-Nava, "Stress and Memory: Behavioral Effects and Neurobiological Mechanisms," *Neural Plasticity* 2007 (2007): 78970, https://doi.org/10.1155/2007/789; Tom Smeets et al., "True or False? Memory Is Differentially Affected by Stress-Induced Cortisol Elevations and Sympathetic Activity at Consolidation and Retrieval," *Psychoneuroendocrinology* 33, no. 10 (November 2008): 1378–86; Susanne Vogel and Lars Schwabe, "True or False? Memory Is Differentially Affected by Stress-Induced Cortisol Elevations and Sympathetic Activity at Consolidation and Retrieval," *Psychoneuroendocrinology* 71 (September 2016): 64–72, https://doi.org/10.1016/j.psyneuen.2016.04.027.

[8] Donald H. Meichenbaum and Jerry L. Deffenbacher, "Stress Inoculation Training," *Counseling Psychologist* 16, no. 1 (1988): 69–90, https://doi.org/10.1177/0011000088161005; Zhanying Sun et al., "Preventing and Mitigating Post-Traumatic Stress: A Scoping Review of Resilience Interventions for Military Personnel in Pre-Deployment," *Psychology Research and Behavior Management* 17 (June 17, 2024): 2377–89, https://doi.org/10.2147/PRBM.S459220.

[9] David M. Lyons et al., "Preliminary Evidence That Hippocampal Volumes in Monkeys Predict Stress Levels of Adrenocorticotropic Hormone," *Biological Psychiatry* 62 (2007): 1171–74, https://doi.org/10.1016/j.biopsych.2007.03.012; Steven F. Maier and Martin E. P. Seligman, "Learned Helplessness at Fifty: Insights from Neuroscience," *Psychological Review* 123, no. 4 (2016): 349–67, https://doi.org/10.1037/rev0000033; Teri Saunders et al., "The Effect of Stress Inoculation Training on Anxiety and Performance," *Journal of Occupational Health Psychology* 1, no. 2 (1996): 170–86, https://doi.org

/10.1037/1076-8998.1.2.170; Glenn E. Richardson, "The Metatheory of Resilience and Resiliency," *Journal of Clinical Psychology* 58, no. 3 (March 2002): 307–21, https://doi.org/10.1002/jclp.10020.

[10] E. Kross et al., "Self-Talk as a Regulatory Mechanism: How You Do It Matters," *Journal of Personality and Social Psychology* 106, no. 2 (2014): 304–24, https://doi.org/10.1037/a0035173; Claire Eagleson et al., "The Power of Positive Thinking: Pathological Worry Is Reduced by Thought Replacement in Generalized Anxiety Disorder," *Behaviour Research and Therapy* 78 (March 2016): 13–18, https://doi .org/10.1016/j.brat.2015.12.017.

[11] Joanne V. Wood et al., "Positive Self-Statements: Power for Some, Peril for Others," *Psychological Science* 20, no. 7 (2009): 860–66, https://doi.org/10.1111/j.1467-9280.2009.02370.x; Eagleson et al., "Power of Positive Thinking."

[12] Elizabeth A. Hoge et al., "The Effect of Mindfulness Meditation Training on Biological Acute Stress Responses in Generalized Anxiety Disorder," *Psychiatry Research* 262 (April 2018): 328–32, https://doi .org/10.1016/j.psychres.2017.01.006.

[13] Julia C. Basso et al., "Brief, Daily Meditation Enhances Attention, Memory, Mood, and Emotional Regulation in Non-Experienced Meditators," *Behavioural Brain Research* 356 (January 1, 2019): 208–20, https://doi.org/10.1016/j.bbr.2018.08.023; Simon B. Goldberg et al., "Testing the Efficacy of a Multicomponent, Self-Guided, Smartphone-Based Meditation App: Three-Armed Randomized Controlled Trial," *JMIR Mental Health* 7, no. 11 (November 2020): e23825, https://doi.org/10.2196 /23825; Melis Yilmaz Balban et al., "Brief Structured Respiration Practices Enhance Mood and Reduce Physiological Arousal," *Cell Reports Medicine* 4, no. 1 (January 2023): 1–15, https://doi.org/10.1016 /j.xcrm.2022.100895.

[14] Daniel Goleman and Richard J. Davidson, *Altered Traits: Science Reveals How Meditation Changes Your Mind, Brain and Body* (Avery, 2017).

[15] Hannes Ernst et al., "Assessment of the Human Response to Acute Mental Stress—an Overview and a Multimodal Study," *PLOS One* 18, no. 11 (2023): e0294069, https://doi.org/10.1371/journal .pone.0294069.

[16] Justina Ngozi Igwe et al., "Effectiveness of Cognitive Behavior Therapy on Occupational Stress Management Among Administrative, Language, Science and Vocational Education Staff Within Open and Distance Learning Centers: A Randomized Controlled Trial Evaluation," *Medicine* 103, no. 9 (2024): e37231, https://pubmed.ncbi.nlm.nih.gov/38428863/.

[17] David H. Barlow et al., "The Unified Protocol for Transdiagnostic Treatment of Emotional Disorders Compared with Diagnosis-Specific Protocols for Anxiety Disorders: A Randomized Clinical Trial," *JAMA Psychiatry* 74, no. 9 (September 2018): 875–84, https://doi.org/10.1001/jamapsychiatry.2017.2164; Beth Fordham et al., "The Evidence for Cognitive Behavioural Therapy in Any Condition, Population or Context: A Meta-Review of Systematic Reviews and Panoramic Meta-Analysis," *Psychological Medicine* 51, no. 1 (January 2021): 21–29, https://doi.org/10.1017/S0033291720005292.

[18] J. N. Langley, *The Autonomic Nervous System, Part I* (W. Heffer & Sons, 1921); Wilfrid Jänig, *The Integrative Action of the Autonomic Nervous System: Neurobiology of Homeostasis* (Cambridge, UK: Cambridge University Press, 2008).

[19] Francesca Baschieri and Pietro Cortelli, "Circadian Rhythms of Cardiovascular Autonomic Function: Physiology and Clinical Implications in Neurodegenerative Diseases," *Autonomic Neuroscience: Basic & Clinical* 217 (March 2019): 91–101, https://doi.org/10.1016/j.autneu.2019.01.009.

[20] Ilaria Barone et al., "Synaptic BMAL1 Phosphorylation Controls Circadian Hippocampal Plasticity," *Science Advances* 9, no. 43 (2023), https://doi.org/10.1126/sciadv.adj1010; Shiyang Xu et al., "Relationship Between Circadian Rhythm and Brain Cognitive Functions," *Frontiers of Optoelectronics* 14, no. 3 (2021): 278–87, https://doi.org/10.1007/s12200-021-1090-y.

[21] Collin M. Douglas et al., "Time of Day and Muscle Strength: A Circadian Output?," *Physiology* 36, no. 1 (2021): 44–51, https://doi.org/10.1152/physiol.00030.2020; Louis Sebastian Gifford, "Circadian

Variation in Human Flexibility and Grip Strength," *Australian Journal of Physiotherapy* 33, no. 1 (1987): 3–9, https://doi.org/10.1016/S0004-9514(14)60579-1.

[22] Aïssatou Bailo Diallo et al., "For Whom the Clock Ticks: Clinical Chronobiology for Infectious Diseases," *Frontiers in Immunology* 11 (July 8, 2020): 1457, https://doi.org/10.3389/fimmu.2020.01457; Gareth B. Kitchen et al., "The Clock Gene *Bmal1* Inhibits Macrophage Motility, Phagocytosis, and Impairs Defense Against Pneumonia," *Proceedings of the National Academy of Sciences* 117, no. 3 (2020): 1543–51, https://doi.org/10.1073/pnas.1915932117.

[23] Thomas Steckler et al., *Stress and the Brain Part 1: The Neurobiology of Stress* (Elsevier Sciences, 2005); Thomas Steckler et al., *Stress and the Brain Part 2: Integrative and Clinical Aspects* (Elsevier Sciences, 2005).

[24] Neal L. Benowitz et al., "Sympathomimetic Effects of Paraxanthine and Caffeine in Humans," *Clinical Pharmacology & Therapeutics* 58, no. 6 (1995): 684–91, https://doi.org/10.1016/0009-9236(95)90025-X.

[25] Ilse C. Schrieks et al., "The Biphasic Effects of Moderate Alcohol Consumption with a Meal on Ambiance-Induced Mood and Autonomic Nervous System Balance: A Randomized Crossover Trial," *PLOS One* 9, no. 1 (2014): e86199, https://doi.org/10.1371/journal.pone.0086199.

[26] Daniel J. Kramer and Adiv A. Johnson, "Apigenin: A Natural Molecule at the Intersection of Sleep and Aging," *Frontiers in Nutrition* 11 (February 26, 2024): 1359176, https://doi.org/10.3389/fnut.2024.1359176.

[27] Florent Besnier et al., "Exercise Training-Induced Modification in Autonomic Nervous System: An Update for Cardiac Patients," *Annals of Physical and Rehabilitation Medicine* 60, no. 1 (2017): 27–35, https://doi.org/10.1016/j.rehab.2016.07.002.

[28] Maria Meier et al., "Standardized Massage Interventions as Protocols for the Induction of Psychophysiological Relaxation in the Laboratory: A Block Randomized, Controlled Trial," *Scientific Reports* 10, article no. 14774 (2020), https://doi.org/10.1038/s41598-020-71173-w; Jian Cui et al., "Repeated Warm Water Baths Decrease Sympathetic Activity in Humans," *Journal of Applied Physiology* 133, no. 1 (2022): 234–45, https://doi.org/10.1152/japplphysiol.00684.2021.

[29] Brian Fiani et al., "The Neurophysiology of Caffeine as a Central Nervous System Stimulant and the Resultant Effects on Cognitive Function," *Cureus* 13, no. 5 (2021): e15032, https://doi.org/10.7759/cureus.15032.

[30] Steckler et al., *Stress and the Brain Part 1*; Steckler et al., *Stress and the Brain Part 2*; Task Force of the European Society of Cardiology and the North American Society of Pacing and Electrophysiology, "Heart Rate Variability: Standards of Measurement, Physiological Interpretation and Clinical Use," *Circulation* 93, no. 5 (March 1996): 1043–65, PMID: 8598068.

[31] Georgina Russell and Stafford Lightman, "The Human Stress Response," *Nature Reviews Endocrinology* 15 (June 2019): 525–34, https://doi.org/10.1038/s41574-019-0228-0.

[32] Amy F. T. Arnsten et al., "The Effects of Stress Exposure on Prefrontal Cortex: Translating Basic Research into Successful Treatments for Post-Traumatic Stress Disorder," *Neurobiology of Stress* 1 (January 2015): 89–99, https://doi.org/10.1016/j.ynstr.2014.10.002; Elizabeth Woo et al., "Chronic Stress Weakens Connectivity in the Prefrontal Cortex: Architectural and Molecular Changes," *Chronic Stress* 5 (August 2021), https://doi.org/10.1177/24705470211029254.

[33] Kai A. Schüren et al., "Stress Disrupts Hippocampal Integration of Overlapping Events and Memory Inference in Humans," *Science Advances* 12, no. 21 (May 2026): eaea5496, https://doi.org/10.1126/sciadv.aea5496.

[34] Andrea Zaccaro et al., "How Breath-Control Can Change Your Life: A Systematic Review on Psycho-Physiological Correlates of Slow Breathing," *Frontiers in Human Neuroscience* 12 (September 2018): 353, https://doi.org/10.3389/fnhum.2018.00353.

[35] Balban et al., "Brief Structured Respiration Practices"; Christina Zelano et al., "Nasal Respiration Entrains Human Limbic Oscillations and Modulates Cognitive Function," *Journal of Neuroscience* 36,

no. 49 (December 2016): 12448–67, https://doi.org/10.1523/JNEUROSCI.2586-16.2016; Peng Li et al., "The Peptidergic Control Circuit for Sighing," *Nature* 530 (February 2016): 293–97, https://doi.org/10.1038/nature16964; Loren Toussaint et al., "Effectiveness of Progressive Muscle Relaxation, Deep Breathing, and Guided Imagery in Promoting Psychological and Physiological States of Relaxation," *Evidence-Based Complementary and Alternative Medicine* 2021 (2021): 5924040, https://doi.org/10.1155/2021/5924040; Kevin Yackle et al., "Breathing Control Center Neurons That Promote Arousal in Mice," *Science* 335, no. 6332 (March 2017): 1411–15, https://doi.org/10.1126/science.aai7984; Sufyan Ashhad et al., "Breathing Rhythm and Pattern and Their Influence on Emotion," *Annual Review of Neuroscience* 45 (July 2022): 223–47, https://doi.org/10.1146/annurev-neuro-090121-014424.

[36] Joshua E. Brinkman et al., "Physiology, Respiratory Drive," StatPearls, last updated June 5, 2023, https://www.ncbi.nlm.nih.gov/books/NBK482414/.

[37] Jänig, *Integrative Action*; Robert Fried, *The Psychology and Physiology of Breathing* (Springer, 1993).

[38] Michael Drechsler and Jason Morris, "Carbon Dioxide Narcosis," StatPearls, last updated January 9, 2023, https://www.ncbi.nlm.nih.gov/books/NBK551620/.

[39] C. Gilbert, "Hyperventilation and the Body," *Accident and Emergency Nursing* 7, no. 3 (1999): 130–40, https://doi.org/10.1016/s0965-2302(99)80072-1.

[40] E. Nattie, "CO_2, Brainstem Chemoreceptors and Breathing," *Progress in Neurobiology* 59, no. 4 (1999): 299–331, https://doi.org/10.1016/s0301-0082(99)00008-8.

[41] Sarah Nadine Meissner et al., "Self-Regulating Arousal via Pupil-Based Biofeedback," *Nature Human Behaviour* 8 (2024): 43–62, https://doi.org/10.1038/s41562-023-01729-z.

[42] Jeffrey C. Smith et al., "Pre-Bötzinger Complex: A Brainstem Region That May Generate Respiratory Rhythm in Mammals," *Science* 254, no. 5032 (1991): 726–29, https://doi.org/10.1126/science.1683005; Paul A. Gray et al., "Normal Breathing Requires Pre-Bötzinger Complex Neurokinin-1 Receptor-Expressing Neurons," *Nature Neuroscience* 4 (2001): 927–30, https://doi.org/10.1038/nn0901-927; Li et al., "Peptidergic Control Circuit."

[43] Andrew Huberman, "Dr. Jack Feldman: Breathing for Mental & Physical Health and Performance," *Huberman Lab* (podcast audio), November 13, 2025, https://www.hubermanlab.com/episode/essentials-breathing-mental-physical-health-performance-jack-feldman.

[44] Alberto Giannoni et al., "Upright Cheyne-Stokes Respiration in Patients with Heart Failure," *JACC* 75, no. 23 (2020): 2934–46, https://doi.org/10.1016/j.jacc.2020.04.033.

[45] R. Doug McEvoy et al., "The Sleep Apnea Cardiovascular Endpoints (SAVE) Trial: Rationale and Start-Up Phase," *Journal of Thoracic Disease* 2, no. 3 (2010): 138–43, https://doi.org/10.3978/j.issn.2072-1439.2010.02.03.5; R. Doug McEvoy et al., "Erratum to the Sleep Apnea Cardiovascular Endpoints (SAVE) Trial," *Journal of Thoracic Disease* 8, no. 8 (2016): E850, https://doi.org/10.21037/jtd.2016.07.79.

[46] Heidi L. Grabenstatter, "Irregular Respiratory Rhythm: A Physiological Biomarker of SUDEP Risk in Patients with Nocturnal Seizures?," *Epilepsy Currents* 16, no. 5 (2016): 327–29, https://doi.org/10.5698/1535-7511-16.5.327; Rup K. Sainju et al., "Interictal Respiratory Variability Predicts Severity of Hypoxemia After Generalized Convulsive Seizures," *Epilepsia* 64, no. 9 (2023): 2373–84, https://doi.org/10.1111/epi.17691.

[47] V. L. Schechtman et al., "Dynamics of Respiratory Patterning in Normal Infants and Infants Who Subsequently Died of the Sudden Infant Death Syndrome," *Pediatric Research* 40, no. 4 (1996): 571–77, https://doi.org/10.1203/00006450-199610000-00010.

[48] Xiaolu Sun et al., "Opioids Modulate an Emergent Rhythmogenic Process to Depress Breathing," *eLife* 8 (2019): e50613, https://doi.org/10.7554/eLife.50613.

[49] Jan-Marino Ramirez, "The Integrative Role of the Sigh in Psychology, Physiology, Pathology, and Neurobiology," *Progress in Brain Research* 209 (2014): 91–129, https://doi.org/10.1016/B978-0-444-63274-6.00006-0.

[50] Anna S. Lijowska et al., "Sequential Arousal and Airway-Defensive Behavior of Infants in Asphyxial Sleep Environments," *Journal of Applied Physiology* 83, no. 1 (1997): 219–28, https://doi.org/10.1152/jappl.1997.83.1.219.

[51] Stefan Soltysik and Piotr Jelen, "In Rats, Sighs Correlate with Relief," *Physiology & Behavior* 85, no. 5 (2005): 598–602, https://doi.org/10.1016/j.physbeh.2005.06.008.

[52] Karolyne S. Magalhães et al., "*Locus Coeruleus* as a Vigilance Centre for Active Inspiration and Expiration in Rats," *Scientific Reports* 8, article no. 15654 (2018), https://doi.org/10.1038/s41598-018-34047-w.

[53] Elke Vlemincx et al., "A Sigh Following Sustained Attention and Mental Stress: Effects on Respiratory Variability," *Physiology & Behavior* 107, no. 1 (2012): 1–6, https://doi.org/10.1016/j.physbeh.2012.05.013.

[54] Rogelio Perez-Padilla et al., "Sighs During Sleep in Adult Humans," *Sleep* 6, no. 3 (1983): 234–43, https://doi.org/10.1093/sleep/6.3.234.

[55] Liza J. Severs et al., "The Psychophysiology of the Sigh: I: The Sigh from the Physiological Perspective," *Biological Psychology* 170, article no. 108313 (April 2022), https://doi.org/10.1016/j.biopsycho.2022.108313.

[56] Gray et al., "Normal Breathing Requires Pre-Bötzinger Complex."

[57] Annette Pisanski and Silvia Pagliardini, "The Parafacial Respiratory Group and the Control of Active Expiration," *Respiratory Physiology & Neurobiology* 265 (July 2019): 153–60, https://doi.org/10.1016/j.resp.2018.06.010; Robert T. R. Huckstepp et al., "Role of Parafacial Nuclei in Control of Breathing in Adult Rats," *Journal of Neuroscience* 35, no. 3 (2015): 1052–67, https://doi.org/10.1523/JNEUROSCI.2953-14.2015; Li et al., "Peptidergic Control Circuit."

[58] Elke Vlemincx et al., "Why Do You Sigh? Sigh Rate During Induced Stress and Relief," *Psychophysiology* 46, no. 5 (2009): 1005–13, https://doi.org/10.1111/j.1469-8986.2009.00842.x.

[59] Balban et al., "Brief Structured Respiration Practices."

[60] Jackson J. Fyfe et al., "Cold Water Immersion Attenuates Anabolic Signaling and Skeletal Muscle Fiber Hypertrophy, but Not Strength Gain, Following Whole-Body Resistance Training," *Journal of Applied Physiology* 127, no. 5 (2019): 1403–18, https://doi.org/10.1152/japplphysiol.00127.2019.

[61] Fyfe et al., "Cold Water Immersion Attenuates"; Elvis S. Malta et al., "The Effects of Regular Cold-Water Immersion Use on Training-Induced Changes in Strength and Endurance Performance: A Systematic Review with Meta-Analysis," *Sports Medicine* 51, no. 1 (January 2021): 161–74, https://doi.org/10.1007/s40279-020-01362-0; Llion A. Roberts et al., "Post-Exercise Cold Water Immersion Attenuates Acute Anabolic Signalling and Long-Term Adaptations in Muscle to Strength Training," *Journal of Physiology* 593, no. 18 (September 2015): 4285–301, https://doi.org/10.1113/JP270570; Jozo Grgic, "Effects of Post-Exercise Cold-Water Immersion on Resistance Training–Induced Gains in Muscular Strength: A Meta-Analysis," *European Journal of Sport Science* 23, no. 3 (March 2023): 372–80; Alec Piñero et al., "Throwing Cold Water on Muscle Growth: A Systematic Review with Meta-Analysis of the Effects of Postexercise Cold Water Immersion on Resistance Training–Induced Hypertrophy," *European Journal of Sport Science* 24, no. 2 (February 2024): 177–89.

[62] Milda Eimonte et al., "Residual Effects of Short-Term Whole-Body Cold-Water Immersion on the Cytokine Profile, White Blood Cell Count, and Blood Markers of Stress," *International Journal of Hyperthermia* 38, no. 1 (2021): 696–707, https://doi.org/10.1080/02656736.2021.1915504; E. E. Hill et al., "Exercise and Circulating Cortisol Levels: The Intensity Threshold Effect," *Journal of Endocrinological Investigation* 31, no. 7 (2008): 587–91, https://doi.org/10.1007/BF03345606.

[63] B. P. O'Malley et al., "Circulating Catecholamine, Thyrotrophin, Thyroid Hormone and Prolactin Responses of Normal Subjects to Acute Cold Exposure," *Clinical Endocrinology* 21, no. 3 (1984): 285–91, https://doi.org/10.1111/j.1365-2265.1984.tb03471.x.

[64] P. Šrámek et al., "Human Physiological Responses to Immersion into Water of Different Temperatures," *European Journal of Applied Physiology* 81 (February 2000): 436–42, https://doi.org/10.1007/s004210050065.

[65] C. P. Arun, "Fight or Flight, Forbearance and Fortitude: The Spectrum of Actions of the Catecholamines and Their Cousins," *Annals of the New York Academy of Sciences* 1018, no. 1 (2004): 137–40, https://doi.org/10.1196/annals.1296.016; Akil, "Stress Fitness."

[66] Crum et al., "Rethinking Stress."

[67] Hans Selye, *Stress Without Distress* (Signet, 1974).

[68] "Hans Selye," Nomination Archive, Nobel Prize, n.d., https://www.nobelprize.org/nomination/archive/show_people.php?id=8395.

[69] Ned H. Kalin, "Prefrontal Cortical and Limbic Circuit Alterations in Psychopathology," *American Journal of Psychiatry* 176, no. 12 (2019): 971–73, https://doi.org/10.1176/appi.ajp.2019.19101036.

[70] Crum et al., "Evaluation of the 'Rethink Stress.'"

[71] Crum et al., "Rethinking Stress"; Crum et al., "Role of Stress Mindset"; Crum et al., "Optimizing Stress"; Crum et al., "Evaluation of the 'Rethink Stress.'"

[72] Linghui Yang et al., "Effects of Stressor Predictability and Controllability on Sleep, Temperature, and Fear Behavior in Mice," *Sleep* 34, no. 6 (2011): 759–71, https://doi.org/10.5665/SLEEP.1044; Chirag Limbachia et al., "Controllability over Stressor Decreases Responses in Key Threat-Related Brain Areas," *Communications Biology* 4, article no. 42 (2021), https://doi.org/10.1038/s42003-020-01537-5; Dakota D. Witzel et al., "Daily Association Between Perceived Control and Resolution of Daily Stressors Strengthens Across a Decade of Adulthood," *Communications Psychology* 3, article no. 130 (2025), https://doi.org/10.1038/s44271-025-00313-7.

[73] Yuval Heled et al., "Heat Acclimation and Performance in Hypoxic Conditions," *Aviation, Space, and Environmental Medicine* 83, no. 7 (2012): 649–53, https://doi.org/10.3357/asem.3241.2012.

[74] C. Mark Harper, "Extreme Preconditioning: Cold Adaptation Through Sea Swimming as a Means to Improving Surgical Outcomes," *Medical Hypotheses* 78, no. 4 (2012): 516–19, https://doi.org/10.1016/j.mehy.2012.01.022.

[75] Cristopher Siegfried Kopplin and Louisa Rosenthal, "The Positive Effects of Combined Breathing Techniques and Cold Exposure on Perceived Stress: A Randomised Trial," *Current Psychology* 42 (October 2022): 27058–70, https://doi.org/10.1007/s12144-022-03739-y.

[76] Heather C. Lunt et al., "'Cross-Adaptation': Habituation to Short Repeated Cold-Water Immersions Affects the Response to Acute Hypoxia in Humans, *Journal of Physiology* 588, pt. 18 (July 2010): 3605–13, https://doi.org/10.1113/jphysiol.2010.193458; Lyudamila T. Kovtun and Mikhail I. Voevoda, Susceptibility to Hypoxia and Breathing Control Changes After Short-Term Cold Exposures," *International Journal of Circumpolar Health* (August 2013): 72, https://doi.org/10.3402/ijch.v72i0.21574; Hitoshi Wakabayashi et al., "Recent Updates on Cold Adaptation in Population and Laboratory Studies, Including Cross-Adaptation With Nonthermal Factors," *Journal of Physiological Anthropology* 44 (February 2025): 7, https://doi.org/10.1186/s40101-025-00387-6.

[77] Nikolai A. Shevchuk, "Adapted Cold Shower as a Potential Treatment for Depression," *Medical Hypotheses* 70, no. 5 (2008): 995–1001, https://doi.org/10.1016/j.mehy.2007.04.052.

[78] Christoffer van Tulleken et al., "Open Water Swimming as a Treatment for Major Depressive Disorder," *BMJ Case Reports* 2018 (August 21, 2018): bcr2018225007, https://doi.org/10.1136/bcr-2018-225007.

[79] K. Overbury et al., "Swimming in Nature: A Scoping Review of the Mental Health and Wellbeing Benefits of Open Water Swimming," *Journal of Environmental Psychology* 90 (September 2023): 102073, https://doi.org/10.1016/j.jenvp.2023.102073.

[80] Pirkko Huttunen et al., "Winter Swimming Improves General Well-Being," *International Journal of Circumpolar Health* 63, no. 2 (2004): 140–44, https://doi.org/10.3402/ijch.v63i2.17700.

[81] Amy Burlingham et al., "Sea Swimming as a Novel Intervention for Depression and Anxiety—a Feasibility Study Exploring Engagement and Acceptability," *Mental Health and Physical Activity* 23 (October 2022), https://doi.org/10.1016/j.mhpa.2022.100472.

[82] John S. Kelly and Ellis Bird, "Improved Mood Following a Single Immersion in Cold Water," *Lifestyle Medicine* 3, no. 1 (2022): e53, https://doi.org/10.1002/lim2.53.

Pirkko Huttunen et al., "Winter Swimming Improves General Well-Being."

[83] Mike Tipton, "Humans: A Homeothermic Animal That Needs Perturbation?," *Experimental Physiology* 104, no. 1 (2019): 1–2, https://doi.org/10.1113/EP087450.

[84] Anne Lembke, *Dopamine Nation: Finding Balance in the Age of Indulgence* (Penguin, 2021).

[85] "Too Much Pleasure Can Lead to Addiction. How to Break the Cycle and Find Balance," *Life Kit*, NPR, April 4, 2022, https://www.npr.org/transcripts/1090009509.

[86] Šrámek et al., "Human Physiological Responses."

[87] J. Daniel Obray et al., "Dopamine D2-Subtype Receptors Outside the Blood-Brain Barrier Mediate Enhancement of Mesolimbic Dopamine Release and Conditioned Place Preference by Intravenous Dopamine," *Frontiers in Cellular Neuroscience* 16 (2022): 944243, https://doi.org/10.3389/fncel.2022.944243; G. Heninger et al., "Plasma and CSF Dopamine Metabolites in Psychiatric Patients: Effects of Probenecid and Haloperidol," *Catecholamines: Basic and Clinical Frontiers* (1979): 1887–89, https://doi.org/10.1016/B978-1-4832-8363-0.50580-2.

[88] Lembke, *Dopamine Nation.*

[89] Geert A. Buijze et al., "The Effect of Cold Showering on Health and Work: A Randomized Controlled Trial," *PLOS One* 11, no. 9 (2016): e0161749, https://doi.org/10.1371/journal.pone.0161749; Geert A. Buijze et al., "Correction: The Effect of Cold Showering on Health and Work," *PLOS One* 13, no. 8 (2018): e0201978, https://doi.org/10.1371/journal.pone.0201978.

[90] Amy F. T. Arnsten, "Stress Signalling Pathways That Impair Prefrontal Cortex Structure and Function," *Nature Reviews Neuroscience* 10, no. 6 (June 2009): 410–22, https://doi.org/10.1038/nrn2648; Shabnam Hossein et al., "Effects of Acute Stress and Depression on Functional Connectivity Between Prefrontal Cortex and the Amygdala," *Molecular Psychiatry* 28, no. 11 (April 2023): 4602–12, https://doi.org/10.1038/s41380-023-02056-5.

[91] Susanna Søberg et al., "Altered Brown Fat Thermoregulation and Enhanced Cold-Induced Thermogenesis in Young, Healthy, Winter-Swimming Men," *Cell Reports Medicine* 2, no. 10 (2021): 100408, https://doi.org/10.1016/j.xcrm.2021.100408.

[92] Balban et al., "Brief Structured Respiration Practices"; Susanna Søberg et al., "Altered Brown Fat Thermoregulation and Enhanced Cold-Induced Thermogenesis in Young, Healthy, Winter-Swimming Men"; Matthijs Kox et al., "Voluntary Activation of the Sympathetic Nervous System and Attenuation of the Innate Immune Response in Humans," *Proceedings of the National Academy of Sciences* 111, no. 20 (May 2014): 7379–84, https://doi.org/10.1073/pnas.1322174111.

[93] Omar Boukhris et al., "The Acute Effects of Nonsleep Deep Rest on Perceptual Responses, Physical, and Cognitive Performance in Physically Active Participants," *Applied Psychology: Health and Well-Being* 16, no. 4 (2024): 1967–87, https://doi.org/10.1111/aphw.12571.

[94] Vaishnu Karthik Kamaraj et al., "Mechanistic Insights from Neurophysiological Studies of OM Chanting, Pranayama and Yoga Nidra on Sleep Quality," *Annals of Neurosciences* (October 29, 2025): 09727531251386644, https://doi.org/10.1177/09727531251386644; Erica Sharpe et al., "A Closer Look at Yoga Nidra—Early Randomized Sleep Lab Investigations," *Journal of Psychosomatic Research* 166 (March 2023): 111169, https://doi.org/10.1016/j.jpsychores.2023.111169.

[95] Abhijit Dutta et al., "Efficacy of Yoga Nidra in Managing Sleep Disorders: A Systematic Review of Randomized Controlled Trials," *Journal of Integrative and Complementary Medicine* 32, no. 3 (2025), https://doi.org/10.1177/27683605251390728.

[96] Shashank Ghai et al., "Effects of Yoga Nidra on Stress, Anxiety, and Depression: A Systematic Review and Meta-Analysis," *Annals of the New York Academy of Sciences* 1556, no. 1 (2026): e70149, https://doi.org/10.1111/nyas.70149; Boukhris et al., "Acute Effects of Nonsleep Deep Rest"; Karuna Datta et al., "Improved Sleep, Cognitive Processing and Enhanced Learning and Memory Task Accuracy with Yoga Nidra Practice in Novices," *PLOS ONE* 18, no. 12 (December 2023): e0294678, https://doi.org/10.1371/journal.pone.0294678.

[97] Prakash Chandra Kavi, "Conscious Entry into Sleep: Yoga Nidra and Accessing Subtler States of Consciousness," *Progress in Brain Research* 280 (2023): 43–60, https://doi.org/10.1016/bs.pbr.2022.12.012; Karuna Datta et al., "Electrophysiological Evidence of Local Sleep During Yoga Nidra Practice," *Frontiers in Neurology* 13 (July 2022): 910794, https://doi.org/10.3389/fneur.2022.910794.

[98] Esther N. Moszeik et al., "The Effects of an Online Yoga Nidra Meditation on Subjective Well-Being and Diurnal Salivary Cortisol: A Randomised Controlled Trial," *Stress & Health* 41, no. 3 (2025): e70049, https://doi.org/10.1002/smi.70049.

[99] Karen R. Konkoly et al., "Real-time Dialogue Between Experimenters and Dreamers During REM Sleep," *Current Biology* 31, no. 7 (April 2021): 1417–27, https://doi.org/10.1016/j.cub.2021.01.026.

[100] Datta et al., "Electrophysiological Evidence of Local Sleep"; Moszeik et al., "Effects of an Online Yoga Nidra Meditation."

[101] Ghalia Akram, "Testing Non-Sleep Deep Rest (NSDR) Protocol to Counter the Cognitive Consequences of Short Sleep in Young Adult Students" (master's thesis, Harvard University Division of Continuing Education, 2024), https://nrs.harvard.edu/URN-3:HUL.INSTREPOS:37378464; Jamie Mobley, "iRest, You Rest: Virtual Yoga Nidra Sessions to Help Fight Stress," VA News, October 23, 2019, https://news.va.gov/67404/irest-rest-virtual-yoga-nidra-sessions-help-fight-stress/; Robert Mays, "The NFL's Mindfulness Movement Is Spreading," *Ringer*, August 15, 2017, https://www.theringer.com/2017/08/15/nfl/mindfulness-training-falcons-colts-49ers-dan-quinn; Lane Florsheim, "Google CEO Sundar Pichai's Vision for Return to Work," *Wall Street Journal*, February 28, 2022, https://www.wsj.com/lifestyle/careers/google-ceo-sundar-pichais-vision-for-return-to-work-11646055640; Adam Wrzeciono et al., "Non-Sleep Deep Rest Relaxation and Virtual Reality Therapy for Psychological Outcomes in Patients with Coronary Artery Disease: A Pilot Randomized Controlled Trial," *Journal of Clinical Medicine* 13, no. 23 (2024): 7178, https://doi.org/10.3390/jcm13237178; Kamalesh K. Gulia and Sapna Erat Sreedharan, "Yogic Sleep and Walking Protocol Induced Improvement in Sleep and Wellbeing in Post-Menopausal Subject: A Longitudinal Case Study During COVID Lockdown," *Sleep Vigil* 6, no. 1 (2022): 229–33, https://doi.org/10.1007/s41782-021-00180-2; L. Stankovic, "Transforming Trauma: A Qualitative Feasibility Study of Integrative Restoration (iRest) Yoga Nidra on Combat-Related Post-Traumatic Stress Disorder," *International Journal of Yoga Therapy* 21 (2011): 23–37, https://doi.org/10.17761/ijyt.21.1.v823454h5v57n160.

[102] Paul Grossman et al., "Mindfulness-Based Stress Reduction and Health Benefits: A Meta-Analysis," *Journal of Psychosomatic Research* 57, no. 1 (2004): 35–43, https://doi.org/10.1016/S0022-3999(03)00573-7; Balban et al., "Brief Structured Respiration Practices."

[103] Fadel Zeidan et al., "Mindfulness Meditation Improves Cognition: Evidence of Brief Mental Training," *Consciousness and Cognition* 19, no. 2 (2010): 597–605, https://doi.org/10.1016/j.concog.2010.03.014.

[104] Basso et al., "Brief, Daily Meditation Enhances Attention."

[105] Andrew Huberman, "Science-Based Meditation Tools to Improve Your Brain and Health | Richard Davidson," *Huberman Lab* (podcast audio), March 6, 2023, https://www.hubermanlab.com/episode/science-based-meditation-tools-to-improve-your-brain-and-health-richard-davidson.

[106] Véronique A. Taylor et al., "Impact of Mindfulness on the Neural Responses to Emotional Pictures in Experienced and Beginner Meditators," *NeuroImage* 57, no. 4 (2011): 1524–33, https://doi.org/10.1016/j.neuroimage.2011.06.001.

[107] Kieran C. R. Fox et al., "Is Meditation Associated with Altered Brain Structure? A Systematic Review and Meta-Analysis of Morphometric Neuroimaging in Meditation Practitioners," *Neuroscience & Biobehavioral Reviews* 43 (June 2014): 48–73, https://doi.org/10.1016/j.neubiorev.2014.03.016.

[108] J. Douglas Bremner et al., "SPECT [I-123]iomazenil Measurement of the Benzodiazepine Receptor in Panic Disorder," *Biological Psychiatry* 47, no. 2 (2000): 96–106, https://doi.org/10.1016/s0006-3223(99)00188-2.

[109] Divya Krishnakumar et al., "Meditation and Yoga can Modulate Brain Mechanisms that Affect Behavior and Anxiety—A Modern Scientific Perspective," *Ancient Science* 2, no. 1 (April 2015): 13–19, https://doi.org/10.14259/as.v2i1.171.

[110] Anna Gavrieli et al., "Caffeinated Coffee Does Not Acutely Affect Energy Intake, Appetite, or Inflammation but Prevents Serum Cortisol Concentrations from Falling in Healthy Men," *Journal of Nutrition* 141, no. 4 (April 2011): 703–7, https://doi.org/10.3945/jn.110.137323; William R. Lovallo et al., "Caffeine Stimulation of Cortisol Secretion Across the Waking Hours in Relation to Caffeine Intake Levels," *Psychosomatic Medicine* 67, no. 5 (2005): 734–39, https://doi.org/10.1097/01.psy.0000181270.20036.06.

[111] Jasleen Kaur et al., "Physiology, Cortisol," StatPearls, last updated December 1, 2025, https://www.ncbi.nlm.nih.gov/books/NBK538239/.

[112] Clara Velazquez Sanchez and Jeffrey W. Dalley, "The Cortisol Awakening Response: Fact or Fiction?," *Brain and Neuroscience Advances* 9 (April 24, 2025), https://doi.org/10.1177/23982128251327712; Tobias Stalder et al., "The Cortisol Awakening Response: Regulation and Functional Significance," *Endocrine Reviews* 46, no. 1 (2025): 43–59, https://doi.org/10.1210/endrev/bnae024; Angela Clow et al., "The Cortisol Awakening Response in Context," *International Review of Neurobiology* 93 (2010): 153–75, https://doi.org/10.1016/S0074-7742(10)93007-9; Nicole P. Bowles et al., "The Circadian System Modulates the Cortisol Awakening Response in Humans," *Frontiers in Neuroscience* 16 (November 2022): 995452, https://doi.org/10.3389/fnins.2022.995452.

[113] Aikaterini Andreadi et al., "Modified Cortisol Circadian Rhythm: The Hidden Toll of Night-Shift Work," *International Journal of Molecular Sciences* 26, no. 5 (February 2025): 2090, https://doi.org/10.3390/ijms26052090; Fadime Ulupinar et al., "The Effect of Single and Double Shift Works on Salivary Cortisol Levels in Nurses," *Nursing Open* 13, no. 4 (April 2026): e70495, https://doi.org/10.1002/nop2.70495.

[114] Andreadi et al., "Modified Cortisol Circadian Rhythm."

[115] Ethan S. Young et al., "The Dual Impact of Early and Concurrent Life Stress on Adults' Diurnal Cortisol Patterns: A Prospective Study," *Psychological Science* 30, no. 5 (2019): 739–47, https://doi.org/10.1177/0956797619833664.

[116] Vittoria Favero et al., "The Degree of Cortisol Secretion Is Associated with Diabetes Mellitus and Hypertension in Patients with Nonfunctioning Adrenal Tumors," *Cardiovascular Diabetology* 22, no. 1 (2023): 102, https://doi.org/10.1186/s12933-023-01836-1; Vittoria Favero et al., "Correction: The Degree of Cortisol Secretion," *Cardiovascular Diabetology* 22, no. 1 (2023): 127, https://doi.org/10.1186/s12933-023-01863-y; Mahmut Cay et al., "Effect of Increase in Cortisol Level Due to Stress in Healthy Young Individuals on Dynamic and Static Balance Scores," *Northern Clinics of Istanbul* 5, no. 4 (2018): 295–301, https://doi.org/10.14744/nci.2017.4210; Eline S. van der Valk et al., "Stress and Obesity: Are There More Susceptible Individuals?," *Current Obesity Reports* 7, no. 2 (2018): 193–203, https://doi.org/10.1007/s13679-018-0306-y; B. R. Walker, "Cortisol—Cause and Cure for Metabolic Syndrome?," *Diabetic Medicine* 23, no. 12 (2006): 1281–88, https://doi.org/10.1111/j.1464-5491.2006.01998.x; Joshua J. Joseph and Sherita H. Golden, "Cortisol Dysregulation: The Bidirectional Link Between Stress, Depression, and Type 2 Diabetes Mellitus," *Annals of the New York Academy of Sciences* 1391, no. 1 (October 2016): 20–34, https://doi.org/10.1111/nyas.13217.

[117] Dominika Borzyszkowska et al., "Evaluation of Hormonal Factors in Acne Vulgaris and the Course of Acne Vulgaris Treatment with Contraceptive-Based Therapies in Young Adult Women," *Cells* 11, no. 24

(2022): 4078, https://doi.org/10.3390/cells11244078; Marzieh Saei Ghare Naz et al., "The Menstrual Disturbances in Endocrine Disorders: A Narrative Review," *International Journal of Endocrinology and Metabolism* 18, no. 4 (2020): e106694, https://doi.org/10.5812/ijem.106694; Christine E. Cherpak, "Mindful Eating: A Review of How the Stress-Digestion-Mindfulness Triad May Modulate and Improve Gastrointestinal and Digestive Function," *Integrative Medicine* 18, no. 4 (2019): 48–53, https://pubmed.ncbi.nlm.nih.gov/32549835/.

118 Matias M. Pulopulos et al., "Relationship Between Cortisol Changes During the Night and Subjective and Objective Sleep Quality in Healthy Older People," *International Journal of Environmental Research and Public Health* 17, no. 4 (2020): 1264, https://doi.org/10.3390/ijerph17041264.

119 C. Martin Beaven et al., "Dose Effect of Caffeine on Testosterone and Cortisol Responses to Resistance Exercise," *International Journal of Sports Nutrition and Exercise Metabolism* 18, no. 2 (April 2008): 131–41, https://doi.org/10.1123/ijsnem.18.2.131.

120 Travis Anderson et al., "The Effect of Acute Exercise on the Cortisol Awakening Response," *European Journal of Applied Physiology* 123 (January 2023): 1027–39, https://doi.org/10.1007/s00421-023-05132-4.

121 Peter Y. Liu, "Rhythms in Cortisol Mediate Sleep and Circadian Impacts on Health," *Sleep* 47, no. 9 (September 2024): zsae151, https://doi.org/10.1093/sleep/zsae151.

122 Petrowski et al., "Effects of Post-Awakening Light"; Brown et al., "Recommendations for Daytime, Evening, and Nighttime Indoor Light."

123 Marjolein Drent et al., "Grapefruit Juice Facilitates Cortisol Replacement Therapy: Role of CYP3A Variant Alleles," *Archives of Clinical and Medical Case Reports* 5, no. 5 (2021): 656–64; Ya-Jie Xiao et al., "Effects of Grapefruit Juice on Cortisol Metabolism in Healthy Male Chinese Subjects," *Food and Chemical Toxicology* 74 (December 2014): 85–90, https://doi.org/10.1016/j.fct.2014.09.012; Christopher Kargl et al., "11β-hydroxysteroid Dehydrogenase Type-II Activity Is Affected by Grapefruit Juice and Intense Muscular Work," *Archives of Endocrinology and Metabolism* 61, no. 6 (2017): 556–61, https://doi.org/10.1590/2359-3997000000296; Y. S. Lee et al., "Grapefruit Juice and Its Flavonoids Inhibit 11 Beta-Hydroxysteroid Dehydrogenase," *Clinical Pharmacology and Therapeutics* 59 (1996): 62–71, https://doi.org/10.1016/S0009-9236(96)90025-9; Y. Kageyama et al., "Glycyrrhizin Induces Mineralocorticoid Activity Through Alterations in Cortisol Metabolism in the Human Kidney," *Journal of Endocrinology* 135, no. 1 (1992): 147–52, https://doi.org/10.1677/joe.0.1350147; M. T. Epstein et al., "Licorice Raises Urinary Cortisol in Man," *Journal of Clinical Endocrinology and Metabolism* 47, no. 2 (August 1978): 397–400, https://doi.org/10.1210/jcem-47-2-397; Yu-Jin Kwon, "A Review of the Pharmacological Efficacy and Safety of Licorice Root from Corroborative Clinical Trial Findings," *Journal of Medicinal Food* 23, no. 1 (January 2020): 12–20, https://doi.org/10.1089/jmf.2019.445; Paal Methlie et al., "Grapefruit Juice and Licorice Increase Cortisol Availability in Patients with Addison's Disease," *European Journal of Endocrinology* 165, no. 5 (November 2011): 761–69, https://doi.org/10.1530/EJE-11-0518.

124 Isabella Robertson-Dixon et al., "The Influence of Light Wavelength on Human HPA Axis Rhythms: A Systematic Review," *Life* 13, no. 10 (2023): 1968, https://doi.org/10.3390/life13101968.

125 Elli L. Cole et al., "Habitual Caffeine Use Is Associated with Heightened Cortisol Reactivity to Lab-Based Stress in Two Samples," *Psychosomatic Medicine* 86, no. 8 (2024): 730–37, https://doi.org/10.1097/PSY.0000000000001334.

126 A. Caplin et al., "The Effects of Exercise Intensity on the Cortisol Response to a Subsequent Acute Psychosocial Stressor," *Psychoneuroendocrinology* 131 (September 2021): 105336, https://doi.org/10.1016/j.psyneuen.2021.105336.

127 Alissa Shida et al., "Cortisol Levels After Cold Exposure Are Independent of Adrenocorticotropic Hormone Stimulation," *PLOS One* 15, no. 2 (2020): e0218910, https://doi.org/10.1371/journal.pone.0218910.

[128] Eva Fries et al., "The Cortisol Awakening Response (CAR): Facts and Future Directions," *International Journal of Psychophysiology* 72, no. 1 (2009): 67–73, https://doi.org/10.1016/j.ijpsycho.2008.03.014.

[129] Daniel J. Powell and Wolff Schlotz, "Daily Life Stress and the Cortisol Awakening Response: Testing the Anticipation Hypothesis," *PLOS One* 7, no. 12 (2012): e52067, https://doi.org/10.1371/journal.pone.0052067.

[130] Adrian L. Lopresti and Stephen J. Smith, "Ashwagandha (*Withania somnifera*) for the Treatment and Enhancement of Mental and Physical Conditions: A Systematic Review of Human Trials," *Journal of Herbal Medicine* 28, article no. 100434 (August 2021), https://doi.org/10.1016/j.hermed.2021.100434.

[131] A. Remenapp et al., "Efficacy of *Withania somnifera* Supplementation on Adults' Cognition and Mood," *Journal of Ayurveda and Integrative Medicine* 13, no. 2 (2022): 100510, https://doi.org/10.1016/j.jaim.2021.08.003.

[132] Adrian L. Lopresti et al., "An Investigation into the Stress-Relieving and Pharmacological Actions of an Ashwagandha (*Withania somnifera*) Extract: A Randomized, Double-Blind, Placebo-Controlled Study," *Medicine* 98, no. 37 (2019): e17186, https://doi.org/10.1097/MD.0000000000017186.

[133] Tobias Backström and Svante Winberg, "Central Corticotropin Releasing Factor and Social Stress," *Frontiers in Neuroscience* 7 (July 2013): 117, https://doi.org/10.3389/fnins.2013.00117; Michał Wiciński et al., "Can Ashwagandha Benefit the Endocrine System? A Review," *International Journal of Molecular Sciences* 24, no. 22 (November 2023); Günter Vollmer and Thomas Brendler, "Evaluation of Potential Hormonal Activities of Ashwagandha (*Withania somnifera*)," *Phytotherapy Research*, December 26, 2025, https://doi.org/10.1002/ptr.70155; Srikanta Pandit et al., "Effects of *Withania somnifera* Extract in Chronically Stressed Adults: A Randomized Controlled Trial," *Nutrients* 16, no. 9 (April 2024): 1293, https://doi.org/10.3390/nu16091293; Mateusz Haber et al., "Ashwagandha as an Adaptogen: Its Influence on Sleep Patterns, Stress Response, and Anxiety in Modern Life," *Journal of Education, Health and Sport* 68 (September 2024): 55327, https://doi.org/10.12775/JEHS.2024.68.55327.

[134] Hyeongyeong Kim et al., "Ashwagandha (*Withania somnifera* [L.] Dunal) Root Extract Containing Withanolide A Alleviates Depression-Like Behavior in Mice by Enhancing the Brain-Derived Neurotrophic Factor Pathway Under Unexpected Chronic Mild Stress," *Journal of Ethnopharmacology* 340 (2025): 119224, https://doi.org/10.1016/j.jep.2024.119224.

[135] Juveria Javid et al., "From Herbal Hope to Hormonal Havoc: Chronic Ashwagandha Use and HPA Axis Suppression," *Endocrinology, Diabetes and Metabolism Case Reports* 2026, no. 1 (January 2026).

[136] Muhammad Saeed et al., "Green Tea (*Camellia sinensis*) and L-Theanine: Medicinal Values and Beneficial Applications in Humans—a Comprehensive Review," *Biomedicine & Pharmacotherapy* 95 (November 2017): 1260–75, https://doi.org/10.1016/j.biopha.2017.09.024.

[137] Raymond Cooper, "Green Tea and Theanine: Health Benefits," *International Journal of Food Sciences and Nutrition* 63, no. S1 (2012): 90–97, https://doi.org/10.3109/09637486.2011.629180.

[138] Sabu M. Chacko et al., "Beneficial Effects of Green Tea: A Literature Review," *Chinese Medicine* 5 (April 6, 2010): 13, https://doi.org/10.1186/1749-8546-5-13.

[139] Kathryn T. Kavanagh et al., "Green Tea Extracts Decrease Carcinogen-Induced Mammary Tumor Burden in Rats and Rate of Breast Cancer Cell Proliferation in Culture," *Journal of Cellular Biochemistry* 82, no. 3 (2001): 387–98, https://doi.org/10.1002/jcb.1164.

[140] Shinsuke Hidese et al., "Effects of L-Theanine Administration on Stress-Related Symptoms and Cognitive Functions in Healthy Adults: A Randomized Controlled Trial," *Nutrients* 11, no. 10 (2019): 2362, https://doi.org/10.3390/nu11102362.

[141] David J. White et al., "Anti-Stress, Behavioural and Magnetoencephalography Effects of an L-Theanine-Based Nutrient Drink: A Randomised, Double-Blind, Placebo-Controlled, Crossover Trial," *Nutrients* 8, no. 1 (2016): 53, https://doi.org/10.3390/nu8010053.

[142] Ryohei Kimura and Toshiro Murata, "Influence of Alkylamides of Glutamic Acid and Related Compounds on the Central Nervous System. I. Central Depressant Effect of Theanine," *Chemical and Pharmaceutical Bulletin* 19, no. 6 (1971): 1257–61, https://doi.org/10.1248/cpb.19.1257.

[143] Hee-Yong Kim et al., "Phosphatidylserine in the Brain: Metabolism and Function," *Progress in Lipid Research* 56 (October 2014): 1–18, https://doi.org/10.1016/j.plipres.2014.06.002.

[144] Palmiero Monteleone et al., "Effects of Phosphatidylserine on the Neuroendocrine Response to Physical Stress in Humans," *Neuroendocrinology* 52, no. 3 (1990): 243–48, https://doi.org/10.1159/000125593.

[145] Katja Schmidt et al., "A Lecithin Phosphatidylserine and Phosphatidic Acid Complex (PAS) Reduces Symptoms of the Premenstrual Syndrome (PMS): Results of a Randomized, Placebo-Controlled, Double-Blind Clinical Trial," *Clinical Nutrition ESPEN* 24 (April 2018): 22–30, https://doi.org/10.1016/j.clnesp.2018.01.067.

[146] J. Hellhammer et al., "Effects of Soy Lecithin Phosphatidic Acid and Phosphatidylserine Complex (PAS) on the Endocrine and Psychological Responses to Mental Stress," *Stress* 7, no. 2 (2004): 119–26, https://doi.org/10.1080/10253890410001728379.

[147] Juliane Hellhammer et al., "Omega-3 Fatty Acids Administered in Phosphatidylserine Improved Certain Aspects of High Chronic Stress in Men," *Nutrition Research* 32, no. 4 (2012): 241–50, https://doi.org/10.1016/j.nutres.2012.03.003.

[148] Elizabeth J. Susman, "Psychobiology of Persistent Antisocial Behavior: Stress, Early Vulnerabilities and the Attenuation Hypothesis," *Neuroscience & Biobehavioral Reviews* 30, no. 3 (2006): 376–89, https://doi.org/10.1016/j.neubiorev.2005.08.002.

[149] Juliane Hellhammer et al., "A Soy-Based Phosphatidylserine/Phosphatidic Acid Complex (PAS) Normalizes the Stress Reactivity of Hypothalamus-Pituitary-Adrenal-Axis in Chronically Stressed Male Subjects: A Randomized, Placebo-Controlled Study," *Lipids in Health and Disease* 13 (July 2014): 121, https://doi.org/10.1186/1476-511X-13-121.

[150] Emilija Ivanova Stojcheva and José Carlos Quintela, "The Effectiveness of *Rhodiola rosea* L. Preparations in Alleviating Various Aspects of Life-Stress Symptoms and Stress-Induced Conditions—Encouraging Clinical Evidence," *Molecules* 27, no. 12 (2022): 3902, https://doi.org/10.3390/molecules27123902.

[151] "Assessment Report on *Rhodiola rosea* L., Rhizoma et Radix," Committee on Herbal Medicinal Products, European Medicines Agency, March 27, 2012, https://www.pharmacompass.com/pAssets/pdf/pubchem/rhodiola-rosea-l.pdf.

[152] V. Darbinyan et al., "*Rhodiola rosea* in Stress-Induced Fatigue—a Double Blind Cross-Over Study of a Standardized Extract SHR-5 with a Repeated Low-Dose Regimen on the Mental Performance of Healthy Physicians During Night Duty," *Phytomedicine* 7, no. 5 (2000): 365–71, https://doi.org/10.1016/S0944-7113(00)80055-0.

[153] V. A. Shevtsov et al., "A Randomized Trial of Two Different Doses of a SHR-5 *Rhodiola rosea* Extract Versus Placebo and Control of Capacity for Mental Work," *Phytomedicine* 10, no. 2–3 (2003): 95–105, https://doi.org/10.1078/094471103321659780.

[154] Erik M. G. Olsson et al., "A Randomised, Double-Blind, Placebo-Controlled, Parallel-Group Study of the Standardised Extract SHR-5 of the Roots of *Rhodiola rosea* in the Treatment of Subjects with Stress-Related Fatigue," *Planta Medica* 75, no. 2 (2009): 105–12, https://doi.org/10.1055/s-0028-1088346.

[155] A. Panossian et al., "Rosenroot (*Rhodiola rosea*): Traditional Use, Chemical Composition, Pharmacology and Clinical Efficacy," *Phytomedicine* 17, no. 7 (2010): 481–93, https://doi.org/10.1016/j.phymed.2010.02.002.

[156] Aaron Hernández-Santana et al., "A *Rhodiola rosea* Root Extract Protects Skeletal Muscle Cells Against Chemically Induced Oxidative Stress by Modulating Heat Shock Protein 70 (HSP70) Expression," *Phytotherapy Research* 28, no. 4 (2014): 623–28, https://doi.org/10.1002/ptr.5046.

[157] Tyler D. Williams et al., "Effects of Short-Term Golden Root Extract (*Rhodiola rosea*) Supplementation on Resistance Exercise Performance," *International Journal of Environmental Research and Public Health* 18, no. 13 (2021): 6953, https://doi.org/10.3390/ijerph18136953.

Chapter 4: Protocols for Nutrition

[1] Ming-Li Sun et al., "Intermittent Fasting and Health Outcomes: An Umbrella Review of Systematic Reviews and Meta-Analyses of Randomised Controlled Trials," *EClinicalMedicine* (Oxford) 70 (April 2024): 102519, https://doi.org/10.1016/j.eclinm.2024.102519.

[2] Andrew Huberman, "How Different Diets Impact Your Health | Dr. Christopher Gardner," *Huberman Lab* (podcast audio), January 29, 2024, https://www.hubermanlab.com/episode/how-different-diets-impact-your-health-dr-christopher-gardner.

[3] Andrew Huberman, "Dr Layne Norton: The Science of Eating for Health, Fat Loss, and Lean Muscle," *Huberman Lab* (podcast audio), November 7, 2022, https://www.hubermanlab.com/episode/dr-layne-norton-the-science-of-eating-for-health-fat-loss-and-lean-muscle; Andrew Huberman, "Dr. Layne Norton: Tools for Nutrition & Fitness," *Huberman Lab* (podcast audio), August 12, 2024, https://www.hubermanlab.com/episode/dr-layne-norton-tools-for-nutrition-fitness; Andrew Huberman, "Alan Aragon: How to Lose Fat and Gain Muscle with Nutrition," *Huberman Lab* (podcast audio), July 7, 2025, https://www.hubermanlab.com/episode/how-to-lose-fat-gain-muscle-with-nutrition-alan-aragon.

[4] Andrew Huberman, "Dr. Gabrielle Lyon: How to Exercise & Eat for Optimal Health & Longevity," *Huberman Lab* (podcast audio), June 24, 2024, https://www.hubermanlab.com/episode/dr-gabrielle-lyon-how-to-exercise-eat-for-optimal-health-longevity; Andrew Huberman, "Dr. Robert Lustig: How Sugar & Processed Foods Impact Your Health," *Huberman Lab* (podcast audio), December 18, 2023, https://www.hubermanlab.com/episode/dr-robert-lustig-how-sugar-processed-foods-impact-your-health.

[5] Andrew Huberman, "Dr. Justin Sonnenburg: How to Build, Maintain & Repair Gut Health," *Huberman Lab* (podcast audio), October 2, 2023, https://www.hubermanlab.com/episode/dr-justin-sonnenburg-how-to-build-maintain-and-repair-gut-health.

[6] Andrew Huberman, "Dr. Chris Palmer: Diet & Nutrition for Mental Health," *Huberman Lab* (podcast audio), November 21, 2022, https://www.hubermanlab.com/episode/dr-chris-palmer-diet-nutrition-for-mental-health.

[7] Andrew Huberman, "Satchin Panda: Intermittent Fasting to Improve Health, Cognition and Longevity," *Huberman Lab* (podcast audio), March 13, 2023, https://www.hubermanlab.com/episode/dr-satchin-panda-intermittent-fasting-to-improve-health-cognition-and-longevity.

[8] Preethi Srikanthan and Arun S. Karlamangla, "Muscle Mass Index as a Predictor of Longevity in Older Adults," *American Journal of Medicine* 127, no. 6 (2014): 547–53, https://doi.org/10.1016/j.amjmed.2014.02.007; Dong Hoon Lee and Edward L. Giovannucci, "Body Composition and Mortality in the General Population: A Review of Epidemiologic Studies," *Experimental Biology and Medicine* 243 (2018): 1273–83, https://doi.org/10.1177/1535370218818161.

[9] National Center for Health Statistics, "Obesity and Overweight," Centers for Disease Control and Prevention (CDC), last reviewed March 6, 2026, https://www.cdc.gov/nchs/fastats/obesity-overweight.htm.

[10] C. Johansson et al., "Bone Mineral Density Is a Predictor of Survival," *Calcified Tissue International* 63, no. 3 (1998): 190–96, https://doi.org/10.1007/s002239900513.

[11] Jay R. Hoffman and Michael J. Falvo, "Protein—Which Is Best?," *Journal of Sports Science & Medicine* 3, no. 3 (2004): 118–30, https://pubmed.ncbi.nlm.nih.gov/24482589/.

[12] "FDA's Updated 'Healthy' Claim Definition—Factsheet," U.S. Food and Drug Administration, December 2024, https://www.fda.gov/media/184535/download?attachment.

[13] T. Brock Symons et al., "A Moderate Serving of High-Quality Protein Maximally Stimulates Skeletal Muscle Protein Synthesis in Young and Elderly Subjects," *Journal of the American Dietetic Association* 109, no. 9 (2009): 1582–86, https://doi.org/10.1016/j.jada.2009.06.369.

[14] Jorn Trommelen et al., "The Anabolic Response to Protein Ingestion During Recovery from Exercise Has No Upper Limit in Magnitude and Duration *In Vivo* in Humans," *Cell Reports Medicine* 4, no. 12 (2023): 101324, https://doi.org/10.1016/j.xcrm.2023.101324.

[15] Brad Jon Schoenfeld and Alan Albert Aragon, "How Much Protein Can the Body Use in a Single Meal for Muscle-Building? Implications for Daily Protein Distribution," *Journal of the International Society of Sports Nutrition* 15, no. 10 (February 2018), https://doi.org/10.1186/s12970-018-0215-1.

[16] Damoon Ashtary-Larky et al., "Effects of Intermittent Fasting Combined with Resistance Training on Body Composition: A Systematic Review and Meta-Analysis," *Physiology & Behavior* 237 (August 2021): 113453, https://doi.org/10.1016/j.physbeh.2021.113453.

[17] Trommelen et al., "Anabolic Response to Protein Ingestion."

[18] Ioannis Delimaris, "Adverse Effects Associated with Protein Intake Above the Recommended Dietary Allowance for Adults," *ISRN Nutrition* 2013 (July 2013): 126929, https://doi.org/10.5402/2013/126929.

[19] Michelle M. Farnfield et al., "Why Protein Ingestion Activates mTOR-dependent Signalling After Resistance Exercise in Young Men: A Double-Blinded Randomized Controlled Trial," *Nutrients* 1, no. 2 (December 2009): 263–75, https://doi.org/10.3390/nu1020263; Grace Y. Liu and David M. Sabatini, "mTOR at the Nexus of Nutrition, Growth, Ageing and Disease," *Nature Reviews Molecular Cell Biology* 21 (January 2020): 183–203, https://doi.org/10.1038/s41580-019-0199-y; Joan B. Mannick and Dudley W. Lamming, "Targeting the Biology of Aging with mTOR Inhibitors," *Nature Aging* 3 (May 2023): 642–60, https://doi.org/10.1038/s43587-023-00416-y.

[20] Liu and Sabatini, "mTOR."

[21] Robert Oh et al., "Low-Carbohydrate Diet," StatPearls (internet) (Treasure Island, FL: StatPearls Publishing, January 2026).

[22] Kirsty J. Martin-McGill et al., "Ketogenic Diets for Drug-Resistant Epilepsy," *Cochrane Database of Systematic Reviews* 6, article no. CD001903 (2020), https://doi.org/10.1002/14651858.CD001903.pub5.

[23] Shebani Sethi et al., "Ketogenic Diet Intervention on Metabolic and Psychiatric Health in Bipolar and Schizophrenia: A Pilot Trial," *Psychiatry Research* 335, article no. 115866 (2024), https://doi.org/10.1016/j.psychres.2024.115866.

[24] Drew D. Decker et al., "A Pilot Study Examining a Ketogenic Diet as an Adjunct Therapy in College Students with Major Depressive Disorder," *Translational Psychiatry* 15, article no. 322 (2025), https://doi.org/10.1038/s41398-025-03544-8.

[25] You can read more about this diet at Paul Saladino, MD, www.paulsaladinomd.com.

[26] A wealth of peer-reviewed literature documents the problems with how starch is consumed in modern Western diets. Here are a few examples for further reading: Erik E. J. G. Aller et al., "Starches, Sugars and Obesity," *Nutrients* 3, no. 3 (2011): 341–69, https://doi.org/10.3390/nu3030341; Tera L. Fazzino et al., "Meal Composition During an Ad Libitum Buffet Meal and Longitudinal Predictions of Weight and Percent Body Fat Change: The Role of Hyper-Palatable, Energy Dense, and Ultra-Processed Foods," *Appetite* 167, article no. 105592 (December 1, 2021), https://doi.org/10.1016/j.appet.2021.105592; Tera L. Fazzino et al., "Hyper-Palatable Foods: Development of a Quantitative Definition and Application to the US Food System Database," *Obesity* 27, no. 11 (2019): 1761–68, https://doi.org/10.1002/oby.22639.

[27] Carlos A. Monteiro et al., "Ultra-Processed Foods: What They Are and How to Identify Them," *Public Health Nutrition* 22, no. 5 (2019): 936–41, https://doi.org/10.1017/S1368980018003762; Kevin D. Hall et al., "Ultra-Processed Diets Cause Excess Calorie Intake and Weight Gain: An Inpatient Randomized Controlled Trial of Ad Libitum Food Intake," *Cell Metabolism* 30, no. 1 (July 2019): 67–77.e3, https://doi.org/10.1016/j.cmet.2019.05.008.

[28] Bob Murray and Christine Rosenbloom, "Fundamentals of Glycogen Metabolism for Coaches and Athletes," *Nutrition Reviews* 76, no. 4 (2018): 243–59, https://doi.org/10.1093/nutrit/nuy001.

[29] Nicola Veronese et al., "The Impact of Dietary Fiber Consumption on Human Health: An Umbrella Review of Evidence from 17,155,277 Individuals," *Clinical Nutrition* 51 (August 2025): 325–33, https://doi.org/10.1016/j.clnu.2025.06.021; Sara B. Seidelmann et al., "Dietary Carbohydrate Intake and Mortality: A Prospective Cohort Study and Meta-Analysis," *Lancet Public Health* 3, no. 9 (2018): E419–28, https://doi.org/10.1016/S2468-2667(18)30135-X.

[30] Masoumeh Akhlaghi, "The Role of Dietary Fibers in Regulating Appetite, an Overview of Mechanisms and Weight Consequences," *Critical Reviews in Food Science and Nutrition* 64, no. 10 (2024): 3139–50, https://doi.org/10.1080/10408398.2022.2130160; Eliana Bistriche Giuntini et al., "The Effects of Soluble Dietary Fibers on Glycemic Response: An Overview and Futures Perspectives," *Foods* 11, no. 23 (2022): 3934, https://doi.org/10.3390/foods11233934.

[31] Pei Qin et al., "Fried-Food Consumption and Risk of Cardiovascular Disease and All-Cause Mortality: A Meta-Analysis of Observational Studies," *Heart* 107 (2021): 1567–75, https://doi.org/10.1136/heartjnl-2020-317883; Taraka V. Gadiraju et al., "Fried Food Consumption and Cardiovascular Health: A Review of Current Evidence," *Nutrients* 7, no. 10 (October 2015): 8424–30, https://doi.org/10.3390/nu7105404; Anli Wang et al., "High Fried Food Consumption Impacts Anxiety and Depression due to Lipid Metabolism Disturbance and Neuroinflammation," *Proceedings of the National Academy of Sciences U.S.A.* 120, no. 18 (2023): e2221097120, https://doi.org/10.1073/pnas.2221097120.

[32] Carole Bartolotto, "Does Consuming Sugar and Artificial Sweeteners Change Taste Preferences?," *Permanente Journal* 19, no. 3 (2015): 81–84, https://doi.org/10.7812/TPP/14-229.

[33] Di Qin et al., "Sugar Addiction: Neural Mechanisms and Health Implications," *Brain and Behavior* 15, no. 7 (2025): e70338, https://doi.org/10.1002/brb3.70338.

[34] Emily J. Endy et al., "Added Sugar Intake Is Associated with Weight Gain and Risk of Developing Obesity over 30 Years: The CARDIA Study," *Nutrition, Metabolism and Cardiovascular Diseases* 34, no. 2 (February 2024), https://doi.org/10.1016/j.numecd.2023.10.022; Quanhe Yang et al., "Added Sugar Intake and Cardiovascular Diseases Mortality Among US Adults," *JAMA Internal Medicine* 174, no. 4 (April 2014): 516–24, https://doi.org/10.1001/jamainternmed.2013.13563.

[35] Anika Knüppel et al., "Sugar Intake from Sweet Food and Beverages, Common Mental Disorder and Depression: Prospective Findings from the Whitehall II Study," *Scientific Reports* 7, no. 1 (2017): 6287, https://doi.org/10.1038/s41598-017-05649-7.

[36] Melissa M. Lane et al., "Ultra-Processed Food Exposure and Adverse Health Outcomes: Umbrella Review of Epidemiological Meta-Analyses," *BMJ* 384 (February 2024): e077310, https://doi.org/10.1136/bmj-2023-077310.

[37] For a helpful review of the data and debates around dietary fat, see Nita G. Forouhi et al., "Dietary Fat and Cardiometabolic Health: Evidence, Controversies, and Consensus for Guidance," *BMJ* 361 (June 2018): k2139, https://doi.org/10.1136/bmj.k2139.

[38] Jade Berg et al., "Saturated Fatty Acid Intake Is Associated with Increased Inflammation, Conversion of Kynurenine to Tryptophan, and Delta-9 Desaturase Activity in Healthy Humans," *International Journal of Tryptophan Research* 13 (January 2020): 117864692098194, https://doi.org/10.1177/1178646920981946; Xiao Ma et al., "Excessive Intake of Sugar: An Accomplice of Inflammation," *Frontiers in Immunology* 13, no. 13 (August 31, 2022), https://doi.org/10.3389/fimmu.2022.988481.

[39] Jibran A. Wali et al., "Cardio-Metabolic Effects of High-Fat Diets and Their Underlying Mechanisms—a Narrative Review," *Nutrients* 12, no. 5 (May 2020): 1505, https://doi.org/10.3390/nu12051505.

[40] Lijuan Han et al., "Environmental Stress-Stable Bigels Structured by Sitosterol–Oryzanol and Guar Gum: Dual-Network Mechanism and Food-Relevant Applications," *Food Hydrocolloids* 173 (April 2026): 112248, https://doi.org/10.1016/j.foodhyd.2025.112248; Dariush Mozaffarian, "Dietary and Policy Priorities for Cardiovascular Disease, Diabetes, and Obesity: A Comprehensive

Review," Circulation 133, no. 2 (January 2016): 187–225, https://doi.org/10.1161/CIRCULATIONAHA.115.018585; Lukas Schwingshackl et al., "Effects of Oils and Solid Fats on Blood Lipids: A Systematic Review and Network Meta-Analysis," *Journal of Lipid Research* 59, no. 9 (July 2018): 1771–82, https://doi.org/10.1194/jlr.P085522; Skaeff C. Murray et al., "Dietary Induced Changes in Fatty Acid Composition of Human Plasma, Platelet, and Erythrocyte Lipids Follow a Similar Time Course," *Journal of Nutrition* 136, no. 3 (March 2006): 565–69, https://doi.org/10.1093/jn/136.3.565.

[41] Marta Guasch-Ferré et al., "Consumption of Olive Oil and Risk of Total and Cause-Specific Mortality Among U.S. Adults," *Journal of the American College of Cardiology* 79, no. 2 (January 18, 2022): 101–12, https://doi.org/10.1016/j.jacc.2021.10.041; Pamela de Aguiar Sobral et al., "Health Outcomes Related to the Consumption of Olive Products: A Brief Review," *Plant Foods for Human Nutrition* 78, no. 4 (November 2023): 643–53, https://doi.org/10.1007/s11130-023-01119-w.

[42] Alexis A. Hung et al., "The Ketogenic Diet: An Anti-Inflammatory Treatment for Schizophrenia?," *Journal of Inflammation Research* 18 (December 2025): 16761–71, https://doi.org/10.2147/JIR.S540859; Carmen Rubio et al., "Impact of the Ketogenic Diet on Neurological Diseases: A Review," *Life* 15, no. 1 (2025): 71, https://doi.org/10.3390/life15010071.

[43] Joyce A. Nettleton et al., "Saturated Fat Consumption and Risk of Coronary Heart Disease and Ischemic Stroke: A Science Update," *Annals of Nutrition & Metabolism* 70, no. 1 (April 1, 2017): 26–33, https://doi.org/10.1159/000455681.

[44] Vicente Javier Clemente-Suárez et al., "The Burden of Carbohydrates in Health and Disease," *Nutrients* 14, no. 18 (2022): 3809, https://doi.org/10.3390/nu14183809.

[45] Herman Pontzer et al., "Daily Energy Expenditure Through the Human Life Course," *Science* 373, no. 6556 (August 2021): 808–12, https://doi.org/10.1126/science.abe5017.

[46] Christian von Loeffelholz and Andreas L. Birkenfeld, "Non-Exercise Activity Thermogenesis in Human Energy Homeostasis," in Endotext (Internet), ed. K. R. Feingold et al. (MDText.com, 2022), https://www.ncbi.nlm.nih.gov/sites/books/NBK279077/.

[47] Gary John Slater et al., "Is an Energy Surplus Required to Maximize Skeletal Muscle Hypertrophy Associated with Resistance Training?" *Frontiers in Nutrition* 6 (August 2019): 131, https://doi.org/10.3389/fnut.2019.00131.

[48] Alex S. Ribeiro et al., "Effects of Different Dietary Energy Intake Following Resistance Training on Muscle Mass and Body Fat in Bodybuilders: A Pilot Study," *Journal of Human Kinetics* 70, no. 1 (November 2019): 125–34, https://doi.org/10.2478/hukin-2019-0038.

[49] John C. Peters et al., "The Effects of Water and Non-Nutritive Sweetened Beverages on Weight Loss and Weight Maintenance: A Randomized Clinical Trial," *Obesity* 24, no. 2 (December 2015): 297–304, https://doi.org/10.1002/oby.21327.

[50] G. Pagliai et al., "Consumption of Ultra-Processed Foods and Health Status: A Systematic Review and Meta-Analysis," *British Journal of Nutrition* 125, no. 3 (2021): 308–18, https://doi.org/10.1017/S0007114520002688.

[51] Melissa M. Lane et al., "Ultra-Processed Food Consumption and Mental Health: A Systematic Review and Meta-Analysis of Observational Studies," *Nutrients* 14, no. 13 (2022): 2568, https://doi.org/10.3390/nu14132568; Lane et al., "Ultra-Processed Food Exposure"; Huiping Li et al., "Association of Ultraprocessed Food Consumption with Risk of Dementia: A Prospective Cohort Study," *Neurology* 99, no. 10 (2022): e1056–66, https://doi.org/10.1212/WNL.0000000000200871; Shenghao Yuan et al., "Associations of Ultra-Processed Food Intake and Its Circulating Metabolomic Signature with Mental Disorders in Middle-Aged and Older Adults," *Nutrients* 17, no. 9 (2025): 1582, https://doi.org/10.3390/nu17091582.

[52] Ryan J. Koene et al., "Shared Risk Factors in Cardiovascular Disease and Cancer," *Circulation* 133, no. 11 (2016): 1104–14, https://doi.org/10.1161/CIRCULATIONAHA.115.020406.

[53] Sonia S. Anand et al., "Food Consumption and Its Impact on Cardiovascular Disease: Importance of Solutions Focused on the Globalized Food System: A Report from the Workshop Convened by the

World Heart Federation," *Journal of the American College of Cardiology* 66, no. 14 (2015): 1590–1614, https://doi.org/10.1016/j.jacc.2015.07.050.

[54] Véronique Bouvard et al., "Carcinogenicity of Consumption of Red and Processed Meat," *Lancet Oncology* 16, no. 16 (2015): 1599–600, https://doi.org/10.1016/S1470-2045(15)00444-1; Renata Micha et al., "Red and Processed Meat Consumption and Risk of Incident Coronary Heart Disease, Stroke, and Diabetes Mellitus: A Systematic Review and Meta-Analysis," *Circulation* 121, no. 21 (2010): 2271–83, https://doi.org/10.1161/CIRCULATIONAHA.109.924977.

[55] Renata Micha et al., "Association Between Dietary Factors and Mortality from Heart Disease, Stroke, and Type 2 Diabetes in the United States," *JAMA* 317, no. 9 (2017): 912–24, https://doi.org/10.1001/jama.2017.0947.

[56] "Why Good Nutrition Is Important," Center for Science in the Public Interest, n.d., https://www.cspi.org/eating-healthy/why-good-nutrition-important.

[57] David J. A. Jenkins et al., "Nibbling Versus Gorging: Metabolic Advantages of Increased Meal Frequency," *New England Journal of Medicine* 321, no. 14 (1989): 929–34, https://doi.org/10.1056/NEJM198910053211403.

[58] Jameason D. Cameron et al., "Increased Meal Frequency Does Not Promote Greater Weight Loss in Subjects Who Were Prescribed an 8-Week Equi-Energetic Energy-Restricted Diet," *British Journal of Nutrition* 103, no. 8 (2010): 1098–1101, https://doi.org/10.1017/S0007114509992984.

[59] Ruth E. Patterson et al., "Intermittent Fasting and Human Metabolic Health," *Journal of the Academy of Nutrition and Dietetics* 115, no. 8 (2015): 1203–12, https://doi.org/10.1016/j.jand.2015.02.018.

[60] Sally Adee, "Does Intermittent Fasting Live Up to the Hype?," *New York Times*, January 26, 2026, https://www.nytimes.com/2026/01/26/well/eat/intermittent-fasting.html.

[61] Deying Liu et al., "Calorie Restriction with or Without Time-Restricted Eating in Weight Loss," *New England Journal of Medicine* 386, no. 16 (2022): 1495–504, https://doi.org/10.1056/NEJMoa2114833.

[62] Fran Smith, "Can Fasting Help You Live Longer? Here's What the Science Says," *National Geographic*, January 17, 2023, https://www.nationalgeographic.com/magazine/article/can-fasting-help-you-live-longer-what-the-science-says.

[63] Arthur V. Everitt and David G. Le Couteur, "Life Extension by Calorie Restriction in Humans," *Annals of the New York Academy of Sciences* 1114, no. 1 (2007): 428–33, https://doi.org/10.1196/annals.1396.005.

[64] Megumi Hatori et al., "Time-Restricted Feeding Without Reducing Caloric Intake Prevents Metabolic Diseases in Mice Fed a High-Fat Diet," *Cell Metabolism* 15, no. 6 (June 2012): 848–60, https://doi.org/10.1016/j.cmet.2012.04.019.

[65] Mark P. Mattson et al., "Meal Frequency and Timing in Health and Disease," *Proceedings of the National Academy of Sciences* 111, no. 47 (November 2014): 16647–53, https://doi.org/10.1073/pnas.1413965111.

[66] Li-Ming Yan et al., "Chronobiological Perspectives: Association Between Meal Timing and Sleep Quality," *PLOS One* 19, no. 8 (2024): e0308172, https://doi.org/10.1371/journal.pone.0308172.

[67] Gabrielle Brandenberger and Laurence Weibel, "The 24-h Growth Hormone Rhythm in Men: Sleep and Circadian Influences Questioned," *Journal of Sleep Research* 13, no. 3 (2004): 251–55, https://doi.org/10.1111/j.1365-2869.2004.00415.x.

[68] Marie-Pierre St-Onge et al., "The Interrelationship Between Sleep, Diet, and Glucose Metabolism," *Sleep Medicine Reviews* 69 (June 2023): 101788, https://doi.org/10.1016/j.smrv.2023.101788.

[69] Arturo Figueroa et al., "Effects of Milk Proteins and Combined Exercise Training on Aortic Hemodynamics and Arterial Stiffness in Young Obese Women with High Blood Pressure," *American Journal of Hypertension* 27, no. 3 (March 2014): 338–44, https://doi.org/10.1093/ajh/hpt224.

[70] Matt Ulgherait et al., "Circadian Autophagy Drives iTRF-Mediated Longevity," *Nature* 598 (2021): 353–58, https://doi.org/10.1038/s41586-021-03934-0.

[71] Sebastian Brandhorst et al., "A Periodic Diet That Mimics Fasting Promotes Multi-System Regeneration, Enhanced Cognitive Performance, and Healthspan," *Cell Metabolism* 22, no. 1 (2015): 86–99, https://doi.org/10.1016/j.cmet.2015.05.012.

[72] Ki Wung Chung and Hae Young Chung, "The Effects of Calorie Restriction on Autophagy: Role on Aging Intervention," *Nutrients* 11, no. 12 (2019): 2923, https://doi.org/10.3390/nu11122923.

[73] Frank Madeo et al., "Essential Role for Autophagy in Life Span Extension," *Journal of Clinical Investigation* 125, no. 1 (2015): 85–93, https://doi.org/10.1172/JCI73946.

[74] Richard Weindruch and Rajindar S. Sohal, "Caloric Intake and Aging," *New England Journal of Medicine* 337, no. 14 (1997): 986–94, https://doi.org/10.1056/NEJM199710023371407.

[75] Jens Frey Halling and Henriette Pilegaard, "Autophagy-Dependent Beneficial Effects of Exercise," *Cold Spring Harbor Perspectives in Medicine* 7, no. 8 (March 2017): a029777, https://doi.org/10.1101/cshperspect.a029777.

[76] Esther Ugo Alum, "Circadian Nutrition and Obesity: Timing as a Nutritional Strategy," *Journal of Health, Population and Nutrition* 44, no. 1 (2025): 367, https://doi.org/10.1186/s41043-025-01102-y.

[77] Monteiro et al., "Ultra-Processed Foods."

[78] National Research Council (US) Committee on Diet, Nutrition, and Cancer, *Diet, Nutrition, and Cancer: Directions for Research* (National Academies Press [US], 1983), chap. 8, https://www.ncbi.nlm.nih.gov/books/NBK216714/.

[79] Djésia Arnone et al., "Sugars and Gastrointestinal Health," *Clinical Gastroenterology and Hepatology* 20, no. 9 (2022): 1912–24.e7, https://doi.org/10.1016/j.cgh.2021.12.011; Fumiaki Imamura et al., "Consumption of Sugar Sweetened Beverages, Artificially Sweetened Beverages, and Fruit Juice and Incidence of Type 2 Diabetes: Systematic Review, Meta-Analysis, and Estimation of Population Attributable Fraction. *BMJ* 351 (2015): h3576, https://doi.org/10.1136/bmj.h3576; Vasanti S. Malik et al., "Sugar-Sweetened Beverages and Risk of Metabolic Syndrome and Type 2 Diabetes: A Meta-Analysis," *Diabetes Care* 33, no. 11 (2010): 2477–83, https://doi.org/10.2337/dc10-1079; Bo Yang et al., "Added Sugar, Sugar-Sweetened Beverages, and Artificially Sweetened Beverages and Risk of Cardiovascular Disease: Findings From the Women's Health Initiative and a Network Meta-Analysis of Prospective Studies," *Nutrients* 14, no. 19 (October 2022): 4226, https://doi.org/10.3390/nu14204226; Quanhe Yang et al., "*Added Sugar Intake and Cardiovascular Diseases Mortality Among US Adults*," *JAMA Internal Medicine* 174, no. 4 (April 2014): 516–24, https://doi.org/10.1001/jamainternmed.2013.13563; Florida Llaha et al., "Consumption of Sweet Beverages and Cancer Risk: A Systematic Review and Meta-Analysis of Observational Studies," *Nutrients* 13, no. 2 (2021): 516, https://doi.org/10.3390/nu13020516; Yuting Li et al., "Consumption of Sugar-Sweetened Beverages and Fruit Juice and Human Cancer: A Systematic Review and Dose-Response Meta-Analysis of Observational Studies," *Journal of Cancer* 12, no. 10 (2021): 3077–88, https://doi.org/10.7150/jca.51322; Yan-Bo Zhang et al., "Association of Consumption of Sugar-Sweetened Beverages or Artificially Sweetened Beverages With Mortality: A Systematic Review and Dose-Response Meta-Analysis of Prospective Cohort Studies," *Advances in Nutrition* 12, no. 2 (2021): 374–83, https://doi:10.1093/advances/nmaa110; Lukas Schwingshackl et al., "Food Groups and Risk of All-Cause Mortality: A Systematic Review and Dose-Response Meta-Analysis of Prospective Studies," *American Journal of Clinical Nutrition* 105, no. 6 (2017): 1462–73, https://doi.org/10.3945/ajcn.117.153148.

[80] Jon Davis, "Hunger, Ghrelin and the Gut," *Brain Research* 1693, Pt. B (2018): 154–58, https://doi.org/10.1016/j.brainres.2018.01.024.

[81] Emeran A. Mayer et al., "The Gut-Brain Axis," *Annual Review of Medicine* 73 (January 2022): 439–53, https://doi.org/10.1146/annurev-med-042320-014032.

[82] C. S. Byrne et al., "The Role of Short Chain Fatty Acids in Appetite Regulation and Energy Homeostasis," *International Journal of Obesity* 39, no. 9 (2015): 1331–38, https://doi.org/10.1038/ijo.2015.84.

[83] Serika Yamada et al., "Immediate Glucose Signaling Transmitted via the Vagus Nerve in Gut–Brain Neural Communication," *iScience* 28, no. 5 (2025), https://doi.org/10.1016/j.isci.2025.112439; Melanie Maya Kaelberer et al., "Neuropod Cells: The Emerging Biology of Gut-Brain Sensory Transduction," Annual Review of Neuroscience 43 (July 2020): 337–53, *https://doi.org/10.1146/annurev-neuro-091619-022657;* Andrew Huberman, "Dr. Diego Bohórquez: The Science of Your Gut Sense & the Gut-Brain Axis," *Huberman Lab* (podcast audio), May 27, 2024, https://hubermanlab.com/episode/dr-diego-bohorquez-the-science-of-your-gut-sense-the-gut-brain-axis.

[84] Hwei-Ee Tan et al., "The Gut–Brain Axis Mediates Sugar Preference," *Nature* 580, no. 7804 (2020): 511–16, https://doi.org/10.1038/s41586-020-2199-7.

[85] Nora D. Volkow et al., "Reward, Dopamine and the Control of Food Intake: Implications for Obesity," *Trends in Cognitive Sciences* 15, no. 1 (2011): 37–46, https://doi.org/10.1016/j.tics.2010.11.001; Ashley N. Gearhardt et al., "Social, Clinical, and Policy Implications of Ultra-Processed Food Addiction," *BMJ* 383 (October 9, 2023): e075354, https://doi.org/10.1136/bmj-2023-075354; Erratum, Gearhardt et al., "Social, Clinical, and Policy Implications," *BMJ* 383 (2023): 2679, https://doi.org/10.1136/bmj.p2679.

[86] Hannah Cory et al., "The Role of Polyphenols in Human Health and Food Systems: A Mini-Review," *Frontiers in Nutrition* 5 (September 21, 2018): 87, https://doi.org/10.3389/fnut.2018.00087.

[87] Konstantinos Mantantzis et al., "Sugar Rush or Sugar Crash? A Meta-Analysis of Carbohydrate Effects on Mood," *Neuroscience & Biobehavioral Reviews* 101 (June 2019): 45–67, https://doi.org/10.1016/j.neubiorev.2019.03.016.

[88] Di Qin et al., "Sugar Addiction."

[89] Le Ma et al., "Beverage Consumption and Mortality Among Adults with Type 2 Diabetes: Prospective Cohort Study," *BMJ* 381 (April 19, 2023): e073406, https://doi.org/10.1136/bmj-2022-073406.

[90] Kristine K. Dennis et al., "Associations of Dietary Sugar Types with Coronary Heart Disease Risk: A Prospective Cohort Study," *American Journal of Clinical Nutrition* 118, no. 5 (2023): 1000–1009, https://doi.org/10.1016/j.ajcnut.2023.08.019.

[91] Victoria Peteliuk et al., "Natural Sweetener *Stevia rebaudiana*: Functionalities, Health Benefits and Potential Risks," *EXCLI Journal* 20 (September 22, 2021): 1412–30, https://doi.org/10.17179/excli2021-4211.

[92] "Aspartame Hazard and Risk Assessment Results Released," World Health Organization, July 14, 2023, https://www.who.int/news/item/14-07-2023-aspartame-hazard-and-risk-assessment-results-released.

[93] Alex Kidangathazhe et al., "Synthetic vs. Non-Synthetic Sweeteners: Their Differential Effects on Gut Microbiome Diversity and Function," *Frontiers in Microbiology* 16 (May 14, 2025): 1531131, https://doi.org/10.3389/fmicb.2025.1531131.

[94] Joanne A. Harrold et al., "Non-Nutritive Sweetened Beverages Versus Water After a 52-Week Weight Management Programme: A Randomised Controlled Trial," *International Journal of Obesity* 48 (2024): 83–93, https://doi.org/10.1038/s41366-023-01393-3.

[95] Sandhya P. Chakravartti et al., "Non-Caloric Sweetener Effects on Brain Appetite Regulation in Individuals Across Varying Body Weights," *Nature Metabolism* 7 (2025): 574–85, https://doi.org/10.1038/s42255-025-01227-8.

[96] Jerry R. Greenfield et al., "Oral Glutamine Increases Circulating Glucagon-Like Peptide 1, Glucagon, and Insulin Concentrations in Lean, Obese, and Type 2 Diabetic Subjects," *American Journal of Clinical Nutrition* 89, no. 1 (2009): 106–13, https://doi.org/10.3945/ajcn.2008.26362.

[97] Hong Lu et al., "Body Water Percentage from Childhood to Old Age," *Kidney Research and Clinical Practice* 42, no. 3 (2023): 340–48, https://doi.org/10.23876/j.krcp.22.062.

[98] Joshua E. Brinkman et al., "Physiology, Body Fluids," StatPearls, last updated January 27, 2023, https://www.ncbi.nlm.nih.gov/books/NBK482447/.

[99] Lawrence W. Judge et al., "Hydration to Maximize Performance and Recovery: Knowledge, Attitudes, and Behaviors Among Collegiate Track and Field Throwers," *Journal of Human Kinetics* 79 (July 2021): 111–22, https://doi.org/10.2478/hukin-2021-0065.

[100] Wisit Cheungpasitporn et al., "Treatment Effect, Adherence, and Safety of High Fluid Intake for the Prevention of Incident and Recurrent Kidney Stones: A Systematic Review and Meta-Analysis," *Journal of Nephrology* 29, no. 2 (2016): 211–19, https://doi.org/10.1007/s40620-015-0210-4.

[101] Jens Jordan et al., "The Pressor Response to Water Drinking in Humans: A Sympathetic Reflex?," *Circulation* 101, no. 5 (2000): 504–9, https://doi.org/10.1161/01.cir.101.5.504.

[102] Paula Booth et al., "Water Supplementation Improves Visual Attention and Fine Motor Skills in Schoolchildren," *Education for Health Change in Learning & Practice* 30, no. 3 (January 2012): 75–79.

[103] Barry M. Popkin et al., "Water, Hydration, and Health," *Nutrition Reviews* 68, no. 8 (2010): 439–58, https://doi.org/10.1111/j.1753-4887.2010.00304.x.

[104] DeAnn Liska et al., "Narrative Review of Hydration and Selected Health Outcomes in the General Population," *Nutrients* 11, no. 1 (2019): 70, https://doi.org/10.3390/nu11010070.

[105] Giuseppe Faraco et al., "Water Deprivation Induces Neurovascular and Cognitive Dysfunction Through Vasopressin-Induced Oxidative Stress," *Journal of Cerebral Blood Flow & Metabolism* 34, no. 5 (2014): 852–60, https://doi.org/10.1038/jcbfm.2014.24.

[106] Naila A. Shaheen et al., "Public Knowledge of Dehydration and Fluid Intake Practices: Variation by Participants' Characteristics," *BMC Public Health* 18 (December 2018): 1346, https://doi.org/10.1186/s12889-018-6252-5.

[107] Tammie R. Ebert et al., "Influence of Hydration Status on Thermoregulation and Cycling Hill Climbing," *Medicine & Science in Sports & Exercise* 39, no. 2 (2007): 323–29, https://doi.org/10.1249/01.mss.0000247000.86847.de.

[108] Daniel A. Judelson et al., "Effect of Hydration State on Strength, Power, and Resistance Exercise Performance," *Medicine & Science in Sports & Exercise* 39, no. 10 (2007): 1817–24, https://doi.org/10.1249/mss.0b013e3180de5f22.

[109] Dmitri Firsov and Oliver Bonny, "Circadian Rhythms and the Kidney," *Nature Reviews Nephrology* 14 (2018): 626–35, https://doi.org/10.1038/s41581-018-0048-9.

[110] Jermaine G. Johnston and David M. Pollock, "Circadian Regulation of Renal Function," *Free Radical Biology and Medicine* 119 (May 1, 2018): 93–107, https://doi.org/10.1016/j.freeradbiomed.2018.01.018.

[111] Mohammad A. Shafiee et al., "Defining Conditions That Lead to the Retention of Water: The Importance of the Arterial Sodium Concentration," *Kidney International* 67, no. 2 (2005): 613–21, https://doi.org/10.1111/j.1523-1755.2005.67117.x.

[112] Guoyao Wu, "Amino Acids: Metabolism, Functions, and Nutrition," *Amino Acids* 37, no. 1 (2009): 1–17, https://doi.org/10.1007/s00726-009-0269-0; National Research Council (US) Subcommittee on the Tenth Edition of the Recommended Dietary Allowances, *Recommended Dietary Allowances*, 10th ed. (National Academies Press [US], 1989), chap. 6, https://www.ncbi.nlm.nih.gov/books/NBK234922/; Richard B. Kreider and Bill Campbell, "Protein for Exercise and Recovery," *Physician and Sportsmedicine* 37, no. 2 (2009): 13–21, https://doi.org/10.3810/psm.2009.06.1705; David D. Church et al., "Essential Amino Acids and Protein Synthesis: Insights into Maximizing the Muscle and Whole-Body Response to Feeding," *Nutrients* 12, no. 12 (2020): 3717, https://doi.org/10.3390/nu12123717.

[113] M. Veldhorst et al., "Protein-Induced Satiety: Effects and Mechanisms of Different Proteins," *Physiology & Behavior* 94, no. 2 (2008): 300–307, https://doi.org/10.1016/j.physbeh.2008.01.003.

[114] Shahab Ur Rehman et al., "Research Progress in the Role and Mechanism of Leucine in Regulating Animal Growth and Development," *Frontiers in Physiology* 14 (November 2023): 1252089, https://doi.org/10.3389/fphys.2023.1252089.

[115] Micah J. Drummond and Blake B. Rasmussen, "Leucine-Enriched Nutrients and the Regulation of Mammalian Target of Rapamycin Signalling and Human Skeletal Muscle Protein Synthesis," *Current Opinion in Clinical Nutrition and Metabolic Care* 11, no. 3 (2008): 222–26, https://doi.org/10.1097/MCO.0b013e3282fa17fb.

[116] Elitsa A. Ananieva et al., "Leucine Metabolism in T Cell Activation: mTOR Signaling and Beyond," *Advances in Nutrition* 7, no. 4 (2016): 798S–805S, https://doi.org/10.3945/an.115.011221.

[117] Rehman et al., "Research Progress in the Role."

[118] Mikhail V. Blagosklonny, "Rapamycin for Longevity: Opinion Article," *Aging* 11, no. 19 (2019): 8048–67, https://doi.org/10.18632/aging.102355.

[119] Douglas Paddon-Jones et al., "Protein, Weight Management, and Satiety," *American Journal of Clinical Nutrition* 87, no. 5 (2008): 1558S–61S, https://doi.org/10.1093/ajcn/87.5.1558S.

[120] Joanne L. Slavin and Beate Lloyd, "Health Benefits of Fruits and Vegetables," *Advances in Nutrition* 3, no. 4 (2012): 506–16, https://doi.org/10.3945/an.112.002154.

[121] Corina-Bianca Ioniță-Mîndrican et al., "Therapeutic Benefits and Dietary Restrictions of Fiber Intake: A State of the Art Review," *Nutrients* 14, no. 13 (2022): 2641, https://doi.org/10.3390/nu14132641.

[122] Mary Ellen Sanders et al., "Probiotics and Prebiotics in Intestinal Health and Disease: From Biology to the Clinic," *Nature Reviews Gastroenterology & Hepatology* 16 (July 2019): 605–16, https://doi.org/10.1038/s41575-019-0173-3; Boushra Dalile et al., "The Role of Short-Chain Fatty Acids in Microbiota–Gut–Brain Communication," *Nature Reviews Gastroenterology & Hepatology* 16, no. 8 (August 2019): 461–78, https://doi.org/10.1038/s41575-019-0157-3; Elizabeth Schneider et al., "Feeding Gut Microbes to Nourish the Brain: Unravelling the Diet–Microbiota–Gut–Brain Axis," *Nature Metabolism* 6 (2024): 1454–78, https://doi.org/10.1038/s42255-024-01108-6; María Aburto and John F. Cryan, "Gastrointestinal and Brain Barriers: Unlocking Gates of Communication Across the Microbiota–Gut–Brain Axis," *Nature Reviews Gastroenterology & Hepatology* 21, no. 4 (April 2024): 222–47, https://doi.org/10.1038/s41575-023-00890-0; Robert Hutkins et al., "Classifying Compounds as Prebiotics—Scientific Perspectives and Recommendations," *Nature Reviews Gastroenterology & Hepatology* 22 (2025): 54–70, https://doi.org/10.1038/s41575-024-00981-6; Yolanda Sanz et al., "The Gut Microbiome Connects Nutrition and Human Health," *Nature Reviews Gastroenterology & Hepatology* 22 (2025): 534–55, https://doi.org/10.1038/s41575-025-01077-5.

[123] Lydia A. Bazzano et al., "Dietary Fiber Intake and Reduced Risk of Coronary Heart Disease in US Men and Women: The National Health and Nutrition Examination Survey I Epidemiologic Follow-Up Study," *Archives of Internal Medicine* 163, no. 16 (2003): 1897–1904, https://doi.org/10.1001/archinte.163.16.1897.

[124] Jun Hu et al., "Use of Dietary Fibers in Reducing the Risk of Several Cancer Types: An Umbrella Review," *Nutrients* 15, no. 11 (2023): 2545, https://doi.org/10.3390/nu15112545.

[125] Eliana Bistriche Giuntini et al., "The Effects of Soluble Dietary Fibers on Glycemic Response: An Overview and Futures Perspectives," *Foods* 11, no. 23 (December 2022): 3934, https://doi.org/10.3390/foods11233934.

[126] Diane Quagliani and Patricia Felt-Gunderson, "Closing America's Fiber Intake Gap," *American Journal of Lifestyle Medicine* 11, no. 1 (July 2016): 80–85, https://doi.org/10.1177/1559827615588079.

[127] Allison W. Peng et al., "Effects of the DASH Diet and Sodium Intake on Bloating: Results from the DASH-Sodium Trial," *American Journal of Gastroenterology* 114, no. 7 (2019): 1109–15, https://doi.org/10.14309/ajg.0000000000000283.

[128] "Magnesium Compounds Statistics and Information," National Minerals Information Center, n.d., https://www.usgs.gov/centers/national-minerals-information-center/magnesium-compounds-statistics-and-information.

[129] "Magnesium: Fact Sheet for Health Professionals," National Institutes of Health Office of Dietary Supplements, updated January 6, 2026, https://ods.od.nih.gov/factsheets/Magnesium-HealthProfessional/.

[130] James J. DiNicolantonio et al., "Subclinical Magnesium Deficiency: A Principal Driver of Cardiovascular Disease and a Public Health Crisis," *Open Heart* 5, no. 1 (January 2018): e000668, https://doi.org/10.1136/openhrt-2017-000668; Erratum, DiNicolantonio et al., "Subclinical Magnesium Deficiency," *Open Heart* 5, no. 1 (April 2018): e000668corr1, https://doi.org/10.1136/openhrt-2017-000668corr1.

[131] Ahmad Hassan Chaudhry et al., "Current Understandings on Magnesium Deficiency and Future Outlooks for Sustainable Agriculture," *International Journal of Molecular Sciences* 22, no. 4 (2021): 1819, https://doi.org/10.3390/ijms22041819.

[132] R. Swaminathan, "Magnesium Metabolism and Its Disorders," *Clinical Biochemist Reviews* 24, no. 2 (2003): 47–66, https://pubmed.ncbi.nlm.nih.gov/18568054/.

[133] Moushumi Sur and Shamim S. Mohiuddin, "Potassium," StatPearls, last updated October 5, 2024, https://www.ncbi.nlm.nih.gov/books/NBK539791/.

[134] Elaine Yu and Sandeep Sharma, "Physiology, Calcium," StatPearls, last updated August 14, 2023, https://www.ncbi.nlm.nih.gov/books/NBK482128/.

[135] A. N. Panche et al., "Flavonoids: An Overview," *Journal of Nutritional Science* 5 (December 29, 2016): e47, https://doi.org/10.1017/jns.2016.41; Panche et al., "Flavonoids: An Overview—CORRIGENDUM in Figure 1," *Journal of Nutritional Science* 14 (January 29, 2025): e11, https://doi.org/10.1017/jns.2024.73.

[136] Jed W. Fahey and Mirran Raphaely, "The Impact of Sulforaphane on Sex-Specific Conditions and Hormone Balance: A Comprehensive Review," *Applied Sciences* 15, no. 2 (January 2025): 522, https://doi.org/10.3390/app15020522.

[137] Ann F. La Berge, "How the Ideology of Low Fat Conquered America," *Journal of the History of Medicine and Allied Sciences* 63, no. 2 (2008): 139–77, https://doi.org/10.1093/jhmas/jrn001.

[138] Dariush Mozaffarian and David S. Ludwig, "The 2015 US Dietary Guidelines: Lifting the Ban on Total Dietary Fat," *JAMA* 313, no. 24 (2015): 2421–22, https://doi.org/10.1001/jama.2015.5941.

[139] James W. Wheless, "History of the Ketogenic Diet," *Epilepsia* 49, no. S8 (2008): 3–5, https://doi.org/10.1111/j.1528-1167.2008.01821.x.

[140] Adam Włodarczyk et al., "Ketogenic Diet for Schizophrenia: Nutritional Approach to Antipsychotic Treatment," *Medical Hypotheses* 118 (September 2018): 74–77, https://doi.org/10.1016/j.mehy.2018.06.022.

[141] Nicole Needham et al., "Pilot Study of a Ketogenic Diet in Bipolar Disorder," *BJPsych Open* 9, no. 6 (2023): e176, https://doi.org/10.1192/bjo.2023.568.

[142] Philip C. Calder, "Functional Roles of Fatty Acids and Their Effects on Human Health," *Journal of Parenteral and Enteral Nutrition* 39, no. 1s (2015): 18S–32S, https://doi.org/10.1177/0148607115595980; Rosanna Chianese et al., "Impact of Dietary Fats on Brain Functions," *Current Neuropharmacology* 16, no. 7 (2018): 1059–85, https://doi.org/10.2174/1570159X15666171017102547.

[143] Chianese et al., "Impact of Dietary Fats."

[144] Richard P. Bazinet and Sophie Layé, "Polyunsaturated Fatty Acids and Their Metabolites in Brain Function and Disease," *Nature Reviews Neuroscience* 15, no. 12 (2014): 771–85, https://doi.org/10.1038/nrn3820; Tommy Cederholm et al., "ω-3 Fatty Acids in the Prevention of Cognitive Decline in Humans," *Advances in Nutrition* 4, no. 6 (2013): 672–76, https://doi.org/10.3945/an.113.004556.

[145] Sean Dornbush and Narothama R. Aeddula, "Physiology, Leptin," StatPearls, last updated April 10, 2023, https://www.ncbi.nlm.nih.gov/books/NBK537038/; M. Romon et al., "Leptin Response to Carbohydrate or Fat Meal and Association with Subsequent Satiety and Energy Intake," *American*

Journal of Physiology-Endocrinology and Metabolism 277, no. 5 (1999): E855–61, https://doi.org/10.1152/ajpendo.1999.277.5.E855.

146 A. M. Salem, "Variation of Leptin During Menstrual Cycle and Its Relation to the Hypothalamic-Pituitary-Gonadal (HPG) Axis: A Systematic Review," *International Journal of Women's Health* 13 (May 2021): 445–58, https://doi.org/10.2147/IJWH.S309299; Pallav Sengupta et al., "Leptin and Male Reproduction," *Asian Pacific Journal of Reproduction* 8, no. 5 (2019): 220–26, https://doi.org/10.4103/2305-0500.268143.

147 Mona A. Hegazy et al., "Hidden Industrial Trans-Fatty Acids: Mechanistic Insights into Dyslipidemia, Cardiovascular Disease, and Metabolic Dysfunction-Associated Steatotic Liver Disease," *International Journal of Molecular Sciences* 26, no. 23 (December 2025): 11715, https://doi.org/10.3390/ijms262311715.

148 Angela Amico et al., "The Demise of Artificial Trans Fat: A History of a Public Health Achievement," *Milbank Quarterly* 99, no. 3 (August 2021): 746–70, https://doi.org/10.1111/1468-0009.12515.

149 Ruth Sander, "Saturated Fat May Not Be as Bad for Us After All," *Nursing Older People* 28, no. 5 (2016): 13, https://doi.org/10.7748/nop.28.5.13.s16.

150 Dariush Mozaffarian et al., "Effects on Coronary Heart Disease of Increasing Polyunsaturated Fat in Place of Saturated Fat: A Systematic Review and Meta-Analysis of Randomized Controlled Trials," *PLOS Medicine* 7, no. 3 (2010): e1000252, https://doi.org/10.1371/journal.pmed.1000252.

151 Zoë Harcombe et al., "Evidence from Prospective Cohort Studies Does Not Support Current Dietary Fat Guidelines: A Systematic Review and Meta-Analysis," *British Journal of Sports Medicine* 51, no. 24 (2017): 1743–49, https://doi.org/10.1136/bjsports-2016-096550; Christopher E. Ramsden et al., "Re-Evaluation of the Traditional Diet-Heart Hypothesis: Analysis of Recovered Data from Minnesota Coronary Experiment (1968–73)," *BMJ* 353 (April 12, 2016): i1246, https://doi.org/10.1136/bmj.i1246; Erratum, Ramsden et al., "Re-Evaluation of the Traditional Diet-Heart Hypothesis," *BMJ* 385 (June 28, 2024): q1450, https://doi.org/10.1136/bmj.q1450.

152 James J. DiNicolantonio et al., "The Evidence for Saturated Fat and for Sugar Related to Coronary Heart Disease," *Progress in Cardiovascular Diseases* 58, no. 5 (2016): 464–72, https://doi.org/10.1016/j.pcad.2015.11.006.

153 Research from the Whitehall II (The Stress and Health Study) is available online here: Whitehall II, UCL Brain Sciences, https://www.ucl.ac.uk/brain-sciences/psychiatry/research/mental-health-older-people/projects/whitehall-ii.

154 Sabita S. Soedamah-Muthu et al., "Consumption of Dairy Products and Associations with Incident Diabetes, CHD and Mortality in the Whitehall II Study," *British Journal of Nutrition* 109, no. 4 (2013): 718–26, https://doi.org/10.1017/S0007114512001845.

155 Matthew R. Hilimire et al., "Fermented Foods, Neuroticism, and Social Anxiety: An Interaction Model," *Psychiatry Research* 228, no. 2 (2015): 203–8, https://doi.org/10.1016/j.psychres.2015.04.023.

156 R. W. Walker et al., "The Prenatal Gut Microbiome: Are We Colonized with Bacteria *in Utero*?," *Pediatric Obesity* 12, no. S1 (2017): 3–17, https://doi.org/10.1111/ijpo.12217.

157 Melissa Lee Phillips, "Gut Reaction: Environmental Effects on the Human Microbiota," *Environmental Health Perspectives* 117, no. 5 (2009): A198–205, https://doi.org/10.1289/ehp.117-a198; Willem M. de Vos et al., "Gut Microbiome and Health: Mechanistic Insights," *Gut* 71, no. 5 (2022): 1020–32, https://doi.org/10.1136/gutjnl-2021-326789.

158 Alexander N. Boytar et al., "The Effect of Exercise Prescription on the Human Gut Microbiota and Comparison Between Clinical and Apparently Healthy Populations: A Systematic Review," *Nutrients* 15, no. 6 (2023): 1534, https://doi.org/10.3390/nu15061534.

159 Vincenzo Monda et al., "Exercise Modifies the Gut Microbiota with Positive Health Effects," *Oxidative Medicine and Cellular Longevity* 2017 (March 2017): 3831972, https://doi.org/10.1155/2017/3831972; Belle Huang et al., "Bidirectional Link Between Exercise and the Gut Microbiota,"

Exercise and Sport Sciences Reviews 52, no. 4 (October 2024): 132–44, https://doi.org/10.1249/JES.0000000000000343; Leizi Min et al., "Effects of Exercise on Gut Microbiota of Adults: A Systematic Review and Meta-Analysis," *Nutrients* 16, no. 7 (April 2024): 1070, https://doi.org/10.3390/nu16071070; Yousra Alsinani et al., "Exercise and the Gut Microbiome: From Mechanisms to Clinical Applications," Nutrients 18, no. 10 (May 2026): 1565, https://doi.org/10.3390/nu18101565.

160 Boytar et al., "Effect of Exercise Prescription"; Muriel Derrien and Johan E. T. van Hylckama Vlieg, "Fate, Activity, and Impact of Ingested Bacteria Within the Human Gut Microbiota," *Trends in Microbiology* 23, no. 6 (June 2015): 354–66, https://doi.org/10.1016/j.tim.2015.03.002; Hilary P. Browne et al., "Transmission of the Gut Microbiota: Spreading of Health," *Nature Reviews Microbiology* 15 (2017): 531–43, https://doi.org/10.1038/nrmicro.2017.50.

161 Jeremy Appleton, "The Gut-Brain Axis: Influence of Microbiota on Mood and Mental Health," *Integrative Medicine* 17, no. 4 (2018): 28–32, https://pubmed.ncbi.nlm.nih.gov/31043907/; John F. Cryan et al., "The Microbiota-Gut-Brain Axis," *Physiological Reviews* 99, no. 4 (2019): 1877–2013, https://doi.org/10.1152/physrev.00018.2018; Magnus Simrén et al., "Intestinal Microbiota in Functional Bowel Disorders: A Rome Foundation Report," *Gut* 62 (2013): 159–76, https://doi.org/10.1136/gutjnl-2012-302167; Alina Janney et al., "Host-Microbiota Maladaptation in Colorectal Cancer," *Nature* 585 (September 2020): 509–17, https://doi.org/10.1038/s41586-020-2729-3.

162 Sauliha R. Alli et al., "The Gut Microbiome in Depression and Potential Benefit of Prebiotics, Probiotics and Synbiotics: A Systematic Review of Clinical Trials and Observational Studies," *International Journal of Molecular Sciences* 23, no. 9 (2022): 4494, https://doi.org/10.3390/ijms23094494.

163 Yu Du et al., "Crosstalk Between the Microbiota-Gut-Brain Axis and Depression," *Heliyon* 6, no. 6 (2020): e04097, https://doi.org/10.1016/j.heliyon.2020.e04097.

164 Rai Khalid Farooq et al., "Role of Inflammatory Cytokines in Depression: Focus on Interleukin-1β," *Biomedical Reports* 6, no. 1 (2017): 15–20, https://doi.org/10.3892/br.2016.807.

165 Cryan et al., "Microbiota-Gut-Brain Axis."

166 Abigail J. Johnson et al., "Daily Sampling Reveals Personalized Diet-Microbiome Associations in Humans," *Cell Host & Microbe* 25, no. 6 (2019): 789–802.e5, https://doi.org/10.1016/j.chom.2019.05.005.

167 Edward C. Deehan and Jens Walter, "The Fiber Gap and the Disappearing Gut Microbiome: Implications for Human Nutrition," *Trends in Endocrinology & Metabolism* 27, no. 5 (2016): 239–42, https://doi.org/10.1016/j.tem.2016.03.001.

168 Hannah C. Wastyk et al., "Gut-Microbiota-Targeted Diets Modulate Human Immune Status," *Cell* 184, no. 16 (2021): 4137–53.e14, https://doi.org/10.1016/j.cell.2021.06.019.

169 Andrew Huberman, "Dr. Sean Mackey: Tools to Reduce and Manage Pain," *Huberman Lab* (podcast audio), January 15, 2024, https://www.hubermanlab.com/episode/dr-sean-mackey-tools-to-reduce-manage-pain.

170 Fereidoon Shahidi and Priyatharini Ambigaipalan, "Omega-3 Polyunsaturated Fatty Acids and Their Health Benefits," *Annual Review of Food Science and Technology* 9 (2018): 345–81, https://doi.org/10.1146/annurev-food-111317-095850.

171 Mauro G. Di Pasquale, "The Essentials of Essential Fatty Acids," *Journal of Dietary Supplements* 6, no. 2 (2009): 143–61, https://doi.org/10.1080/19390210902861841.

172 Ibrahim M. Dighriri et al., "Effects of Omega-3 Polyunsaturated Fatty Acids on Brain Functions: A Systematic Review," *Cureus* 14, no. 10 (2022): e30091, https://doi.org/10.7759/cureus.30091.

173 Yuriko Adkins and Darshan S. Kelley, "Mechanisms Underlying the Cardioprotective Effects of Omega-3 Polyunsaturated Fatty Acids," *Journal of Nutritional Biochemistry* 21, no. 9 (2010): 781–92, https://doi.org/10.1016/j.jnutbio.2009.12.004; Heiner C. Bucher et al., "N-3 Polyunsaturated Fatty

Acids in Coronary Heart Disease: A Meta-Analysis of Randomized Controlled Trials," *American Journal of Medicine* 112, no. 4 (2002): 298–304, https://doi.org/10.1016/s0002-9343(01)01114-7.

[174] Mahin Nomali et al., "Omega-3 Supplementation and Outcomes of Heart Failure: A Systematic Review of Clinical Trials," *Medicine* 103, no. 3 (2024): e36804, https://doi.org/10.1097/MD.0000000000036804.

[175] Yuhua Liao et al., "Efficacy of Omega-3 PUFAs in Depression: A Meta-Analysis," *Translational Psychiatry* 9, no. 1 (2019): 190, https://doi.org/10.1038/s41398-019-0515-5; Erratum, Liao et al., "Efficacy of Omega-3 PUFAs," *Translational Psychiatry* 11, no. 1 (2021): 465, https://doi.org/10.1038/s41398-021-01582-6.

[176] H. O. Bang et al., "Plasma Lipid and Lipoprotein Pattern in Greenlandic West-Coast Eskimos," *Lancet* 297, no. 7710 (1971): 1143–46, https://doi.org/10.1016/S0140-6736(71)91658-8.

[177] Shima Jazayeri et al., "Comparison of Therapeutic Effects of Omega-3 Fatty Acid Eicosapentaenoic Acid and Fluoxetine, Separately and in Combination, in Major Depressive Disorder," *Australian & New Zealand Journal of Psychiatry* 42, no. 3 (2008): 192–98, https://doi.org/10.1080/00048670701827275.

Chapter 5: Protocols for Light

[1] Rana Begum et al., "Near-Infrared Light Increases ATP, Extends Lifespan and Improves Mobility in Aged *Drosophila melanogaster*," *Biology Letters* 11, no. 3 (March 2015): 20150073, https://doi.org/10.1098/rsbl.2015.0073.

[2] Ingrid D. van Iperen et al., "Greenery and Outdoor Facilities to Improve the Wellbeing of Critically Ill Patients, Their Families and Caregivers: Things to Consider," *Intensive Care Medicine* 49, no. 10 (2023): 1229–31, https://doi.org/10.1007/s00134-023-07185-7.

[3] Jesse N. Aronowitz, "The *Other* Radiation Therapy," *International Journal of Radiation Oncology, Biology, Physics* 93, no. 2 (2015): 227–28, https://doi.org/10.1016/j.ijrobp.2015.04.041.

[4] Sherry Ershadi and John S. Barbieri, "At-Home LED Devices for the Treatment of Acne Vulgaris: A Systematic Review and Meta-Analysis," *JAMA Dermatology* 161, no. 5 (2025): 552–55, https://doi.org/10.1001/jamadermatol.2025.0019.

[5] Claudia Dompe et al., "Photobiomodulation—Underlying Mechanism and Clinical Applications," *Journal of Clinical Medicine* 9, no. 6 (2020): 1724, https://doi.org/10.3390/jcm9061724.

[6] Yi-Fan Wang and Yu-Chiao Chen, "Clinical Trial Comparing Three Wavelengths in Photobiomodulation Therapy for Hair Loss," *Photobiomodulation, Photomedicine, and Laser Surgery* 43, no. 7 (2025): 288–93, https://doi.org/10.1089/photob.2025.0020.

[7] Kevin Cheng et al., "Mechanisms and Pathways of Pain Photobiomodulation: A Narrative Review," *Journal of Pain* 22, no. 7 (2021): 763–77, https://doi.org/10.1016/j.jpain.2021.02.005.

[8] Michael B. Powner and Glen Jeffery, "Light Stimulation of Mitochondria Reduces Blood Glucose Levels," *Journal of Biophotonics* 17, no. 5 (2024): e202300521, https://doi.org/10.1002/jbio.202300521.

[9] Harpreet Shinhmar et al., "Weeklong Improved Colour Contrasts Sensitivity After Single 670 nm Exposures Associated with Enhanced Mitochondrial Function," *Scientific Reports* 11, article no. 22872 (2021), https://doi.org/10.1038/s41598-021-02311-1; Cem Küçükerdönmez and Stephanie E. Tedford, "Multiwavelength Photobiomodulation Improves Multiple Aspects of Visual Function in Early-Stage Dry Age-Related Macular Degeneration," *Ophthalmology and Therapy* 14 (June 2025): 1843–53, https://doi.org/10.1007/s40123-025-01183-2.

[10] Venera Berisha-Muharremi et al., "Efficacy of Combined Photobiomodulation Therapy with Supplements Versus Supplements Alone in Restoring Thyroid Gland Homeostasis in Hashimoto Thyroiditis: A Clinical Feasibility Parallel Trial with 6-Months Follow-Up," *Journal of Personalized Medicine* 13, no. 8 (2023): 1274, https://doi.org/10.3390/jpm13081274.

Notes

[11] Elizabeth A. Andraska et al., "Alterations in Visible Light Exposure Modulate Platelet Function and Regulate Thrombus Formation," *Journal of Thrombosis and Haemostasis* 23, no. 1 (2025): 123–38, https://doi.org/10.1016/j.jtha.2024.08.020.

[12] Lee So Maeng et al., "Refined Photobiomodulation Therapy Ameliorates Inflammatory Bowel Disease via Modulation of Immune Pathways and Gut Microbiota," *Journal of Photochemistry and Photobiology B: Biology* 274 (January 2026): 113330, https://doi.org/10.1016/j.jphotobiol.2025.113330.

[13] Osama Fekry Al Balah et al., "Immunomodulatory Effects of Photobiomodulation: A Comprehensive Review," *Lasers in Medical Science* 40, no. 1 (2025): 187, https://doi.org/10.1007/s10103-025-04417-8.

[14] Jun Yang et al., "Chronic Blue Light Leads to Accelerated Aging in *Drosophila* by Impairing Energy Metabolism and Neurotransmitter Levels," *Frontiers in Aging* 3 (August 2022): 983373, https://doi.org/10.3389/fragi.2022.983373; Trevor R. Nash et al., "Daily Blue-Light Exposure Shortens Lifespan and Causes Brain Neurodegeneration in *Drosophila*," *npj Aging and Mechanisms of Disease* 5, article no. 8 (2019), https://doi.org/10.1038/s41514-019-0038-6; Zhaolin Liu et al., "Light-Emitting-Diode-Derived Blue Light Overexposure Accelerates Corneal Endothelial Cell Aging by Inducing Abnormal ROS Accumulation," *Journal of Photochemistry and Photobiology B: Biology* 272 (November 2025): 113252, https://doi.org/10.1016/j.jphotobiol.2025.113252.

[15] Allison M. Kohler et al., "Ultraviolet Fluorescence Discovered in New World Flying Squirrels (*Glaucomys*)," *Journal of Mammalogy* 100, no. 1 (February 2019): 21–30, https://doi.org/10.1093/jmammal/gyy177.

[16] Gerd P. Pfeifer, "Mechanisms of UV-Induced Mutations and Skin Cancer," *Genome Instability & Disease* 1, no. 3 (2020): 99–113, https://doi.org/10.1007/s42764-020-00009-8.

[17] Yu Liu et al., "Vitamin D and Bone Health: From Physiological Function to Disease Association," *Nutrition & Metabolism* 22, article no. 113 (2025), https://doi.org/10.1186/s12986-025-01011-1; Michela Soda et al., "The Impact of Vitamin D on Immune Function and Its Role in Hashimoto's Thyroiditis: A Narrative Review," *Life* 14, no. 6 (2024): 771, https://doi.org/10.3390/life14060771; Ran Zhang and Declan P. Naughton, "Vitamin D in Health and Disease: Current Perspectives," *Nutrition Journal* 9, article no. 65 (2010), https://doi.org/10.1186/1475-2891-9-65.

[18] Chikako Nishigori et al., "Sunlight and Ultraviolet Radiation: Affecting Skin Cancer Incidence in Many Countries," in *World Cancer Report: Cancer Research for Cancer Prevention*, ed. C. P. Wild et al. (International Agency for Research on Cancer, 2020), https://www.ncbi.nlm.nih.gov/books/NBK606489/.

[19] Ethan Waisberg et al., "Near Infrared/Red Light Therapy a Potential Countermeasure for Mitochondrial Dysfunction in Spaceflight Associated Neuro-Ocular Syndrome (SANS)," *Eye* 38 (2024): 2499–501, https://doi.org/10.1038/s41433-024-03091-4; Yiming Shi et al., "Light, Opsins, and Life: Mammalian Photophysiological Functions Beyond Image Perception," *Neuron* 113, no. 19 (October 2025): 3108–28, https://doi.org/10.1016/j.neuron.2025.05.025; Glen Jeffery et al., "Longer Wavelengths in Sunlight Pass Through the Human Body and Have a Systemic Impact Which Improves Vision," *Scientific Reports* 15 (July 2025): 24435, https://doi.org/10.1038/s41598-025-09785-3; Joseph Tafur et al., "Low-Intensity Light Therapy: Exploring the Role of Redox Mechanisms," *Photobiomodulation, Photomedicine, and Laser Surgery* 26, no. 4 (July 2008): 323–28, https://doi.org/10.1089/pho.2007.2184.

[20] Lucas Freitas de Freitas and Michael R. Hamblin, "Proposed Mechanisms of Photobiomodulation or Low-Level Light Therapy," *IEEE Journal of Selected Topics in Quantum Electronics* 22, no. 3 (2016): 7000417, https://doi.org/10.1109/JSTQE.2016.2561201; Shijun Wang et al., "Therapeutic Potential of Nitric Oxide and Its Donors in Hemorrhagic and Ischemic Stroke: A Systematic Review," *Medical Gas Research* 16, no. 3 (September 2026): 241–57, https://doi.org/10.4103/mgr.MEDGASRES-D-25-00161.

[21] Rachel Leproult et al., "Transition from Dim to Bright Light in the Morning Induces an Immediate Elevation of Cortisol Levels," *Journal of Clinical Endocrinology & Metabolism* 86, no. 1 (January 2001): 151–57, https://doi.org/10.1210/jcem.86.1.7102.

[22] Aikaterini Andreadi et al., "Modified Cortisol Circadian Rhythm: The Hidden Toll of Night-Shift Work," *International Journal of Molecular Sciences* 26, no. 5 (2025): 2090, https://doi.org/10.3390/ijms26052090.

[23] Shazia Jehan et al., "Shift Work and Sleep: Medical Implications and Management," *Sleep Medicine and Disorders* 1, no. 2 (2017): 00008, https://pubmed.ncbi.nlm.nih.gov/29517053/; Diane B. Boivin et al., "Disturbance of the Circadian System in Shift Work and Its Health Impact," *Journal of Biological Rhythms* 37, no. 1 (2022): 3–28, https://doi.org/10.1177/07487304211064218.

[24] Emma K. Adam et al., "Diurnal Cortisol Slopes and Mental and Physical Health Outcomes: A Systematic Review and Meta-Analysis," *Psychoneuroendocrinology* 83 (September 2017): 25–41, https://doi.org/10.1016/j.psyneuen.2017.05.018; Lisa R. Starr et al., "Chronic Stress Exposure, Diurnal Cortisol Slope, and Implications for Mood and Fatigue: Moderation by Multilocus HPA-Axis Genetic Variation," *Psychoneuroendocrinology* 100 (February 2019): 156–63, https://doi.org/10.1016/j.psyneuen.2018.10.003.

[25] Emilija Knezevic et al., "The Role of Cortisol in Chronic Stress, Neurodegenerative Diseases, and Psychological Disorders," *Cells* 12, no. 23 (2023): 2726, https://doi.org/10.3390/cells12232726.

[26] L. T. Hoyt et al., "Positive Upshots of Cortisol in Everyday Life," *Emotion* 16, no. 4 (2016): 431–35, https://doi.org/10.1037/emo0000174; Jasleen Kaur et al., "Physiology, Cortisol," StatPearls, last updated December 1, 2025, https://www.ncbi.nlm.nih.gov/books/NBK538239/.

[27] Stafford L. Lightman et al., "Dynamics of ACTH and Cortisol Secretion and Implications for Disease," *Endocrine Reviews* 41, no. 3 (2020): bnaa002, https://doi.org/10.1210/endrev/bnaa002.

[28] Wade S. Warren et al., "The Suprachiasmatic Nucleus Controls the Circadian Rhythm of Heart Rate via the Sympathetic Nervous System," *Physiology & Behavior* 55, no. 6 (June 1994): 1091–99, https://doi.org/10.1016/0031-9384(94)90392-1; Thomas Dickmeis, "Glucocorticoids and the Circadian Clock," *Journal of Endocrinology* 200, no. 1 (2009): 3–22, https://doi.org/10.1677/JOE-08-0415; Atsushi Ishida et al., "Light Activates the Adrenal Gland: Timing of Gene Expression and Glucocorticoid Release," *Cell Metabolism* 2, no. 5 (November 2005): 297–307, https://doi.org/10.1016/j.cmet.2005.09.009; Yvonne M. Ulrich-Lai et al., "Adrenal Splanchnic Innervation Contributes to the Diurnal Rhythm of Plasma Corticosterone in Rats by Modulating Adrenal Sensitivity to ACTH," *American Journal of Physiology—Regulatory, Integrative and Comparative Physiology* 290, no. 4 (April 2006): R1128–35, https://doi.org/10.1152/ajpregu.00042.2003; Ruud M. Buijs et al., "Anatomical and Functional Demonstration of a Multisynaptic Suprachiasmatic Nucleus Adrenal (Cortex) Pathway," *European Journal of Neuroscience* 11 (1999): 1535–44, https://doi.org/10.1046/j.1460-9568.1999.00575.x.

[29] Sadaf Munir et al., "Seasonal Affective Disorder," StatPearls, last updated April 20, 2024, https://www.ncbi.nlm.nih.gov/books/NBK568745/.

[30] Gagan Virk et al., "Short Exposure to Light Treatment Improves Depression Scores in Patients with Seasonal Affective Disorder: A Brief Report," *International Journal on Disability and Human Development* 8, no. 3 (2009): 283–86, https://doi.org/10.1901/jaba.2009.8-283.

[31] Cecilia Rastad et al., "Improvement in Fatigue, Sleepiness, and Health-Related Quality of Life with Bright Light Treatment in Persons with Seasonal Affective Disorder and Subsyndromal SAD," *Depression Research and Treatment* 2011 (June 2011): 543906, https://doi.org/10.1155/2011/543906; Stephen J. Lurie et al., "Seasonal Affective Disorder," *American Family Physician* 74, no. 9 (2006): 1521–24, https://pubmed.ncbi.nlm.nih.gov/17111890/.

[32] Timothy M. Brown et al. "Recommendations for Daytime, Evening, and Nighttime Indoor Light Exposure to Best Support Physiology, Sleep, and Wakefulness in Healthy Adults," *PLOS Biology* 20, no. 3 (2022): e3001571, https://doi.org/10.1371/journal.pbio.3001571.

[33] Palmiero Monteleone et al., "Temporal Relationship Between Melatonin and Cortisol Responses to Nighttime Physical Stress in Humans," *Psychoneuroendocrinology* 17, no. 1 (1992): 81–86, https://doi.org/10.1016/0306-4530(92)90078-l.

[34] Joshua J. Gooley et al., "Exposure to Room Light Before Bedtime Suppresses Melatonin Onset and Shortens Melatonin Duration in Humans," *Journal of Clinical Endocrinology & Metabolism* 96, no. 3 (2011): E463–72, https://doi.org/10.1210/jc.2010-2098.

[35] Marc Hébert et al., "The Effects of Prior Light History on the Suppression of Melatonin by Light in Humans," *Journal of Pineal Research* 3, no. 4 (2002): 198–203, https://doi.org/10.1034/j.1600-079x.2002.01885.x.

[36] Marije te Kulve et al., "Early Evening Light Mitigates Sleep Compromising Physiological and Alerting Responses to Subsequent Late Evening Light," *Scientific Reports* 9, article no. 16064 (2019), https://doi.org/10.1038/s41598-019-52352-w.

[37] Rafael Lazar et al., "Afternoon to Early Evening Bright Light Exposure Reduces Later Melatonin Production in Adolescents," *npj Biological Timing and Sleep* 2, article no. 25 (2025), https://doi.org/10.1038/s44323-025-00040-6.

[38] Tracy A. Bedrosian et al., "Dim Light at Night Provokes Depression-Like Behaviors and Reduces CA1 Dendritic Spine Density in Female Hamsters," *Psychoneuroendocrinology* 36, no. 7 (2011): 1062–69, https://doi.org/10.1016/j.psyneuen.2011.01.004.

[39] Yujiro Yamanaka et al., "Hypothalamic-Pituitary-Adrenal Axis Differentially Responses to Morning and Evening Psychological Stress in Healthy Subjects," *Neuropsychopharmacology Reports* 39, no. 1 (2019): 41–47, https://doi.org/10.1002/npr2.12042.

[40] Subha Nasir-Ahmad et al., "Melanopsin-Expressing Ganglion Cells in Human Retina: Morphology, Distribution, and Synaptic Connections," *Journal of Comparative Neurology* 527, no. 1 (January 2019): 312–27, https://doi.org/10.1002/cne.24176.

[41] Gooley et al., "Exposure to Room Light."

[42] Ana Sanchez-Cano et al., "Comparative Effects of Red and Blue LED Light on Melatonin Levels During Three-Hour Exposure in Healthy Adults," *Life* 15, no. 5 (2025): 715, https://doi.org/10.3390/life15050715; Isabella Robertson-Dixon et al., "The Influence of Light Wavelength on Human HPA Axis Rhythms: A Systematic Review," *Life* 13, no. 10 (2023): 1968, https://doi.org/10.3390/life13101968.

[43] Ari Shechter et al., "Blocking Nocturnal Blue Light for Insomnia: A Randomized Controlled Trial," *Journal of Psychiatric Research* 96 (January 2018): 196–202, https://doi.org/10.1016/j.jpsychires.2017.10.015.

[44] Manuel Spitschan and Nayantara Santhi, "Individual Differences and Diversity in Human Physiological Responses to Light," *eBioMedicine* 75 (January 2022): 103640, https://doi.org/10.1016/j.ebiom.2021.103640.

[45] Ivy C. Mason et al., "Light Exposure During Sleep Impairs Cardiometabolic Function," *Proceedings of the National Academy of Sciences* 119, no. 12 (2022): e2113290119, https://doi.org/10.1073/pnas.2113290119.

[46] Daniel P. Windred et al., "Light Exposure at Night and Cardiovascular Disease Incidence," *JAMA Network Open* 8, no. 10 (2025): e2539031, https://doi.org/10.1001/jamanetworkopen.2025.39031.

[47] Ivy N. Cheung et al., "Morning and Evening Blue-Enriched Light Exposure Alters Metabolic Function in Normal Weight Adults," *PLOS One* 11, no. 5 (2016): e0155601, https://doi.org/10.1371/journal.pone.0155601; Yong-Moon Mark Park et al., "Association of Exposure to Artificial Light at Night While Sleeping with Risk of Obesity in Women," *JAMA Internal Medicine* 179, no. 8 (2019): 1061–71, https://doi.org/10.1001/jamainternmed.2019.0571.

[48] Altug Didikoglu et al., "Relationships Between Light Exposure and Aspects of Cognitive Function in Everyday Life," *Communications Psychology* 4, article no. 5 (2026), https://doi.org/10.1038/s44271-025-00373-9.

[49] Angus C. Burns et al., "Day and Night Light Exposure Are Associated with Psychiatric Disorders: An Objective Light Study in over 85,000 People," *Nature Mental Health* 1 (2023): 853–62, https://doi.org/10.1038/s44220-023-00135-8.

[50] Shi et al., "Light, Opsins, and Life."

[51] Sarah Cameron et al., "The Disappointment Centre of the Brain Gets Exciting: A Systematic Review of Habenula Dysfunction in Depression," *Translational Psychiatry* 14, no. 1 (December 2024), https://doi.org/10.1038/s41398-024-03199-x; Diego Carlos Fernandez et al., "Light Affects Mood and Learning Through Distinct Retina-Brain Pathways," *Cell* 175, no. 1 (September 2018): 71–84.e18, https://doi.org/10.1016/j.cell.2018.08.004.

[52] Daniel P. Windred et al., "Brighter Nights and Darker Days Predict Higher Mortality Risk: A Prospective Analysis of Personal Light Exposure in over 88,000 Individuals," *Proceedings of the National Academy of Sciences* 121, no. 43 (2024): e2405924121, https://doi.org/10.1073/pnas.2405924121.

[53] Max Bell et al., "Individual and Neighborhood Risk Factors of Hospital Admission and Death During the COVID-19 Pandemic: A Population-Based Cohort Study," *BMC Medicine* 21, article no. 1 (2023), https://doi.org/10.1186/s12916-022-02715-4; Shengzhi Sun et al., "Outdoor Light at Night and Risk of Coronary Heart Disease Among Older Adults: A Prospective Cohort Study," *European Heart Journal* 42, no. 8 (2021): 822–30, https://doi.org/10.1093/eurheartj/ehaa846; P. G. Lindqvist et al., "Avoidance of Sun Exposure Is a Risk Factor for All-Cause Mortality: Results from the Melanoma in Southern Sweden Cohort," *Journal of Internal Medicine* 276, no. 1 (2014): 77–86, https://doi.org/10.1111/joim.12251.

[54] Burns et al., "Day and Night Light Exposure."

[55] David G. Hoel and Allen Miller, "Are Vitamin D Supplements an Adequate Substitute for Sun Exposure?," *Medical Research Archives* 11, no. 3 (2023), https://doi.org/10.18103/mra.v11i3.3635; Roger Bouillon et al., "The Health Effects of Vitamin D Supplementation: Evidence from Human Studies," *Nature Reviews Endocrinology* 18, no. 2 (November 2021): 96–110, https://doi.org/10.1038/s41574-021-00593-z; Michael F. Holick, "Health Benefits of Vitamin D and Sunlight: A D-bate," *Nature Reviews Endocrinology* 7 (January 2011): 73–75, https://doi.org/10.1038/nrendo.2010.234.

[56] Roma Parikh et al., "Skin Exposure to UVB Light Induces a Skin-Brain-Gonad Axis and Sexual Behavior," *Cell Reports* 36, no. 8 (2021): 109579, https://doi.org/10.1016/j.celrep.2021.109579.

[57] Cezary Skobowiat et al., "Skin Exposure to Ultraviolet B Rapidly Activates Systemic Neuroendocrine and Immunosuppressive Responses," *Photochemistry and Photobiology* 93, no. 4 (2017): 1008–15, https://doi.org/10.1111/php.12642.

[58] Catherine J. Dunlavey, "Introduction to the Hypothalamic-Pituitary-Adrenal Axis: Healthy and Dysregulated Stress Responses, Developmental Stress and Neurodegeneration," *Journal of Undergraduate Neuroscience Education* 16, no. 2 (2018): R59–60, https://pubmed.ncbi.nlm.nih.gov/30057514/; Frauke Nees et al., "Hypothalamic-Pituitary-Adrenal Axis Feedback Sensitivity in Different States of Back Pain," *Psychoneuroendocrinology* 101 (March 2019): 60–66, https://doi.org/10.1016/j.psyneuen.2018.10.026.

[59] Tobias Backström and Svante Winberg, "Central Corticotropin Releasing Factor and Social Stress," *Frontiers in Neuroscience* 7 (July 2013): 117, https://doi.org/10.3389/fnins.2013.00117.

[60] Adam S. Sprouse-Blum et al., "Understanding Endorphins and Their Importance in Pain Management," *Hawaii Medical Journal* 69, no. 3 (2010): 70–71, https://pubmed.ncbi.nlm.nih.gov/20397507/.

[61] Lindqvist et al., "Avoidance of Sun Exposure."

[62] Ling Yang et al., "Ultraviolet Exposure and Mortality Among Women in Sweden," *Cancer Epidemiology, Biomarkers & Prevention* 20, no. 4 (2011): 683–90, https://doi.org/10.1158/1055-9965.EPI-10-0982; Erratum, Yang et al., "Ultraviolet Exposure," *Cancer Epidemiology, Biomarkers & Prevention* 20, no. 6 (2011): 1259.

[63] Lynne Peeples, "The Surprising Science Behind Red-Light Therapy—and How It Really Works," *Nature* 651, no. 8107 (March 2026): 871–74, https://doi.org/10.1038/d41586-026-00878-1.

64 Nancy B. Lipko, "Photobiomodulation: Evolution and Adaptation," *Photobiomodulation: Evolution and Adaptation* 40, no. 4 (2022): 213–33, https://doi.org/10.1089/photob.2021.0145; Powner and Jeffery, "Light Stimulation of Mitochondria."

65 Waisberg et al., "Near Infrared/Red Light Therapy."

66 Edio Maldonado et al., "Aging Hallmarks and the Role of Oxidative Stress," *Antioxidants* 12, no. 3 (2023): 651, https://doi.org/10.3390/antiox12030651.

67 Jeffery et al., "Longer Wavelengths in Sunlight."

68 Rodrigo Noseda et al., "Migraine Photophobia Originating in Cone-Driven Retinal Pathways," *Brain* 139, no. 7 (2016): 1971–86, https://doi.org/10.1093/brain/aww119; Sabrina Rohringer et al., "The Impact of Wavelengths of LED Light-Therapy on Endothelial Cells," *Scientific Reports* 7, no. 1 (2017): 10700, https://doi.org/10.1038/s41598-017-11061-y; Laurent F. Martin et al., "Green Light Exposure Elicits Anti-Inflammation, Endogenous Opioid Release and Dampens Synaptic Potentiation to Relieve Post-Surgical Pain," *Journal of Pain* 24, no. 3 (2023): 509–29, https://doi.org/10.1016/j.jpain.2022.10.011.

69 Eva Chamorro et al., "Effects of Light-Emitting Diode Radiations on Human Retinal Pigment Epithelial Cells In Vitro," *Photochemistry and Photobiology* 89, no. 2 (October 2012): 468–73, https://doi.org/10.1111/j.1751-1097.2012.01237.x; Edward M. Barrett and Glen Jeffery, "LED Lighting (350–650nm) Undermines Human Visual Performance Unless Supplemented by Wider Spectra (400–1500nm+) like Daylight," *Scientific Reports* 16, no. 3061 (January 2026), https://doi.org/10.1038/s41598-026-35389-6; Bernard F. Godley et al., "Blue Light Induces Mitochondrial DNA Damage and Free Radical Production in Epithelial Cells," *Journal of Biological Chemistry* 280, no. 22 (June 2005): 21061–66, https://doi.org/10.1074/jbc.M502194200.

70 Tatsiana Mironava et al., "The Effects of UV Emission from Compact Fluorescent Light Exposure on Human Dermal Fibroblasts and Keratinocytes In Vitro," *Photochemistry and Photobiology* 88, no. 6 (July 20, 2012): 1497–1506, https://doi.org/10.1111/j.1751-1097.2012.01192.x; T. A. Kalajian et al., "Ultraviolet B Light Emitting Diodes (LEDs) Are More Efficient and Effective in Producing Vitamin D_3 in Human Skin Compared to Natural Sunlight," *Scientific Reports* 7, no. 1 (September 2017), https://doi.org/10.1038/s41598-017-11362-2.

71 Jeffrey M. Walch et al., "The Effect of Sunlight on Postoperative Analgesic Medication Use: A Prospective Study of Patients Undergoing Spinal Surgery," *Psychosomatic Medicine* 67, no. 1 (2005): 156–63, https://doi.org/10.1097/01.psy.0000149258.42508.70.

72 Helen J. Burgess et al., "Morning Versus Evening Bright Light Treatment at Home to Improve Function and Pain Sensitivity for Women with Fibromyalgia: A Pilot Study," *Pain Medicine* 18, no. 1 (2017): 116–23, https://doi.org/10.1093/pm/pnw160.

73 John W. Burns et al., "Morning Bright Light Treatment for Chronic Low Back Pain: Potential Impact on the Volatility of Pain, Mood, Function, and Sleep," *Pain Medicine* 21, no. 6 (2020): 1153–61, https://doi.org/10.1093/pm/pnz235.

74 Zhengfang Hu et al., "A Visual Circuit Related to the Periaqueductal Gray Area for the Antinociceptive Effects of Bright Light Treatment," *Neuron* 110, no. 10 (2022): 1712–27.e7, https://doi.org/10.1016/j.neuron.2022.02.009.

75 G. Vandewalle et al., "Spectral Quality of Light Modulates Emotional Brain Responses in Humans," *Proceedings of the National Academy of Sciences* 107, no. 45 (2010): 19549–54, https://doi.org/10.1073/pnas.1010180107.

76 Ci-Wen Luo et al., "Association Between Ultraviolet B Exposure Levels and Depression in Taiwanese Adults: A Nested Case-Control Study," *International Journal of Environmental Research and Public Health* 19, no. 11 (2022): 6846, https://doi.org/10.3390/ijerph19116846.

77 Bistra I. Veleva et al., "Effect of Ultraviolet Light on Mood, Depressive Disorders and Well-Being," *Photodermatology, Photoimmunology & Photomedicine* 34, no. 5 (2018): 288–97, https://doi.org/10.1111/phpp.12396.

[78] Ershadi and Barbieri, "At-Home LED Devices for the Treatment of Acne Vulgaris: A Systematic Review and Meta-Analysis"; Le Thi Nhu Ngoc et al., "Utilization of Light-Emitting Diodes for Skin Therapy: Systematic Review and Meta-Analysis," *Photodermatology, Photoimmunology & Photomedicine* 39, no. 4 (2023): 303–17, https://doi.org/10.1111/phpp.12841; Jing Zhang et al., "Efficacy and Safety of Red and Infrared Light in the Adjunctive Treatment on Diabetic Foot Ulcers: A Systematic Review and Meta-Analysis," *Complementary Therapies in Clinical Practice* 57, article no. 101906 (November 2024), https://doi.org/10.1016/j.ctcp.2024.101906.

[79] S. V. K. R. Rajeswari et al., "Development of a Near Infrared Region Based Non-Invasive Therapy Device for Diabetic Peripheral Neuropathy," *Scientific Reports* 14, article no. 27993 (2024), https://doi.org/10.1038/s41598-024-78144-5; Ming Li et al., "A Wearable and Stretchable Dual-Wavelength LED Device for Home Care of Chronic Infected Wounds," *Nature Communications* 15, no. 1 (2024): 9380, https://doi.org/10.1038/s41467-024-53579-6.

[80] Hoon Chung et al., "The Nuts and Bolts of Low-Level Laser (Light) Therapy," *Annals of Biomedical Engineering* 40, no. 2 (November 2011): 516–33, https://doi.org/10.1007/s10439-011-0454-7; Evan Austin et al., "Visible Light. Part I: Properties and Cutaneous Effects of Visible Light," *Journal of the American Academy of Dermatology* 84, no. 5 (May 2021): 1219–31, https://doi.org/10.1016/j.jaad.2021.02.048.

[81] Jeffery et al., "Longer Wavelengths in Sunlight."

[82] David M. Harris, "Editorial Comment Biomolecular Mechanisms of Laser Biostimulation," *Journal of Clinical Laser Medicine & Surgery* 9, no. 4 (1991): 277–80, https://doi.org/10.1089/clm.1991.9.277.

[83] Michael B. Powner and Glen Jeffery, "Systemic Glucose Levels Are Modulated by Specific Wavelengths in the Solar Light Spectrum That Shift Mitochondrial Metabolism," *PLOS One* 17, no. 11 (November 2022): e0276937, https://doi.org/10.1371/journal.pone.0276937.

[84] Russel J. Reiter et al., "Melatonin: A Mitochondrial Resident with a Diverse Skill Set," *Life Sciences* 301, article no. 120612 (July 15, 2022), https://doi.org/10.1016/j.lfs.2022.120612.

[85] Jesus A. Simon et al., "Beyond Sleeping Disorders, the Role of Melatonin in Skin Diseases and Emerging Applications in Dermatology and Topical Therapy," *Gels* 11, no. 11 (2025): 860, https://doi.org/10.3390/gels11110860.

[86] Graeme Ewan Glass, "Photobiomodulation: The Clinical Applications of Low-Level Light Therapy," *Aesthetic Surgery Journal* 41, no. 6 (2021): 723–38, https://doi.org/10.1093/asj/sjab025; Erratum, Glass, "Photobiomodulation," *Aesthetic Surgery Journal* 42, no. 5 (2022): 566, https://doi.org/10.1093/asj/sjab396.

[87] Robert A. Weiss et al., "A Novel Non-Thermal Non-Ablative Full Panel LED Photomodulation Device for Reversal of Photoaging: Digital Microscopic and Clinical Results in Various Skin Types," *Journal of Drugs in Dermatology* 3, no. 6 (2004): 605–10, https://pubmed.ncbi.nlm.nih.gov/15624743/; B. A. Russell et al., "A Study to Determine the Efficacy of Combination LED Light Therapy (633 nm and 830 nm) in Facial Skin Rejuvenation," *Journal of Cosmetic and Laser Therapy* 7, no. 3–4 (2005): 196–200, https://doi.org/10.1080/14764170500370059.

[88] Robert A. Weiss et al., "Clinical Trial of a Novel Non-Thermal LED Array for Reversal of Photoaging: Clinical, Histologic, and Surface Profilometric Results," *Lasers in Surgery and Medicine* 36, no. 2 (February 2005): 85–91, https://doi.org/10.1002/lsm.20107.

[89] B. A. Russell et al., "A Study to Determine the Efficacy of Combination LED Light Therapy (633 nm and 830 nm) in Facial Skin Rejuvenation," *Journal of Cosmetic and Laser Therapy* 7, no. 3–4 (2005): 196–200, https://doi.org/10.1080/14764170500370059.

[90] David J. Goldberg and Bruce A. Russell, "Combination Blue (415 nm) and Red (633 nm) LED Phototherapy in the Treatment of Mild to Severe Acne Vulgaris," *Journal of Cosmetic and Laser Therapy* 8, no. 2 (2006): 71–75, https://doi.org/10.1080/14764170600735912.

[91] P. Papageorgiou et al., "Phototherapy with Blue (415 nm) and Red (660 nm) Light in the Treatment of Acne Vulgaris," *British Journal of Dermatology* 142, no. 5 (2000): 973–78, https://doi.org/10.1046/j.1365-2133.2000.03481.x.

[92] Powner and Jeffery, "Light Stimulation of Mitochondria."

[93] Shaopeng Yang et al., "Photoreceptor Metabolic Window Unveils Eye–Body Interactions," *Nature Communications* 16, article no. 697 (2025), https://doi.org/10.1038/s41467-024-55035-x.

[94] John M. Ball et al., "Mitochondria in Cone Photoreceptors Act as Microlenses to Enhance Photon Delivery and Confer Directional Sensitivity to Light," *Science Advances* 8, no. 9 (2022): eabn2070, https://doi.org/10.1126/sciadv.abn2070; M. Wong-Riley, "Energy Metabolism of the Visual System," *Eye and Brain* 2 (July 2010): 99–116, https://doi.org/10.2147/EB.S9078.

[95] Christin Henein and David H. W. Steel, "Photobiomodulation for Non-Exudative Age-Related Macular Degeneration," *Cochrane Database of Systematic Reviews* 2018, no. 5 (2018): CD013029, https://doi.org/10.1002/14651858.CD013029.

[96] Harpreet Shinhmar et al., "Optically Improved Mitochondrial Function Redeems Aged Human Visual Decline," *Journals of Gerontology: Series A* 75, no. 9 (2020): e49–52, https://doi.org/10.1093/gerona/glaa155.

[97] Harpreet Shinhmar et al., "Weeklong Improved Colour Contrasts Sensitivity After Single 670 nm Exposures Associated with Enhanced Mitochondrial Function," *Scientific Reports 11* (November 2021): 22872, https://doi.org/10.1038/s41598-021-02311-1.

[98] Ahmed Abdelsalam et al., "Drusen in Age-Related Macular Degeneration: Pathogenesis, Natural Course, and Laser Photocoagulation-Induced Regression," *Survey of Ophthalmology* 44, no. 1 (1999): 1–29, https://doi.org/10.1016/s0039-6257(99)00072-7.

[99] Patricia T. Harvey, "Common Eye Diseases of Elderly People: Identifying and Treating Causes of Vision Loss," *Gerontology* 49, no. 1 (2003): 1–11, https://doi.org/10.1159/000066507.

[100] Glynis Ablon, "Phototherapy with Light Emitting Diodes: Treating a Broad Range of Medical and Aesthetic Conditions in Dermatology," *Journal of Clinical and Aesthetic Dermatology* 11, no. 2 (2018): 21–27, https://pubmed.ncbi.nlm.nih.gov/29552272/.

[101] Jessica K. Atencio et al., "Comparison of Thermoregulatory, Cardiovascular, and Immune Responses to Different Passive Heat Therapy Modalities," *American Journal of Physiology-Regulatory, Integrative and Comparative Physiology* 329, no. 1 (2025): R20–35, https://journals.physiology.org/doi/abs/10.1152/ajpregu.00012.2025.

Chapter 6: Protocols for Focus, Motivation, and Learning

[1] Geraldine Gvozdanovic et al., "Experimental Trauma Rapidly Modifies Functional Connectivity," *Brain Imaging and Behavior* 15 (2021): 2017–30, https://doi.org/10.1007/s11682-020-00396-2; Xin Wang et al., "Preliminary Study of Acute Changes in Emotion Processing in Trauma Survivors with PTSD Symptoms," *PLOS One* 11, no. 7 (2016): e0159065, https://doi.org/10.1371/journal.pone.0159065.

[2] Felicia A. Hardi et al., "Trauma-Predictive Brain Network Connectivity Adaptively Responds to Mild Acute Stress," *Proceedings of the National Academy of Sciences* 122, no. 31 (2025): e2505965122, https://doi.org/10.1073/pnas.2505965122; Dongju Seo et al., "Limbic Response to Stress Linking Life Trauma and Hypothalamus-Pituitary-Adrenal Axis Function," *Psychoneuroendocrinology* 99 (January 2019): 38–46, https://doi.org/10.1016/j.psyneuen.2018.08.023.

[3] Mark A. Lumley et al., "Trauma Matters: Psychological Interventions for Comorbid Psychosocial Trauma and Chronic Pain," *Pain* 163, no. 4 (2022): 599–603, https://doi.org/10.1097/j.pain.0000000000002425.

[4] Neslihan Cansel et al., "The Role of Childhood Trauma in Patients with Chronic Urticaria," *Northern Clinics of Istanbul* 10, no. 1 (2023): 79–86, https://doi.org/10.14744/nci.2021.10170.

[5] Shanlin Ke et al., "The Emerging Role of the Gut Microbiome in Posttraumatic Stress Disorder," *Brain, Behavior, and Immunity* 114 (November 2023): 360–70, https://doi.org/10.1016/j.bbi.2023.09.005.

[6] Brianna Chu et al., "Physiology, Stress Reaction," StatPearls, last updated May 7, 2024, https://www.ncbi.nlm.nih.gov/books/NBK541120/.

[7] Amy F. T. Arnsten, "Stress Signalling Pathways That Impair Prefrontal Cortex Structure and Function," *Nature Reviews Neuroscience* 10, no. 6 (2009): 410–22, https://doi.org/10.1038/nrn2648.

[8] Michael C. Avery and Jeffrey L. Krichmar, "Neuromodulatory Systems and Their Interactions: A Review of Models, Theories, and Experiments," *Frontiers in Neural Circuits* 11 (December 21, 2017): 108, https://doi.org/10.3389/fncir.2017.00108.

[9] Adrian J. Duszkiewicz et al., "Novelty and Dopaminergic Modulation of Memory Persistence: A Tale of Two Systems," *Trends in Neurosciences* 42, no. 2 (2019): 102–14, https://doi.org/10.1016/j.tins.2018.10.002.

[10] Vinay Parikh and Debra A. Bangasser, "Cholinergic Signaling Dynamics and Cognitive Control of Attention," in *Behavioral Pharmacology of the Cholinergic System*, ed. M. Shoaib and T. Wallace (Springer Nature Switzerland, 2020), 71–87, https://doi.org/10.1007/7854_2020_133.

[11] Liqun Luo, *Principles of Neurobiology* (CRC Press, 2020).

[12] Matt Puderbaugh and Prabhu D. Emmady, "Neuroplasticity," StatPearls, last updated May 1, 2023, https://www.ncbi.nlm.nih.gov/books/NBK557811/.

[13] Joshua P. Rising et al., "United States Trends in Non-Prescribed Use of Adderall and Ritalin: Population Assessment of Tobacco and Health (PATH) Study Estimates from 2013 to 2022," *Addiction* 120, no. 11 (2025): 2348–54, https://doi.org/10.1111/add.70123; Justine W. Welsh et al., "Substance Use Among College Students," *Focus* 17, no. 2 (2019): 117–27, https://doi.org/10.1176/appi.focus.20180037; Christian J. Teter et al., "Nonmedical Use of Prescription Stimulants Among US High School Students to Help Study: Results from a National Survey," *Journal of Pharmacy Practice* 33, no. 1 (2020): 38–47, https://doi.org/10.1177/0897190018783887.

[14] Diane C. Mitchell et al., "An Update on Beverage Consumption Patterns and Caffeine Intakes in a Representative Sample of the US Population," *Food and Chemical Toxicology* 196 (February 2025): 115237, https://doi.org/10.1016/j.fct.2025.115237.

[15] Mohamad Awada et al., "Cognitive Performance, Creativity and Stress Levels of Neurotypical Young Adults Under Different White Noise Levels," *Scientific Reports* 12, article no. 14566 (2022), https://doi.org/10.1038/s41598-022-18862-w; Anthony J. Angwin et al., "White Noise Enhances New-Word Learning in Healthy Adults," *Scientific Reports* 7, article no. 13045 (2017), https://doi.org/10.1038/s41598-017-13383-3; Elza Othman et al., "Low Intensity White Noise Improves Performance in Auditory Working Memory Task: An fMRI Study," *Heliyon* 5, no. 9 (2019): e02444, https://doi.org/10.1016/j.heliyon.2019.e02444.

[16] Liqun Luo, *Principles of Neurobiology* (CRC Press, 2020); Patrícia Marzola et al., "Exploring the Role of Neuroplasticity in Development, Aging, and Neurodegeneration," Brain Sciences 13, no. 12 (2023), https://doi.org/10.3390/brainsci13121610; Alvaro Pascual-Leone et al., "The Plastic Human Brain Cortex," Annual Review of Neuroscience 28 (July 2005): 377–401, https://doi.org/10.1146/annurev.neuro.27.070203.144216; Pasko Rakic, "Limits of Neurogenesis in Primates," *Science* 227, no. 4690 (1985): 1054–56, https://doi.org/10.1126/science.3975601; Beatrix P. Rubin, "Changing Brains: The Emergence of the Field of Adult Neurogenesis," *BioSocieties* 4 (December 2009): 407–24, https://doi.org/10.1017/S1745855209990330; Michael M. Merzenich et al., "Brain Plasticity-Based Therapeutics," *Frontiers in Human Neuroscience* 8 (2014): 385, https://doi.org/10.3389/fnhum.2014.00385.

[17] Marzola et al., "Exploring the Role of Neuroplasticity"; Merzenich et al., "Brain Plasticity-Based Therapeutics."

[18] Chiara La Rosa et al., "Brain Structural Plasticity: From Adult Neurogenesis to Immature Neurons," *Frontiers in Neuroscience* 14 (2020): 75, https://doi.org/10.3389/fnins.2020.00075.

[19] Jeanette Skowronek et al., "The Mere Presence of a Smartphone Reduces Basal Attentional Performance," *Scientific Reports* 13, article no. 9363 (2023), https://doi.org/10.1038/s41598-023-36256-4.

[20] Adrian M. Haith and John W. Krakauer, "The Multiple Effects of Practice: Skill, Habit and Reduced Cognitive Load," *Current Opinion in Behavioral Sciences* 20 (April 2018): 196–201, https://doi.org/10.1016/j.cobeha.2018.01.015.

[21] Dinara Talypova et al., "Are Six Minutes of Focus Enough? An Exploratory Study of Multitasking Patterns in Workplace Environments," *Proceedings of the 4th Annual Symposium on Human-Computer Interaction for Work, CHIWORK 2025*, Amsterdam, Netherlands, June 23–25, 2025.

[22] David Adam, "Are Attention Spans Really Shrinking? What the Science Says," *Nature* 653 (2026): 20–22, https://doi.org/10.1038/d41586-026-01407-w.

[23] Hugo Gernsback, "The Isolator," *Science and Invention* 13, no. 3 (July 1925).

[24] Helmfon, Hochu-rayu, n.d., https://hochurayu.com/product_design/helmfon/.

[25] Zofia Kobylińska et al., "Coffee as a Source of Antioxidants and an Elixir of Youth," *Antioxidants* 14, no. 3 (2025): 285, https://doi.org/10.3390/antiox14030285; "China-England Tea Trade," EBSCO, 2022, https://www.ebsco.com/research-starters/history/china-england-tea-trade.

[26] Gabriela F. Gil et al., "Health Effects Associated with Chewing Tobacco: A Burden of Proof Study," *Nature Communications* 15, no. 1 (February 2024): 1082, https://doi.org/10.1038/s41467-024-45074-9; Alpana K. Gupta et al., "Oral Cancer Risk Assessment for Different Types of Smokeless Tobacco Products Sold Worldwide: A Review of Reviews and Meta-Analyses," *Cancer Prevention Research* 15, no. 11 (September 2022): 733–46, https://doi.org/10.1158/1940-6207.capr-21-0567.

[27] S. M. Berman et al., "Potential Adverse Effects of Amphetamine Treatment on Brain and Behavior: A Review," *Molecular Psychiatry* 14, no. 2 (2009): 123–42, https://doi.org/10.1038/mp.2008.90; Erratum, Berman et al., "Potential Adverse Effects of Amphetamine Treatment," *Molecular Psychiatry* 15, no. 11 (2010): 1121, https://doi.org/10.1038/mp.2010.39.

[28] David J. Heal et al., "Amphetamine, Past and Present—a Pharmacological and Clinical Perspective," *Journal of Psychopharmacology* 27, no. 6 (2013): 479–96, https://doi.org/10.1177/0269881113482532.

[29] Madeleine P. Strohl, "Bradley's Benzedrine Studies on Children with Behavioral Disorders," *Yale Journal of Biology and Medicine* 84, no. 1 (2011): 27–33, https://pubmed.ncbi.nlm.nih.gov/21451781/; Stanley C. Harris et al., "The Mechanism of Amphetamine-Induced Loss of Weight: A Consideration of the Theory of Hunger and Appetite," *JAMA* 134, no. 17 (1947): 1468–75, https://doi.org/10.1001/jama.1947.02880340022005.

[30] Nicolas Rasmussen, "America's First Amphetamine Epidemic 1929–1971: A Quantitative and Qualitative Retrospective with Implications for the Present," *American Journal of Public Health* 98, no. 6 (2008): 974–85, https://doi.org/10.2105/AJPH.2007.110593.

[31] Rasmussen, "America's First Amphetamine Epidemic 1929–1971."

[32] Florence T. Bourgeois et al., "Premarket Safety and Efficacy Studies for ADHD Medications in Children," *PLOS One* 9, no. 7 (2014): e102249, https://doi.org/10.1371/journal.pone.0102249.

[33] Amber N. Edinoff et al., "Prescription Stimulants in College and Medical Students: A Narrative Review of Misuse, Cognitive Impact, and Adverse Effects," *Psychiatry International* 3, no. 3 (July 2022): 221–35, https://doi.org/10.3390/psychiatryint3030018.

[34] Larry Cahill and James L. McGaugh, "Mechanisms of Emotional Arousal and Lasting Declarative Memory," *Trends in Neurosciences* 21, no. 7 (1998): 294–99, https://doi.org/10.1016/s0166-2236(97)01214-9.

[35] Sereena Pigeon et al., "Impairing Memory Reconsolidation with Propranolol in Healthy and Clinical Samples: A Meta-Analysis," *Journal of Psychiatry and Neuroscience* 47, no. 2 (2022): E109–22, https://doi.org/10.1503/jpn.210057.

[36] Keith Tully and Vadim Y. Bolshakov, "Emotional Enhancement of Memory: How Norepinephrine Enables Synaptic Plasticity," *Molecular Brain* 3, article no. 15 (2010), https://doi.org/10.1186/1756-6606-3-15; Larry Cahill et al., "Enhanced Human Memory Consolidation with Post-Learning Stress: Interaction with the Degree of Arousal at Encoding," *Learning & Memory* 10, no. 4 (2003): 270–74, https://doi.org/10.1101/lm.62403.

[37] Tom Smeets et al., "True or False? Memory Is Differentially Affected by Stress-Induced Cortisol Elevations and Sympathetic Activity at Consolidation and Retrieval," *Psychoneuroendocrinology* 33, no. 10 (2008): 1378–86, https://doi.org/10.1016/j.psyneuen.2008.07.009.

[38] "Classics in the History of Psychology," Christopher D. Green, York University, n.d., https://psychclassics.yorku.ca/Yerkes/Law/; Lola Beerendonk et al., "A Disinhibitory Circuit Mechanism Explains a General Principle of Peak Performance During Mid-Level Arousal," *Proceedings of the National Academy of Sciences* 121, no. 5 (2024): e2312898121, https://doi.org/10.1073/pnas.2312898121.

[39] Jeanne Nakamura and Mihaly Csikszentmihalyi, "The Concept of Flow," in *Handbook of Positive Psychology*, ed. C. R. Snyder and Shane J. Lopez (Oxford University Press, 2002), 89–105.

[40] Mihaly Csikszentmihalyi, *Flow: The Psychology of Optimal Experience* (Harper & Row, 1990); Roberta Antonini Philippe et al., "Achieving Flow: An Exploratory Investigation of Elite College Athletes and Musicians," *Frontiers in Psychology* 13 (March 29, 2022): 831508, https://doi.org/10.3389/fpsyg.2022.831508.

[41] Twyla Tharp, *The Creative Habit: Learn It and Use It for Life* (Simon & Schuster, 2006).

[42] Dean V. Buonomano and Michael M. Merzenich, "Cortical Plasticity: From Synapses to Maps," *Annual Review of Neuroscience* 21 (1998): 149–86, https://doi.org/10.1146/annurev.neuro.21.1.149.

[43] G. H. Recanzone et al., "Topographic Reorganization of the Hand Representation in Cortical Area 3b of Owl Monkeys Trained in a Frequency-Discrimination Task," *Journal of Neurophysiology* 67, no. 5 (1992): 1031–56, https://doi.org/10.1152/jn.1992.67.5.1031; G. H. Rencanzone et al., "Plasticity in the Frequency Representation of Primary Auditory Cortex Following Discrimination Training in Adult Owl Monkeys," *Journal of Neuroscience* 13, no. 1 (1993): 87–103, https://doi.org/10.1523/JNEUROSCI.13-01-00087.1993; Nancy N. Byl et al., "A Primate Genesis Model of Focal Dystonia and Repetitive Strain Injury: I. Learning-Induced Dedifferentiation of the Representation of the Hand in the Primary Somatosensory Cortex in Adult Monkeys," *Neurology* 47, no. 2 (1996): 508–20, https://doi.org/10.1212/wnl.47.2.508.

[44] Eleanor A. Maguire et al., "London Taxi Drivers and Bus Drivers: A Structural MRI and Neuropsychological Analysis," *Hippocampus* 16, no. 12 (2006): 1091–1101, https://doi.org/10.1002/hipo.20233; Alvaro Pascual-Leone and Fernando Torres, "Plasticity of the Sensorimotor Cortex Representation of the Reading Finger in Braille Readers," *Brain* 116, no. 1 (February 1993): 39–52, https://doi.org/10.1093/brain/116.1.39; Thomas Elbert et al., "Increased Cortical Representation of the Fingers of the Left Hand in String Players," *Science* 270, no. 5234 (October 1995): 305–07, https://doi.org/10.1126/science.270.5234.305; Friederike Spengler et al., "Learning Transfer and Neuronal Plasticity in Humans Trained in Tactile Discrimination," *Neuroscience Letters* 232, no. 3 (September 1997): 151–54, https://doi.org/10.1016/S0304-3940(97)00602-2; A. Karni and D. Sagi, "Where Practice Makes Perfect in Texture Discrimination: Evidence for Primary Visual Cortex Plasticity," *Proceedings of the National Academy of Sciences* 88, no. 11 (June 1991): 4966–70, https://doi.org/10.1073/pnas.88.11.496; Pascual-Leone et al., "The Plastic Human Brain Cortex."

[45] M. Lotze et al., "The Musician's Brain: Functional Imaging of Amateurs and Professionals During Performance and Imagery," *NeuroImage* 20, no. 3 (2003): 1817–29, https://doi.org/10.1016/j.neuroimage.2003.07.018.

[46] Bogdan Draganski et al., "Changes in Grey Matter Induced by Training," *Nature* 427 (2004): 311–12, https://doi.org/10.1038/427311a.

[47] Robert J. Zatorre et al., "Plasticity in Gray and White: Neuroimaging Changes in Brain Structure During Learning," *Nature Neuroscience* 15, no. 4 (March 2012): 528–36, https://doi.org/10.1038/nn.3045; Eran Dayan and Leonardo G. Cohen, "Neuroplasticity Subserving Motor Skill Learning," *Neuron* 72, no. 3 (November 2011): 443–54, https://doi.org/10.1016/j.neuron.2011.10.008; Yongmin Chang, "Reorganization and Plastic Changes of the Human Brain Associated with Skill Learning and Expertise," *Frontiers in Human Neuroscience* 8 (2014), https://doi.org/10.3389/fnhum.2014.00035.

[48] M. Ahissar and S. Hochstein, "Attentional Control of Early Perceptual Learning," *Proceedings of the National Academy of Sciences* 90, no. 12 (1993): 5718–22, https://doi.org/10.1073/pnas.90.12.5718.

[49] Carla J. Shatz, "The Developing Brain," *Scientific American*, September 1, 1992, https://www.scientificamerican.com/article/the-developing-brain/.

[50] Shatz, "Developing Brain."

[51] Stephen P. J. Goodman et al., "The Effect of Active Hypohydration on Cognitive Function: A Systematic Review and Meta-Analysis," *Physiology & Behavior* 204 (May 15, 2019): 297–308, https://doi.org/10.1016/j.physbeh.2019.03.008.

[52] Roy F. Baumeister et al., "Self-Control and Limited Willpower: Current Status of Ego Depletion Theory and Research," *Current Opinion in Psychology* 60, article no. 101882 (December 2024), https://doi.org/10.1016/j.copsyc.2024.101882.

[53] B. J. Schmeichel et al., "Intellectual Performance and Ego Depletion: Role of the Self in Logical Reasoning and Other Information Processing," *Journal of Personality and Social Psychology* 85, no. 1 (2003): 33–46, https://doi.org/10.1037/0022-3514.85.1.33; Christoph Lindner et al., "A New Perspective on the Interplay Between Self-Control and Cognitive Performance: Modeling Progressive Depletion Patterns," *PLOS One* 12, no. 6 (2017): e0180149, https://doi.org/10.1371/journal.pone.0180149.

[54] Julia C. Basso et al., "Brief, Daily Meditation Enhances Attention, Memory, Mood, and Emotional Regulation in Non-Experienced Meditators," *Behavioural Brain Research* 356 (January 1, 2019): 208–20, https://doi.org/10.1016/j.bbr.2018.08.023.

[55] Marius Golubickis et al., "Brief Mindfulness-Based Meditation Enhances the Speed of Learning Following Positive Prediction Errors," *Quarterly Journal of Experimental Psychology* 77, no. 11 (January 2024): 2312–24, https://doi.org/10.1177/17470218241228859.

[56] Jonathan M. Lieberman et al., "Neurophysiological Mechanisms of Focused Attention Meditation: A Scoping Systematic Review," *Imaging Neuroscience* 3 (2025): IMAG.a.14, https://doi.org/10.1162/IMAG.a.14.

[57] Yi-Yuan Tang et al., "Short-Term Meditation Training Improves Attention and Self-Regulation," *Proceedings of the National Academy of Sciences* 104, no. 43 (2007): 17152–56, https://doi.org/10.1073/pnas.0707678104.

[58] Basso et al., "Brief, Daily Meditation Enhances Attention."

[59] Heather L. Rusch et al., "The Effect of Mindfulness Meditation on Sleep Quality: A Systematic Review and Meta-Analysis of Randomized Controlled Trials," *Annals of the New York Academy of Sciences* 1445, no. 1 (2019): 5–16, https://doi.org/10.1111/nyas.13996.

[60] Daniel Goleman and Richard J. Davidson, *Altered Traits: Science Reveals How Meditation Changes Your Mind, Brain, and Body* (Avery, 2017); Bryce A. Keating et al., "Neurofluid Circulation Changes During a Focused Attention Style of Mindfulness Meditation," *Proceedings of the National Academy of Sciences U.S.A.* 122, no. 49 (December 2025): e2504961122, https://doi.org/10.1073/pnas.2504961122.

[61] Melis Yilmaz Balban et al., "Brief Structured Respiration Practices Enhance Mood and Reduce Physiological Arousal," *Cell Reports Medicine* 4, no. 1 (2023): 100895, https://doi.org/10.1016/j.xcrm.2022.100895.

[62] Gary Elkins, "Hypnotherapy for Smoking Cessation, Sleep, Pain, and the Potential of Hypnosis Apps," *International Journal* of *Clinical* and *Experimental Hypnosis* 73, no. 1 (2025): 1–3, https://doi.org/10.1080/00207144.2024.2432843; Ernil Hansen et al., "Editorial: Clinical Hypnosis," *Frontiers in Psychology* 15 (August 21, 2024): 1464449, https://doi.org/10.3389/fpsyg.2024.1464449; Jenny Rosendahl et al., "Meta-Analytic Evidence on the Efficacy of Hypnosis for Mental and Somatic Health Issues: A 20-Year Perspective," *Frontiers in Psychology* 14 (2024): 1330238, https://doi.org/10.3389/fpsyg.2023.1330238; Leonard S. Milling et al., "A Meta-Analysis of Hypnotic Interventions for Depression Symptoms: High Hopes for Hypnosis?," *American Journal of Clinical Hypnosis* 61, no. 3 (2019): 227–43, https://doi.org/10.1080/00029157.2018.1489777; Winfried Häuser, "Gut-Directed Hypnosis and Hypnotherapy for Irritable Bowel Syndrome: A Mini-Review," *Frontiers in Psychology* 15 (2024): 1389911, https://doi.org/10.3389/fpsyg.2024.1389911.

[63] Heidi Jiang et al., "Brain Activity and Functional Connectivity Associated with Hypnosis," *Cerebral Cortex* 27, no. 8 (2017): 4083–93, https://doi.org/10.1093/cercor/bhw220.

[64] Lorenza S. Colzato et al., "More Attentional Focusing Through Binaural Beats: Evidence from the Global-Local Task," *Psychological Research* 81, no. 1 (2017): 271–77, https://doi.org/10.1007/s00426-015-0727-0; Nantawachara Jirakittayakorn and Yodchanan Wongsawat, "Brain Responses to 40-Hz Binaural Beat and Effects on Emotion and Memory," *International Journal of Psychophysiology* 120 (October 2017): 96–107, https://doi.org/10.1016/j.ijpsycho.2017.07.010.

[65] Jung M. Park and Li-Huei Tsai, "Innovations in Noninvasive Sensory Stimulation Treatments to Combat Alzheimer's Disease," *PLOS Biology* 23, no. 2 (2025): e3003046, https://doi.org/10.1371/journal.pbio.3003046; Lee Bartel and Abdullah Mosabbir, "Possible Mechanisms for the Effects of Sound Vibration on Human Health," *Healthcare* 9, no. 5 (2021): 597, https://doi.org/10.3390/healthcare9050597.

[66] Xixi Chen et al., "Gamma Oscillations and Application of 40-Hz Audiovisual Stimulation to Improve Brain Function," *Brain and Behavior* 12, no. 12 (2022): e2811, https://doi.org/10.1002/brb3.2811.

[67] Artemis Traikapi and Nikos Konstantinou, "Gamma Oscillations in Alzheimer's Disease and Their Potential Therapeutic Role," *Frontiers in Systems Neuroscience* 15 (December 12, 2021): 782399, https://doi.org/10.3389/fnsys.2021.782399.

[68] Susan A. Reedijk et al., "Eliminating the Attentional Blink Through Binaural Beats: A Case for Tailored Cognitive Enhancement," *Frontiers in Psychiatry* 6 (June 3, 2015): 82, https://doi.org/10.3389/fpsyt.2015.00082.

[69] Colzato et al., "More Attentional Focusing."

[70] Michèle Moessinger et al., "Auditive Beta Stimulation as a Countermeasure Against Driver Fatigue," *PLOS One* 16, no. 1 (2021): e0245251, https://doi.org/10.1371/journal.pone.0245251;

Anastasiia Melnichuk et al., "A Parametric Investigation of Binaural Beats for Brain Entrainment and Enhancing Sustained Attention," *Scientific Reports* 15, no. 4308 (2025), https://doi.org/10.1038/s41598-025-88517-z; Ruth Maria Ingendoh et al., "Binaural Beats to Entrain the Brain? A Systematic Review of the Effects of Binaural Beat Stimulation on Brain Oscillatory Activity, and the Implications for Psychological Research and Intervention," PLOS One 18, no. 5 (2023): e0286023, https://doi.org/10.1371/journal.pone.0286023.

[71] Othman et al., "Low Intensity White Noise"; Junhong Zhou et al., "Pink Noise: Effect on Complexity Synchronization of Brain Activity and Sleep Consolidation," *Journal of Theoretical Biology* 306 (August 7, 2012): 68–72, https://doi.org/10.1016/j.jtbi.2012.04.006.

[72] Alessandra S. Souza and Luís Carlos Leal Barbosa, "Should We Turn Off the Music? Music with Lyrics Interferes with Cognitive Tasks," *Journal of Cognition* 6, no. 1 (2023): 24, https://doi.org/10.5334/joc.273; Lucia De Francesco et al., "What You Listen to Makes a Difference: The Impact of Music on Attention and Well-Being," *Annals of the New York Academy of Sciences* 1552, no. 1 (2025): 273–83, https://doi.org/10.1111/nyas.70049.

[73] Kai Chen et al., "Exercise Training Improves Motor Skill Learning via Selective Activation of mTOR," *Science Advances* 5, no. 7 (2019): eaaw1888, https://doi.org/10.1126/sciadv.aaw1888; H. G. Laurie Rauch et al., "Neural Correlates of Motor Vigour and Motor Urgency During Exercise," *Sports Medicine* 43, no. 4 (2013): 227–41, https://doi.org/10.1007/s40279-013-0025-1; Travis Anderson et al., "Exercise and the Hypothalamic-Pituitary-Adrenal Axis: A Special Focus on Acute Cortisol and Growth Hormone Responses," *Current Opinion in Endocrine and Metabolic Research* 9 (2019): 74–77, https://doi.org/10.1016/j.coemr.2019.08.002; Cristina Mennitti et al., "How Does Physical Activity Modulate Hormone Responses?," *Biomolecules* 14, no. 11 (2024): 1418, https://doi.org/10.3390/biom14111418; Richard P. Dum et al., "The Mind-Body Problem: Circuits That Link the Cerebral Cortex to the Adrenal Medulla," *Proceedings of the National Academy of Sciences* 116, no. 51 (2019): 26321–28, https://doi.org/10.1073/pnas.1902297116.

[74] T. Miyashita and C. L. Williams, "Epinephrine Administration Increases Neural Impulses Propagated Along the Vagus Nerve: Role of Peripheral β-Adrenergic Receptors," *Neurobiology of Learning and Memory* 85, no. 2 (2006): 116–24, https://doi.org/10.1016/j.nlm.2005.08.013.

[75] Dona Lee Wong et al., "Epinephrine: A Short- and Long-Term Regulator of Stress and Development of Illness: A Potential New Role for Epinephrine in Stress," *Cellular and Molecular Neurobiology* 32, no. 5 (2012): 737–48, https://doi.org/10.1007/s10571-011-9768-0.

[76] Kirk I. Erickson et al., "Physical Activity, Cognition, and Brain Outcomes," *Medicine & Science in Sports & Exercise* 51, no. 6 (June 2019): 1242–51, https://doi.org/10.1249/mss.0000000000001936.

[77] Neil L. Coplan et al., "Exercise-Related Changes in Serum Catecholamines and Potassium: Effect of Sustained Exercise Above and Below Lactate Threshold," *American Heart Journal* 117, no. 5 (1989): 1070–75, https://doi.org/10.1016/0002-8703(89)90864-8; Mennitti et al., "How Does Physical Activity Modulate Hormone Responses?"

[78] Anna Abbasi et al., "A Comprehensive Review of Obstructive Sleep Apnea," *Sleep Science* 14, no. 2 (2021): 142–54, https://doi.org/10.5935/1984-0063.20200056.

[79] Ju-Yeon Jung and Chang-Ki Kang, "Investigation on the Effect of Oral Breathing on Cognitive Activity Using Functional Brain Imaging," *Healthcare* 9, no. 6 (2021): 645, https://doi.org/10.3390/healthcare9060645.

[80] D. A. Werntz et al., "Alternating Cerebral Hemispheric Activity and the Lateralization of Autonomic Nervous Function," *Human Neurobiology* 2, no. 1 (1983): 39–43, https://pubmed.ncbi.nlm.nih.gov/6874437/; David Shannahoff-Khalsa, "Lateralized Rhythms of the Central and Autonomic Nervous Systems," *International Journal of Psychophysiology* 11, no. 3 (1991): 225–51, https://doi.org/10.1016/0167-8760(91)90017-r; Maria Elide Vanutelli et al., "Breathing Right . . . or Left! The Effects of Unilateral Nostril Breathing on Psychological and Cognitive Wellbeing: A Pilot Study," *Brain Sciences* 14, no. 4 (2024): 302, https://doi.org/10.3390/brainsci14040302.

[81] Christina Zelano et al., "Nasal Respiration Entrains Human Limbic Oscillations and Modulates Cognitive Function," *Journal of Neuroscience* 36, no. 49 (2016): 12448–67, https://doi.org/10.1523/JNEUROSCI.2586-16.2016.

[82] Jacek Sein Anand et al., "Hyperventilation with Maintenance of Isocapnia. An 'Old New' Method in Carbon Monoxide Intoxication," *PLOS One* 12, no. 1 (2017): e0170621, https://doi.org/10.1371/journal.pone.0170621.

[83] Omar Almahayni and Lucy Hammond, "Does the Wim Hof Method Have a Beneficial Impact on Physiological and Psychological Outcomes in Healthy and Non-Healthy Participants? A Systematic Review," *PLOS One* 19, no. 3 (March 2024): e0286933, https://doi.org/10.1371/journal.pone.0286933; Sascha Ketelhut et al., "The Effectiveness of the Wim Hof Method on Cardiac Autonomic Function, Blood Pressure, Arterial Compliance, and Different Psychological Parameters," *Scientific Reports* 13, no. 1 (October 2023): 17517, https://doi.org/10.1038/s41598-023-44902-0.

[84] Marika Falla et al., “The Effect of Cold Exposure on Cognitive Performance in Healthy Adults: A Systematic Review,” *International Journal of Environmental Research and Public Health* 18, no. 18 (2021): 9725, https://doi.org/10.3390/ijerph18189725.

[85] T. E. Graham and L. L. Spriet, “Metabolic, Catecholamine, and Exercise Performance Responses to Various Doses of Caffeine,” *Journal of Applied Physiology* 78, no. 3 (1995): 867–74, https://doi.org/10.1152/jappl.1995.78.3.867; Christos Papadelis et al., “Effects of Mental Workload and Caffeine on Catecholamines and Blood Pressure Compared to Performance Variations,” *Brain and Cognition* 51, no. 1 (2003): 143–54, https://doi.org/10.1016/s0278-2626(02)00530-4.

[86] David Robertson et al., “Effects of Caffeine on Plasma Renin Activity, Catecholamines and Blood Pressure,” *New England Journal of Medicine* 298, no. 4 (January 1978): 181–86, https://doi.org/10.1056/nejm197801262980403.

[87] N. D. Volkow et al., “Caffeine Increases Striatal Dopamine D_2/D_3 Receptor Availability in the Human Brain,” *Translational Psychiatry* 5, no. 4 (2015): e549, https://doi.org/10.1038/tp.2015.46.

[88] Gayani S. Nawarathna et al., “High-Dose L-Theanine-Caffeine Combination Improves Neurobehavioural and Neurophysiological Measures of Selective Attention in Acutely Sleep-Deprived Young Adults: A Double-Blind, Placebo-Controlled Crossover Study,” *British Journal of Nutrition* 134, no. 3 (2025): 195–204, https://doi.org/10.1017/S0007114525104169.

[89] Suzanne J. L. Einöther et al., “L-Theanine and Caffeine Improve Task Switching but Not Intersensory Attention or Subjective Alertness,” *Appetite* 54, no. 2 (2010): 406–9, https://doi.org/10.1016/j.appet.2010.01.003.

[90] Simon P. Kelly et al., “L-Theanine and Caffeine in Combination Affect Human Cognition as Evidenced by Oscillatory Alpha-Band Activity and Attention Task Performance,” *Journal of Nutrition* 138, no. 8 (2008): 1572S–77S, https://doi.org/10.1093/jn/138.8.1572S.

[91] Ai Yoto et al., “Effects of L-Theanine or Caffeine Intake on Changes in Blood Pressure Under Physical and Psychological Stresses,” *Journal of Physiological Anthropology* 31, no. 1 (2012): 28, https://doi.org/10.1186/1880-6805-31-28.

[92] T. Giesbrecht et al., “The Combination of L-Theanine and Caffeine Improves Cognitive Performance and Increases Subjective Alertness,” *Nutritional Neuroscience* 13, no. 6 (2010): 283–90, https://doi.org/10.1179/147683010X12611460764840.

[93] Inge Klinkenberg et al., “Acetylcholine and Attention,” *Behavioural Brain Research* 221, no. 2 (2011): 430–42, https://doi.org/10.1016/j.bbr.2010.11.033.

[94] Yasuhisa Tamura et al., “Alpha-Glycerylphosphorylcholine Increases Motivation in Healthy Volunteers: A Single-Blind, Randomized, Placebo-Controlled Human Study,” *Nutrients* 13, no. 6 (2021): 2091, https://doi.org/10.3390/nu13062091.

[95] Chad M. Kerksick, “Acute Alpha-Glycerylphosphorylcholine Supplementation Enhances Cognitive Performance in Healthy Men,” *Nutrients* 16, no. 23 (2024): 4240, https://doi.org/10.3390/nu16234240.

[96] Getu Gamo Sagaro et al., “Activity of Choline Alphoscerate on Adult-Onset Cognitive Dysfunctions: A Systematic Review and Meta-Analysis,” *Journal of Alzheimer’s Disease* 92, no. 1 (2023): 59–70, https://doi.org/10.3233/JAD-221189.

[97] Adam G. Parker et al., “The Effects of Alpha-Glycerylphosphorylcholine, Caffeine or Placebo on Markers of Mood, Cognitive Function, Power, Speed, and Agility,” *Journal of the International Society of Sports Nutrition* 12, no. S1 (2015): P41, https://doi.org/10.1186/1550-2783-12-S1-P41.

[98] Elise Demeter and Martin Sarter, “Leveraging the Cortical Cholinergic System to Enhance Attention,” *Neuropharmacology* 64 (January 2013): 294–304, https://doi.org/10.1016/j.neuropharm.2012.06.060.

[99] Zeneng Wang et al., “The Nutritional Supplement *L*-Alpha Glycerylphosphorylcholine Promotes Atherosclerosis,” *International Journal of Molecular Sciences* 22, no. 24 (2021): 13477, https://doi.org/10.3390/ijms222413477.

[100] Wei-Kai Wu et al., "Dietary Allicin Reduces Transformation of L-Carnitine to TMAO Through Impact on Gut Microbiota," *Journal of Functional Foods* 15 (2015): 408–17, https://doi.org/10.1016/j.jff.2015.04.001.

[101] Toshiharu Nagatsu, "The Catecholamine System in Health and Disease—Relation to Tyrosine 3-Monooxygenase and Other Catecholamine-Synthesizing Enzymes," *Proceedings of the Japan Academy, Series B* 82, no. 10 (2006): 388–415, https://doi.org/10.2183/pjab.82.388.

[102] S. Colette Daubner et al., "Tyrosine Hydroxylase and Regulation of Dopamine Synthesis," *Archives of Biochemistry and Biophysics* 508, no. 1 (2011): 1–12, https://doi.org/10.1016/j.abb.2010.12.017.

[103] Bryant J. Jongkees et al., "Effect of Tyrosine Supplementation on Clinical and Healthy Populations Under Stress or Cognitive Demands—a Review," *Journal of Psychiatric Research* 70 (November 2015): 50–57, https://doi.org/10.1016/j.jpsychires.2015.08.014.

[104] Simon N. Young, "L-Tyrosine to Alleviate the Effects of Stress?," *Journal of Psychiatry & Neuroscience* 32, no. 3 (2007): 224, https://pubmed.ncbi.nlm.nih.gov/17476368/.

[105] Gema Aonso-Diego et al., "Prevalence of Energy Drink Consumption World-Wide: A Systematic Review and Meta-Analysis," *Addiction* 119, no. 3 (2024): 438–63, https://doi.org/10.1111/add.16390.

[106] Lyndsey D. Ruiz and Rachel E. Scherr, "Risk of Energy Drink Consumption to Adolescent Health," *American Journal of Lifestyle Medicine* 13, no. 1 (2018): 22–25, https://doi.org/10.1177/1559827618803069.

[107] "The Buzz on Energy Drinks," School Nutrition, CDC, July 22, 2024, https://www.cdc.gov/school-nutrition/energy-drinks/index.html.

[108] Zhong Ming Qian and Ya Ke, "Huperzine A: Is It an Effective Disease-Modifying Drug for Alzheimer's Disease?," *Frontiers in Aging Neuroscience* 6 (August 18, 2014): 216, https://doi.org/10.3389/fnagi.2014.00216.

[109] Ryusei Satoh et al., "Effects of Smart Drugs on Cholinergic System and Non-Neuronal Acetylcholine in the Mouse Hippocampus: Histopathological Approach," *Journal of Clinical Medicine* 11, no. 12 (2022): 3310, https://doi.org/10.3390/jcm11123310.

[110] Anna Gawron-Gzella et al., "Yerba Mate—a Long but Current History," *Nutrients* 13, no. 11 (2021): 3706, https://doi.org/10.3390/nu13113706.

[111] "Life at the Front in Objects," Imperial War Museums, n.d., https://www.iwm.org.uk/history/life-at-the-front-in-14-objects; "Collection: World War I," Stanford Research into the Impact of Tobacco Advertising, n.d., https://tobacco.stanford.edu/cigarettes/war-aviation/world-war-i/.

[112] National Center for Chronic Disease Prevention and Health Promotion (US) Office on Smoking and Health, "Fifty Years of Change 1964–2014," in *The Health Consequences of Smoking—50 Years of Progress: A Report of the Surgeon General* (Centers for Disease Control and Prevention, 2014), https://www.ncbi.nlm.nih.gov/books/NBK294310/.

[113] William S. Griesar et al., "Nicotine Effects on Alertness and Spatial Attention in Non-Smokers," *Nicotine & Tobacco Research* 4, no. 2 (2002): 185–94, https://doi.org/10.1080/14622200210123617; Leonie R. Price and Javier Martinez, "Cardiovascular, Carcinogenic and Reproductive Effects of Nicotine Exposure: A Narrative Review of the Scientific Literature," *F1000Research* 8 (September 4, 2019): 1586, https://doi.org/10.12688/f1000research.20062.2.

[114] Marina R. Picciotto et al., "Effect of Nicotine and Nicotinic Receptors on Anxiety and Depression," *NeuroReport* 13, no. 9 (2002): 1097–1106, https://doi.org/10.1097/00001756-200207020-00006; Price and Martinez, "Cardiovascular, Carcinogenic and Reproductive Effects"; A. C. Parrott, "Nesbitt's Paradox Resolved? Stress and Arousal Modulation During Cigarette Smoking," Addiction 93, no. 1 (1998): 27–39, https://doi.org/10.1046/j.1360-0443.1998.931274.x.

[115] Reena S. Shah and John W. Cole, "Smoking and Stroke: The More You Smoke the More You Stroke," *Expert Review of Cardiovascular Therapy* 8, no. 7 (2010): 917–32, https://doi.org/10.1586/erc.10.56.

[116] John A. Dani and David J. K. Balfour, "Historical and Current Perspective on Tobacco Use and Nicotine Addiction," *Trends in Neurosciences* 34, no. 7 (2011): 383–92, https://doi.org/10.1016/j.tins.2011.05.001.

[117] Juan S. Izquierdo-Condoy et al., "Direct Health Implications of E-Cigarette Use: A Systematic Scoping Review with Evidence Assessment," *Frontiers in Public Health* 12 (July 29, 2024): 1427752, https://doi.org/10.3389/fpubh.2024.1427752.

[118] Jessica L. Reid et al., "Awareness and Use of Oral Nicotine Pouches Among Youth and Young Adults, 2022–2024: Repeat Cross-Sectional Surveys in Canada, England, the USA and New Zealand," *BMJ Public Health* 3, no. 2 (2025): e003457, https://doi.org/10.1136/bmjph-2025-003457; Dae-Hee Han et al., "Nicotine Pouch and E-Cigarette Use and Co-Use Among US Youths in 2023 and 2024," *JAMA Network Open* 8, no. 4 (2025): e256739, https://doi.org/10.1001/jamanetworkopen.2025.6739.

[119] Ahmad Alhowail, "Molecular Insights into the Benefits of Nicotine on Memory and Cognition (Review)," *Molecular Medicine Reports* 23, no. 6 (2021): 398, https://doi.org/10.3892/mmr.2021.12037.

[120] Chih-Hung Liang et al., "Nicotine Therapy for Parkinson's Disease: A Meta-Analysis of Randomized Controlled Trials," *Biomedicines* 13, no. 8 (2025): 1814, https://doi.org/10.3390/biomedicines13081814.

[121] Qi Sun and Chunyuan Jin, "Cell Signaling and Epigenetic Regulation of Nicotine-Induced Carcinogenesis," *Environmental Pollution* 345 (January 2024): 123426, https://doi.org/10.1016/j.envpol.2024.123426; Courtney Schaal and Srikumar P. Chellappan, "Nicotine-Mediated Cell Proliferation and Tumor Progression in Smoking-Related Cancers," *Molecular Cancer Research* 12, no. 1 (2014): 14–23, https://doi.org/10.1158/1541-7786.MCR-13-0541.

[122] Anna K. Whitehead et al., "Nicotine and Vascular Dysfunction," *Acta Physiologica* 231, no. 4 (2021): e13631, https://doi.org/10.1111/apha.13631; Christopher B. Harte and Cindy M. Meston, "Acute Effects of Nicotine on Physiological and Subjective Sexual Arousal in Nonsmoking Men: A Randomized, Double-Blind, Placebo-Controlled Trial," *Journal of Sexual Medicine* 5, no. 1 (2008): 110–21, https://doi.org/10.1111/j.1743-6109.2007.00637.x; Erratum, Harte and Meston, "Acute Effects of Nicotine," *Journal of Sexual Medicine* 7, no. 11 (2010): 3803, https://doi.org/10.1111/j.1743-6109.2010.02112_3.x.

[123] Laurent Misery, "Nicotine Effects on Skin: Are They Positive or Negative?," *Experimental Dermatology* 13, no. 11 (2004): 665–70, https://doi.org/10.1111/j.0906-6705.2004.00274.x.

[124] Paulina Natalia Kopa-Stojak and Rafał Pawliczak, "Comparison of Carcinogenic Potential of Alternative Tobacco Products. A Systematic Review," *Toxicology Mechanisms and Methods* 35, no. 9 (July 2025): 1161–75, https://doi.org/10.1080/15376516.2025.2536664.

[125] Stephen V. Faraone, "The Pharmacology of Amphetamine and Methylphenidate: Relevance to the Neurobiology of Attention-Deficit / Hyperactivity Disorder and Other Psychiatric Comorbidities," *Neuroscience & Biobehavioral Reviews* 87 (April 2018): 255–70, https://doi.org/10.1016/j.neubiorev.2018.02.001; Mehmet Sofuoglu and R. Andrew Sewell, "Norepinephrine and Stimulant Addiction," *Addiction Biology* 14, no. 2 (2009): 119–29, https://doi.org/10.1111/j.1369-1600.2008.00138.x; Benjamin P. Kay et al., "Stimulant Medications Affect Arousal and Reward, Not Attention Networks," *Cell* 188, no. 26 (2025): 7529–46.e20, https://doi.org/10.1016/j.cell.2025.11.039.

[126] Preeti Patel et al., "Dextroamphetamine-Amphetamine," StatPearls, last updated April 6, 2025, https://www.ncbi.nlm.nih.gov/books/NBK507808/.

[127] A. Abdul-Sattar et al., "Adderall Laced with Fentanyl: The Epidemic Is Killing Our Youth," *Internet Journal of Public Health* 9, no. 1 (2023), https://ispub.com/doi/10.5580/IJPH.56911.

[128] Wayne C. Drevets et al., "Amphetamine-Induced Dopamine Release in Human Ventral Striatum Correlates with Euphoria," *Biological Psychiatry* 49, no. 2 (2001): 81–96, https://doi.org/10.1016/s0006-3223(00)01038-6.

[129] Bahadar S. Srichawla et al., "Attention Deficit Hyperactivity Disorder and Substance Use Disorder: A Narrative Review," *Cureus* 14, no. 4 (2022): e24068, https://doi.org/10.7759/cureus.24068.

[130] Erin Richardson et al., "Growth Perturbations from Stimulant Medications and Inhaled Corticosteroids," *Translational Pediatrics* 6, no. 4 (2017): 237–47, https://doi.org/10.21037/tp.2017.09.14.

[131] J. A. Santisteban et al., "Effect of Extended-Release Dexmethylphenidate and Mixed Amphetamine Salts on Sleep: A Double-Blind, Randomized, Crossover Study in Youth with Attention-Deficit Hyperactivity Disorder," *CNS Drugs* 28, no. 9 (2014): 825–33, https://doi.org/10.1007/s40263-014-0181-3.

[132] Lauren V. Moran et al., "Risk of Incident Psychosis and Mania with Prescription Amphetamines," *American Journal of Psychiatry* 181, no. 10 (2024): 901–9, https://doi.org/10.1176/appi.ajp.20230329.

[133] L. L. Weyandt et al., "Prescription Stimulant Medication Misuse: Where Are We and Where Do We Go from Here?," *Experimental and Clinical Psychopharmacology* 24, no. 5 (2016): 400–414, https://doi.org/10.1037/pha0000093.

[134] Dusan Kolar et al., "Treatment of Adults with Attention-Deficit / Hyperactivity Disorder," *Neuropsychiatric Disease and Treatment* 4, no. 2 (2008): 389–403, https://doi.org/10.2147/ndt.s6985.

[135] Benjamin P. Kay et al., "Stimulant Medications Affect Arousal and Reward, Not Attention Networks," *Cell* 188, no. 26 (December 2025): 7529–46, https://doi.org/10.1016/j.cell.2025.11.039.

[136] Stephen M. Stahl, "Norepinephrine and Dopamine Regulate Signals and Noise in the Prefrontal Cortex," *Journal of Clinical Psychiatry* 70, no. 5 (2009): 617–18, https://doi.org/10.4088/jcp.09bs05143.

[137] Anna Moszczynska and Sean Patrick Callan, "Molecular, Behavioral, and Physiological Consequences of Methamphetamine Neurotoxicity: Implications for Treatment," *Journal of Pharmacology and Experimental Therapeutics* 362, no. 3 (2017): 474–88, https://doi.org/10.1124/jpet.116.238501.

[138] IQVIA, "Stimulant Prescription Trends in the United States from 2012–2023," November 13, 2024, https://www.deadiversion.usdoj.gov/pubs/docs/IQVIA-Report-on-Stimulant-Trends-2024.pdf.

[139] Brian J. Piper et al., "Trends in Use of Prescription Stimulants in the United States and Territories, 2006 to 2016," *PLOS One* 13, no. 11 (2018): e0206100, https://doi.org/10.1371/journal.pone.0206100.

[140] Thomas Roth et al., "Evaluation of the Safety of Modafinil for Treatment of Excessive Sleepiness," *Journal of Clinical Sleep Medicine* 3, no. 6 (2007): 595–602, https://pubmed.ncbi.nlm.nih.gov/17993041/.

[141] Reyna Lamas-Aguilar et al., "Armodafinil as a Potential Pharmacological Treatment for Attention Deficit Hyperactivity Disorder in Adults: A Review," *Current Neuropharmacology* 22, no. 11 (2024): 1899–908, https://doi.org/10.2174/1570159X22666240131121642; Erratum, Lamas-Aguilar et al., "Armodafinil as a Potential Pharmacological Treatment," *Current Neuropharmacology* 23, no. 14 (2025): 2004, https://doi.org/10.2174/1570159X23999250210110914; R. M. Battleday and A.-K. Brem, "Modafinil for Cognitive Neuroenhancement in Healthy Non-Sleep-Deprived Subjects: A Systematic Review," *European Neuropsychopharmacology* 25, no. 11 (2015): 1865–81, https://doi.org/10.1016/j.euroneuro.2015.07.028.

[142] Ahmed Dahir Mohamed, "The Effects of Modafinil on Convergent and Divergent Thinking of Creativity: A Randomized Controlled Trial," *Journal of Creative Behavior* 50, no. 4 (2016): 252–67, https://doi.org/10.1002/jocb.73.

[143] Vivien C. Abad, "Profile of Solriamfetol in the Management of Excessive Daytime Sleepiness Associated with Narcolepsy or Obstructive Sleep Apnea: Focus on Patient Selection and Perspectives," *Nature and Science of Sleep* 13 (January 2021): 75–91, https://doi.org/10.2147/NSS.S245020.

[144] Megan C. Cuomo et al., "Solriamfetol for the Management of Excessive Daytime Sleepiness," *Journal of Pharmacy Practice* 35, no. 6 (2022): 963–70, https://doi.org/10.1177/08971900211009080; Sheridan M. Hoy, "Solriamfetol: A Review in Excessive Daytime Sleepiness Associated with Narcolepsy and Obstructive Sleep Apnoea," *CNS Drugs* 37, no. 11 (2023): 1009–20, https://doi.org/10.1007/s40263-023-01040-5.

[145] Ruta Nonacs, "Solriamfetol (Sunosi): Another Option for the Treatment of Adult ADHD?," *MGH Psychiatry News*, November 17, 2023, https://m7ghpsychnews.org/solriamfetol-sunosi-another-option-for-adhd/.

[146] Maurizio Fava et al., "15 Years of Clinical Experience with Bupropion HCl: From Bupropion to Bupropion SR to Bupropion XL," *Primary Care Companion to The Journal of Clinical Psychiatry* 7, no. 3 (2005): 106–13, https://doi.org/10.4088/pcc.v07n0305; Barrett R. Cooper et al., "Evidence That the Acute Behavioral and Electrophysiological Effects of Bupropion (Wellbutrin®) Are Mediated by a Noradrenergic Mechanism," *Neuropsychopharmacology* 11 (1994): 133–41, https://doi.org/10.1038/npp.1994.43; Jianming Dong and Pierre Blier, "Modification of Norepinephrine and Serotonin, but Not Dopamine, Neuron Firing by Sustained Bupropion Treatment," *Psychopharmacology* 155 (March 2001): 52–57, https://doi.org/10.1007/s002130000665.

[147] Wim Verbeeck et al., "Bupropion for Attention Deficit Hyperactivity Disorder (ADHD) in Adults," *Cochrane Database of Systematic Reviews* 10, no. 10 (2017): CD009504, https://doi.org/10.1002/14651858.CD009504.pub2.

[148] "Wellbutrin (Bupropion Hydrochloride) Tablets" (label), Drugs@FDA: FDA-Approved Drugs, revised May 2017, https://www.accessdata.fda.gov/drugsatfda_docs/label/2017/018644s052lbl.pdf.

[149] Skowronek et al., "Mere Presence of a Smartphone."

[150] Josef Parvizi et al., "The Will to Persevere Induced by Electrical Stimulation of the Human Cingulate Gyrus," *Neuron* 80, no. 6 (2013): 1359–67, https://doi.org/10.1016/j.neuron.2013.10.057.

[151] Alia Crum, "#1 Mindset Expert: Simple Mindset Shifts That Transform Your Body, Energy, & Life," interview by Mel Robbins, December 20, 2025, YouTube, https://www.youtube.com/watch?v=oJAV0rtSrFc.

[152] Alia J. Crum and Ellen J. Langer, "Mind-Set Matters: Exercise and the Placebo Effect," *Psychological Science* 18, no. 2 (2007): 165–71, https://doi.org/10.1111/j.1467-9280.2007.01867.x.

[153] Carol S. Dweck and David S. Yeager, "Mindsets: A View from Two Eras," *Perspectives on Psychological Science* 14, no. 3 (2019): 481–96, https://doi.org/10.1177/1745691618804166.

[154] J. L. Burnette et al., "A Systematic Review and Meta-Analysis of Growth Mindset Interventions: For Whom, How, and Why Might Such Interventions Work?," *Psychological Bulletin* 149, no. 3–4 (2023): 174–205, https://doi.org/10.1037/bul0000368; Victoria F. Sisk et al., "To What Extent and Under Which Circumstances Are Growth Mind-Sets Important to Academic Achievement? Two Meta-Analyses," *Psychological Science* 29, no. 4 (2018): 549–71, https://doi.org/10.1177/0956797617739704; A. J. Crum et al., "Rethinking Stress: The Role of Mindsets in Determining the Stress Response," *Journal of Personality and Social Psychology* 104, no. 4 (2013): 716–33, https://doi.org/10.1037/a0031201.

[155] Friedrich Nietzsche, *The Case of Wagner, Nietzsche Contra Wagner, The Twilight of the Idols, The Antichrist*, trans. Thomas Common (H. Henry and Company, 1896), 100.

[156] Viktor E. Frankl, *Man's Search for Meaning*, trans. Ilse Lasch (Rider, 2004), 84.

[157] Chu et al., "Physiology, Stress Reaction."

[158] Andrew Westbrook and Todd S. Braver, "Dopamine Does Double Duty in Motivating Cognitive Effort," *Neuron* 89, no. 4 (2016): 695–710, https://doi.org/10.1016/j.neuron.2015.12.029.

[159] Gabriele Oettingen et al., "Mental Contrasting and Goal Commitment: The Mediating Role of Energization," *Personality and Social Psychology Bulletin* 35, no. 5 (2009): 608–22, https://doi.org/10.1177/0146167208330856.

[160] Angel D. Prabakar, "The Power of Thought: The Role of Psychological Attentiveness and Emotional Support in Patient Trajectories," *Yale Journal of Biology and Medicine* 97, no. 3 (2024): 335–47, https://doi.org/10.59249/CPTG1770.

[161] Gabriele Oettingen and Doris Mayer, "The Motivating Function of Thinking About the Future: Expectations Versus Fantasies," *Journal of Personality and Social Psychology* 83, no. 5 (2002): 1198–1212, https://pubmed.ncbi.nlm.nih.gov/12416922/.

[162] Gabriele Oettingen, "Future Thought and Behaviour Change," *European Review of Social Psychology* 23, no. 1 (2012): 1–63, https://doi.org/10.1080/10463283.2011.643698.

[163] Anne Lembke, *Dopamine Nation: Finding Balance in the Age of Indulgence* (Penguin, 2021).

[164] John P. Grogan et al., "Dopamine Promotes Instrumental Motivation, but Reduces Reward-Related Vigour," *eLife* 9 (October 1, 2020): e58321, https://doi.org/10.7554/eLife.58321.

[165] Lembke, *Dopamine Nation.*

[166] Gabriele Oettingen's Publications, https://wp.nyu.edu/motivationlab/publications/gabriele-oettingen/.

[167] Andreas Kappes et al., "Mental Contrasting Instigates Goal Pursuit by Linking Obstacles of Reality with Instrumental Behavior," *Journal of Experimental Social Psychology* 48, no. 4 (2012): 811–18, https://doi.org/10.1016/j.jesp.2012.02.002.

[168] Gabriele Oettingen, *Rethinking Positive Thinking: Inside the New Science of Motivation* (Current, 2015).

[169] Alexandra Touroutoglou et al., "The Tenacious Brain: How the Anterior Mid-Cingulate Contributes to Achieving Goals," *Cortex* 123 (February 2020): 12–29, https://doi.org/10.1016/j.cortex.2019.09.011.

[170] Yuri Miyamoto et al., "Cultural Variation in the Focus on Goals Versus Processes of Actions," *Personality and Social Psychology Bulletin* 39, no. 6 (2013): 707–19, https://doi.org/10.1177/0146167213483579.

[171] Archy O. de Berker et al., "Computations of Uncertainty Mediate Acute Stress Responses in Humans," *Nature Communications* 7 (2016): 10996, https://doi.org/10.1038/ncomms10996.

[172] Abdullahi Ali et al., "Predictive Coding Is a Consequence of Energy Efficiency in Recurrent Neural Networks," *Patterns* 3, no. 12 (2022): 100639, https://doi.org/10.1016/j.patter.2022.100639.

[173] Mitsuko Watabe-Uchida et al., "Neural Circuitry of Reward Prediction Error," *Annual Review of Neuroscience* 40 (July 25, 2017): 373–94, https://doi.org/10.1146/annurev-neuro-072116-031109.

[174] James B. Heald et al., "The Computational and Neural Bases of Context-Dependent Learning," *Annual Review of Neuroscience* 46 (2023): 233–58, https://doi.org/10.1146/annurev-neuro-092322-100402; Thomas M. Tzschentke, "Review on CPP: Measuring Reward with the Conditioned Place Preference (CPP) Paradigm: Update of the Last Decade," *Addiction Biology* 12, no. 3–4 (September 2007): 227–462, https://doi.org/10.1111/j.1369-1600.2007.00070.x.

[175] Sebastian Rumpf et al., "Energy Metabolic Pathways in Neuronal Development and Function," *Oxford Open Neuroscience* 2 (March 21, 2023): kvad004, https://doi.org/10.1093/oons/kvad004.

[176] Preeti Rishi et al., "Errorless and Errorful Learning in People with Aphasia Across Novel-Object Pairing and Word Retrieval Tasks," *Aphasiology* 39, no. 10 (2025): 1381–1413, https://doi.org/10.1080/02687038.2024.2432022; Josie Briscoe et al., "Errorful Learning Improves Recognition Memory for New Vocabulary for People Living with Memory and Dysexecutive Impairment Following Brain Injury," *Neuropsychological Rehabilitation* 34, no. 7 (2024): 974–1004, https://doi.org/10.1080/09602011.2023.2259017; Steven C. Pan and Faria Sana, "Pretesting Versus Posttesting: Comparing the Pedagogical Benefits of Errorful Generation and Retrieval Practice," *Journal of Experimental Psychology: Applied* 27, no. 2 (2021): 237–52, https://doi.org/10.1037/xap0000345; Yeray Mera et al., "Unraveling the Benefits of Experiencing Errors During Learning: Definition, Modulating Factors, and Explanatory Theories," *Psychonomic Bulletin & Review* 29 (2022): 753–65, https://doi.org/10.3758/s13423-021-02022-8; Naser Al-Fawakhiri et al., "Evidence of an Optimal Error Rate for Motor Skill Learning," preprint, *bioRxiv* (July 2023): 549705, https://doi.org/10.1101/2023.07.19.549705.

[177] Robert C. Wilson et al., "The Eighty-Five Percent Rule for Optimal Learning," *Nature Communications* 10, article no. 4646 (2019), https://doi.org/10.1038/s41467-019-12552-4.

[178] Manu Kapur and Katerine Bielaczyc, "Designing for Productive Failure," *Journal of the Learning Sciences* 21, no. 1 (2012): 45–83, https://doi.org/10.1080/10508406.2011.591717.

[179] Adrien F. Baranes et al., "The Effects of Task Difficulty, Novelty and the Size of the Search Space on Intrinsically Motivated Exploration," *Frontiers in Neuroscience* 8 (October 13, 2014): 317, https://doi.org/10.3389/fnins.2014.00317.

[180] Hans S. Schroder et al., "Neural Evidence for Enhanced Attention to Mistakes Among School-Aged Children with a Growth Mindset," *Developmental Cognitive Neuroscience* 24 (April 2017): 42–50, https://doi.org/10.1016/j.dcn.2017.01.004.

[181] Scott T. Albert and Reza Shadmehr, "The Neural Feedback Response to Error as a Teaching Signal for the Motor Learning System," *Journal of Neuroscience* 36, no. 17 (2016): 4832–45, https://doi.org/10.1523/JNEUROSCI.0159-16.2016; Dominique L. Pritchett and Megan R. Carey, "A Matter of Trial and Error for Motor Learning," *Trends in Neurosciences* 37, no. 9 (2014): 465–66, https://doi.org/10.1016/j.tins.2014.08.001.

[182] Jean-Baptiste Eichenlaub et al., "Replay of Learned Neural Firing Sequences During Rest in Human Motor Cortex," *Cell Reports* 31, no. 5 (2020): 107581, https://doi.org/10.1016/j.celrep.2020.107581.

[183] Matthew P. Walker, "The Role of Slow Wave Sleep in Memory Processing," *Journal of Clinical Sleep Medicine* 5, no. S2 (2009): S20–26, https://pubmed.ncbi.nlm.nih.gov/19998871/.

[184] Jaap M. J. Murre and Joeri Dros, "Replication and Analysis of Ebbinghaus' Forgetting Curve," *PLOS One* 10, no. 7 (2015): e0120644, https://doi.org/10.1371/journal.pone.0120644.

[185] Marlene Bönstrup et al., "A Rapid Form of Offline Consolidation in Skill Learning," *Current Biology* 29, no. 8 (2019): 1346–51.e4, https://doi.org/10.1016/j.cub.2019.02.049.

[186] Ethan R. Buch et al., "Consolidation of Human Skill Linked to Waking Hippocampo-Neocortical Replay," *Cell Reports* 35, no. 10 (2021): 109193, https://doi.org/10.1016/j.celrep.2021.109193.

[187] Patricia Albulescu et al., "'Give Me a Break!' A Systematic Review and Meta-Analysis on the Efficacy of Micro-Breaks for Increasing Well-Being and Performance," *PLOS One* 17, no. 8 (2022): e0272460, https://doi.org/10.1371/journal.pone.0272460; Bönstrup et al., "Rapid Form of Offline Consolidation."

[188] Elisabeth Wenger et al., "Expansion and Renormalization of Human Brain Structure During Skill Acquisition," *Trends in Cognitive Sciences* 21, no. 12 (2017): 930–39, https://doi.org/10.1016/j.tics.2017.09.008.

[189] Christa K. McIntyre et al., "Interacting Brain Systems Modulate Memory Consolidation," *Neuroscience & Biobehavioral Reviews* 36, no. 7 (2012): 1750–62, https://doi.org/10.1016/j.neubiorev.2011.11.001; K. C. Liang et al., "Involvement of Amygdala Pathways in the Influence of Post-Training Intra-Amygdala Norepinephrine and Peripheral Epinephrine on Memory Storage," *Brain Research* 508, no. 2 (1990): 225–33, https://doi.org/10.1016/0006-8993(90)90400-6.

[190] Henry L. Roediger III and Jeffrey D. Karpicke, "Test-Enhanced Learning: Taking Memory Tests Improves Long-Term Retention," *Psychological Science* 17, no. 3 (2006): 249–55, https://doi.org/10.1111/j.1467-9280.2006.01693.x.

[191] Roediger and Karpicke, "Test-Enhanced Learning"; Cynthia J. Brame and Rachel Biel, "Test-Enhanced Learning: The Potential for Testing to Promote Greater Learning in Undergraduate Science Courses," *CBE—Life Sciences Education* 14, no. 2 (June 2015), https://doi.org/10.1187/cbe.14-11-0208; Christopher A. Rowland, "The Effect of Testing Versus Restudy on Retention: A Meta-Analytic Review of the Testing Effect," *Psychological Bulletin* 140, no. 6 (2014): 1432–63, https://doi.org/10.1037/a0037559; Jeffrey D. Karpicke and Janell R. Blunt, "Retrieval Practice Produces More Learning than Elaborative Studying with Concept Mapping," Science 331, no. 6018 (January 2011): 772–75, https://doi.org/10.1126/science.1199327; Khalil A. Bin Abdulrahman et al., "Study Habits of Highly Effective Medical Students," *Advances in Medical Education and Practice* 12 (2021): 627–33, https://pmc.ncbi.nlm.nih.gov/articles/PMC8197661/pdf/amep-12-627.pdf; Sally Binks, "Testing Enhances Learning: A Review of the Literature," *Journal of Professional Nursing* 34, no. 3 (May–June 2018): 205–10, https://doi.org/10.1016/j.profnurs.2017.08.008.

Chapter 7: Protocols for Personal Growth

[1] Julianne Holt-Lunstad, "Social Connection as a Critical Factor for Mental and Physical Health: Evidence, Trends, Challenges, and Future Implications," *World Psychiatry* 23, no. 3 (September 2024): 312–32, https://doi.org/10.1002/wps.21224.

[2] Anne E. Storey and Toni E. Ziegler, "Primate Paternal Care: Interactions Between Biology and Social Experience," *Hormones and Behavior* 77 (August 2015): 260–71, https://doi.org/10.1016/j.yhbeh.2015.07.024; Allan Schore, *Right Brain Psychotherapy* (W. W. Norton & Company): 2019.

[3] George M. Slavich, "Social Safety Theory: A Biologically Based Evolutionary Perspective on Life Stress, Health, and Behavior," *Annual Review of Clinical Psychology* 16 (March 2020), https://doi.org/10.1146/annurev-clinpsy-032816-045159.

[4] Marcus Aurelius, *Meditations*.

[5] René Descartes, *Discourse on the Method* (1637) ("I think, therefore I am").

[6] Buddha, *The Dhammapada*, chap. 1, verses 1–2 ("What you think, you become").

[7] "Ralph Waldo Emerson: 'A Man Is What He Thinks About All Day Long,'" The Socratic Method, September 21, 2023, https://www.socratic-method.com/quote-meanings/ralph-waldo-emerson-a-man-is-what-he-thinks-about-all-day-long.

[8] William Shakespeare, *Hamlet*, act 2, scene 2 ("There is nothing either good or bad but thinking makes it so").

[9] Proverbs 4:23 ("Be careful how you think; your life is shaped by your thoughts"); Proverbs 23:7 ("For as a man thinks in his heart, so he is").

[10] Jennifer M. Groh, *Making Space: How the Brain Knows Where Things Are* (Belknap Press of Harvard University, 2014).

[11] Jennifer M. Groh et al., "Signal Switching May Enhance Processing Power of the Brain," *Trends in Cognitive Sciences* 28, no. 7 (2024): 600–613, https://doi.org/10.1016/j.tics.2024.04.008.

[12] Guozhang Chen and Pulin Gong, "A Spatiotemporal Mechanism of Visual Attention: Superdiffusive Motion and Theta Oscillations of Neural Population Activity Patterns," *Science Advances* 8, no. 16 (2022): eabl4995, https://doi.org/10.1126/sciadv.abl4995; Edmund T. Rolls, "Attractor Network Dynamics, Transmitters, and Memory and Cognitive Changes in Aging," in *Cognitive Changes and the Aging Brain*, ed. Kenneth M. Heilman and Stephen E. Nadeau (Cambridge University Press, 2019), 203–25; Robert Englert et al., "Functional Connectivity-Based Attractor Dynamics of the Human Brain in Rest, Task, and Disease," *eLife* 13 (2026): RP98725, https://doi.org/10.7554/eLife.98725.3; Edmund T. Rolls, "Attractor Cortical Neurodynamics, Schizophrenia, and Depression," *Translational Psychiatry* 11, article no. 215 (2021), https://doi.org/10.1038/s41398-021-01333-7; Samming Song et al., "A Modular Latching Chain," *Cognitive Neurodynamics* 8 (2014): 37–46, https://doi.org/10.1007/s11571-013-9261-1.

[13] Andrew Huberman, "Dr. James Hollis: How to Find Your True Purpose & Create Your Best Life," *Huberman Lab* (podcast audio), May 13, 2024, https://www.hubermanlab.com/episode/dr-james-hollis-how-to-find-your-true-purpose-create-your-best-life.

[14] Radwa Khalil et al., "The Link Between Creativity, Cognition, and Creative Drives and Underlying Neural Mechanisms," *Frontiers in Neural Circuits* 13 (March 21, 2019): 18, https://doi.org/10.3389/fncir.2019.00018; Gerald L. Clore and Jeffrey R. Huntsinger, "How Emotions Inform Judgment and Regulate Thought," *Trends in Cognitive Sciences* 11, no. 9 (2007): 393–99, https://doi.org/10.1016/j.tics.2007.08.005; Kostadin Kushlev et al., "Does Happiness Improve Health? Evidence from a Randomized Controlled Trial," *Psychological Science* 31, no. 7 (2020): 807–21, https://doi.org/10.1177/0956797620919673.

[15] Jamil Zaki, *Hope for Cynics: The Surprising Science of Human Goodness* (New York: Grand Central Publishing, 2024).

[16] Bernard A. Nijstad et al., "The Dual Pathway to Creativity Model: Creative Ideation as a Function of Flexibility and Persistence," *European Review of Social Psychology* 21, no. 1 (2010): 34–77, https://doi.org/10.1080/10463281003765323; Arthur M. Nezu et al., "Social Problem Solving as a Risk Factor for Depression," in *Risk Factors in Depression*, ed. Keith S. Dobson and David J. A. Dozois (Amsterdam: Elsevier, 2008), 263–86; Nathan Ridout et al., "The Influence of Induced Dysphoria on Autobiographical Memory Specificity and Social Problem Solving: Examining the Role of Executive Function," *Behaviour Research and Therapy* 169 (October 2023): 104404, https://doi.org/10.1016/j.brat.2023.104404; C. Donaldson and D. Lam, "Rumination, Mood and Social Problem-Solving in Major Depression," *Psychological Medicine* 34, no. 7 (October 2004): 1309–18.

[17] Daniel Kahneman and Angus Deaton, "High Income Improves Evaluation of Life but Not Emotional Well-Being," *Proceedings of the National Academy of Sciences* 107, no. 38 (2010): 16489–93, https://doi.org/10.1073/pnas.1011492107.

[18] Anuradha Baminiwatta and Indrajith Solangaarachchi, "Trends and Developments in Mindfulness Research over 55 Years: A Bibliometric Analysis of Publications Indexed in Web of Science," *Mindfulness* 12, no. 9 (2021): 2099–116, https://doi.org/10.1007/s12671-021-01681-x.

[19] Laura G. Kiken et al., "Being Present and Enjoying It: Dispositional Mindfulness and Savoring the Moment Are Distinct, Interactive Predictors of Positive Emotions and Psychological Health," *Mindfulness* 8, no. 5 (2017): 1280–90, https://doi.org/10.1007/s12671-017-0704-3; E. S. Blanke et al., "Pathways to Happiness Are Multidirectional: Associations Between State Mindfulness and Everyday Affective Experience," *Emotion* 18, no. 2 (2018): 202–11, https://doi.org/10.1037/emo0000323.

[20] Matthew A. Killingsworth and Daniel T. Gilbert, "A Wandering Mind Is an Unhappy Mind," *Science* 330, no. 6006 (2010): 932, https://doi.org/10.1126/science.1192439.

[21] Killingsworth and Gilbert, "Wandering Mind Is an Unhappy Mind."

[22] B. Q. Ford et al., "The Psychological Health Benefits of Accepting Negative Emotions and Thoughts: Laboratory, Diary, and Longitudinal Evidence," *Journal of Personality and Social Psychology* 115, no. 6 (2018): 1075–92, https://doi.org/10.1037/pspp0000157.

[23] Benjamin P. Chapman et al., "Emotion Suppression and Mortality Risk over a 12-Year Follow-Up," *Journal of Psychosomatic Research* 75, no. 4 (2013): 381–85, https://doi.org/10.1016/j.jpsychores.2013.07.014; Alexandra T. Tyra et al., "Emotion Suppression and Acute Physiological Responses to Stress in Healthy Populations: A Quantitative Review of Experimental and Correlational Investigations," *Health Psychology Review* 18, no. 2 (2024): 396–420, https://doi.org/10.1080/17437199.2023.2251559; Jainish Patel and Prittesh Patel, "Consequences of Repression of Emotion: Physical Health, Mental Health and General Well-Being," *International Journal of Psychotherapy Practice and Research* 1, no. 3 (2019): 16–21, https://doi.org/10.14302/issn.2574-612X.ijpr-18-2564.

[24] Shaghayegh Konjedi and Reza Maleeh, "A Closer Look at the Relationship Between the Default Network, Mind Wandering, Negative Mood, and Depression," *Cognitive, Affective, & Behavioral Neuroscience* 17, no. 4 (2017): 697–711, https://doi.org/10.3758/s13415-017-0506-z.

[25] Osman Ulvi et al., "Social Media Use and Mental Health: A Global Analysis," *Epidemiologia* 3, no. 1 (2022): 11–25, https://doi.org/10.3390/epidemiologia3010002; Bdour Alwuqaysi, "A Systematic Review and Meta-Analysis of Social Media's Influence on Mental Health, Family Functioning, and Visual Content," *Social Sciences & Humanities Open* 12 (2025): 101793, https://doi.org/10.1016/j.ssaho.2025.101793.

[26] Diana Kwon, "How Your Brain Controls Ageing—and Why Zombie Cells Could Be Key," *Nature* 642, no. 8068 (2025): 563–65, https://doi.org/10.1038/d41586-025-01886-3; Ming Xu et al., "Senolytics Improve Physical Function and Increase Lifespan in Old Age," *Nature Medicine* 24, no. 8 (2018): 1246–56, https://doi.org/10.1038/s41591-018-0092-9.

[27] Enzo Tedone et al., "Telomere Length and Telomerase Activity in T Cells Are Biomarkers of High-Performing Centenarians," *Aging Cell* 18, no. 1 (2019): e12859, https://doi.org/10.1111/acel.12859.

[28] Elissa S. Epel et al., "Accelerated Telomere Shortening in Response to Life Stress," *Proceedings of the National Academy of Sciences* 101, no. 49 (2004): 17312–15, https://doi.org/10.1073/pnas.0407162101.

[29] Andy Stumpf, *Drownproof: Eight Life Lessons to Keep Your Head Above Water* (St. Martin's Press, 2026).

[30] Monika Sohal et al., "Efficacy of Journaling in the Management of Mental Illness: A Systematic Review and Meta-Analysis," *Family Medicine and Community Health* 10, no. 1 (2022): e001154, https://doi.org/10.1136/fmch-2021-001154; Wang He and Jun Gan, "The Relationship Between Self-Reflection and Mental Health: A Meta-Analysis Review," *Current Psychology* 44 (2025): 3899–913, https://doi.org/10.1007/s12144-025-07415-9; Christoph Flückiger et al., "Psychotherapy Works—an Inclusive and Affirming View to a Modern Mental Health Treatment," *Clinical Psychology in Europe* 6 (April 2024): e11971, https://doi.org/10.32872/cpe.11971.

[31] Vinod Menon, "20 Years of the Default Mode Network: A Review and Synthesis," *Neuron* 111, no. 16 (2023): 2469–87, https://doi.org/10.1016/j.neuron.2023.04.023; Wei Luo et al., "Rest to Promote Learning: A Brain Default Mode Network Perspective," *Behavioral Sciences* 14, no. 4 (2024): 349, https://doi.org/10.3390/bs14040349.

[32] Hui-Xia Zhou et al., "Rumination and the Default Mode Network: Meta-Analysis of Brain Imaging Studies and Implications for Depression," *NeuroImage* 206 (February 1, 2020): 116287, https://doi.org/10.1016/j.neuroimage.2019.116287; Sahar Riaz et al., "Functional Connectivity in the Default Mode Network During Rumination in Depression: A Systematic Review," *BJPsych Open* 11, no. S1 (2025): S62–63, https://doi.org/10.1192/bjo.2025.10214; L. L. Beason-Held, "Dementia and the Default Mode," *Current Alzheimer Research* 8, no. 4 (2011): 361–65, https://doi.org/10.2174/156720511795745294; Vincent Malotaux et al., "Default-Mode Network Connectivity Changes During the Progression Toward Alzheimer's Dementia: A Longitudinal Functional Magnetic Resonance Imaging Study," *Brain Connectivity* 13, no. 5 (2023): 287–96, https://doi.org/10.1089/brain.2022.0008; Tina Chou et al., "The Default Mode Network and Rumination in Individuals at Risk for Depression," *Social Cognitive and Affective Neuroscience* 18, no. 1 (2023): nsad032, https://doi.org/10.1093/scan/nsad032.

[33] Jonathan Posner et al., "Antidepressants Normalize the Default Mode Network in Patients with Dysthymia," *JAMA Psychiatry* 70, no. 4 (2013): 373–82, https://doi.org/10.1001/jamapsychiatry.2013.455; Guido A. van Wingen et al., "Short-Term Antidepressant Administration Reduces Default Mode and Task-Positive Network Connectivity in Healthy Individuals During Rest," *NeuroImage* 88 (March 2014): 47–53, https://doi.org/10.1016/j.neuroimage.2013.11.022.

[34] Marjo Kullberg-Turtiainen et al., "Individualized Goal Directed Dance Rehabilitation in Chronic State of Severe Traumatic Brain Injury: A Case Study," *Heliyon* 5, no. 2 (2019): e01184, https://doi.org/10.1016/j.heliyon.2019.e01184; Young-woo Ko et al., "Changes in Functional Connectivity Between Default Mode Network and Attention Network in Response to Changes in Aerobic Exercise Intensity," *Psychiatry Investigation* 20, no. 1 (2023): 27–34, https://doi.org/10.30773/pi.2022.0245; Yaara Yeshurun et al., "The Default Mode Network: Where the Idiosyncratic Self Meets the Shared Social World," *Nature Reviews Neuroscience* 22, no. 3 (2021): 181–92, https://doi.org/10.1038/s41583-020-00420-w.

[35] Cátia Ribeiro da Costa et al., "Interplay Between the Salience and the Default Mode Network in a Social-Cognitive Task Toward a Close Other," *Frontiers in Psychiatry* 12 (February 6, 2022): 718400, https://doi.org/10.3389/fpsyt.2021.718400.

[36] Trenton D. Mize and Reilly Kincaid, "Role-Accumulation and Mental Health Across the Life Course," *American Sociological Review* 90, no. 2 (2025): 226–56, https://doi.org/10.1177/00031224241313394.

[37] Robert A. Emmons and Michael E. McCullough, "Counting Blessings Versus Burdens: An Experimental Investigation of Gratitude and Subjective Well-Being in Daily Life," *Journal of Personality and Social Psychology* 84, no. 2 (2003): 377–89, https://greatergood.berkeley.edu/pdfs/GratitudePDFs/6Emmons-BlessingsBurdens.pdf.

[38] Yukako Tani et al., "Association Between Gratitude, the Brain and Cognitive Function in Older Adults: Results from the NEIGE Study," *Archives of Gerontology and Geriatrics* 100 (May–June 2022): 104645, https://doi.org/10.1016/j.archger.2022.104645; Sunghyon Kyeong et al., "Effects of Gratitude

Meditation on Neural Network Functional Connectivity and Brain-Heart Coupling," *Scientific Reports* 7, no. 1 (2017): 5058, https://doi.org/10.1038/s41598-017-05520-9.

[39] M. E. McCullough et al., "The Grateful Disposition: A Conceptual and Empirical Topography," *Journal of Personality and Social Psychology* 82, no. 1 (2002): 112–27, https://doi.org/10.1037/0022-3514.82.1.112.

[40] Emmons and McCullough, "Counting Blessings Versus Burdens."

[41] Stephen Gallagher et al., "State, but Not Trait Gratitude Is Associated with Cardiovascular Responses to Acute Psychological Stress," *Physiology & Behavior* 221 (July 1, 2020): 112896, https://doi.org/10.1016/j.physbeh.2020.112896.

[42] Xiaoxiao Wang and Chunli Song, "The Impact of Gratitude Interventions on Patients with Cardiovascular Disease: A Systematic Review," *Frontiers in Psychology* 14 (September 20, 2023): 1243598, https://doi.org/10.3389/fpsyg.2023.1243598.

[43] McCullough et al., "Grateful Disposition."

[44] Gewnhi Park et al., "The Benefit of Gratitude: Trait Gratitude Is Associated with Effective Economic Decision-Making in the Ultimatum Game," *Frontiers in Psychology* 12 (April 19, 2021): 590132, https://doi.org/10.3389/fpsyg.2021.590132; Kai Zhao and Wenna Ji, "The Influence of Gratitude and Personality Traits on Career Resilience and Career Success Among College Students," *Frontiers in Psychology* 15 (April 23, 2024): 1340200, https://doi.org/10.3389/fpsyg.2024.1340200.

[45] Ying Chen et al., "Gratitude and Mortality Among Older US Female Nurses," *JAMA Psychiatry* 81, no. 10 (2024): 1030–38, https://doi.org/10.1001/jamapsychiatry.2024.1687.

[46] Glenn R. Fox et al., "Neural Correlates of Gratitude," *Frontiers in Psychology* 6 (September 29, 2015): 1491, https://doi.org/10.3389/fpsyg.2015.01491.

[47] Daisuke Hori et al., "Prefrontal Activation While Listening to a Letter of Gratitude Read Aloud by a Coworker Face-to-Face: A NIRS Study," *PLOS One* 15, no. 9 (2020): e0238715, https://doi.org/10.1371/journal.pone.0238715.

[48] Hori et al., "Prefrontal Activation."

[49] Tobias Egner, "Principles of Cognitive Control over Task Focus and Task Switching," *Nature Reviews Psychology* 2, no. 11 (2023): 702–14, https://doi.org/10.1038/s44159-023-00234-4; Lena Rademacher et al., "Individual Differences in Resilience to Stress Are Associated with Affective Flexibility," *Psychological Research* 87, no. 6 (2023): 1862–79, https://doi.org/10.1007/s00426-022-01779-4.

[50] J. S. Rubinstein et al., "Executive Control of Cognitive Processes in Task Switching," *Journal of Experimental Psychology: Human Perception and Performance* 27, no. 4 (2001): 763–97, https://doi.org/10.1037/0096-1523.27.4.763.

[51] Michèle C. Muhmenthaler and Beat Meier, "Task Switching Hurts Memory Encoding," *Experimental Psychology* 66, no. 1 (2019): 58–67, https://doi.org/10.1027/1618-3169/a000431; Kamrul Hasan, "Digital Multitasking and Hyperactivity: Unveiling the Hidden Costs to Brain Health," *Annals of Medicine & Surgery* 86, no. 11 (2024): 6371–73, https://doi.org/10.1097/MS9.0000000000002576.

[52] Simone Montuori et al., "Executive Functioning Profiles in Elite Volleyball Athletes: Preliminary Results by a Sport-Specific Task Switching Protocol," *Human Movement Science* 63 (February 2019): 73–81, https://doi.org/10.1016/j.humov.2018.11.011; Enrico Premi et al., "Enhanced Dynamic Functional Connectivity (Whole-Brain Chronnectome) in Chess Experts," *Scientific Reports* 10, no. 1 (2020): 7051, https://doi.org/10.1038/s41598-020-63984-8.

[53] Andrew D. Huberman, "Dorian Yates: Build Muscle & Strength & Forge Your Life Path," *Huberman Lab* (podcast audio), January 19, 2026, https://www.hubermanlab.com/episode/build-muscle-and-strength-and-forge-your-life-path-dorian-yates.

[54] As one example, see the following: Leon Bax, *Building Performance Routines: Empowering Habits Toward Impact* (2Mynds, 2025).

[55] Michael Falkenstein et al., "Action Monitoring, Error Detection, and the Basal Ganglia: An ERP Study," *NeuroReport* 12, no. 1 (2001): 157–61, https://doi.org/10.1097/00001756-200101220-00039.

[56] Richard Feloni, "A Retired Navy SEAL Commander Does 2 Things Every Night Before Bed So He Can Attack the Next Day the Minute He Wakes Up," *Business Insider*, November 10, 2017, https://finance.yahoo.com/news/retired-navy-seal-commander-does-141500339.html.

[57] Twyla Tharp, *The Creative Habit: Learn It and Use It for Life* (Simon & Schuster, 2006).

[58] Tobias Egner and Audrey Siqi-Liu, "Insights into Control over Cognitive Flexibility from Studies of Task-Switching," *Current Opinion in Behavioral Sciences* 55 (February 2024): 101342, https://doi.org/10.1016/j.cobeha.2023.101342; Rademacher et al., "Individual Differences in Resilience to Stress"; Bettina Wollesen et al., "Effects of Cognitive-Motor Dual Task Training on Cognitive and Physical Performance in Healthy Children and Adolescents: A Scoping Review," *Acta Psychologica* 224 (April 2022): 103498, https://doi.org/10.1016/j.actpsy.2022.103498; Laurence Desjardins-Crepeau et al., "Effects of Combined Physical and Cognitive Training on Fitness and Neuropsychological Outcomes in Healthy Older Adults," *Clinical Interventions in Aging* 11 (September 2016): 1287–99, https://doi.org/10.2147/cia.s115711.

[59] C. G. Jung, *Letters Vol 1, 1906–1950*, ed. Gerhard Adler (Routledge, 1973), https://jungiancenter.org/wp-content/uploads/2023/09/letters-of-c-g-jung-vol-1-1906-1950.pdf.

[60] Mary C. McCluskey, "Revitalizing Alfred Adler: An Echo for Equality," *Clinical Social Work Journal* 50, no. 4 (2022): 387–99, https://doi.org/10.1007/s10615-021-00793-0.

[61] Rommy Cedeno and Tyler J. Torrico, "Adlerian Therapy," StatPearls, last updated January 11, 2024, https://www.ncbi.nlm.nih.gov/books/NBK599518/.

[62] Christian Roesler, "Evidence for the Effectiveness of Jungian Psychotherapy: A Review of Empirical Studies," *Behavioral Sciences* 3, no. 4 (2013): 562–75, https://doi.org/10.3390/bs3040562.

[63] Netta Weinstein et al., "Balance Between Solitude and Socializing: Everyday Solitude Time Both Benefits and Harms Well-Being," *Scientific Reports* 13, article no. 21160 (2023), https://doi.org/10.1038/s41598-023-44507-7.

[64] Hei Wan Mak et al., "Hobby Engagement and Mental Wellbeing Among People Aged 65 Years and Older in 16 Countries," *Nature Medicine* 29 (2023): 2233–40, https://doi.org/10.1038/s41591-023-02506-1.

[65] Huberman, "Dr. James Hollis: How to Find Your True Purpose."

[66] Vincent J. Felitti et al., "Relationship of Childhood Abuse and Household Dysfunction to Many of the Leading Causes of Death in Adults," *American Journal of Preventive Medicine* 14, no. 4 (May 1998): 245–58, https://doi.org/10.1016/S0749-3797(98)00017-8.

[67] Paul Conti, *Trauma: The Invisible Epidemic* (St. Martin's Essentials, 2021).

[68] Kathryn L. Humphreys et al., "Stressful Life Events, ADHD Symptoms, and Brain Structure in Early Adolescence," *Journal of Abnormal Child Psychology* 47, no. 3 (May 2018): 421–32, https://doi.org/10.1007/s10802-018-0443-5.

[69] J. W. Pennebaker and S. K. Beall, "Confronting a Traumatic Event: Toward an Understanding of Inhibition and Disease," *Journal of Abnormal Psychology* 95, no. 3 (1986): 274–81, https://doi.org/10.1037/0021-843X.95.3.274.

[70] J. W. Pennebaker et al., "Disclosure of Traumas and Immune Function: Health Implications for Psychotherapy," *Journal of Consulting and Clinical Psychology* 56, no. 2 (1988): 239–45, https://doi.org/10.1037/0022-006X.56.2.239.

[71] Xiaojuan Gao, "Research on Expressive Writing in Psychology: A Forty-Year Bibliometric Analysis and Visualization of Current Status and Research Trends," *Frontiers in Psychology* 13 (October 2022): 825626, https://doi.org/10.3389/fpsyg.2022.825626.

[72] Pasquale G. Frisina et al., "A Meta-Analysis of the Effects of Written Emotional Disclosure on the Health Outcomes of Clinical Populations," *Journal of Nervous and Mental Disease* 192, no. 9 (September 2004): 629–34, https://doi.org/10.1097/01.nmd.0000138317.30764.63.

[73] Michel André Maréchal et al., "Increasing Honesty in Humans with Noninvasive Brain Stimulation," *Proceedings of the National Academy of Sciences U.S.A.* 114, no. 17 (April 2017): 4360–64, https://doi.org/10.1073/pnas.1614912114.

[74] Kerry J. Ressler, "Amygdala Activity, Fear, and Anxiety: Modulation by Stress," *Biological Psychiatry* 67, no. 12 (2010): 1117–19, https://doi.org/10.1016/j.biopsych.2010.04.027.

[75] Benno Roozendaal et al., "Adrenal Stress Hormones, Amygdala Activation, and Memory for Emotionally Arousing Experiences," *Progress in Brain Research* 167 (2007): 79–97, https://doi.org/10.1016/S0079-6123(07)67006-X.

[76] Jennifer N. Morey et al., "Current Directions in Stress and Human Immune Function," *Current Opinion in Psychology* 5 (October 2015): 13–17, https://doi.org/10.1016/j.copsyc.2015.03.007.

[77] Hua Tang et al., "Prefrontal Cortical Plasticity During Learning of Cognitive Tasks," *Nature Communications* 13, article no. 90 (2022), https://doi.org/10.1038/s41467-021-27695-6.

[78] Hayley Phelan, "What's All This About Journaling?," *New York Times*, October 25, 2018, https://www.nytimes.com/2018/10/25/style/journaling-benefits.html.

[79] Donna M. Wilson et al., "What Exactly Is 'Complicated' Grief? A Scoping Research Literature Review to Understand Its Risk Factors and Prevalence," *OMEGA* 86, no. 2 (December 1, 2020): 471–87, https://doi.org/10.1177/0030222820977305.

[80] K. B. Komischke-Konnerup et al., "Grief-Focused Cognitive Behavioral Therapies for Prolonged Grief Symptoms: A Systematic Review and Meta-Analysis," *Journal of Consulting and Clinical Psychology* 92, no. 4 (2024): 236–48, https://doi.org/10.1037/ccp0000884.

[81] János Pilling et al., "Alcohol Use in the First Three Years of Bereavement: A National Representative Survey," *Substance Abuse Treatment, Prevention, and Policy* 7, article no. 3 (2012), https://doi.org/10.1186/1747-597X-7-3.

[82] "Coping with Grief and Loss," National Institute on Aging, content reviewed July 15, 2024, https://www.nia.nih.gov/health/grief-and-mourning/coping-grief-and-loss.

[83] Mary-Frances O'Connor et al., "Craving Love? Enduring Grief Activates Brain's Reward Center," *NeuroImage* 42, no. 2 (2008): 969–72, https://doi.org/10.1016/j.neuroimage.2008.04.256.

[84] Anne F. Pierce et al., "Nucleus Accumbens Dopamine Release Reflects the Selective Nature of Pair Bonds," *Current Biology* 34, no. 3 (2024): 519–30.e5, https://doi.org/10.1016/j.cub.2023.12.041.

[85] Edvard I. Moser et al., "Place Cells, Grid Cells, and the Brain's Spatial Representation System," *Annual Review of Neuroscience* 31 (July 2008): 69–89, https://doi.org/10.1146/annurev.neuro.31.061307.090723; Valeria C. Caruso et al., "Compensating for a Shifting World: Evolving Reference Frames of Visual and Auditory Signals Across Three Multimodal Brain Areas," *Journal of Neurophysiology* 126, no. 1 (April 2021): 82–94, https://doi.org/10.1152/jn.00385.2020; Russell A. Epstein et al., "The Cognitive Map in Humans: Spatial Navigation and Beyond," *Nature Neuroscience* 20, no. 11 (November 2017): 1504–13, https://doi.org/10.1038/nn.4656.

[86] Michael Peer et al., "Brain System for Mental Orientation in Space, Time, and Person," *Proceedings of the National Academy of Sciences* 112, no. 35 (2015): 11072–77, https://doi.org/10.1073/pnas.1504242112.

[87] Carolyn Parkinson et al., "A Common Cortical Metric for Spatial, Temporal, and Social Distance," *Journal of Neuroscience* 34, no. 5 (2014): 1979–87, https://doi.org/10.1523/JNEUROSCI.2159-13.2014.

[88] Mary-Frances O'Connor and Saren H. Seeley, "Grieving as a Form of Learning: Insights from Neuroscience Applied to Grief and Loss," *Current Opinion in Psychology* 43 (February 2022): 317–22, https://doi.org/10.1016/j.copsyc.2021.08.019.

[89] Amanda W. Baker et al., "The Role of Avoidance in Complicated Grief: A Detailed Examination of the Grief-Related Avoidance Questionnaire (GRAQ) in a Large Sample of Individuals with Complicated Grief," *Journal of Loss and Trauma* 21, no. 6 (February 2016): 533–47, https://doi.org/10.1080/15325024.2016.1157412.

[90] O'Connor and Seeley, "Grieving as a Form of Learning."

[91] Joanna Wojtkowiak et al., "Ritual in Therapy for Prolonged Grief: A Scoping Review of Ritual Elements in Evidence-Informed Grief Interventions," *Frontiers in Psychiatry* 11 (February 2021): 623835, https://doi.org/10.3389/fpsyt.2020.623835.

[92] Maarten C. Eisma et al., "Upward and Downward Counterfactual Thought After Loss: A Multiwave Controlled Longitudinal Study," *Behavioral Therapy* 52, no. 3 (2021): 577–93, https://doi.org/10.1016/j.beth.2020.07.007.

Index

About the Author

Andrew D. Huberman, PhD, is a neuroscientist and tenured professor in the departments of neurobiology and ophthalmology and, by courtesy, psychiatry and behavioral sciences at Stanford School of Medicine. He has made numerous significant contributions to the fields of brain development, brain function, and neural plasticity. His laboratory at Stanford School of Medicine has published work in top journals such as *Nature*, *Science*, and *Cell* and in top media outlets like the BBC, *Time*, *Scientific American*, and Discover. Huberman is a McKnight Foundation and Pew Foundation Fellow and was awarded the Association for Research in Vision and Ophthalmology's Cogan Award in 2017, given to the scientist making the most significant discoveries in the study of vision. In 2021, Andrew launched the *Huberman Lab* podcast, which consistently ranks as the top health and fitness podcast in the world and has consistently ranked in the top ten podcasts globally.